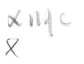

X 114 c
X

D1758818

# CLINICAL DISSECTION GUIDE FOR LARGE ANIMALS

## Horse and Large Ruminants

### Second Edition

*To our children with love, for their support and sweet memories*

*To all veterinary students in the dissection laboratory*

# CLINICAL DISSECTION GUIDE FOR LARGE ANIMALS

## Horse and Large Ruminants

### Second Edition

Gheorghe M. Constantinescu
Ileana A. Constantinescu

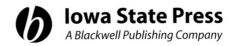

**Iowa State Press**
*A Blackwell Publishing Company*

**GHEORGHE M. CONSTANTINESCU, D.V.M., Ph.D., Dr.h.c.,** is a Professor of Veterinary Anatomy and Medical Illustrator, Department of Biomedical Sciences, College of Veterinary Medicine, University of Missouri-Columbia. Dr. Constantinescu is also a professional member of the Association of Medical Illustrators and a Diplomate of the Romanian College of Veterinary Pathologists.

**ILEANA A. CONSTANTINESCU, B.V.Sc., D.V.M., M.S.,** is a Clinical Instructor of Veterinary Anatomy, Department of Biomedical Sciences, College of Veterinary Medicine, University of Missouri-Columbia.

© 2004 Iowa State Press
A Blackwell Publishing Company
All rights reserved

Iowa State Press
2121 State Avenue, Ames, Iowa 50014

Orders:  1-800-862-6657      Fax:        1-515-292-3348
Office:   1-515-292-0140      Web site:  www.iowastatepress.com

Figures R5.12–R5.17, R6.31–R6.35, H7.25, H7.26, R7.21, and R7.22 reprinted from *The Merck Veterinary Manual,* CD-ROM version. S.E. Aiello, editor. Copyright 2000 by Merck and Co., Inc., Whitehouse Station, NJ. Used with permission of the publisher.

Figures H3.1, H4.4, H5.2A-F, H5.3, R2.1A, R3.1, R4.2, R4.3, R5.1A-D, R5.2, R5.3A,C,D, R5.4, and R6.2A-C are redrawn in halftone from Barone, 1999.

Figure R6.27 was redrawn in halftone from Habel, 1989.

Figures H4.5A,B, H5.6B,C, H6.8, R6.7, R6.8, and R6.9 are redrawn in halftone from Barone, 2000.

Figures H6.3B,E,F and H6.10 are redrawn from figures 15-33, 15-35, 15-36, 16-7 to 10 from *Getty - Sisson and Grossman's The Anatomy of the Domestic Animals 5th ed*. 1975, W. B. Saunders Company, with permission of the publisher.

Cover and text illustrations by Gheorghe M. Constantinescu

Authorization to photocopy items for internal or personal use, or the internal or personal use of specific clients, is granted by Iowa State Press, provided that the base fee of $.10 per copy is paid directly to the Copyright Clearance Center, 222 Rosewood Drive, Danvers, MA 01923. For those organizations that have been granted a photocopy license by CCC, a separate system of payments has been arranged. The fee code for users of the Transactional Reporting Service is 0-8138-0319-5/2004 $.10.

Printed on acid-free paper in the United States of America

First edition, 1991 (© Mosby–Yearbook, Inc.)
Second edition, 2004

Library of Congress Cataloging-in-Publication Data

Constantinescu, Gheorghe M., 1932–
    Clinical dissection guide for large animals : horse and large ruminants/ Gheorghe M. Constantinescu, Ileana A. Constantinescu.—2nd ed.
         p. cm.
Includes bibliographic references (p.    )
    ISBN 0-8138-0319-5 (alk. paper)
    1. Veterinary dissection—Laboratory manuals. 2. Veterinary anatomy—Laboratory manuals. 3. Veterinary dissection—Atlases. 4. Veterinary anatomy—Atlases. I. Constantinescu, Ileana A. II. Title.
SF762.C66 2003
636.089′1—dc22        2003020720

The last digit is the print number:  9  8  7  6  5  4  3  2  1

# Contents

Contributors . . . . . . . . . . . vi

Foreword to the First Edition . . . . . vii

Preface to the First Edition. . . . . . viii

Preface to the Second Edition . . . . . ix

Acknowledgments . . . . . . . . . . x

Introduction: How to Use This Book . xi

Abbreviations . . . . . . . . . . . xii

**Horse**
Chapter H1
The Neck. . . . . . . . . . . . . 3

Chapter H2
The Thorax and Thoracic
Viscera . . . . . . . . . . . . . 23

Chapter H3
The Abdomen and Abdominal
Viscera . . . . . . . . . . . . . 49

Chapter H4
The Pelvis, Pelvic Viscera, Tail,
and External Genitalia . . . . . . . 75

Chapter H5
The Pelvic Limb. . . . . . . . . 117

Chapter H6
The Thoracic Limb . . . . . . . 155

Chapter H7
The Head. . . . . . . . . . . 207

**Large Ruminants**
Chapter R1
The Neck. . . . . . . . . . . . 267

Chapter R2
The Thorax and Thoracic
Viscera . . . . . . . . . . . . 273

Chapter R3
The Abdomen and Abdominal
Viscera . . . . . . . . . . . . 289

Chapter R4
The Pelvis, Pelvic Viscera, Tail,
and External Genitalia . . . . . . . 313

Chapter R5
The Pelvic Limb. . . . . . . . . 339

Chapter R6
The Thoracic Limb . . . . . . . 359

Chapter R7
The Head. . . . . . . . . . . 397

References . . . . . . . . . 427

Index . . . . . . . . . . 433

# Contributors*
(in Alphabetical Order)

Johnson, Philip J., B.V.Sc., M.R.C.V.S., M.S., Diplomate of the American College of Veterinary Internal Medicine, Professor of Equine Internal Medicine

Kramer, Joanne, D.V.M., Diplomate of the American College of Veterinary Surgeons, Clinical Assistant Professor of Equine Medicine and Surgery

Lakritz, Jeffrey, D.V.M., Ph.D., Dipolomate of the American College of Veterinary Internal Medicine, Assistant Professor of Large Animal Medicine and Surgery

Wilson, David. A., D.V.M., M.S., Diplomate of the American College of Veterinary Surgeons, Associate Professor of Equine Medicine and Surgery

*College of Veterinary Medicine, University of Missouri-Columbia.

# Foreword to the First Edition

It is a pleasure and an honor for me, as the former professor of Veterinary Anatomy of Dr. Gheorghe M. Constantinescu, to write the foreword for his *Clinical Dissection Guide for Large Animals.*

A short biographic sketch about Dr. Constantinescu seems relevant. Dr. Constantinescu was born in Bucharest, Romania, on January 20, 1932. His father was an M.D., and his mother earned a B.L. (Bachelor of Letters in Romanian, French, and German) and a B.A.Ed. He graduated from the Faculty of Veterinary Medicine in Bucharest in 1955 (with a D.V.M.) and received his Ph.D. in Veterinary Anatomy in 1964. During his first and second years, he was the only student who earned the highest grade in Anatomy: 10. He was a brilliant student, and I asked him to be an honorary preparator—to help me with teaching and in the laboratory for the last four years out of the five years of the D.V.M. program.

After graduation, Dr. Constantinescu worked for three years as a laboratory chief in Veterinary Anatomy in Bucharest, then as a researcher in the Zootechnical Institute and was the first Veterinarian of the Zoological Park in Bucharest. After three years as a veterinarian and Vice-President of the Agricultural Council of the Panciu county, he was named Associate Professor of Veterinary Anatomy of the Faculty of Veterinary Medicine in Timisoara, Romania, from 1965 to 1982. During this last period, he was Scientific Secretary of the Agronomic Institute in Timisoara and Associate Dean. He was appointed as an Associate Professor of Veterinary Anatomy at the College of Veterinary Medicine, University of Missouri-Columbia, U.S.A., in 1984, where he is presently employed.

Dr. Constantinescu is the author or coauthor of more than 200 publications, including more than 30 books and chapters. He is a talented anatomical and medical illustrator, as well as a sculptor. He is married and has a son and a daughter.

The *Clinical Dissection Guide for Large Animals* that I am presenting is a remarkable work—a world premiere in Veterinary Anatomy, which accumulates the author's knowledge, experience, and talent and which is the first dissection guide to discuss all the large domestic animals in one volume. It is one of the few examples in which the author of a veterinary anatomical book is also the illustrator. All of the illustrations are original; they cannot be seen in any other book.

The style of the text is vivid and original, filled both with practical directions on using specimens and, especially, with sentences that serve to reinforce the importance of major anatomical structures. This saves students time, because they will not have to return to descriptive anatomy discussion during a dissection. The impressive number of illustrations (504) printed by Mosby-Year Book, Inc., in an excellent manner contributes to the high quality of this guide.

I warmly recommend the *Clinical Dissection Guide for Large Animals* to students, practitioners, and breeders. My most sincere congratulations to Dr. Gheorghe M. Constantinescu and to Mosby-Year Book, Inc., for this superb work.

Vasile Ghetie, D.V.M., Ph.D., Dr.h.c.,
Member of the Romanian Academy
Professor Emeritus of Veterinary Anatomy
Faculty of Veterinary Medicine
Bucharest, Romania

# Preface to the First Edition

*"Hic locus est ubi mors gaudet succurrere vitae."* *

This book is directed principally to professional students in colleges of veterinary medicine. The purpose of this text is to provide the student with a self-directed and detailed guide for the anatomic dissection of the major species of large domestic animals—the horse, ox, sheep, goat, and pig.

The guide to large animal dissection is organized as a progressive series of anatomical illustrations, accompanied by keyed descriptive text. The impetus to prepare such a profusely illustrated guide came from questions and concerns raised by veterinary students during anatomy teaching laboratories. The book's organizational format reflects the presentation techniques that have proven to be most helpful to the student (and the teacher) during the author's 30 years of experience in teaching professional level veterinary anatomy.

This guide presents regional and topographical dissection approaches; it starts with surface features and progresses to deeper structures, stopping along the way for appropriate comments on principal anatomical entities for each region. All of the anatomical drawings and accompanying descriptions are original to this text and are based on specimens dissected personally by the author.

The primary dissection models are the horse and the ox, but appropriate attention is paid to other species when important interspecific anatomical differences are encountered. Although elements of clinical anatomy are mentioned throughout the entire book, the "clinical" anatomy of the horse is especially well developed, with one chapter devoted to structural landmarks and approaches to major structures that are subject to clinical intervention.

The nomenclature used in this guide generally conforms to the most recent edition of *Nomina Anatomica Veterinaria* (1983). For structures not included in the *Nomina Anatomica Veterinaria,* the author has provided especially detailed descriptions and illustrations.

Although this dissection guide is dedicated principally to the veterinary student, it also provides relevant anatomical information that will prove helpful to other groups. Students and veterinarians in meat inspection and necropsy services will find details about the location, relationships (topography), and shape of lymph nodes, of the structures of the digestive, respiratory, and urogenital apparatuses, and of the cardiovascular and central nervous systems. The chapter on clinical anatomy of the horse is dedicated primarily to students in equine clinical rotations and to veterinarians in equine practice. They will find detailed landmarks and approaches for nerve block or local anesthesia, for collection of blood samples, for rectal exploration, for percussion and auscultation of the lungs and heart, and for other structures subject to clinical intervention. Likewise, undergraduate-school and graduate-school educators in veterinary science, biomedical science, and animal science can gain extensive familiarity with the anatomy of large domestic animals through this guide. Finally, the professional equine breeder and cattle breeder will discover in this book new and useful information about the anatomy of large animals.

---

* "Here is the place where the death is glad to be of use to the life."

# Preface to the Second Edition

The concept of a dissection guide is to give students the directions to self-perform the "act of cutting apart or separating the tissues (structures) of the body for anatomical study." The text should be accompanied by as many original illustrations as possible, preferably illustrations that have as a model prosected specimens dissected by the authors themselves. The best way to dissect fresh or embalmed specimens is by using the scalpel and the forceps, and sometimes the scissors. Before the dissection starts, the students should read the text to be familiar with the given directions.

The improved second edition of the *Clinical Dissection Guide for Large Animals: Horse and Large Ruminants* includes only these two groups of animals. A guide for the small ruminants has already been published under the title *Guide to Regional Ruminant Anatomy Based on the Dissection of the Goat.** 

Based on our experience in the anatomy laboratory, the best results are achieved by students who start by studying the bones before dissecting the specimens. In this way, the joints, the attachments of the muscles and their actions; the radiographic, MRI, CT-scan and other interpretations; and the relationships of any structure to the bones can be better understood.

In addition to the first edition, the second edition introduces all the bones (only illustrations with legends) and the most important clinical correlations with the anatomical structures exposed during the dissection. The clinical correlations were provided by clinicians from our Veterinary Medical Teaching Hospital and are printed in bold. Also printed in bold are the names of all the structures when they are first introduced.

Details of descriptive anatomy of the thoracic and abdominopelvic viscera, tables with the systematization of the muscles, arteries, and nerves, and detailed illustrations are provided to contribute to the basic knowledge necessary in surgery (including endoscopic procedures), for physical examination, clinical approach, and in the necropsy room.

The book is organized into two parts of seven chapters each and includes 658 illustrations on 326 plates. The first part covers the horse, the second the ruminants, and the chapters on the ruminants parallel those on the horse. Chapter, figure, and table numbers in the section on horses are preceded by an H; those in the section on ruminants are preceded by an R. The official nomenclature from the *Nomina Anatomica Veterinaria* (fourth edition, 1994) and the *Illustrated Veterinary Anatomical Nomenclature* (1992) is used. Some synonyms used by clinicians are mentioned within parentheses. Unlike the first edition, modlabs for horses and large ruminants are presented at the end of each chapter, except the first three chapters on large ruminants. Remarks following words like ***Remember! Caution,*** and ***Notice*** or *Note* throughout the guide are intended to be of use for refreshing the students' memory and to emphasize the importance of some structures. The authors will be grateful for any suggestions, comments, or criticism for improving the book.

Gheorghe M. Constatinescu
Ileana A. Constantinescu
Columbia, Missouri

---

*Gheorghe M. Constantinescu, Iowa State Press, 2001.

# Acknowledgments

The authors first thank the contributors, who added the "salt and pepper" to the book. The comments on clinical correlations based on their own experience correspond to the trend of Anatomy—the Clinical Anatomy.

The authors also thank all VM 1 students of the Class of 2006 who made comments and suggestions, especially to Betsy Bialon.

High appreciation and gratitude go to Ms. Gretchen Van Houten, former Publishing Director of the Iowa State Press (a Blackwell Publishing Company), and especially to Mr. Dave Rosenbaum, former Senior Publisher of the same company, who without reservation suggested and encouraged the project of this second edition. Dave Rosenbaum, with his experience and professionalism, was in permanent contact with the authors, who, despite a heavy teaching load throughout the entire academic year, were able to deliver the manuscript on time. Thanks also goes to Lynne Bishop, the project managing editor of the book; to Bonnie Harmon, the copyeditor; to Justin Eccles, the designer; to Jamie Johnson, the prepress computer specialist; and the whole team at the Iowa State Press involved in publishing the book.

(such as the need for ventral drainage). *The guttural pouch, specific for the horse, is a diverticulum of the mucosa of the pharyngotympanic (auditory) tube, known also as the Eustachian tube.*

The linguofacial V. is also used as a landmark for the commonly used modified Whitehouse approach to the guttural pouch. The incision is made along the ventral border of the linguofacial V. and continues through the fascial plane above the larynx to the guttural pouch.

The sites for intramuscular (i.m.) injections should avoid the nuchal ligament and the crest of fat and the accessory N. A recommended site is within a triangular area shown in Figure H1.3.

## THE DISSECTION TECHNIQUE OF THE NECK

*Caution.* Because there is only a small amount of subcutaneous loose connective tissue, skin the neck carefully.

Cut off the **mane**. Make an incision of the skin at the edge of the mane from the **poll** to the cranial extent of the **withers**. From both ends of this incision extend ventral incisions to the ventral midline of the neck: from the poll caudal to the **base of the ear** and over the **caudal border of the mandible**, and from the withers parallel to the cranial border of the **shoulder** up to the **manubrium sterni**, respectively. Leaving 2–3 cm of skin on the dorsal midline, reflect the skin ventrally. Another technique uses the incision of the skin on the ventral midline and the reflection of the skin dorsally, as shown in Figure H1.5.

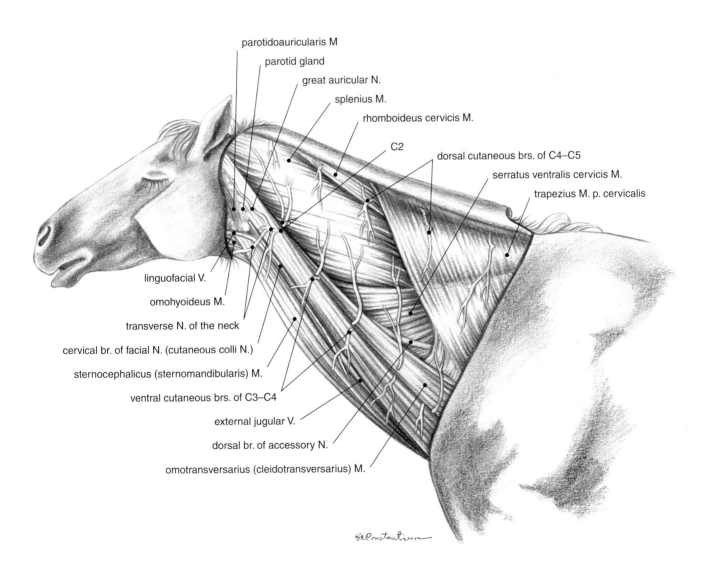

Fig. H1.5. Superficial structures of the neck, horse, lateral aspect.

The following is a short presentation of the distribution of the cutaneous nerves in the neck, in comparison to the cutaneous nerves in the thoracic and lumbar regions (Fig. H1.8). All these cutaneous nerves originate from, and are branches of, **spinal nerves**. The major difference between the cervical spinal nerves and the thoracic and lumbar spinal nerves is the distribution of the **dorsal branch**: the **cutaneous branch** is the continuation of the **medial branch of the dorsal branch** of a cervical spinal nerve, while the exclusive **muscular branch is the lateral branch of the dorsal branch**. The cutaneous branch of the dorsal branch of a thoracic and/or a lumbar spinal nerve is the continuation of the lateral branch, while the muscular branch is the medial branch of the dorsal branch. In addition, the dorsal cutaneous branch of the thoracic and lumbar spinal nerves branch again into lateral and medial branches. Another difference is the fact that the **ventral cutaneous branch** of a cervical spinal nerve is the only continuation of the **ventral branch**. The thoracic and lumbar spinal nerves send ventral *and* lateral cutaneous branches from the ventral branch.

The muscles of the neck located dorsal to the cervical vertebrae are supplied by the dorsal branches of the spinal nerves, whereas the muscles located ventral to the cervical vertebrae are innervated by the ventral branches, before they reach the skin. There are some exceptions: the trapezius, sternocephalicus, cleidomastoideus, and omotransversarius Mm. are supplied by the accessory N., and the cleidobrachialis is supplied by the axillary N.

**Bilateral neurectomy of the ventral branch of the accessory N. is sometimes advocated for management of stereotypical aerophagia in horses (windsucking, cribbing). The same nerve is biopsied to support diagnosis of equine motor neuron disease (Lou Gehrig's disease).**

Palpate the ventral extent of the border of the wing of the atlas, where the ventral branch of the second spinal N. emerges. Dissect the **great auricular N.** along the border of the wing of the atlas and the **transverse N. of the neck (transverse cervical N.)** in a rostroventral direction to the intermandibular space (Figs. H1.5 and H1.9). The apparent origin of the cervical spinal nerves 3–5 (C3–C5) will

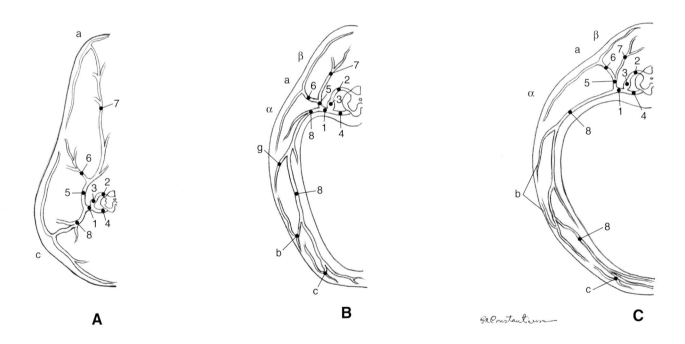

Fig. H1.8. The distribution of the cutaneous spinal nerves. **A.** Cervical spinal nerves. **B.** Thoracic spinal nerves. **C.** Lumbar spinal nerves. *Key:* 1-**spinal N.:** 2-*dorsal root:* 3-spinal ganglion; 4-*ventral root.* 5-**dorsal branch:** 6-lateral branch: a-*dorsal cutaneous branch:* α-lateral branch, β-medial branch. 7-medial branch. 8-**ventral branch:** b-*lateral cutaneous branches,* c-*ventral cutaneous branch.* g-*branch to intercostal Mm.*

(such as the need for ventral drainage). *The guttural pouch, specific for the horse, is a diverticulum of the mucosa of the pharyngotympanic (auditory) tube, known also as the Eustachian tube.*

The linguofacial V. is also used as a landmark for the commonly used modified Whitehouse approach to the guttural pouch. The incision is made along the ventral border of the linguofacial V. and continues through the fascial plane above the larynx to the guttural pouch.

The sites for intramuscular (i.m.) injections should avoid the nuchal ligament and the crest of fat and the accessory N. A recommended site is within a triangular area shown in Figure H1.3.

## THE DISSECTION TECHNIQUE OF THE NECK

*Caution.* Because there is only a small amount of subcutaneous loose connective tissue, skin the neck carefully.

Cut off the **mane**. Make an incision of the skin at the edge of the mane from the **poll** to the cranial extent of the **withers**. From both ends of this incision extend ventral incisions to the ventral midline of the neck: from the poll caudal to the **base of the ear** and over the **caudal border of the mandible**, and from the withers parallel to the cranial border of the **shoulder** up to the **manubrium sterni**, respectively. Leaving 2–3 cm of skin on the dorsal midline, reflect the skin ventrally. Another technique uses the incision of the skin on the ventral midline and the reflection of the skin dorsally, as shown in Figure H1.5.

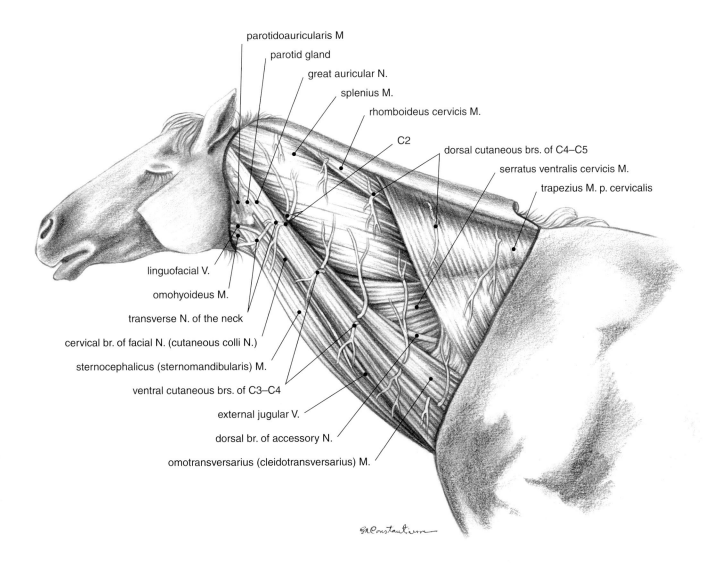

Fig. H1.5. Superficial structures of the neck, horse, lateral aspect.

Lymph vessels, arterial and nervous cutaneous branches, and the **cutaneous colli M.** are the first structures encountered after skinning. The cutaneous muscles of the entire body including the cutaneous colli M. are shown in Figure H1.6.

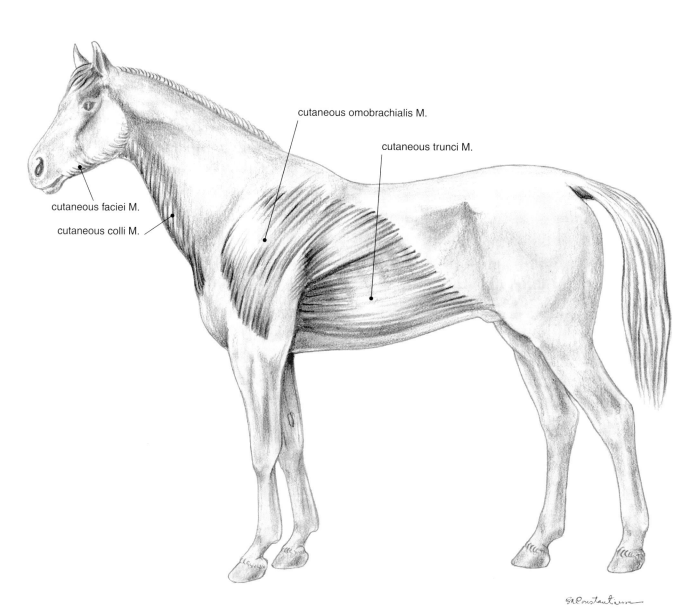

Fig. H1.6. Cutaneous muscles of the horse.

*Note.* The cutaneous muscles develop within superficial fasciae. There are three fasciae in the neck: superficial, middle, and deep (listed in the *N.A.V.* as **laminae of the cervical fascia**). The **superficial lamina** blends its fibers with the cutaneous colli M. The **middle (pretracheal) lamina** surrounds and protects the esophagus and trachea, and extends as the **carotid sheath**; it continues at the tho-racic inlet with the endothoracic fascia, which lines the thoracic cavity. The **deep (prevertebral) lamina** sur-rounds the intimate muscles lying against the cervical ver-tebrae. The three cervical fasciae and their relationship with the surrounding structures are illustrated on a cross section (Fig. H1.7).

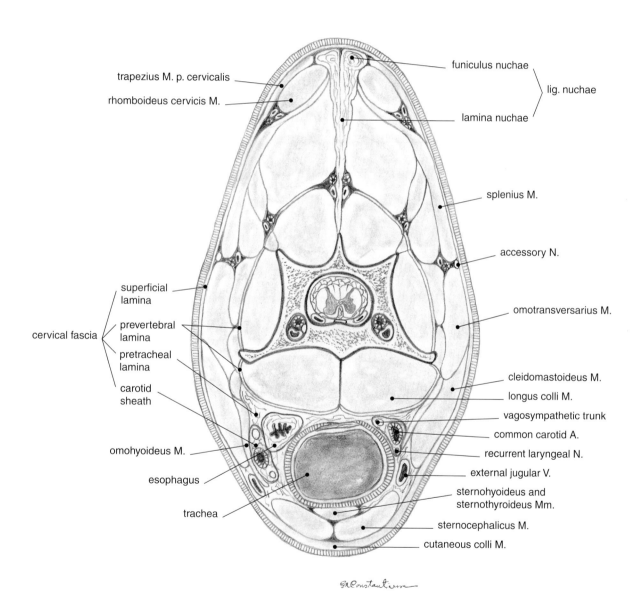

Fig. H1.7. Transverse section through the neck of the horse at the level of the fourth cervical vertebra (caudal view).

The following is a short presentation of the distribution of the cutaneous nerves in the neck, in comparison to the cutaneous nerves in the thoracic and lumbar regions (Fig. H1.8). All these cutaneous nerves originate from, and are branches of, **spinal nerves**. The major difference between the cervical spinal nerves and the thoracic and lumbar spinal nerves is the distribution of the **dorsal branch**: the **cutaneous branch** is the continuation of the **medial branch of the dorsal branch** of a cervical spinal nerve, while the exclusive **muscular branch is the lateral branch of the dorsal branch**. The cutaneous branch of the dorsal branch of a thoracic and/or a lumbar spinal nerve is the continuation of the lateral branch, while the muscular branch is the medial branch of the dorsal branch. In addition, the dorsal cutaneous branch of the thoracic and lumbar spinal nerves branch again into lateral and medial branches. Another difference is the fact that the **ventral cutaneous branch** of a cervical spinal nerve is the only continuation of the **ventral branch**. The thoracic and lumbar spinal nerves send ventral *and* lateral cutaneous branches from the ventral branch.

The muscles of the neck located dorsal to the cervical vertebrae are supplied by the dorsal branches of the spinal nerves, whereas the muscles located ventral to the cervical vertebrae are innervated by the ventral branches, before they reach the skin. There are some exceptions: the trapezius, sternocephalicus, cleidomastoideus, and omotransversarius Mm. are supplied by the accessory N., and the cleidobrachialis is supplied by the axillary N.

**Bilateral neurectomy of the ventral branch of the accessory N. is sometimes advocated for management of stereotypical aerophagia in horses (windsucking, cribbing). The same nerve is biopsied to support diagnosis of equine motor neuron disease (Lou Gehrig's disease).**

Palpate the ventral extent of the border of the wing of the atlas, where the ventral branch of the second spinal N. emerges. Dissect the **great auricular N.** along the border of the wing of the atlas and the **transverse N. of the neck (transverse cervical N.)** in a rostroventral direction to the intermandibular space (Figs. H1.5 and H1.9). The apparent origin of the cervical spinal nerves 3–5 (C3–C5) will

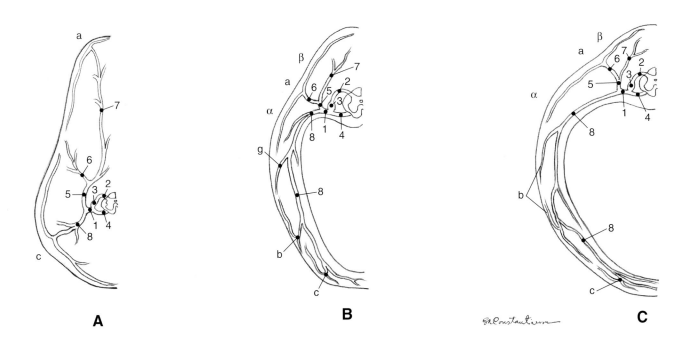

**A**     **B**     **C**

Fig. H1.8. The distribution of the cutaneous spinal nerves. **A.** Cervical spinal nerves. **B.** Thoracic spinal nerves. **C.** Lumbar spinal nerves. *Key:* 1-**spinal N.:** 2-*dorsal root:* 3-spinal ganglion; 4-*ventral root.* 5-**dorsal branch:** 6-lateral branch: a-*dorsal cutaneous branch:* α-lateral branch, β-medial branch. 7-medial branch. 8-**ventral branch:** b-*lateral cutaneous branches,* c-*ventral cutaneous branch.* g-*branch to intercostal Mm.*

be exposed later at the level of the intervertebral foramina, between the dorsal and middle fascicles of the intertransversarii Mm. The ventral branches of C6–C8, together with the ventral branches of T1 and T2 (thoracic spinal nerves) build up the **brachial plexus**. In addition, the ventral branches of C5–C7 are the origin of the **phrenic N.**

Dissect and reflect the cutaneous colli M. ventrally. Carefully separate it from the **external jugular V.** Isolate the vein from the surrounding structures.

*Caution.* Dissect carefully the **cervical branch of the facial N.** over the lateral aspect of the cranial half of the external jugular V. (Fig. H1.5).

Based on our experience, before starting the dissection of the muscles, students should know the systematization of the cervical muscles, which is presented in the Table H1.1

Outline the superficial muscles shown in Figure H1.5 and separate them from each other. Leave a portion of the superficial fascia connecting the **trapezius M. pars cervicalis** to the **omotransversarius M.** 10 cm cranial to the scapula. In the angle between these two muscles and the fascia, the dorsal branch of the **accessory N.** is exposed. Locate the ventral cutaneous branches of the C2–C6 Nn. They indicate the border between the **cleidomastoideus** and omotransversarius Mm. Make only a superficial incision on the line that unites the origins of these nerves, to mark the difference between the two muscles (Fig. H1.9).

*Note.* Do not separate the cleidomastoideus M. from the omotransversarius M.

Back to the superficial lamina of the cervical fascia, make an incision parallel to the trapezius M. and observe the duplication of the fascia into a superficial and a deep layer. Extend the exploration of the area by identifying the **rhomboideus cervicis M.** Dissect it and **notice** that the muscle is totally surrounded by a fascia.

Locate the **linguofacial V.**, and the **parotid gland** covered by the **parotidoauricularis M.**

Move to the ventral aspect of the neck. Dissect the common origin of the **sternocephalicus Mm.** on the manubrium sterni, covered only by the cutaneous colli M. The symmetrical sternocephalicus Mm. extend cranially in a common mass up to the middle of the neck, where they separate from each other, become thinner, and end with tendinous attachments on the caudal borders of the mandibular rami. The attachment is crossed on the deep side by the mandibular attachment of the **occipito-mandibular part of the digastricus M.** In its way to the mandible, the tendon of the sternocephalicus M. is crossed obliquely by the linguofacial V.

*Note.* Because in the horse the sternocephalicus is not divided in parts, it is called by some anatomists the "**sternomandibularis.**"

## Table H1.1. Muscles of the Neck, Horse and Large Ruminants

**Dorsal Muscles of the Neck** (dorsal to the cervical vertebrae)

*1st layer*
 – trapezius p. cervicalis
 – omotransversarius
   (cleidotransversus in Eq.)
*2nd layer*
 – rhomboideus cervicis
 – splenius
 – serratus ventralis cervicis
*3rd layer*
 – iliocostalis cervicis (from
    iliocostalis thoracis)          ⎤ (erector spinae)
 – longissimus cervicis
 – longissimus atlantis (from
    longissimus thoracis)
 – longissimus capitis
 – semispinalis capitis (from
    semispinalis thoracis)          ⎦ (transversospinalis)
*4th layer*
 – multifidi cervicis
 – spinalis cervicis (from spinalis
    thoracis)                       ⎤ (erector spinae)
 – intertransversarii cervicis      ⎦
 – rectus capitis dorsalis major
    (superficial and deep fascicles)
 – rectus capitis dorsalis minor
 – obliquus capitis cranialis
 – obliquus capitis caudalis

**Ventral Muscles of the Neck** (ventral to the cervical vertebrae)

*Superficial muscles*
 – cleidobrachialis
 – cleidocephalicus
  • mastoid part (cleidomastoideus)
  • occipital part (cleidooccipitalis—only in Ru.)
 – clavicular intersection
 – sternocephalicus
  • mandibular part (sternomandibularis)
  • mastoid part (sternomastoideus—only in Ru.)
 – sternohyoideus and sternothyroideus
 – omohyoideus
*Deep muscles*
 – longus capitis
 – longus colli
 – rectus capitis ventralis
 – rectus capitis lateralis
 – scalenus dorsalis (only in Ru.)
 – scalenus medius
 – scalenus ventralis

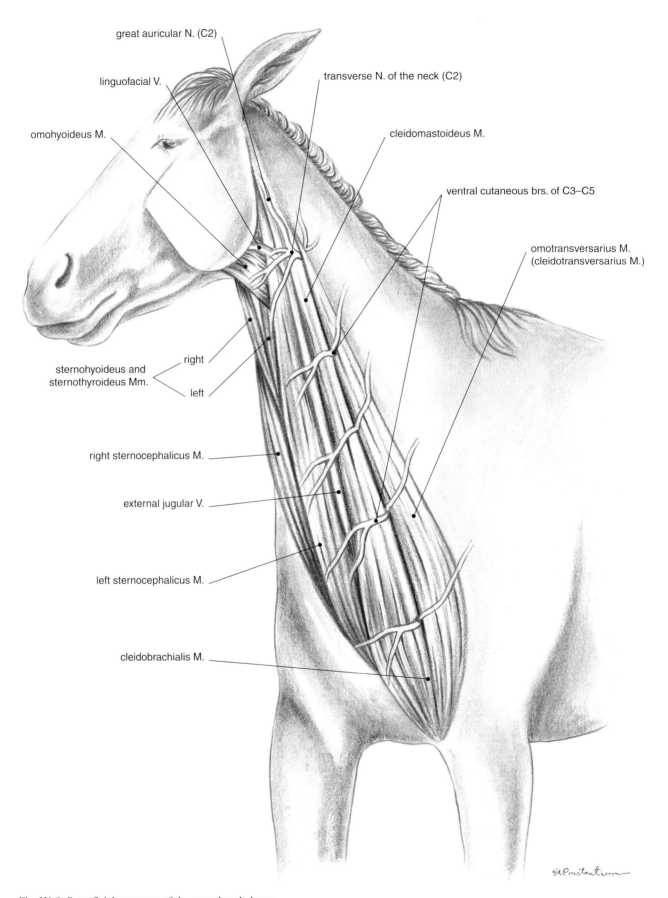

great auricular N. (C2)

linguofacial V.

omohyoideus M.

transverse N. of the neck (C2)

cleidomastoideus M.

ventral cutaneous brs. of C3–C5

omotransversarius M.
(cleidotransversarius M.)

right

sternohyoideus and
sternothyroideus Mm.

left

right sternocephalicus M.

external jugular V.

left sternocephalicus M.

cleidobrachialis M.

Fig. H1.9. Superficial structures of the ventral neck, horse.

Reflect the sternocephalicus M. and find on its deep aspect, close to the terminal tendon, the ventral branch of the accessory N. which supplies this muscle exclusively.

Toward the head, the space left open between the two sternocephalicus Mm. is filled by the symmetrical **sternohyoideus and sternothyroideus Mm.** These four muscles have a common origin from the manubrium sterni. In the middle of the neck, the common body of these four muscles continues with a short and thin tendon. From this tendon, the four muscles separate from each other. The identification of these four muscles is easy: in the middle the sternohyoideus Mm. (attached to the basihyoid bone) and laterally the sternothyroideus Mm. (attached to the two wings of the thyroid cartilage of the larynx). The **tracheal rings** can be distinguished in this area on the midline.

**The sternohyoideus and sternothyroideus Mm. are often either transected or removed (in large part) for management of stereotypical aerophagia.**

**Partial removal of the sternomandibularis, sternothyroideus, sternohyoideus, and omohyoideus Mm. is known as the "Forssell's procedure" in cribbiting or cribbing. With another technique (which is very ineffective on its own), only the sectioning of the accessory N. is performed (Adams 1999).**

**A modification of the Forssell's procedure has also been recommended for treatment of dorsal displacement of the soft palate. The sternohyoideus, sternothyroideus, and omohyoideus Mm. are transected (Harrison 1988). The ventral branch of the accessory N. is left intact in this procedure. In a more recent report, only the tendon of insertion of the sternothyroideus M. has been transected for treatment of soft palate displacement (Bonen et al. 1999).**

**Partial removal of the sternothyroideus and sternohyoideus Mm. is performed to reduce caudal retraction of the larynx as a treatment for intermittent dorsal displacement of the soft palate. The procedure involves tenectomy** *(removal of a tendon, or a portion of a tendon)* **of the sternothyroid M. at its insertion on the lateral aspect of the thyroid cartilage.**

Remove the pretracheal lamina to expose all the tracheal rings and the **esophagus** running dorsal to and slightly on the left side of the trachea. Make a cross section in the trachea and one in the esophagus and examine the relationship between the mucosa, the cartilages, and the **trachealis M.**, and between the mucosa and the muscular coat, respectively.

At the origin of the trachea, identify the **cricoid cartilage of the larynx** and the right and/or the left **lobe of the thyroid gland**, lying on the lateral aspect of the first three to four tracheal cartilages.

In the cranial third of the neck the **omohyoideus M.** is shortly exposed. It extends from the basihyoid bone to the shoulder, lies deep to the sternocephalicus M., separates the external jugular V. from the carotid sheath, and ends on the **axillary fascia**. The axillary fascia covers the medial muscles of the shoulder. Dissect the omohyoideus M. and preserve the transverse N. of the neck crossing it on its way toward the intermandibular space (see Figs. H1.5 and H1.9).

Incise the superficial lamina of the cervical fascia at the dorsal border of the omotransversarius M. and reflect it dorsally and ventrally. Deep to the omotransversarius, identify the **splenius M.** Between the two above mentioned muscles identify the dorsal branch of the accessory N. in its way to supply the trapezius M. (see Fig. H1.5).

Transect the cleidomastoideus and the omotransversarius Mm. 10 cm cranial to the shoulder, separate them from the omohyoideus M., and reflect the stumps. The **superficial cervical lnn.** lie superficial to the omohyoideus M. and deep to the cleidomastoideus and omotransversarius Mm. The 20–40 small lymph nodes are imbedded in fat, cranial to the **subclavius M.** They are supplied by the **prescapular branch of the superficial cervical A.** Transect the omohyoideus and reflect it (Fig. H1.10).

Reflect the external jugular V., open the carotid sheath, and dissect **the common carotid A.**, the **vagosympathetic trunk** (dorsal to the artery), and the **recurrent laryngeal N.** (ventral to the artery) (Fig. H1.10). The **cranial** and **middle deep cervical lnn.** and the **tracheal duct** are now exposed. The vagosympathetic trunk consists of the **vagus N.** (with parasympathetic fibers) and the **cervical sympathetic trunk**. They run together but do not exchange fibers. The paired recurrent laryngeal Nn. are branches of the vagus N. The two nerves, right and left, have different origins and topographies: the right nerve courses around the **right subclavian A.**, while the left courses around the **ligamentum arteriosum** (between the **aorta** and the **pulmonary trunk**).

The cleidomastoideus and omotransversarius Mm. run side by side and continue caudally as the **cleidobrachialis M.;** they are separated by the fibrous intersection of the **clavicle**. Because of its position, the omotransversarius, in the horse only, was formerly called **cleidotransversus M.** According to some authors, only the cleidomastoideus ends at the fibrous intersection of the clavicle and then continues as the cleidobrachialis M. The omotransversarius, like cleidobrachialis attaches caudally to the scapular spine and the humeral crest. Therefore, in the horse, the

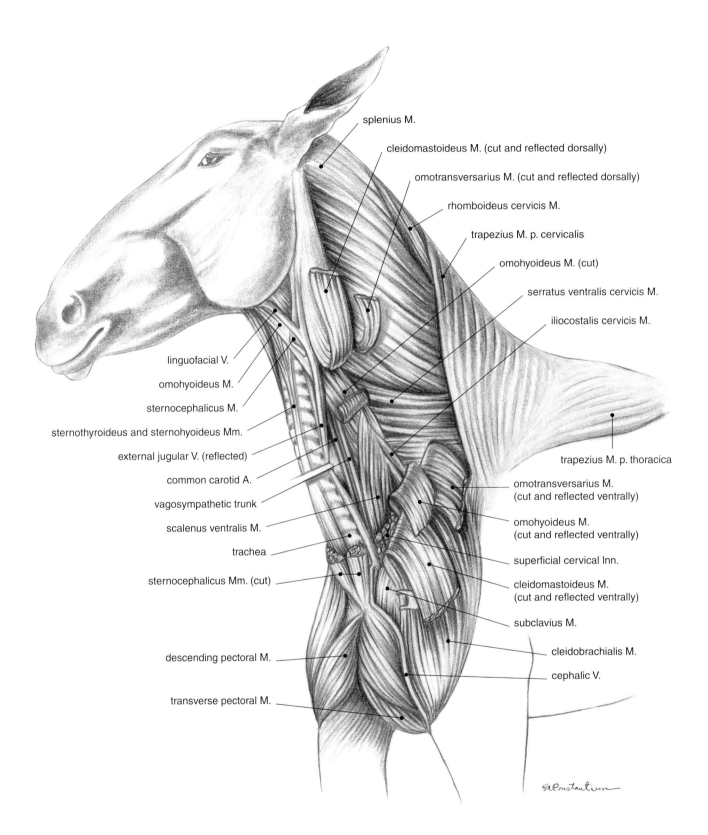

splenius M.

cleidomastoideus M. (cut and reflected dorsally)

omotransversarius M. (cut and reflected dorsally)

rhomboideus cervicis M.

trapezius M. p. cervicalis

omohyoideus M. (cut)

serratus ventralis cervicis M.

iliocostalis cervicis M.

linguofacial V.

omohyoideus M.

sternocephalicus M.

sternothyroideus and sternohyoideus Mm.

external jugular V. (reflected)

common carotid A.

vagosympathetic trunk

scalenus ventralis M.

trachea

sternocephalicus Mm. (cut)

trapezius M. p. thoracica

omotransversarius M.
(cut and reflected ventrally)

omohyoideus M.
(cut and reflected ventrally)

superficial cervical lnn.

cleidomastoideus M.
(cut and reflected ventrally)

subclavius M.

cleidobrachialis M.

cephalic V.

descending pectoral M.

transverse pectoral M.

Fig. H1.10. Deep structures of the neck, horse, lateroventral aspect.

brachiocephalicus is represented either by the cleido-brachialis, cleidomastoideus, and omotransversarius (cleidotransversus) or by the cleidobrachialis and the cleidomastoideus. Dissect them and decide which version is the right one. The authors support the first version, verified in the dissection room.

Between the cleidobrachialis M. and the **descending pectoral M.,** identify the **cephalic V.** accompanied by the **deltoid branch of the superficial cervical A.,** located in the **lateral pectoral groove.**

Make an incision in the **splenius M.** parallel and 2 cm ventral to the rhomboideus cervicis M. followed by a vertical incision ventrally, from the caudal end of the first one. Another option is to first transect the trapezius M. pars cervicalis and widen the area of the two incisions in

the splenius M. On the deep aspect of splenius find **lateral branches of the dorsal branches of the spinal cervical Nn.** accompanied by the **deep cervical A.** and **V.** The nerve branches intermingle in a plexus. The **semispinalis capitis, longissimus capitis,** and **longissimus atlantis Mm.** are also exposed.

Make an incision in the semispinalis capitis M. parallel and 2 cm ventral to the splenius M. and isolate it from the **ligamentum nuchae.** The ligamentum nuchae is made up of the **funiculus nuchae** and the **lamina nuchae** (Fig. H1.11).

Transect the trapezius M. pars cervicalis and extend the incisions of the splenius M. as far caudally as possible to widen the area of exposure of the deepest structures (the **longissimus cervicis** and the **spinalis cervicis Mm.**).

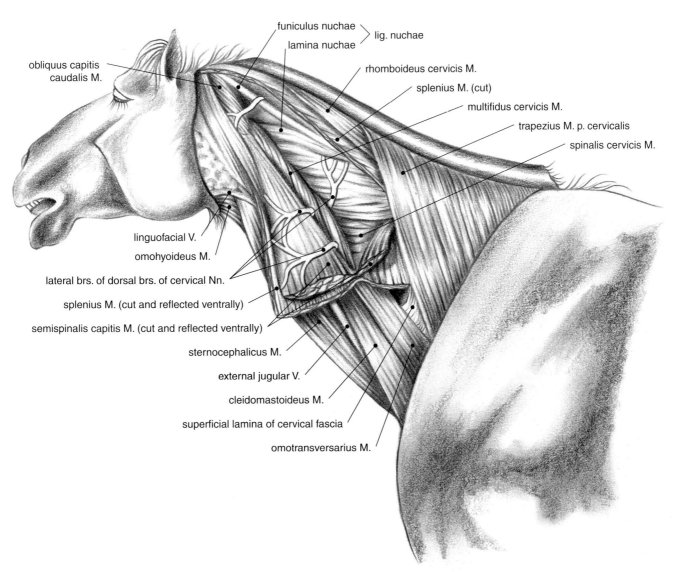

Fig. H1.11. Deep structures of the neck, horse, lateral aspect.

Extend the incision of the semispinalis capitis M. caudally, make a vertical incision through the cranial aponeurosis of this muscle and reflect it ventrally. Identify the **obliquus capitis caudalis** and the **multifidi cervicis Mm.** In Figures H1.12 and H1.13A the **obliquus capitis cranialis**, the **rectus capitis dorsalis major** and the **rectus capitis dorsalis minor** are illustrated.

*Notice* that the semispinalis capitis M. has two portions: **biventer cervicis** (dorsally) and **complexus** (ventrally) (Fig. H1.12).

*Notice* that the rectus capitis dorsalis major has a superficial and a deep portion.

Palpate the atlas and locate the **lateral vertebral** and **alar foramina** (see Fig. H1.1). Make a longitudinal incision through the obliquus capitis caudalis M. over the two foramina and expose the **dorsal branch of the first cervical spinal N. (C1)** and the **occipital branch of the occipital A.** Locate the transverse foramen of the atlas and make a similar incision to expose the vertebral A. (Fig. H1.13B). The **cranial** and **caudal nuchal bursae** are also shown in Figure H1.13B.

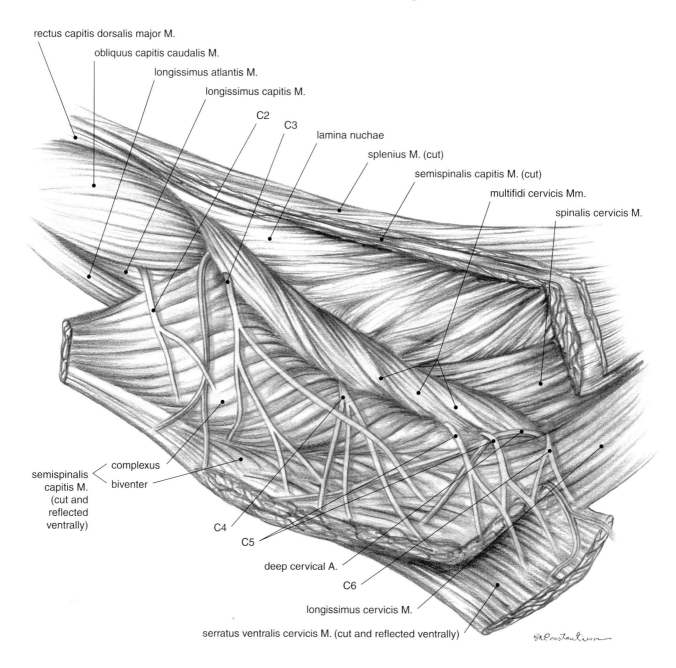

Fig. H1.12. Deepest structures of the neck, horse, left lateral aspect (the head is toward the left side).

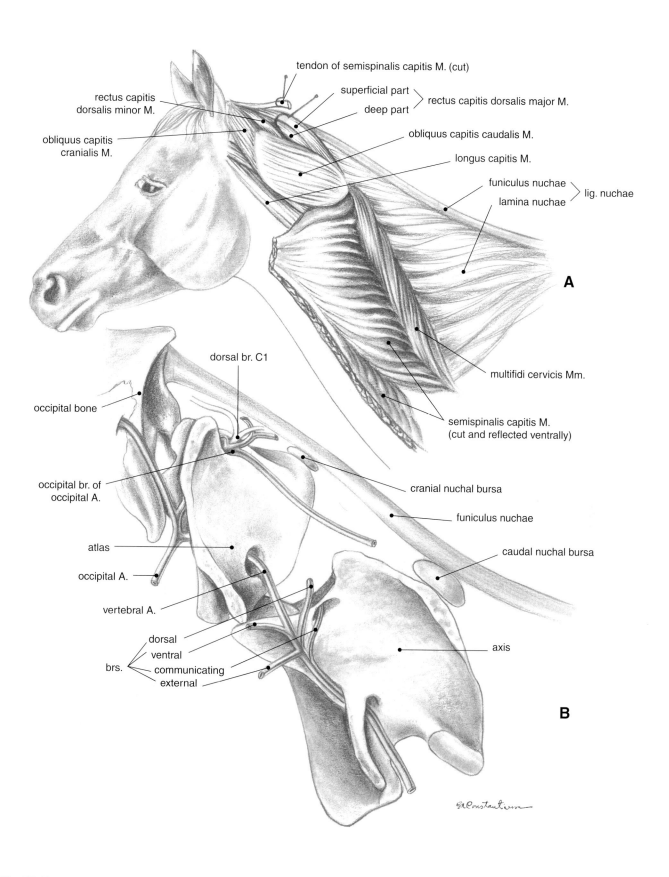

tendon of semispinalis capitis M. (cut)

superficial part
rectus capitis dorsalis major M.
deep part

rectus capitis dorsalis minor M.

obliquus capitis cranialis M.

obliquus capitis caudalis M.

longus capitis M.

funiculus nuchae
lig. nuchae
lamina nuchae

**A**

multifidi cervicis Mm.

semispinalis capitis M. (cut and reflected ventrally)

dorsal br. C1

occipital bone

cranial nuchal bursa

occipital br. of occipital A.

funiculus nuchae

atlas

caudal nuchal bursa

occipital A.

vertebral A.

dorsal
ventral
brs.
communicating
external

axis

**B**

Fig. H1.13. Deepest structures of the cranial half of the neck, horse, lateral aspect. **A.** Muscles. **B.** Arteries and nuchal bursae.

Figure H1.14 shows the deep muscles, vessels, nerves, trachea, and esophagus after the **serratus ventralis cervicis M.** has been removed, the splenius and the semispinalis capitis Mm. have been transected, and the thoracic limb with cervical muscles attached has been removed. If the thoracic limb has not yet been removed, cut off the cervical attachments of the serratus ventralis cervicis, splenius, and semispinalis capitis Mm.

The caudal extent of **longus capitis M.** crosses the cranial extent of the **scalenus M.** In the horse, the scalenus M. has only two parts: the **scalenus ventralis** and the **scalenus medius**. The brachial plexus emerges from the space between the two parts. Preserve the branches of the phrenic N., which passes over the scalenus ventralis M. and runs toward the **thoracic inlet**. Between the scalenus M. and the longissimus cervicis M. find the **iliocostalis**

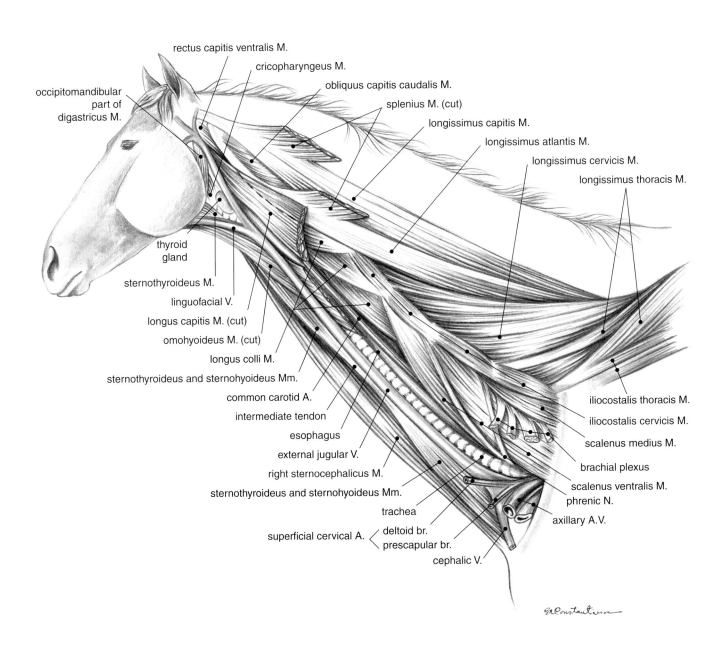

Fig. H1.14. Deepest structures of the neck, horse, left lateral aspect, after removing the thoracic limb.

cervicis M. (Fig. H1.14). On the ventral aspect of the cervical vertebrae and in intimate relation to them, identify the V-shaped fasciculated **longus colli M.**

*Notice* that the longus colli M. replaces the ventral longitudinal lig. all the way to the level of $T_6$.

Two small muscles, the **rectus capitis ventralis** and **rectus capitis lateralis,** can be identified between the atlas and the skull.

**These two muscles, when traumatically avulsed from their origin, produce heavy hemorrhage following certain types of skull trauma.**

The esophagus lies dorsal to the trachea and is slightly deviated to the left side. It makes contact with the longus colli M. dorsally (Fig. H1.14).

The deepest muscles of the neck located on the dorsal and lateral sides of the cervical vertebrae (the multifidi and intertransversarii cervicis Mm., respectively) are shown in Figure H1.15. *It is suggested that the dissection of these muscles be performed by the instructor, as a demonstration.* Remove all muscles from the transverse processes of $C_2$–$C_4$. Remove the prevertebral lamina of the cervical fascia from the **intertransversarii cervicis Mm.** Carefully separate the three fascicles of these muscles, taking as landmarks the nerves and the vessels shown in Figure H1.15. Move dorsal to the intertransversarii and isolate the three parts of the **multifidi cervicis Mm.** (sing. multifidus) from each other, according to Figure H1.15.

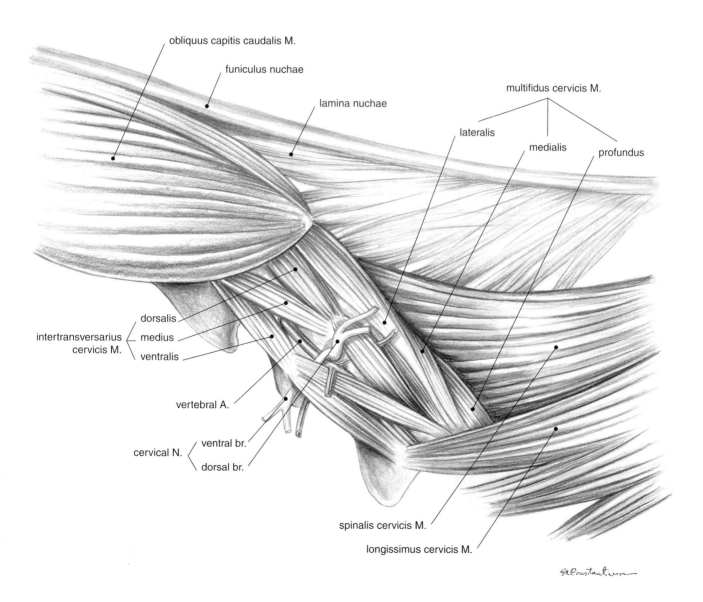

Fig. H1.15. Intertransversarii and multifidi cervicis Mm.

# MODLAB H1

On a living horse, under the supervision of your instructor and taking all the necessary precautions, attempt to palpate all those structures listed at the very beginning of this chapter.

The next step is the identification of the *landmarks* and *approaches* of the clinically important structures of the neck, such as bones, joints, arteries, veins, nerves, lymph nodes, viscera, and so on.

1. **External jugular V., common carotid A., vagosympathetic trunk, and recurrent laryngeal N.** (Fig. H1.16A)
   A. *Landmarks*: jugular groove (bordered dorsally by the cleidomastoideus and ventrally by the sternocephalicus)
   B. *Approach*:
      a. In the middle third of the groove for the external jugular V., deep to the cutaneous colli M. and the superficial lamina of the cervical fascia. The vein is separated from the common carotid A. by the omohyoideus M.
      b. In the caudal third of the groove for the rest of the structures, deep and within the carotid sheath
2. **Superficial cervical A. and the cephalic V. (the brachial segment)** (Fig. H1.16B)
   A. *Landmarks*: lateral pectoral groove (outlined laterally by the cleidobrachialis M. and medially by the descending pectoral M.)
   B. *Approach*: through the skin and cutaneous colli M. at any point within the groove
3. **Superficial cervical lnn.** (Fig. H1.16A,B)
   A. *Landmarks*: shoulder joint, subclavius M., jugular groove, lateral pectoral groove, jugular fossa, and omotransversarius and cleidomastoideus Mm.
   B. *Approach*: midway between the following landmarks at the cranial border of subclavius M.: a point 10 cm dorsal to the shoulder joint or the merge of jugular groove with the lateral pectoral groove (jugular fossa), deep to omotransversarius and cleidomastoideus Mm., and at the cranial border of subclavius M. Press the fingertips of both hands in front of the subclavius M. and roll them deeply forward. A chain of 20–40 lymph nodes will be felt.
4. **Trachea and esophagus** (Fig. H1.16B)
   A. *Landmarks*: the two symmetrical sternocephalicus Mm.
   B. *Approach*: through the ventral midline of the neck and between the two sternocephalicus Mm. The trachea is superficial and easily palpable in the cranial two-thirds of the neck. (The sternothyroideus and sternohyoideus Mm. lie on the ventral aspect of the trachea.) The esophagus accompanies the trachea dorsally and slightly toward the left side.
   *Caution.* The external jugular V. lies superficially in the jugular groove, whereas the common carotid A., the vagosympathetic trunk, and the recurrent laryngeal N. lie deep in that groove, within the carotid sheath, along the lateral aspect of the trachea (see Modlab no. 1).
5. **Atlantooccipital space** (Fig. H1.17)
   A. *Landmarks:* wing of atlas, nuchal crest, and funiculus nuchae
   B. *Approach*: between these three landmarks
6. **Cranial nuchal (atlantal) bursa** (Fig. H1.17)
   A. *Landmarks*: wing of atlas and funiculus nuchae
   B. *Approach*: midway between the cranial and caudal limits of the wing of atlas, between the funiculus nuchae and the dorsal arch of the atlas
7. **Caudal nuchal bursa** (Fig. H1.17)
   A. *Landmarks*: transverse process of axis and funiculus nuchae
   B. *Approach*: at a point 5 cm dorsocranial to the transverse process of the axis and between the funiculus nuchae and the spinous process of the axis.

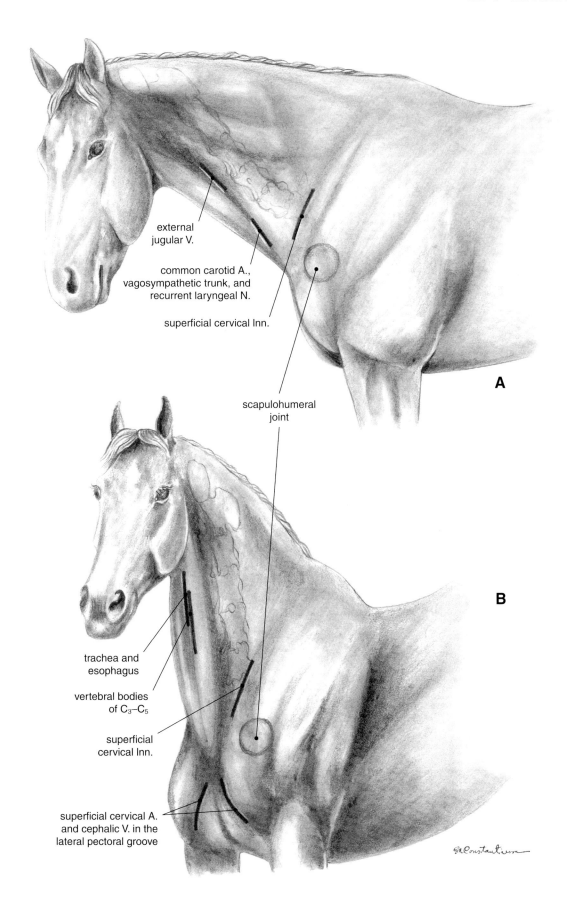

external
jugular V.

common carotid A.,
vagosympathetic trunk, and
recurrent laryngeal N.

superficial cervical lnn.

scapulohumeral
joint

**A**

**B**

trachea and
esophagus

vertebral bodies
of C$_3$–C$_5$

superficial
cervical lnn.

superficial cervical A.
and cephalic V. in the
lateral pectoral groove

Fig. H1.16. Landmarks and approaches on the neck, horse. **A.** Lateral aspect. **B.** Lateroventral aspect.

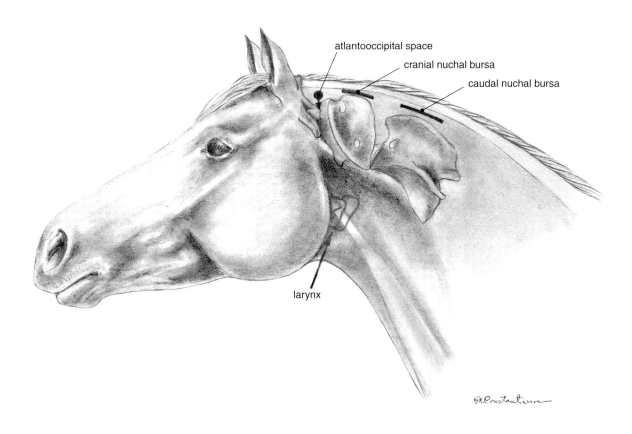

atlantooccipital space

cranial nuchal bursa

caudal nuchal bursa

larynx

Fig. H1.17. Landmarks and clinical approaches, horse. Nuchal bursae and atlantooccipital space.

# H 2

## The Thorax and Thoracic Viscera

The **thoracic vertebrae** are illustrated from the lateral and dorsal perspectives in Figure H2.1A,B. The proximal part of a **rib** is illustrated from the lateral perspective in Figure H2.1C. Details about the **articular surfaces of the ribs** are shown in Figure H2.1D. The **sternum** is illustrated from the lateral and dorsal perspectives in Figure H2.2A,B.

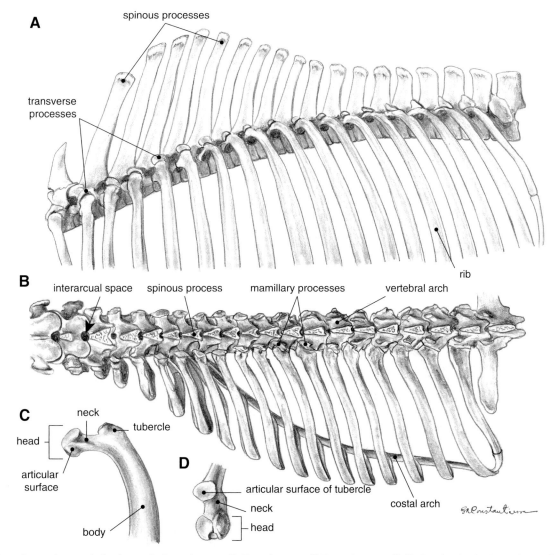

Fig. H2.1. Thoracic vertebrae and ribs, horse. **A.** Lateral aspect. **B.** Dorsal aspect. **C.** Lateral aspect, rib. **D.** Proximal articular surfaces, rib.

23

The **costovertebral** and **sternocostal joints** are illustrated in Figures H2.2A,C,D and H2.2A,B, respectively.

*Outline and/or palpate the following structures: the withers, the ribs, the costal arch, the tips of the spinous processes of the thoracic vertebrae, the triceps brachii M., the olecranon, the caudal angle of scapula, the shoulder joint, the tuber of the scapular spine, and the tuber coxae* (**Fig. H2.3**).

The ribs are landmarks for the sites of pleurocentesis and for auscultation and percussion of the lungs and the heart.

The last rib, the costal arch, and the olecranon are important landmarks for assessing the pleural reflection. The tuber coxae, the tuber of scapular spine and the caudal border of triceps brachii M. are landmarks for the maximal areas of auscultation and percussion of the lungs. The last rib also outlines the cranial border of the lateral abdominal region, while the costal arch outlines the dorsal extent of the xiphoid region.

The triceps brachii M., the olecranon, the caudal angle of the scapula, and the shoulder joint are landmarks for the auscultation and percussion of the heart.

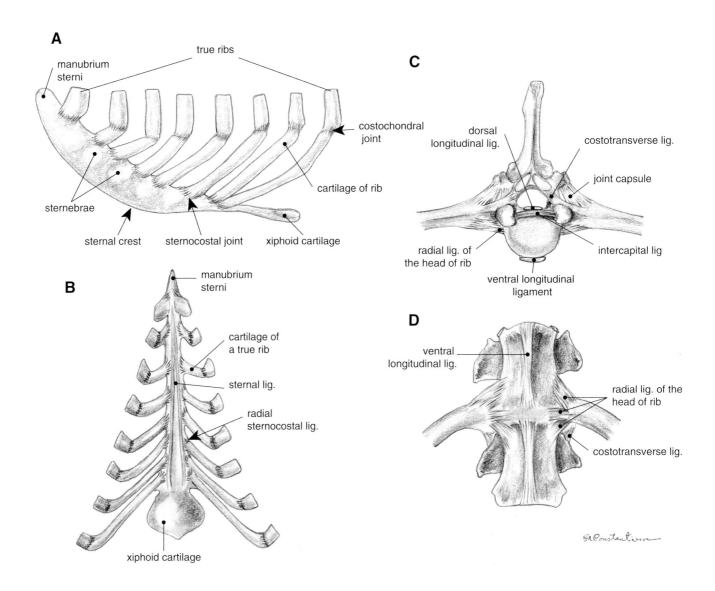

Fig. H2.2. Sternum, costovertebral, and sternocostal joints, horse. **A.** Sternum and joints, left lateral aspect. **B.** Sternum and joints, dorsal aspect. **C.** Costovertebral joints, cranial aspect. **D.** Costovertebral joints, ventral aspect.

Continue the incision of the skin from the cranial extent of the withers to the **spinous process of the last thoracic vertebra**, following the dorsal midline of the specimen. Use the last rib as a landmark. Make a transverse incision through the skin along the last rib to the corresponding **costochondral junction**, and continue the incision ventrally and perpendicularly to the ventral midline. Extend the incision of the skin from the cranial border of the withers to the **manubrium sterni** and then on the midline to the ventral border of the pectoral region. Reflect the skin from the pectoral region, shoulder, arm, thorax, and abdomen, ventrally, to the midline. Skin the area carefully to separate the skin from the cutaneous muscles and the superficial fasciae.

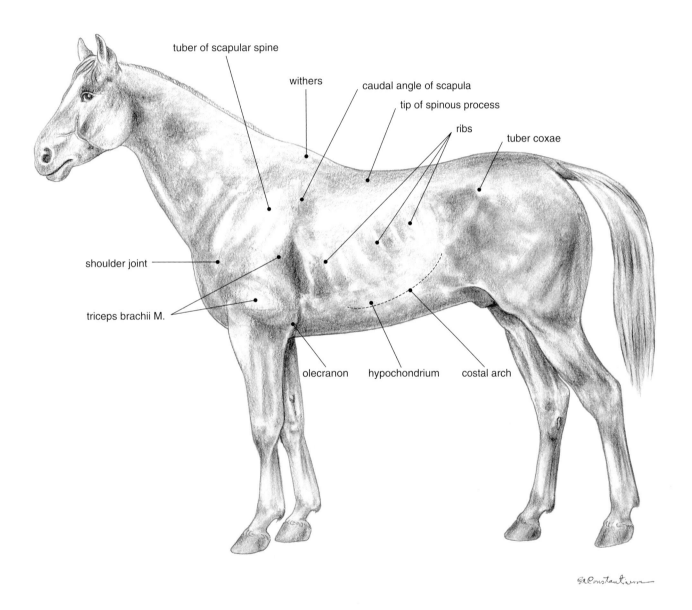

Fig. H2.3. Landmarks for physical examination and/or clinical approach, lateral thorax, horse.

Dissect the **cutaneous omobrachialis** and the **cutaneous trunci Mm.** (see Fig. H1.6) and reflect them ventrally. Outline and dissect the muscles shown in Figure H2.4.

The systematization of the muscles of the dorsal aspect of the body and the thorax is shown in the Table H2.1.

*Notice* the **cutaneous branches of the thoracic nerves** that pierce the **thoracolumbar fascia** and the **latissimus dorsi M.**, the **intercostal** and **external abdominal oblique Mm.** Identify the **intercostobrachial N.** at the intersection of the ventral border of the latissimus dorsi M. and **triceps brachii M.** (Fig. H2.5).

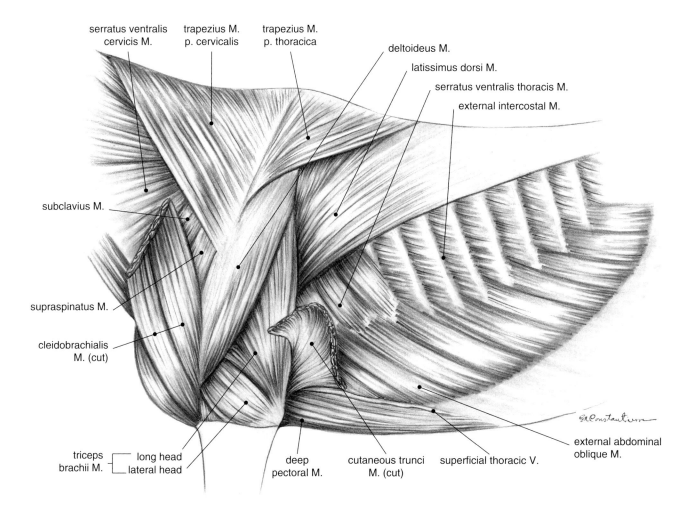

Fig. H2.4. Superficial muscles of the thorax, horse, left aspect.

Table H2.1. Muscles of the Dorsal Aspect of the Body and Thorax, Horse and Large Ruminants

**Dorsal Muscles**

*(Extrinsic muscles of thoracic limb and epaxial muscles)*

– trapezius p. thoracica (+ cervical part)
– latissimus dorsi
– rhomboideus thoracis (+ cervicis)
– serratus dorsalis cranialis
– serratus dorsalis caudalis

    *Erector spinae M.*

– iliocostalis
  • iliocostalis thoracis and lumborum (+ cervicis)
– longissimus
  • longissimus thoracis and lumborum (+ atlantis + capitis)
– spinalis
  • spinalis thoracis (+ cervicis)

    *Transversospinalis M.*

– semispinalis
  • semispinalis thoracis (+ capitis – biventer and complexus)
– multifidi
– rotatores

    *Interspinales Mm.*

    *Intertransversarii Mm.*

– intertransversarii thoracis and lumborum (+ cervicis)

**Muscles of the Thorax**

– superficial pectoral
  • descending pectoral
  • transverse pectoral
– deep pectoral (ascending pectoral)
– subclavius
– serratus ventralis thoracis (+ serratus ventralis cervicis)
– levatores costarum
– external intercostal Mm.
– internal intercostal Mm.
– retractor costae
– transversus thoracis
– rectus thoracis

    *Diaphragm*

– pars lumbalis
  • crus dextrum
  • crus sinistrum
– pars costalis
– pars sternalis
  • aortic hiatus
  • esophageal hiatus
  • diaphragmatic cupula
  • tendinous center (centrum tendineum)
  • foramen of caudal vena cava

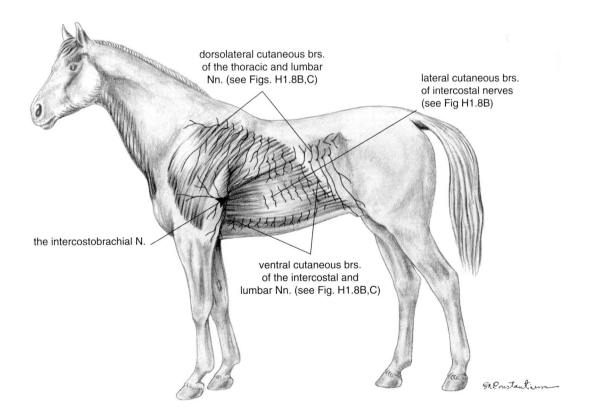

Fig. H2.5. Cutaneous branches of the thoracic nerves, horse, lateral aspect.

Palpate the **scapular spine and tuberosity (tuber of scapular spine)** and make an incision to separate the two parts of the **trapezius M. (the cervical and thoracic parts)**, starting from the tuberosity of the scapular spine to the withers. Reflect the two parts dorsally. However, as another technique, you may choose to transect the vertebral attachment of the trapezius M. and reflect it ventrally (Fig. H2.6). The **scapular cartilage** is now exposed; its caudal extent is overlapped by the aponeurosis of the latissimus dorsi M. Choosing the second technique, both **rhomboideus cervicis and thoracis Mm.**, as well as part of the splenius, serratus ventralis cervicis, **supraspinatus, and infraspinatus Mm.** are now exposed (Fig. H2.6).

At about 10 cm ventral to the junction of the ventral border of the latissimus dorsi and the triceps brachii Mm., find the apparent origin of the **superficial thoracic V. (the spur vein)**, specific to the horse. Together with the **lateral thoracic N.**, the vein parallels the dorsal border of the **deep pectoral M.** Between the latissimus dorsi and the ascending pectoral two other muscles are exposed: the **serratus ventralis thoracis** and the external abdominal oblique. The former is protected by a tough fascia, whereas the latter is covered by the **tunica flava abdominus (abdominal tunic)**. The intercostal Mm. are metamerically spread and fill the intercostal spaces. The **external intercostal Mm.** are oriented caudoventrally,

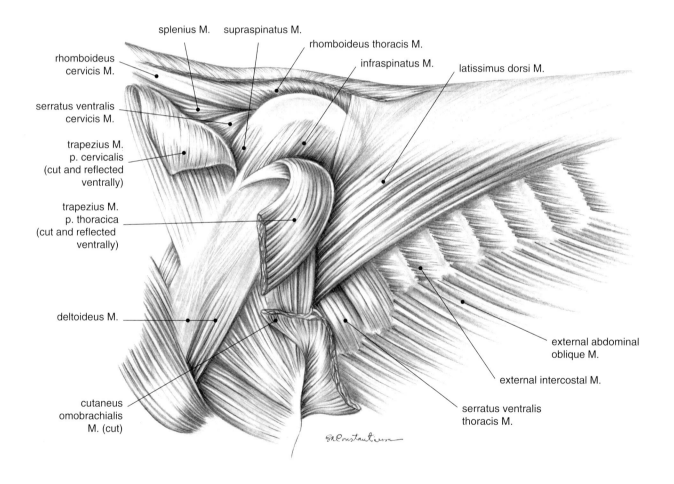

Fig. H2.6. Deep dorsoscapular structures, horse, left side.

while the **internal intercostal Mm.** are oriented cranioventrally. Transect the latissimus dorsi close to the caudal border of the triceps brachii M., dissect it, and reflect it dorsally. The **serratus dorsalis cranialis** and **serratus dorsalis caudalis Mm.** are now exposed (Fig. H2.7).

*Notice* that the serratus dorsalis Mm. have a muscular portion (ventrally) and an aponeurosis (dorsally), which are in continuation with each other; the muscle fibers are differently oriented (dorsocranially for the serratus dorsalis cranialis, and dorsocaudally for the serratus dorsalis caudalis).

Make two parallel incisions 10–15 cm apart through the serratus dorsalis M. to expose its attachment on the ribs. The attachment separates the **iliocostalis thoracis M.** from the **longissimus, semispinalis, and spinalis thoracis Mm.** altogether. Make the incision deeper through the last three muscles to expose the **multifidus thoracis, levatores costarum** (Fig. H2.7), **and intertransversarii thoracis Mm.**

In the shoulder area identify the following muscles: subclavius, cleidobrachialis, descending pectoral, and **deltoideus**.

Two different techniques for removing the thoracic limb are suggested.

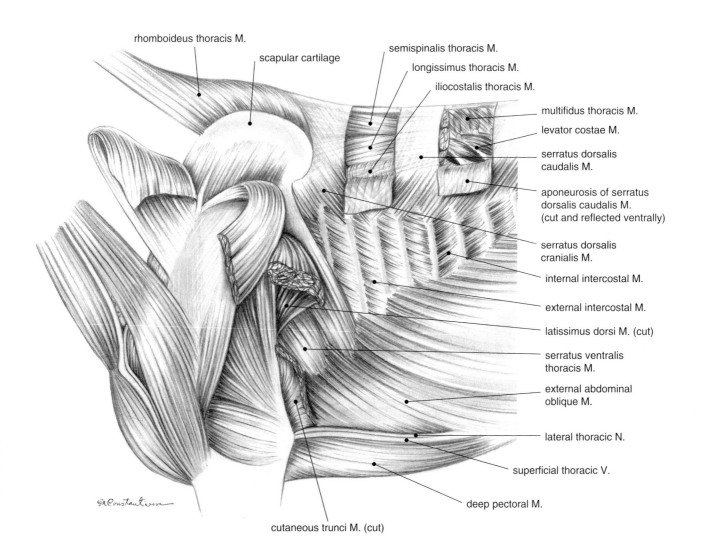

Fig. H2.7. Deep muscles of the thorax, horse, left aspect.

## The First Technique

Transect the scapula and the corresponding muscles transversely with a saw, dorsal to the tuberosity of the spine. Cut through the subclavius, supraspinatus, infraspinatus, deltoideus, triceps brachii (on the lateral aspect of the shoulder), and **subscapularis, tensor fasciae antebrachii,** and **serratus ventralis Mm.** (on the medial aspect of the shoulder). Separate the forelimb from the scapular attachment of the serratus ventralis (Fig. H2.8). There is an abundance of loose connective tissue between the limb and the serratus ventralis thoracis M., therefore blunt dissection is suggested. For an easier procedure, push the free end of the limb medially.

Expose the **brachial plexus** between the **scalenus medius** (dorsally) and the **scalenus ventralis** (ventrally) (Fig. H2.8). Identify and isolate the **axillary A. and V.** Transect the brachial plexus and the axillary vessels as close as possible to the body.

Transect the descending, transverse and deep pectoral Mm., and the subclavius M. 10 cm dorsal to the **sternal crest.**

Remove the thoracic limb, wrap and store it in the cold room for a later dissection.

## The Second Technique

Transect the rhomboideus cervicis and thoracis Mm. around the free edge of the scapular cartilage. Expose the **dorsoscapular lig.** with all the connections and *notice* its yellow color due to the abundance of elastic fibers. Transect the ligament and the serratus ventralis M. from their attachments on the base of the scapula. Follow the same procedure already conducted on the other limb for the ventral structures.

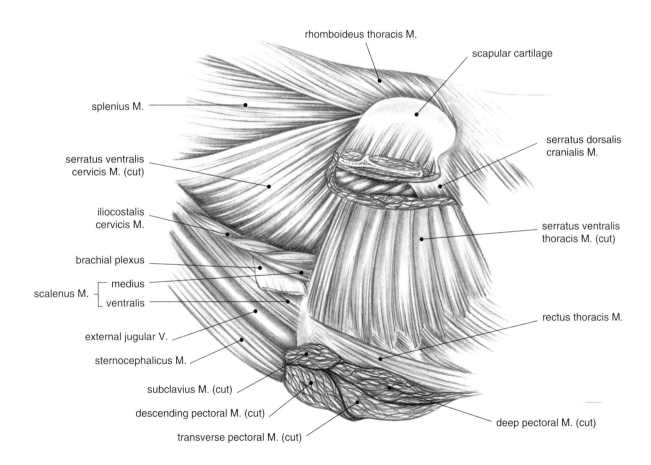

Fig. H2.8. Deep muscles of the cervicothoracic area after removing the forelimb, horse, left aspect.

*If the first technique was chosen*, reflect the remnant of the scapula with the scapular cartilage dorsally to expose the dorsoscapular lig. This structure is the result of the intermingling aponeuroses of the splenius, semispinalis capitis and serratus dorsalis cranialis Mm. (Fig. H2.9A). The elastic component comes from the **supraspinous lig.** and the **funiculus nuchae** (Fig. H2.9B; see Figs. H1.11 and H1.13A).

Before exploring the deep structures of the thoracic inlet and the transition of some structures from the neck into the thoracic cavity, identify the superficial structures of the thoracic inlet after removing the thoracic limb (Fig. H2.10). Identify the origin of the **long thoracic and lateral thoracic Nn.** from the brachial plexus.

*If the second technique was your choice*, dissect the deep aspect of the dorsoscapular lig., reflect the

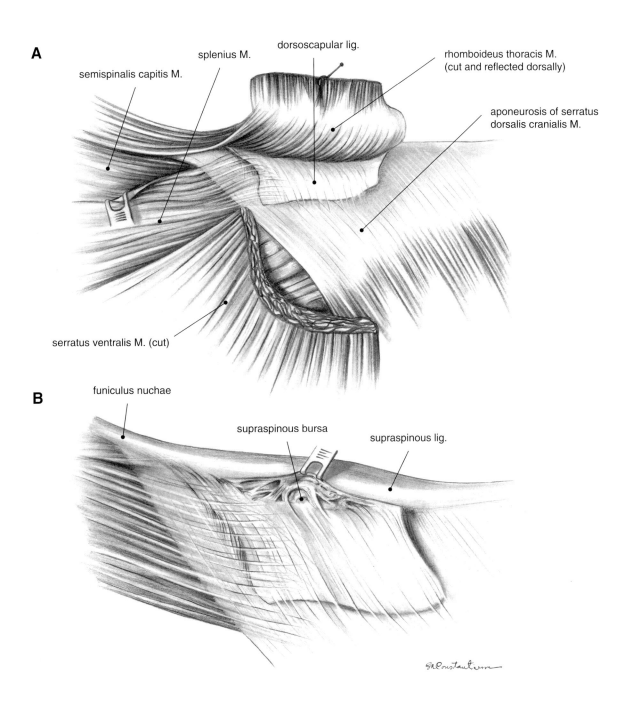

Fig. H2.9. Structures in the withers area, horse, left aspect. **A.** The dorsoscapular ligament. **B.** The supraspinous bursa.

supraspinous lig. dorsally and expose the **supraspinous bursa**. This structure is surrounded by a large amount of connective tissue and is located over the tips of the **spinous processes of T₂ and T₃** (Fig. H2.9B).

By lateral approach continue to open the **carotid sheath** toward the thoracic inlet and isolate the **common carotid A.**, the **vagosympathetic trunk** and the **recurrent laryngeal N.**

*Notice* the separation of the **cervical sympathetic trunk** from the **vagus N.** The sympathetic trunk joins the **middle cervical ggl.** in a slightly dorsal direction, while the vagus continues its course within the thoracic cavity (Fig. H2.11). Dissect the **common carotid A.** and *notice*

the common origin of both right and left arteries from **truncus bicaroticus**.

Continue to dissect the external jugular V. to the point where the cephalic and axillary (**subclavian**) Vv. join it. Here is the origin of the **bijugular trunk**, the origin of the **cranial vena cava**.

The axillary and the **superficial cervical Aa.** exit through the thoracic inlet.

Dissect the roots of the brachial plexus, the scalenus ventralis and medius and the iliocostalis cervicis Mm., saving the **phrenic N.** already identified. Transect both scaleni Mm. from the first rib. Leaving intact the origins of the phrenic N., transect and remove most of the

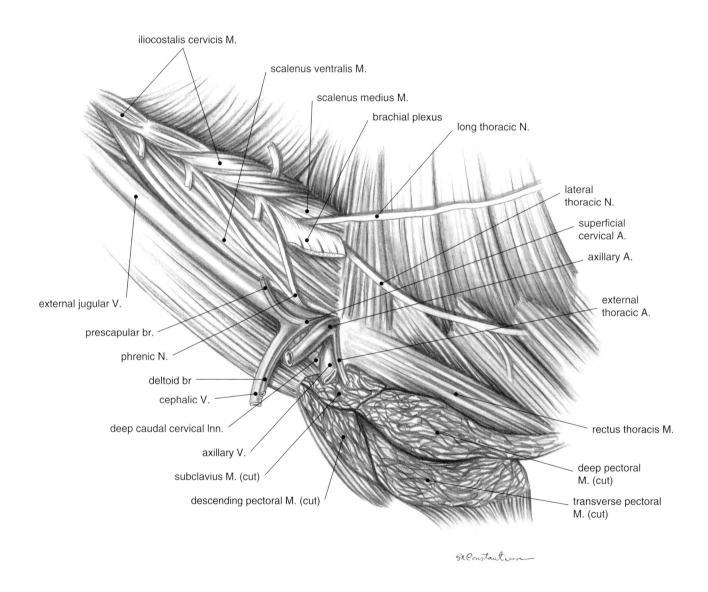

Fig. H2.10. Superficial structures of the thoracic inlet, horse, left aspect, after removing the thoracic limb.

scalenus ventralis M. to allow dissection deep to the first rib, to better expose the middle cervical ggl.

Dissect the recurrent laryngeal N., the **trachea**, the **esophagus** and the **caudal deep cervical lnn.** that surround the vessels, nerves and viscera at the thoracic inlet, as they are shown in Fig. H2.11A (on the left side) and Fig. H2.11B (on the right side).

Dissect the **rectus thoracis M.** (see Figs. H2.8 and H2.10) and the cranial aponeurosis of **the rectus abdominis M.** They appear almost in continuation with each other. Remove a 5 × 5 cm strip from the abdominal tunic and check its elasticity. It is very adherent to the external abdominal oblique M.

Remove the serratus ventralis thoracis M. from the ribs, and the serratus ventralis cervicis M., leaving 1–2 cm of this muscle attached to the cervical vertebrae.

Dissect the external and internal intercostal Mm. and the **intercostal A.V.N.** running in the **costal sulcus/groove** at the caudal border of each rib. Remove all the muscles from the lateral aspect of the thoracic wall starting from the next to the last intercostal space and continue cranially. Penetrate the thorax in the middle third of an intercostal

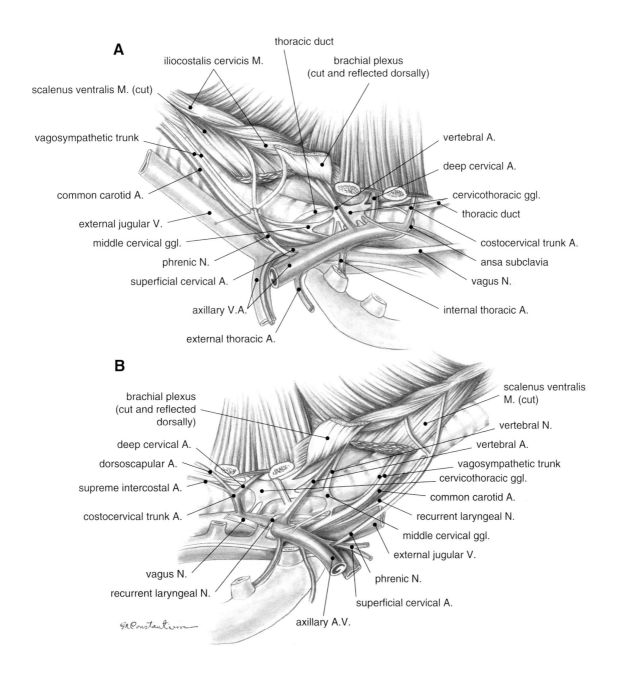

Fig. H2.11. Deep structures of the thoracic inlet, horse. **A.** Left aspect. **B.** Right aspect.

space and make an incision in the **endothoracic fascia** lined by the **costal pleura**. Continue the incision in a ventral direction and carefully check with the finger the point where the costal pleura reflects onto the **diaphragm** as the **diaphragmatic pleura**. This is the **costodiaphragmatic recess**, the maximal extent of the **pleural cavity**. Along the entire pleural cavity the reflection of the costal pleura on the diaphragm is known as the **line of pleural reflection**, an anatomical structure with clinical importance (Fig. H2.12).

**When performing pleurocentesis, the cranial border of a rib is used as a landmark, thus avoiding the intercostal A., V., and N., which run along the caudal border of the rib.**

The endothoracic fascia is the continuation of the pretracheal lamina of the cervical fascia and will continue with the **endoabdominal (transverse) fascia** through the three openings of the diaphragm.

*Caution.* While removing the intercostal Mm. do not exceed the line of pleural reflection.

In the following steps, examine the **lungs** and the **heart** enclosed within the **pericardium**. Identify the lobes of the lungs and the wide **cardiac notches**.

Carefully remove all the ribs except the 5th, 9th, 10th, 17th, and 18th (Fig. H2.12). Direct the rib cutter with your finger on the medial aspect of each rib dorsally and then ventrally, and transect it. The use of a large, flat rib cutter for this operation is recommended. It is also suggested to disarticulate the **costal cartilages** from the **costochondral joints** of all the **sternal ribs**. Remove the **asternal ribs** by transecting them dorsal to the pleural reflection.

*Caution.* The **ansa subclavia** (the communicating loop between the middle cervical ggl. and the **cervicothoracic ggl.—the stellate ggl.**), and the **cardiac Nn.** are sometimes very fine structures and, in addition, they are embed-

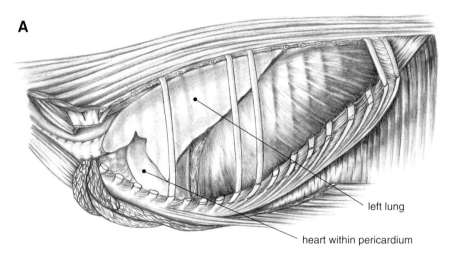

**A**

left lung

heart within pericardium

Interrupted line, line of pleural reflection

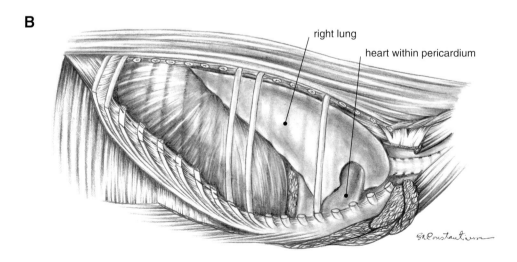

**B**

right lung

heart within pericardium

Fig. H2.12. The thoracic cavity with the lungs and the heart in situ, horse. **A.** Left aspect. **B.** Right aspect.

ded in fat or loose connective tissue. Dissect them cautiously.

Carefully dissect the arteries, veins and nerves within the thoracic inlet, including the sympathetic ganglia and their branches. Continue the dissection inside of the thoracic cavity, in the **cranial mediastinum**, the **middle mediastinum** and the **caudal mediastinum**.

*Note.* The "mediastinum" is defined as the connective tissue septum and the corresponding **pleurae** separating the right from the left **pleural cavities**. It contains most of the structures in the thoracic cavity, except the lungs. The "cranial mediastinum" is located cranial to the pericardium and contains great vessels and nerves, the **thoracic duct**, trachea and esophagus. The "middle mediastinum" contains the heart (and the pericardium). The middle mediastinum has two divisions: the "dorsal mediastinum," between the pericardium and the vertebrae, and the "ventral mediastinum," between the pericardium and the sternum. The "caudal mediastinum," between the heart and the diaphragm, contains the aorta and the esophagus, vessels and nerves.

Remove the left lung by transecting the **primary bronchus** and the **pulmonary vessels** and save it for further examination.

Figure H2.13 shows the structures within the thoracic cavity after removal of the left lung. In the cranial mediastinum identify in a craniocaudal direction the **vertebral A., deep cervical A.,** and the **costocervical trunk (A.)**

oriented dorsally. The costocervical trunk branches into the **dorsoscapular** and the **supreme intercostal Aa.** They are overlapped by veins with similar names, as follows: the vertebral, deep cervical, dorsoscapular and supreme intercostal Vv. *Notice* that there is no costocervical trunk V. on the left side in the horse. The homologous veins of the superficial cervical, axillary, and **external and internal thoracic Aa.** are deep to the arteries. Identify the cranial mediastinal lnn.

The cranial vena cava, **bicarotid and brachiocephalic trunks (Aa.),** trachea and esophagus are large and visible structures (given here in a ventrodorsal order). The thoracic duct is observed crossing the esophagus and the trachea cranioventrally toward the **left venous angle**.

*Remember!* The venous angle (right and left) is located in the horse (and ruminants) at the confluence of the subclavian V. with the bijugular trunk (V.).

Continue the dissection of the vagus N. dorsal to, and the phrenic N. ventral to the cranial vena cava, and passing over the **pulmonary trunk**. The vagus N. travels toward the **aortic arch** and gives off the left recurrent laryngeal N. The latter surrounds the aorta just ventral to the **lig. arteriosum**.

*Remember!* The lig. arteriosum joins the aorta to the pulmonary trunk and is the remnant of the patent **ductus arteriosus** from the developmental life.

After surrounding the **aortic arch** the recurrent laryngeal N. turns back to the neck and will take a parallel

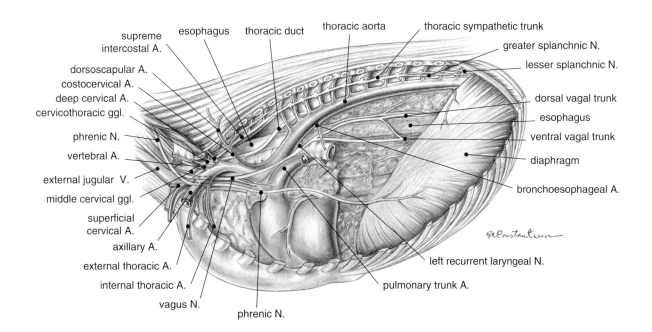

Fig. H2.13. Heart, vessels, and nerves within the thoracic cavity, horse, left side.

course to, and ventral to the vagosympathetic trunk. The vagus continues to travel caudally toward the esophagus and splits into two branches, one dorsal and one ventral. The contralateral vagus N. also splits into two branches. The symmetrical dorsal branches join and form the **dorsal vagal trunk**. The symmetrical ventral branches form the **ventral vagal trunk**. The vagal trunks run parallel with each other, dorsal and ventral to the esophagus, respectively, and exit the thoracic cavity with the esophagus through the esophageal hiatus.

*Notice* that there are three foramina of the diaphragm: the **aortic hiatus,** the **esophageal hiatus** and the **foramen of the caudal vena cava.**

The phrenic N. travels along the lateral aspect of the **left auricula** toward the diaphragm and supplies its left half.

Return to the cervicothoracic ggl. and continue the dissection of the **thoracic sympathetic trunk**, which is close to the **costovertebral joints** and parallel to the supreme intercostal A.; dissect the **thoracic ganglia** and their **communicating branches** in relationship with the **dorsal intercostal Aa.** Toward the caudal end of the thoracic cavity dissect the **greater and lesser splanchnic Nn.**

*Remember.* In the horse, the greater splanchnic N. is the result of the communication between the T7 through T15 sympathetic fibers, whereas the lesser splanchnic N. arises from T16 through T18. They leave the thoracic cavity to reach the **celiac and the cranial mesenteric/renal ganglia**, respectively.

Identify the **bronchoesophageal A.**, which supplies the lungs and the esophagus.

*Caution.* The **caudal cardiac Nn.** originate from the stellate ggl., while the **middle cardiac Nn.** are branches of the middle cervical ggl. (sympathetic postganglionic branches). Dissect the cardiac Nn. branching off the vagus N. (parasympathetic preganglionic branches).

Remove the same ribs on the right side and dissect the similar structures as those already dissected on the left side. Differences observed on the right side in comparison to the left side are as follows (Fig. H2.14):

- The deep cervical and the costocervical trunk Aa. and Vv. originate from a common trunk.
- The **azygos V.**, present only on the right side courses along the roof of the thoracic cavity, dorsal to the thoracic duct. At the level of the eighth and seventh ribs it bends ventrally, opening into the dorsal wall of the cranial vena cava. At the same level, the thoracic duct crosses the medial aspect of the azygos V. and then the esophagus, and passes into the left half of the thoracic cavity.
- The right recurrent laryngeal N. originates from the vagus N. and turns around the right subclavian A. and costocervical trunk A.
- Locate the caudal vena cava and the **plica venae cavae**, a fold of pleura enclosing the right phrenic N.
- Identify the **accessory lobe of the right lung.**

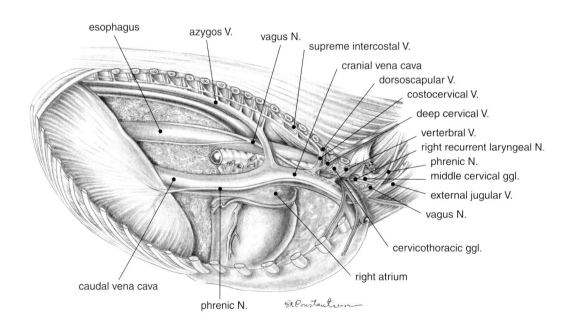

Fig. H2.14. Heart, vessels, and nerves within the thoracic cavity, horse, right side.

Remove the right lung by transecting the right primary bronchus and the right pulmonary vessels. Examine the **right tracheobronchial lnn.** and dissect the **right pulmonary ln.**

After removing the right lung, *notice* the fenestration of the caudal mediastinum and the possibility of communication between the right and the left pleural cavities.

**Make certain you understand the difference between the thoracic cavity and the pleural cavities.**

Examine the removed lungs and observe the wide cardiac notches, the absence of the cranial and caudal parts of the cranial lobes, the absence of the polyhedral design, and of a tracheal bronchus. Identify the grooves or so-called **impressions** of other structures on the medial and costal surfaces of the lungs.

Examine the left removed lung on both lateral aspect (Fig. H2.15A) and medial aspect (Fig. H2.15B).

**A**

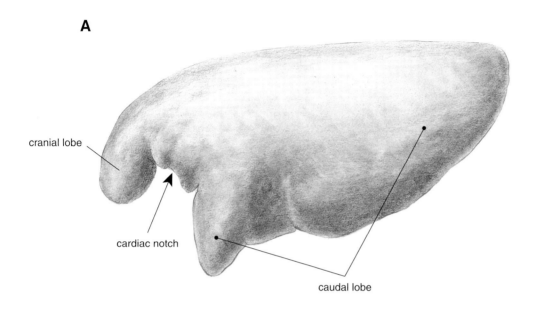

**B**

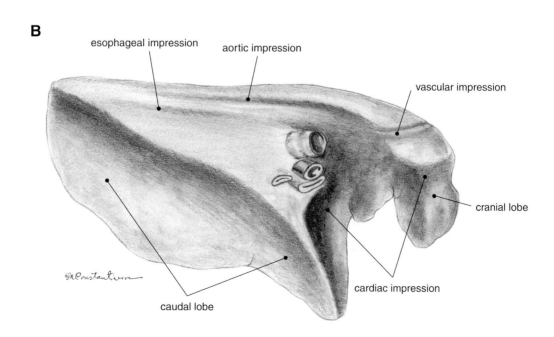

Fig. H2.15. Lungs of the horse. **A.** Left lung, lateral aspect. **B.** Left lung, medial aspect.

Examine the right removed lung on both lateral aspect (Fig. H2.16A) and medial aspect (Fig. H2.16B), and *notice* the presence of the accessory lobe (from the caudal lobe) and the absence of the middle lobe.

Examine the heart and transect the **sternopericardial lig.**, which connects the fibrous pericardium to the sternum. Transect the cranial and caudal venae cavae, the azygos V., and the brachiocephalic trunk A. Remove the heart with the pericardium and place it on a tray.

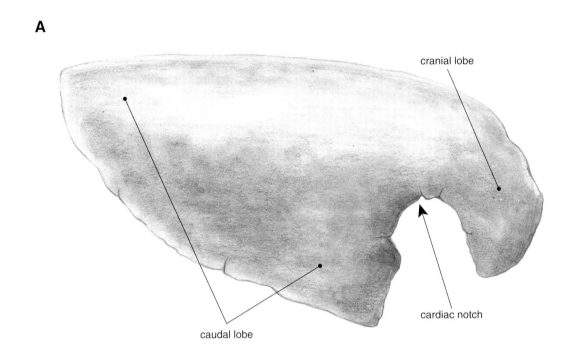

A

cranial lobe

cardiac notch

caudal lobe

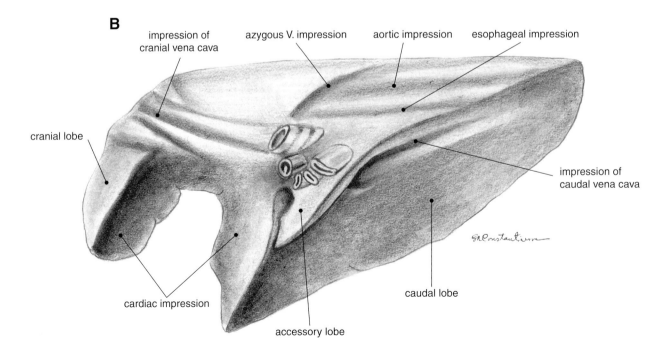

B

impression of cranial vena cava

azygous V. impression

aortic impression

esophageal impression

cranial lobe

impression of caudal vena cava

cardiac impression

accessory lobe

caudal lobe

Fig. H2.16. Lungs of the horse. **A.** Right lung, lateral aspect. **B.** Right lung, medial aspect.

Open the pericardium, examine the **fibrous and the serous pericardium** and remove it by cutting off the attachments of the fibrous pericardium to the great vessels of the heart.

Examine the left (auricular) aspect of the heart (Fig. H2.17A) and the right (atrial) aspect (Fig. H2.17B) with the following grooves:

- The **coronary groove** separating the **atrial mass** (dorsally) from the **ventricular mass** (ventrally). The **right coronary A.** runs in the coronary groove on the atrial side; the **circumflex branch of the left coronary A.** lies in the coronary groove on the auricular side, accompanied by the **great cardiac V.**

- The **paraconal interventricular groove** (on the auricular side), with the **paraconal interventricular branch of the left coronary A.**, accompanied by the great cardiac V.

- The **subsinuosal groove** (on the atrial side), with the **subsinuosal interventricular branch of the right coronary A.**, accompanied by the **middle cardiac V.**

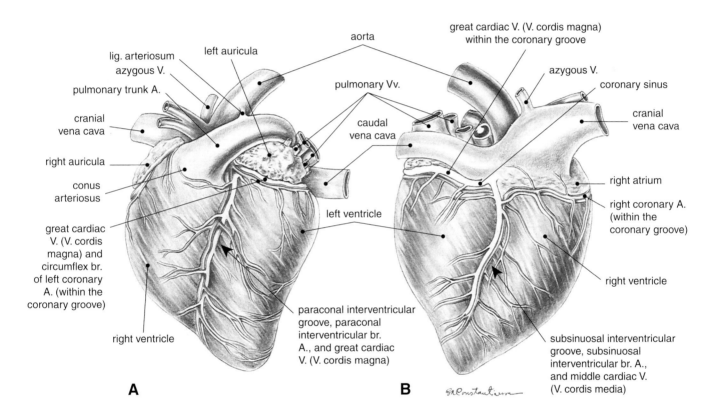

Fig. H2.17. Heart of the horse. **A.** Left (auricular) aspect. **B.** Right (atrial) aspect.

*Notice* that the horse has a **bilateral coronary type of supply to the heart**, by both right and left coronary Aa., in comparison to the large ruminants, which have a left type of supply (both paraconal and subsinuosal interventricular branches originate from the left coronary A.).

To prove that, separate the atria from the ventricles through the coronary groove and examine the **atrioven-**tricular (AV), aortic and pulmonary valves (Fig. H2.18A). Remove the right ventricular wall sectioning through the two interventricular grooves saving the arteries and the veins within the grooves. Examine the **interventricular septum** (Fig. H2.18B), showing the bilateral type of supply to the heart.

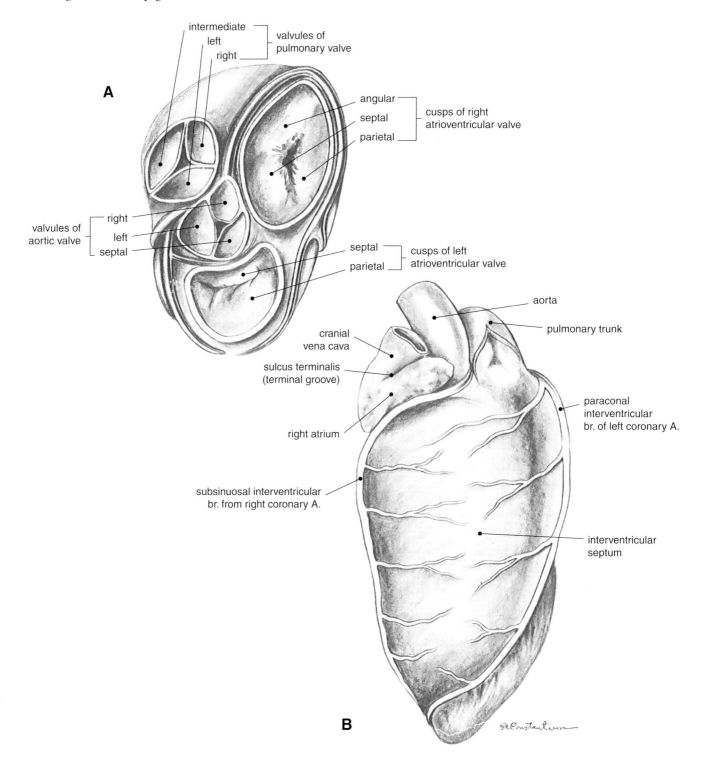

Fig. H2.18. Heart of the horse. **A.** Atrioventricular and arterial valves of heart. **B.** Interventricular septum. Right ventricle is removed.

Make an incision in the long axis of the cranial vena cava and continue throughout the caudal vena cava. The entire **right atrium** is opened and ready for identification of structures, such as the **right auricula** provided with the **pectinate Mm.**, the **interatrial septum** with the **fossa ovalis** in the middle and the opening of the **coronary sinus** ventrally, the **intervenous tubercle**, the **crista terminalis (terminal crest)**, and the **right atrioventricular (AV) valve** with its three **cusps** (angular, parietal, and septal) (Fig. H2.19).

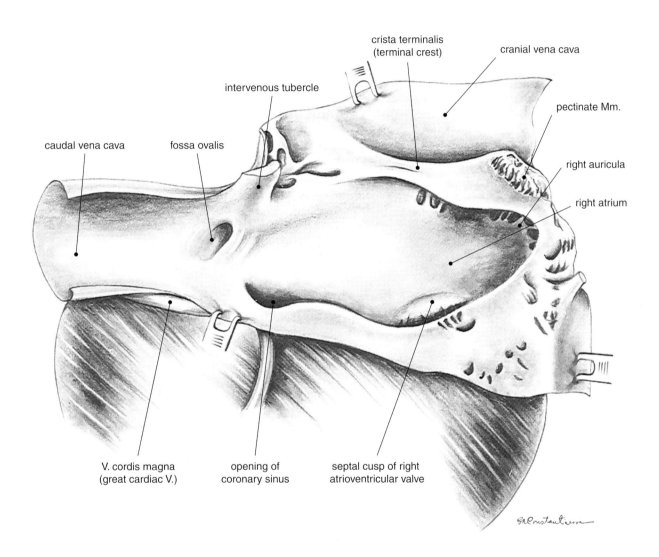

Fig. H2.19. Heart of the horse, right atrium opened.

Turn the heart auricular side up. Identify the **conus arteriosus** as the basal segment of the right ventricle at the origin of the pulmonary trunk. Make an incision in the long axis of the conus arteriosus and the pulmonary trunk. Open up the right ventricle and the origin of the pulmonary trunk. Examine the interventricular septum and the following structures: the three cusps of the right AV valve connected to the **papillary Mm.** by **chordae tendineae**, the **trabeculae septomarginalis**, the **trabeculae carneae,** and the **pulmonary valve** with its three **semilunar valvules** (right, left, and intermediate) (Fig. H2.20).

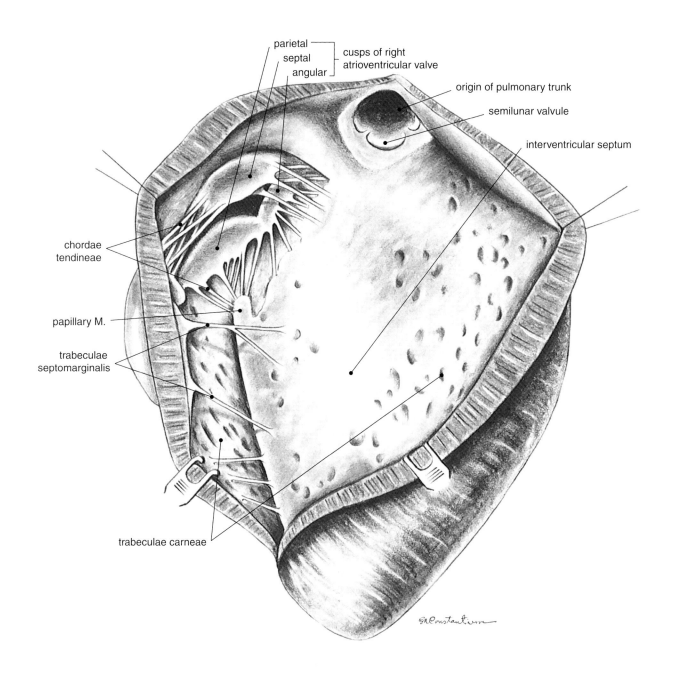

Fig. H2.20. Heart of the horse, right ventricle opened.

Focus your attention on the left atrium and ventricle. Make an incision in the long axis of one of the pulmonary veins and continue it into the left atrium. Examine the **left auricula** with the pectinate Mm., and the **left AV valve** with its two cusps (parietal and septal). Continue the incision through the left ventricle, examine the two cusps, the chordae tendineae and the papillary Mm. Look for the origin of the aorta and identify the three **semilunar valvules of the aortic valve** (right, left, and septal). Locate the origin of the coronary Aa. from the ascending aorta and examine the trabeculae carneae within the ventricle (Fig. H2.21).

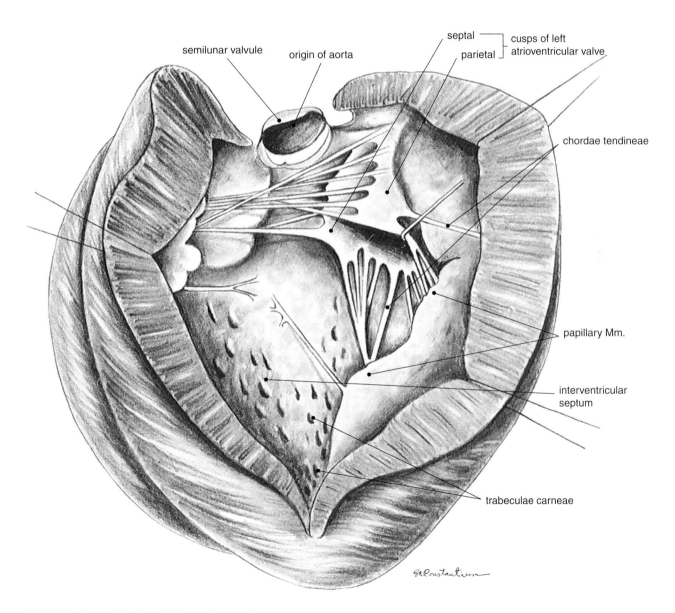

Fig. H2.21. Heart of the horse, left ventricle opened.

*Notice* that the two coronary arteries originate from the **aortic sinuses**, three dilations of the aortic wall, located dorsal to the corresponding semilunar valvules. The sinuses occupy entirely the **aortic bulb**, the dilation of the origin of the aorta.

In domestic animals, (in quadrupeds in general), there is no joint between the thoracic limbs and the body wall, as it is in humans. The liaison between these body parts is accomplished by muscles, aponeuroses, and fasciae. The body is suspended between the two thoracic limbs by the serratus ventralis thoracis Mm., which act like a hinge, but the body weight is supported mainly by the dorsoscapular ligg., the fasciae of the serratus ventralis thoracis Mm., and the tunica flava abdominis (abdominal tunic). In addition, the fasciae of the trapezius Mm. and even the aponeuroses of the serratus dorsalis Mm. help in supporting the body weight. (Fig. H2.22).

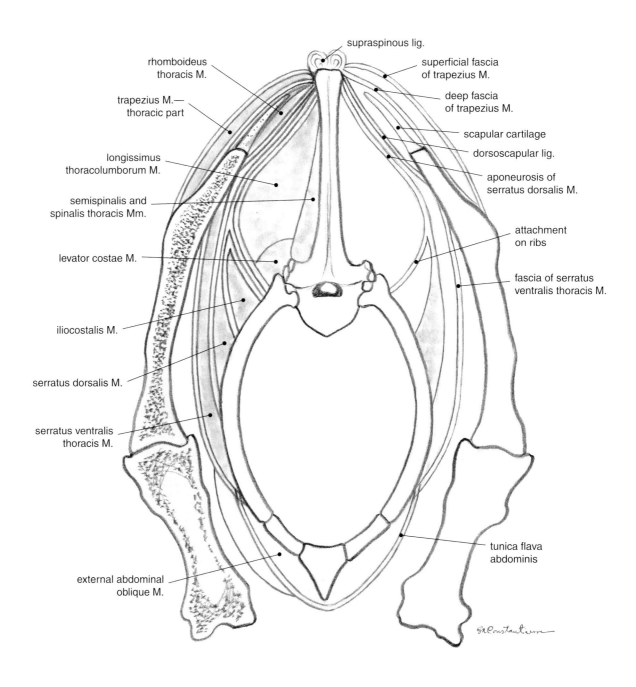

Fig. H2.22. Suspensory apparatus of the body, transverse section through the withers, horse.

# MODLAB H2

Similar to the exercise you did on the neck, attempt to palpate those structures listed at the beginning of this chapter on a living horse.

Then, identify the **landmarks** and **approaches** of the clinically important structures listed as follows.

1. **Superficial thoracic (spur) V.** (Fig. H2.23A)
   A. *Landmarks*: olecranon and dorsal border of deep pectoral M.
   B. *Approach*: on a line starting from the olecranon caudally along the dorsal border of deep pectoral M.
   ***Caution.*** The vein runs parallel to the lateral thoracic N. and is covered by cutaneous trunci.
2. **Supraspinous bursa** (Fig. H2. 23A)
   A. *Landmarks*: supraspinous lig. and the highest point of withers, which corresponds to the spinous processes of $T_2$ to $T_4$
   B. *Approach*: between the two above listed landmarks
3. **Intercostal A.V.N.** (Fig. H2.23A)
   A. *Landmarks*: caudal border of ribs
   B. *Approach*:
      a. At the caudal border of one rib, between the internal intercostal M. and the endothoracic fascia along the entire costal area in a dorsoventral direction (for the intercostal A.V.N.)
      b. In the middle of an intercostal space, between the two intercostal Mm. (the lateral cutaneous branches are found in the proximal half, and the ventral cutaneous branches are found in the distal half of the intercostal N.)
4. **Line of pleural reflection** (Fig. H2.23B)
   A. *Landmarks*: the ribs and the costal cartilages; the costochondral joints; the tuber coxae; the tuber of scapular spine (the projection of the roof of the thoracic cavity is outlined between the tuber coxae and the tuber of scapular spine)
   B. *Approach*: From the 6th costochondral joint trace a line with the convexity oriented caudally through all costochondral joints to the intersection of the 17th rib with the projection of the roof of the thoracic cavity.
5. **Area of auscultation and percussion of the lungs** (see Fig. H2.23B)
   A. *Landmarks*: the projection of the roof of the thoracic cavity; the ribs and costal cartilages; the caudal border of the triceps brachii M.

   B. *Approach*: from a point 10 cm dorsal to the 6th costochondral joint trace a slight ventrocaudal convex line to the intersection of the 16th intercostal space with the projection of the roof of the thoracic cavity; then, along the projection of the roof of the thoracic cavity and the caudal border of the triceps brachii M.
6. **Auscultation of the heart** (Fig. H2.24)
   A. *Landmarks*: intercostal spaces III–V; a horizontal line passing through the shoulder joint; the caudal border of the triceps brachii M.; the olecranon
   ***Caution.*** To have access to all sounds of the heart you have to move the limb as much forward as possible and introduce the stethoscope as deep as possible under the triceps brachii M.
   B. *Approach*:
      a. The pulmonary valve at the level of the left third intercostal space (a hand ventral to the horizontal line passing through the shoulder joint)
      b. The aortic valve on, or ventral to, the horizontal line of the shoulder joint, in the left fourth intercostal space
      c. The left atrioventricular (AV) valve in the fifth intercostal space, and one and one-half hand (12–15 cm) dorsal to the olecranon, or one hand ventral to the horizontal line of the shoulder joint
      d. The right AV valve in the fourth intercostal space and one hand dorsal to the olecranon; on the left side, in the third intercostal space and one hand dorsal to the olecranon
7. **Percussion of the heart** (Fig. 2.24)
   A. *Landmarks*: the second to sixth intercostal spaces; the line passing through the shoulder joint; the caudal border of the triceps brachii M.; the olecranon; the sternum
   B. *Approach*:
      a. The area of relative dullness extends between the second and sixth intercostal spaces, one hand dorsal to the line of shoulder joint, and the sternum.
      b. The area of absolute dullness extends on the left side between the third and fifth intercostal spaces, one hand dorsal to the olecranon in the fourth space, and 2–3 cm dorsal to the olecranon in the fifth space, and the sternum. On the right side, the area of absolute dullness extends between the third and fourth intercostal spaces, 2–3 cm dorsal to the olecranon in the fourth space, and the sternum.

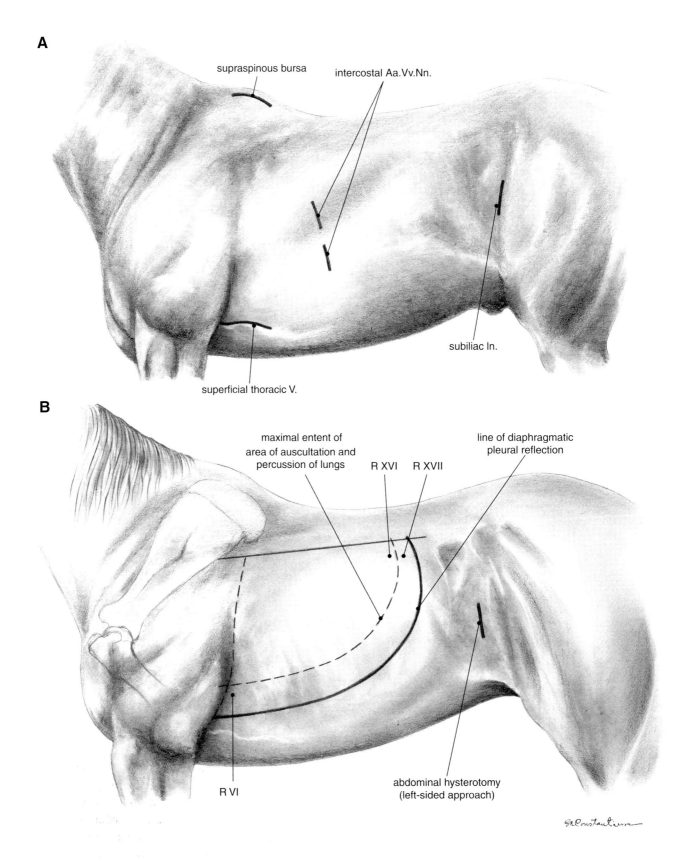

**A**

supraspinous bursa

intercostal Aa.Vv.Nn.

subiliac ln.

superficial thoracic V.

**B**

maximal entent of
area of auscultation and
percussion of lungs

R XVI   R XVII

line of diaphragmatic
pleural reflection

R VI

abdominal hysterotomy
(left-sided approach)

Fig. H2.23. Landmarks and approaches on the thorax, horse. **A.** Structures on lateral aspect. **B.** Auscultation and percussion of lungs and surgical approach in left flank.

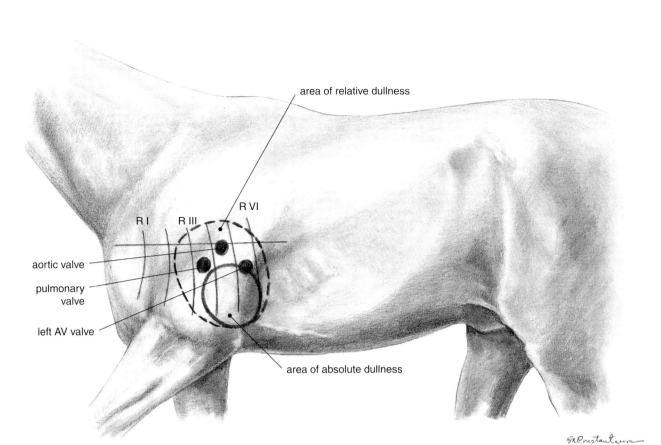

Fig. H2.24. Auscultation and percussion areas of the heart, horse, left aspect.

# H 3

## The Abdomen and Abdominal Viscera

The **lumbar vertebrae** are the only bones of the abdomen. They are illustrated in Figure H3.1.

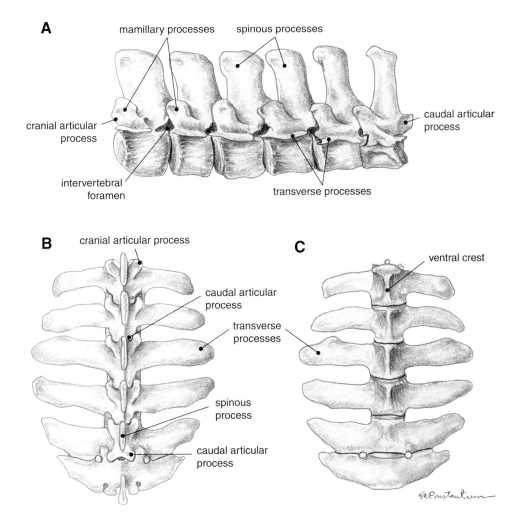

Fig. H3.1. Lumbar vertebrae, horse. **A.** Left lateral aspect. **B.** Dorsal aspect. **C.** Ventral aspect.

*Before starting the dissection, outline and palpate the following structures for physical examination and/or clinical approach: the last rib and costal cartilage, the hypochondrium (the band of abdominal wall over the costal cartilages), the tuber coxae, the patella, and the fold of the flank. In the horse it is difficult to palpate the tips of the transverse processes of the lumbar vertebrae. Therefore, to outline the dorsal border of the paralumbar fossa, trace a horizontal line from the tuber coxae to the last rib. The entire area outlined by all the above-mentioned landmarks is called the "flank." During expiration observe a prominent bridge between tuber coxae and the last costochondral joint; this is part of the internal abdominal oblique muscle and is called the "cord of the flank." Ventral to it, the rest of the area is called the "slope of the flank." The paralumbar fossa is also called the "hole of the flank" (Fig. H3.2).*

These three divisions of the flank are important landmarks for assessing the normal topography of the abdominal viscera by means of palpation, percussion, auscultation, ultrasonography, and even rectal exploration.

The flank consists of the external and internal abdominal oblique and the transversus abdominis Mm. The flank is the access site for celiotomy, for performing correction of uterine torsion (on either side), for cecocentesis and cecotomy (in the hole of the right flank and the slope of the right flank, respectively), for laparoscopy and laparotomy (on either side), for biopsy of the liver (either the caudate process, on the right side, or the left lobe), spleen (on the left side), and both right and left kidneys.

Skin the abdomen up to the **tuber coxae** and the **fold of the flank** and reflect the skin ventrally.

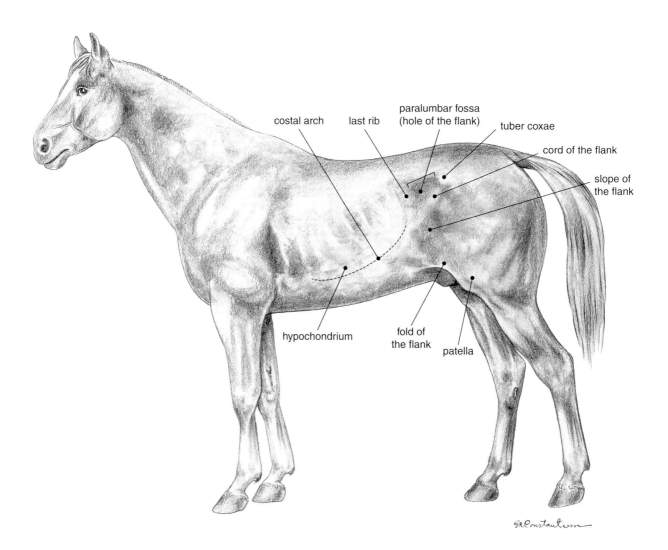

Fig. H3.2. Landmarks for physical examination and/or clinical approach, horse.

*Caution.* Skin carefully, identify and dissect the **dorso-lateral cutaneous branches of the costoabdominal** and **lumbar Nn.**

*Notice* that these branches become superficial upon emerging from beneath the **retractor costae M.** (the costoabdominal N.) and from between the lumbar origin of the **gluteus medius M.** and the **iliocostalis thoracolumborum M.** (the lumbar Nn.). They can be identified at the ventral edge of the aponeurosis of the **latissimus dorsi M.**, which is fused with the **thoracolumbar fascia.** This edge corresponds to a line from tuber coxae to the **tuberosity of the scapular spine.**

*Caution.* When dissecting the **ventral cutaneous branches** of the same nerves, use care at the level of a line from the tuber coxae to the **olecranon.** This line separates the dorsolateral cutaneous branches from the ventral cutaneous branches of these nerves (Fig. H3.3).

The systematization of the abdominal muscles is shown in the Table H3.1.

Continue the dissection of the **cutaneous trunci M.** and reflect it ventrally. The most caudoventral attachment (the origin) of this muscle is located within the fold of the flank. At the cranial border of the **tensor fasciae latae M.,**

Table H3.1. Abdominal Muscles, Horse and Large Ruminants

**Ventral Abdominal Muscles**
– rectus abdominis
  • rectus sheath
    ○ external lamina
    ○ internal lamina
– external abdominal oblique
  • superficial inguinal ring
  • arcus inguinalis
  • deep inguinal ring
  • femoral lamina
– internal abdominal oblique
  • deep inguinal ring
  • cremaster M.
– transversus abdominis
– tunica flava abdominis (abdominal tunic)
– linea alba
  • umbilical ring

**Dorsal Abdominal Muscles**
– quadratus lumborum
– intertransversarii lumborum
– iliopsoas
  • iliacus
  • psoas major
– psoas minor

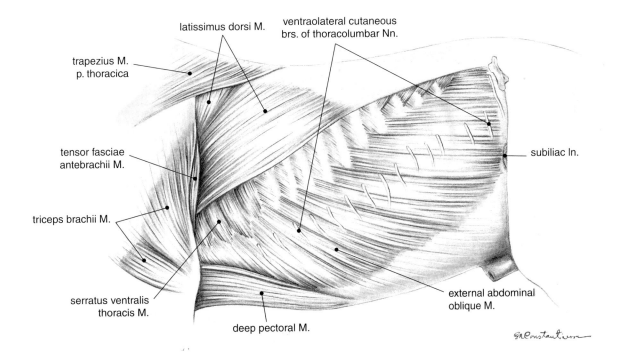

latissimus dorsi M.

ventraolateral cutaneous brs. of thoracolumbar Nn.

trapezius M. p. thoracica

tensor fasciae antebrachii M.

triceps brachii M.

serratus ventralis thoracis M.

deep pectoral M.

subiliac ln.

external abdominal oblique M.

Fig. H3.3. Superficial structures on the left abdominal wall, horse.

slightly ventral to the middistance between the tuber coxae and the **patella,** the following structures are exposed: the **subiliac ln., lateral cutaneous femoral N.** (ventral branches of L3 and L4), and **caudal branches of the deep circumflex iliac A.V.** Dissect them carefully.

The **abdominal tunic (tunica flava abdominis)** is an elastic structure adhering to the **external abdominal oblique M.** Dissect and reflect a small area of the tunic and check its elasticity. Dissect the muscular fibers of the external abdominal oblique M. from the **last rib,** thoracolumbar fascia, and tuber coxae.

*Remember!* The external abdominal oblique M. attaches to the ribs starting from the fifth rib caudally; the first four attachments interdigitate with the last four attachments of the **serratus ventralis thoracis M.** (see Fig. H3.3).

Continue to dissect the aponeurosis of the external abdominal oblique M. from the tuber coxae to the patella and reflect the whole muscle ventrally. The muscle is still anchored by the perforating ventral cutaneous branches of nerves T18, L1, and L2; transect them to liberate the mus-

cle and to better and more easily examine the **internal abdominal oblique M.** (Fig. H3.4A).

The reflection of the external abdominal oblique M. reveals, in a dorsoventral direction, the retractor costae, **transversus abdominis,** and internal abdominal oblique Mm. Identify the ventral branches of the costoabdominal and first two lumbar nerves. Observe the prominent part of the internal abdominal oblique M. running from the tuber coxae to the last costochondral joint, and corresponding to the "cord of the flank" (Fig. H3.4A). Transect the origin and the insertions of this muscle from the tuber coxae, the last rib, and the **costal arch**; then transect and reflect the muscle from the tuber coxae to the patella ventrally. The transversus abdominis and rectus abdominis Mm. are now exposed (Fig. H3.4B).

Close to the lateral border of the **rectus abdominis M.,** the aponeurosis of the internal abdominal oblique M. splits into lateral and medial laminae. The lateral lamina fuses with the aponeurosis of the external abdominal oblique M. to form the **external rectus sheath**.

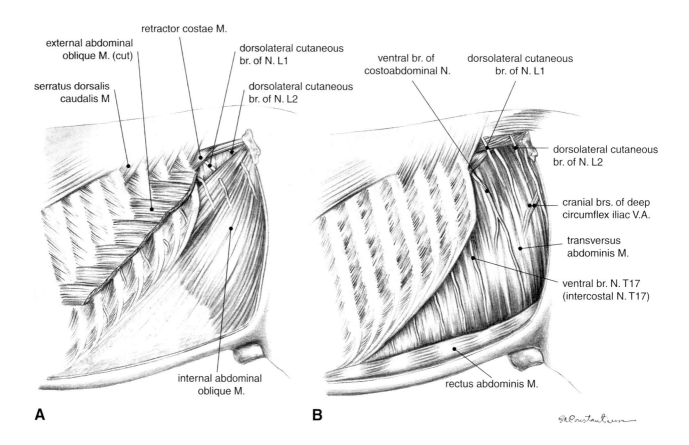

Fig. H3.4. Deep structures of the left abdominal wall, horse. **A.** Second level. **B.** Third level.

On the lateral aspect of the transversus abdominis M., in a vertical position, lie the ventral branches of the last six thoracic Nn. (12–17), the costoabdominal N., and the first two lumbar Nn. Between the internal abdominal oblique and transversus abdominis Mm., the **cranial branches of the deep circumflex iliac A.V.** are visible, ventral to the tuber coxae (see Fig. H3.4B).

Transect the transversus abdominis M. from the **transverse processes of the lumbar vertebrae** and the medial aspect of the last rib and costal arch and reflect it ventrally. On the medial aspect of the rectus abdominis M., the aponeurosis of the transversus abdominis M. fused with the medial lamina of the internal abdominal oblique M. represents the cranial part of the **internal rectus sheath**. The caudal part of the rectus sheath is represented by the **transverse fascia**.

*Note.* The transverse fascia, or the endoabdominal fascia, is the fibrous structure intimately lining the abdominal cavity. It continues cranially with the endothoracic fascia through the three orifices of the diaphragm.

*Remember!* The aponeuroses of the external and internal abdominal oblique and the transversus abdominis Mm. fuse with each other and with their symmetrical fellows in a strong structure called "**linea alba**."

*Caution.* The transversus abdominis M. is lined by the transverse (endoabdominal) fascia and the **parietal peritoneum**.

To penetrate the **peritoneal cavity**, transect the transverse fascia and the parietal peritoneum together, starting at the tuber coxae and continuing cranially on the transverse processes of the lumbar vertebrae, the last rib, and the costal arch, and ventrally toward the patella. Cranial to the last rib, the transverse fascia and parietal peritoneum line the diaphragm; do not displace them from this position.

Remove the **intercostal Mm.** from the last **intercostal space** (right and left).

A brief description of the postdiaphragmatic digestive viscera may help in their identification in situ and after removal from the peritoneal cavity.

The postdiaphragmatic digestive viscera consist of the abdominal portion of the esophagus, the stomach, the small intestines, the large intestines, the liver, and the pancreas.

The *esophagus* enters the peritoneal cavity through the esophageal hiatus, runs over the dorsal border of the liver (the esophageal impression), and opens within the stomach through the cardia, on the lesser curvature. The opening is called cardiac ostium.

The *stomach* has a parietal surface (facing the liver) and a visceral surface (facing the intestines), a lesser curvature oriented dorsally and a greater curvature oriented ven-

trally, a body, a fundus (on the left side), and a pyloric part (on the right side). The highest part of the fundus is called saccus cecus (the blind sac) and is present only in the horse. The cardia is separated from the body by the angular notch and from the fundus by the cardiac notch.

Inside the stomach, the cardiac ostium is provided by a sphincter (of circular muscular fibers) and a cardiac loop (of internal oblique muscular fibers). Between cardia and pylorus, the gastric groove follows the lesser curvature. The pyloric part consists of an antrum and a pyloric canal leading to the pylorus—provided with a sphincter. The pyloric ostium outlines the transition between the stomach and the duodenum. The margo plicatus is an irregular thick border between the nonglandular (on the left) and glandular (on the right) parts of the stomach.

The small intestines consist of duodenum, jejunum, and ileum.

The *duodenum* has several parts and flexures. The cranial part starts with a dilation (bulb, ampulla) and is provided with a sigmoid loop. The descending part, craniocaudally oriented, starts from the cranial flexure and lasts up to the caudal flexure, while surrounding the right kidney. From the caudal flexure, a short transverse part continues with the ascending part up to the duodenojejunal flexure. The duodenum is attached to several structures in its long way, collectively called mesoduodenum. Inside, the duodenum is provided with the major and minor duodenal papillae, opposite to each other, 12–15 cm from the pylorus. The major duodenal papilla is located inside the hepatopancreatic ampulla. There is a sphincter associated with this ampulla. Both the choledochus (bile duct) and pancreatic duct open on the major duodenal papilla. The accessory pancreatic duct opens on the minor duodenal papilla.

The *jejunum,* up to 25 m long starts at the duodenojejunal flexure and continues with the ileum at the level of the ileocecal fold. The mesojejunum, as part of the mesentery, suspends the jejunum from the lesser curvature.

The *ileum,* which averages 70 cm long, is suspended by the mesoileum, also part of the mesentery from the lesser curvature, but after surrounding the ileum the mesoileum continues from the greater curvature of the ileum to the lesser curvature of the cecum as the ileocecal fold. The ileum opens into the cecum.

The large intestines consist of the cecum, colon, and rectum.

The *cecum,* located on the right side of the body, has haustrae (sacculations) and longitudinal bands on its surface. The bands are longitudinal agglomerated muscle fibers. With an average capacity of 40–50 l, it has a base, a body, and an apex. The bands are called dorsal, lateral, ventral, and medial. The ventral and medial bands meet with each other before the apex. The ileocecal fold is attached on the dorsal band, whereas the cecocolic fold is attached to the lateral band.

There are two openings inside the cecum: the ileocecal ostium and the cecocolic ostium. The former opens in the tip of the ileal papilla, provided with the ileal sphincter, and the latter is provided with the cecocolic valve and cecal sphincter. Semilunar folds of the mucosa correspond to the grooves separating the sacculations.

The colon is divided into the ascending, transverse, and descending colons.

The *ascending colon* has sacculations and bands and is folded twice on itself, producing four segments of about 1 m each, called the "colon": the right ventral, the left ventral, the left dorsal, and the right dorsal colons. The four colons are provided with the following numbers of bands: four, four, one, and three. The bands of the ventral colon are concentrated, two dorsally and two ventrally, medial and lateral. The band of the left dorsal colon is ventrally located and continues to the right dorsal colon. The other two bands of the right dorsal colon are dorsally located. Between the ventral colon and the dorsal colon, the ascending mesocolon, or intercolic fold, is attached to the same bands along which the arteries run. Folding the 4 m long ascending colon, the pelvic flexure separates the ventral colon from the dorsal colon. Folding of the ventral and dorsal colons together creates two more flexures: the sternal flexure and the diaphragmatic flexure. The former runs from right to left, dorsal to the xiphoid cartilage. The latter runs from left to right, in contact with the diaphragm and dorsal to the previous flexure. The pelvic flexure is vertically oriented and runs ventrodorsally. The origin of the right ventral colon has a reduced lumen and is called the neck of the colon. The right dorsal colon ends with a dilation called the colic ampulla. The ventral colon has an average diameter of 25 cm, the left dorsal colon less than 10 cm, and the right dorsal colon increases to 35–50 cm. Semilunar folds of the mucosa correspond to the grooves separating the sacculations. The left dorsal colon has no sacculations. One usually talks about the ventral colon and the dorsal colon when the blood supply is described: the former is supplied by the colic branch, whereas the latter is supplied by the right colic A., both from the ileocolic A. (the colic branch runs along the dorsomedial band of the ventral colon, whereas the right colic A. runs along the ventral band of the dorsal colon).

The *transverse colon* follows the colic ampulla. It is transversely oriented, from right to left, and suffers a sudden reduction in lumen. No sacculations and only one band are the characteristics of this colon. The transverse mesocolon anchors it to the origin of the mesentery.

The *descending colon* is located on the left side of the body and has sacculations, two opposite bands (on the lesser and greater curvature), and a constant diameter of 7–10 cm. It is suspended from the lesser curvature by the descending mesocolon. Semilunar folds of the mucosa correspond to the grooves separating the sacculations.

The *liver* has a parietal aspect facing the diaphragm, a visceral aspect facing the stomach, duodenum, cecum, and ascending colon, and a contour. Five lobes are present in the horse: left lateral, left medial, quadrate, right, and caudate, but no gall bladder.

The *pancreas* has a body, a right lobe, and a left lobe. It is pushed against the roof of the abdominal cavity by the pressure of the digestive viscera. The pancreatic ring allows the portal V. to pass through, on its way to the liver. Both pancreatic duct and accessory pancreatic duct are present in the horse.

Before the viscera from the abdominal cavity are removed, here is a short summary of the topographic anatomy of the projection of the viscera on the lateral and ventral walls of the abdomen.

*In embalmed specimens the topography of abdominal viscera looks different than that of live horses. The euthanasia and the embalming process disturb the relationship between viscera. One has to take into account this difference while in the dissection room and make the necessary adjustment toward live individuals. The topography we are learning corresponds to live horses. There are still differences in live horses, related to*

- *The plenitude of the digestive viscera (before, during, or after meals),*
- *Pregnancy,*
- *Abnormal relationships that may occur as a result of*
  - *Congenital abnormalities or*
  - *A specific pathological status.*

*The viscera that are not in intimate contact with the lateral and/or ventral walls of the abdominal cavity, such as the liver, the stomach, the spleen, and part of the duodenum are still mentioned as subjects of clinical investigations and procedures. Those viscera are in contact with the diaphragm, and in order to reach them from a lateral perspective, one has to penetrate the pleural cavity and the diaphragm.*

The caudal extent of the abdominal cavity communicates with the pelvic cavity through the pelvic inlet.

*Note.* The pelvic inlet is outlined by the terminal line (see Fig. H4.1, Chapter H4, and Fig. R4.4, Chapter R4,).

The viscera located caudally within the abdominal cavity cannot be approached directly from the lateral walls because the cranial muscles of the thigh overlap the area of projection for some viscera. These viscera are part of the cecum, the pelvic flexure, the last part of the left ventral colon, the initial part of the left dorsal colon, and part of the descending colon.

*The endoscopic investigations and/or procedures don't require the perforation of the pleural cavity and*

*diaphragm. The endoscope can be introduced within the peritoneal cavity through a small incision in the abdominal wall.*

The following viscera may be identified on the *right lateral wall of the abdomen*: cecum, liver, right kidney, right ventral and right dorsal colon, pancreas, and duodenum (Fig. H3.5A).

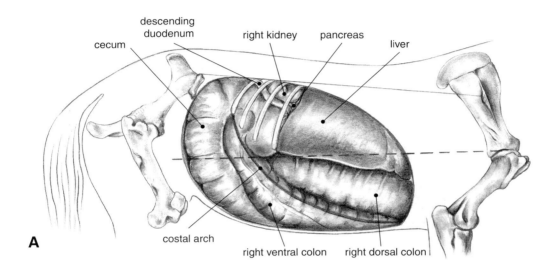

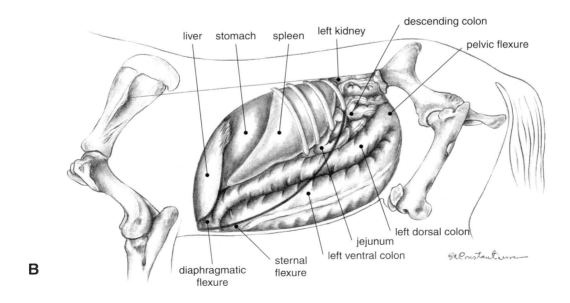

Fig. H3.5. Topography of abdominal viscera, horse. **A.** Right side. **B.** Left side.

The **cecum** is positioned with the base in the hole of the flank, exceeding the last rib, cranially to the third intercostal space (from caudal to cranial), and ventrally to a horizontal line between the **shoulder joint** and **hip joint**. Its body continues ventrally in the cord and slope of the flank, one hand caudal to the costal arch, and deep to the **thigh** up to the **pelvic inlet**. This part can be partially palpated from outside, because it is overlapped caudally by the tensor fasciae latae M. The cecum can also be examined by per rectum abdominal palpation.

The **right lobe of the liver** is located between the **centrum tendineum (the tendinous center) of the diaphragm**, the third or fourth intercostal space (from caudal to cranial) to the base of the cecum, and along an oblique line to the olecranon.

The **right kidney** is located at the level of the last two to three intercostal spaces (the last four ribs), between the **caudate lobe of the liver** and the base of the cecum, and on the roof of the abdominal cavity (the sublumbar area).

The **right ventral colon** and the **right dorsal colon** are located between the body of the cecum, liver, centrum tendineum of diaphragm, and floor of the abdominal cavity. The costal arch separates their area of projection. The right dorsal colon insinuates deep to the right lobe of the liver.

The **pancreas** lies in contact with the liver, descending duodenum, and kidney.

The **descending part of the duodenum** is located between the liver and the base of the cecum, surrounding the lateral border of the kidney.

On the *left side of the abdomen*, the spleen; liver; stomach; left kidney; left ventral and left dorsal colon; diaphragmatic, sternal, and pelvic flexures of the ascending colon; descending colon; jejunum; and pancreas can be identified (Fig. H3.5B).

The **spleen** reaches the roof of the abdominal cavity with its **base** at the level of the last three to four ribs. The concave **cranial border** extends from the cranial end of the base, whereas the convex **caudal border** runs from the caudal end of the base. They meet at the **apex** toward the costal arch (one hand dorsal to it), between the 9th and 11th intercostal spaces.

The **liver** is the closest organ to the diaphragm. Its caudal border starts at the 10th rib dorsally and ends at the 7th rib ventrally, at the level of the costal arch.

The **stomach** fills the space between the spleen and the liver. It never reaches the floor of the abdominal cavity, but makes contact with the diaphragmatic flexure of the ascending colon.

The **left kidney** is supported by the base of the spleen at the level of the last three ribs; it exceeds the last rib caudally.

The **left ventral colon** lies on the floor of the abdominal cavity, 5–10 cm dorsal to the costal arch, and continues in the slope of the flank up to the pelvic inlet (this last part can only be approached by rectal palpation).

The **diaphragmatic flexure of the ascending colon** is oriented from the right to the left, from the right ventral colon to the left ventral colon.

The **left dorsal colon** is located dorsal to the ventral colon at the level of the costal arch and the cord of the flank. The transition between the ventral and the dorsal colon is represented by the **pelvic flexure**, which reaches the pelvic inlet.

The **sternal flexure of the ascending colon** is oriented from the left to the right, from the left dorsal colon to the right dorsal colon.

The **descending colon** fills the hole of the flank.

The **jejunum** is located deep to, and between the descending colon, spleen, and left dorsal colon.

The **pancreas** follows the cranial extremity of the kidney, lying between the base of the spleen and the stomach.

**The projection of the viscera on the lateral wall of the abdomen is clinically very important for three reasons: physical examination, exploratory techniques, and surgical approach. Inspection, palpation, percussion, and auscultation can be performed as part of physical examination, and ultrasound and endoscopy as exploratory techniques, whereas the projection *and* the relationship of the viscera are helpful in surgery (and in the autopsy room).**

The *ventral wall* (the floor) of the abdomen is divided into the following regions (Fig. H3.6):

* Cranial abdominal region
  – hypochondriac region
  – xiphoid region
* Middle abdominal region
  – lateral abdominal region (the flank)
    ○ paralumbar fossa (the hole of the flank)
    ○ the cord of the flank
    ○ the slope of the flank (the only part of the lateral abdominal region exposed on the ventral aspect)
    ○ umbilical region
* Caudal abdominal region
  – inguinal region
  – pubic region
    ○ preputial region
* Inguinal mammary region

On the floor of the abdominal cavity, the following viscera and structures can be identified: the right ventral colon, sternal flexure, left ventral colon, cecum, and occa-

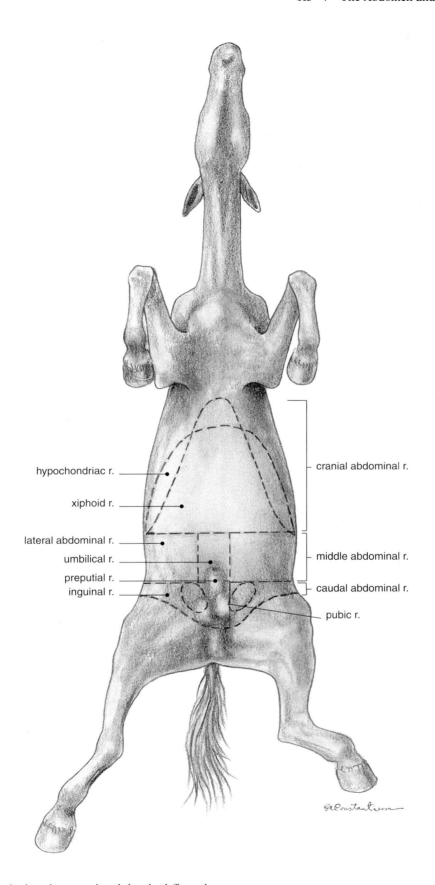

hypochondriac r.

xiphoid r.

lateral abdominal r.

umbilical r.

preputial r.

inguinal r.

cranial abdominal r.

middle abdominal r.

caudal abdominal r.

pubic r.

Fig. H3.6. The anatomical regions on the abdominal floor, horse.

sionally the diaphragmatic flexure and jejunal ansae (loops) (Fig. H3.7).

The **right ventral colon** is located on the right side of the abdominal cavity, between the hypochondrium and the body of the cecum.

The **sternal flexure** lies on the xiphoid cartilage surrounding the apex of the cecum.

The **left ventral colon** is located on the left side of the abdominal cavity, between the hypochondrium and the body of the cecum.

The **body of the cecum** lies between the right and left ventral colons, with the apex positioned toward the sternal flexure.

The **diaphragmatic flexure** is sometimes located cranial to the sternal flexure.

The **jejunal ansae** can be observed on the left caudal side, either between the left ventral colon and the left wall of the abdominal cavity, or between the left ventral colon and the cecum.

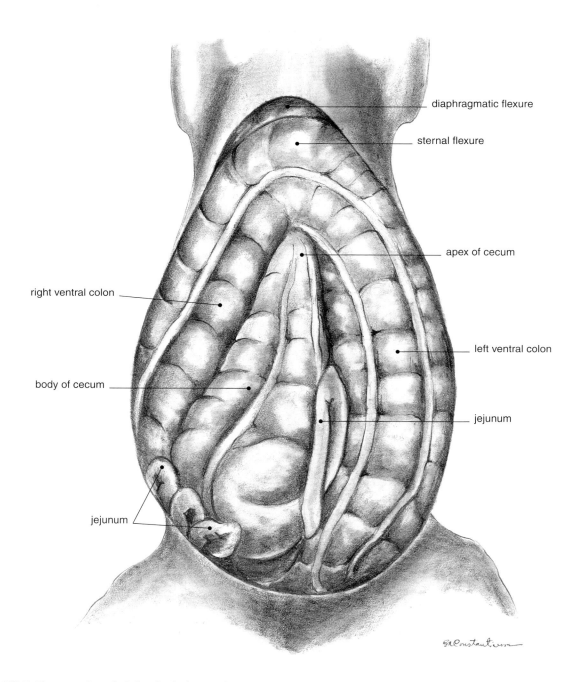

Fig. H3.7. Topography of abdominal viscera, horse, ventral aspect.

**The projection of the viscera on the floor of the abdomen is helpful for physical examination, in surgery, and in the necropsy room.**

An important characteristic of the horse is the lack of any contact of the **stomach** and liver with the floor of the abdominal cavity, such as exists in other species; and this is because of the enormous size and development of the cecum and ascending colon. The apex of the spleen often extends to the floor of the abdominal cavity in vivo.

Slide your hand inside the peritoneal cavity and palpate the **triangular ligg. of the liver**. The right lig. connects the dorsal border of the **right lobe of the liver** to the costal part of the diaphragm (Fig. H3.8), whereas the left lig. connects the dorsal border of the **left lateral lobe of the liver** to the tendinous center of the diaphragm. *Note.* The liver is obliquely oriented, with the left lateral lobe located ventrally and to the left side, and the right lobe located dorsally and to the right side. Palpate the **coronary lig.**, which is attached between the right side of the tendinous center of the diaphragm and the diaphragmatic (cranial)

aspect of the liver, surrounding the **caudal vena cava**. Palpate and preserve the **gastrophrenic lig.** between the stomach and the **crura of the diaphragm**.

On the right side of the specimen palpate the following peritoneal structures: the **hepatorenal lig.** (between the caudate lobe of the liver and the right kidney—there is a renal impression on the caudate lobe), the **ascending mesocolon (intercolic fold)**, the **mesoduodenum** (connecting the duodenum to different other viscera, such as the right kidney, descending and transverse colon), and the adherence of the base of the cecum to the dorsal wall of the abdominal cavity (Fig. H3.8).

Trace the different parts of the duodenum exiting from under the right lobe of the liver: the descending part, connected to the right kidney by the **duodenorenal lig.**, the **caudal flexure**, the **transverse part**, and the **ascending part**. The ascending part is attached to the descending colon by the **duodenocolic fold**, and to the transverse colon by the **duodenotransverse lig.**, both parts of the mesoduodenum. The duodenum continues with the **duo-**

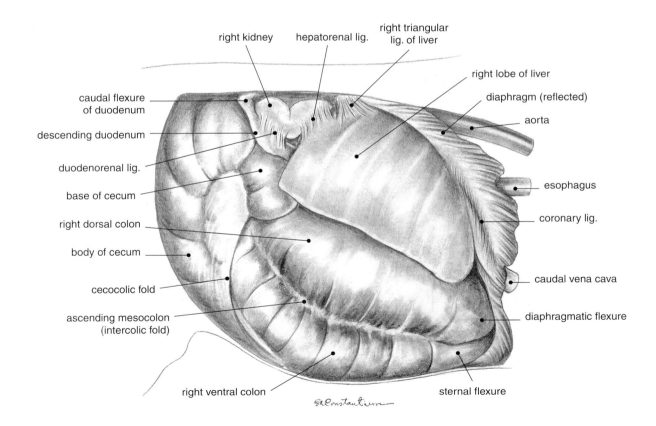

Fig. H3.8. Right abdominal viscera in situ, horse.

**denojejunal flexure**, and from here the jejunum starts. The jejunum is suspended by the **mesojejunum**.

Reflect the right lobe of the liver as far cranially as possible and follow the descending part of the duodenum in a cranial direction up to the **cranial flexure** and the **cranial part**. *Remember!* The cranial part of the duodenum originates from the pylorus and is provided with the **duodenal ampulla** and the **sigmoid loop**.

The cranial part and flexure run along the visceral aspect of the liver, and they are attached to it by the **hepatoduodenal lig.**, as part of the **lesser omentum**.

*Remember!* The lesser omentum consists of the hepatogastric and hepatoduodenal ligg.

To reach the **hepatogastric lig.,** continue to palpate the lesser omentum up to its attachment to the cranial aspect of the stomach. The hepatogastric and the hepatoduodenal ligg. are in continuation with each other.

Locate the pancreas, which is attached to the base of the cecum, and *notice* its relationships with the surrounding viscera. Identify the **portal V.**, which lies between the pancreas, liver, and caudal vena cava (Fig. H3.9). Attempt to introduce a finger between the caudate lobe of the liver (cranially), the pancreas (caudally), the caudal vena cava (dorsally), and the portal V. (ventrally). Here is a narrow foramen called **omental (epiploic) foramen**, which is the passage between the peritoneal cavity and the **omental bursa**.

**Small intestinal loops and, much less commonly, ascending and descending colons can penetrate the omental foramen from the peritoneal cavity into the omental bursa. This condition is called omental (epiploic) hernia.**

*Note.* **The old idea that the epiploic foramen "enlarges" with age (due to atrophy of caudate lobe of liver) has been recently diminished.**

On the left side of the specimen palpate the base of the spleen, the left kidney, the **phrenicosplenic** and the **splenorenal (or renosplenic, or nephrosplenic) ligg.**, which belong to the **greater omentum**.

*Note.* The splenorenal lig. is the former (still in use) name for the phrenicosplenic lig. In the horse, the ventral portion of the phrenicosplenic lig. is attached to the left

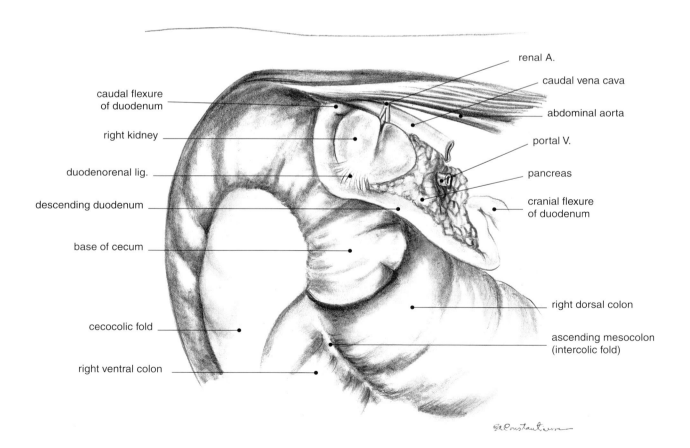

Fig. H3.9. Upper right abdominal viscera, horse, after removing the liver.

kidney (according to the *Illustrated Veterinary Anatomical Nomenclature*), under the unofficial name of splenorenal lig.

*Note.* Clinicians tend to refer to the splenorenal lig. as either the renosplenic lig., or the nephrosplenic lig.

Trace the ascending mesocolon between the left ventral and left dorsal colon in a craniocaudal direction and *notice* that it broadens toward the **pelvic flexure**. Reflect the spleen caudally to liberate the greater curvature of the stomach and the attachment of the **gastrosplenic lig.**, also part of the greater omentum. *Notice* the hilus on the visceral side of the spleen, which is both the place of attachment of the gastrosplenic lig. and the groove in which the **splenic A.** runs. Between the two laminae of the gastrosplenic lig., observe **short gastric Aa.**, supplying the greater curvature of the stomach. After sending the gastrosplenic lig., the greater omentum continues in a caudal direction to the pelvic inlet as the **superficial wall**. The superficial wall returns to the stomach as the **deep wall** and ends on the transverse colon and pancreas. Slip a hand

dorsal to the base of the spleen, between it and the **left crus of the diaphragm**, and palpate the **gastrophrenic lig.**, cranial to the phrenicosplenic lig. The gastrophrenic lig. is the last component of the greater omentum, located between the dorsal extent of the greater curvature of the stomach and the crura of the diaphragm.

*Remember!* The greater omentum consists of the gastrophrenic, gastrosplenic, phrenicosplenic, and (in the horse only) splenorenal ligg., and the superficial and deep walls.

Locate the **abdominal aorta** and push the hand deeper toward the dorsal wall of the abdominal cavity to palpate the **root of the mesentery**, on the left side of the aorta. Slip your hand ventrally over the mesojejunum, which is attached to the **lesser curvature of the jejunum**. Caudal to the mesojejunum, and still on the dorsal wall of the abdominal cavity, palpate the origin of the **descending mesocolon**, attached to the lesser curvature of the descending colon (Fig. H3.10).

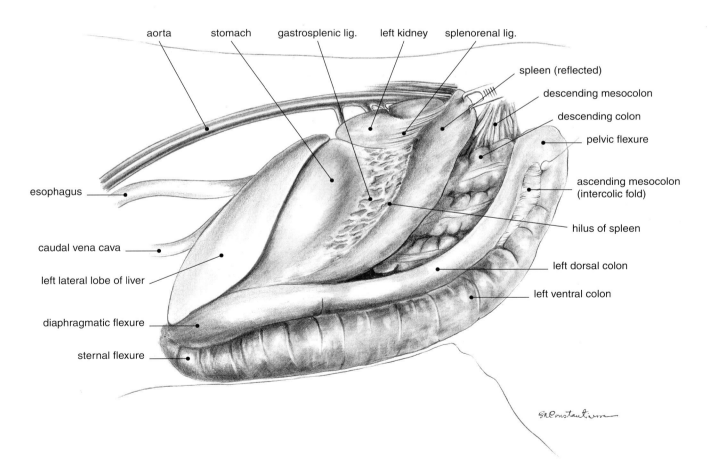

Fig. H3.10. Left abdominal viscera in situ, horse.

The following dissection steps describe the removal of the abdominal viscera. Two techniques are suggested. In *the first technique,* all of the large intestine (except the rectum—that is, the cecum and the ascending, transverse, and descending colons), the ileum, the jejunum, and the caudal segment of the duodenum are removed as a unit, followed by the stomach and spleen together, and finally by the liver with the cranial segment of the duodenum and the pancreas, or, if possible, all of the viscera, starting with the stomach and ending with the pancreas, together. *The second technique* starts with the removal of the liver, continues with the stomach, the duodenum, the spleen, the rest of the small intestine, and the descending colon, and ends with the cecum, the ascending colon, and the transverse colon. A detailed description of each technique follows.

The authors suggest the first technique as the method of choice.

## *The First Technique*

Free the cecum from the attachment on the dorsal wall of the abdominal cavity. Isolate the descending part of the duodenum from the base of the cecum. Double ligate the duodenum caudal to the pancreas, and transect it between the two ligatures. Identify the **caudal mesenteric A.** and the **testicular/ovarian A.** Double ligate the descending colon caudal to the kidneys and transect it in a manner similar to that described for the duodenum. On the left side, introduce a hand and palpate the root of the mesentery. Transect it together with the **cranial mesenteric A.** as far as possible from the abdominal aorta, to preserve the **cranial mesenteric ggl.** and **plexus**. Separate the greater omentum from its attachments. Remove the entire intestinal mass, except the cranial part of the duodenum, and place it on the table for later examination.

A variant of this technique may be utilized, leaving the transverse colon and the entire duodenum attached to the greater omentum and to the mesoduodenum, respectively. To accomplish this, transect, between double ligatures, the transverse colon in the middle and the duodenum at the duodenojejunal flexure.

Double ligate the esophagus, either in the thoracic or in the abdominal cavity, and transect it between the two ligatures. Identify and transect the **celiac A.** far enough from the aorta in order to preserve the **celiac ganglia** and **plexus**. Retain the cranial part of the duodenum, cranial flexure, and part of the descending part of the duodenum with the stomach, pancreas, and liver for examination of the **bile** and **pancreatic ducts**. Transect the splenorenal and gastrophrenic ligg.

Transect the triangular ligg., the coronary lig., the **falciform lig.** and the caudal vena cava as close as possible to the **foramen of the caudal vena cava** of the diaphragm and 5 cm caudal to the dorsal border of the liver. Remove the spleen, stomach, and liver with the duodenum and pancreas and place them together on the table.

Examine the continuity of the falciform lig. on the floor of the abdominal cavity toward the **umbilicus** (Fig. H3.11), where it meets the **median vesical lig.**

Examine the two **adrenal glands**, the two kidneys surrounded by the **retroperitoneal fat** (adipose capsule) and **renal fascia**, and the **visceral peritoneum** covering only the ventral aspect of the kidneys. Because of the uncomfortable position for examining the sublumbar structures, transect the abdominal aorta caudal to the **aortic hiatus** of the diaphragm. Transect both the abdominal aorta and caudal vena cava caudal to the kidneys and cranial to the caudal mesenteric A. Transect the **lumbar Aa.,** freeing the great vessels from any other attachment to the sublumbar area, and liberate the kidneys from the adipose capsule, renal fascia, and peritoneum. Transect the **ureters** a short distance from where they leave the kidneys, and place all these structures on a tray.

Examine the relationship between the kidneys, adrenal glands, **renal lnn.,** vessels supplying the kidneys (the **renal A.V.**), and the origin of each ureter. Identify the **hilus** of the kidneys, and *notice* the position of the hilus and the shape of each kidney (Fig. H3.12A,B).

Make a longitudinal section in each kidney from the lateral border toward the hilus and remove the **renal capsule**. The **renal sinus** (including the two **terminal recesses**, specific to the horse), lined by the **renal pelvis**, and the **renal crest** are surrounded by the **medulla** and the **renal cortex**. Identify the macroscopic structures as they are shown in Figure H3.12C.

Make a longitudinal section in an adrenal gland and examine the capsule, cortex, and medulla.

*Notice* that the horse has a smooth unipyramidal type of kidney.

Identify and dissect the celiac ganglia and plexus around the origin of the celiac A., the cranial mesenteric ggl. and plexus around the origin of the cranial mesenteric A., and the **renal gan-** **glia and plexuses**, between the renal Aa. and the hilus of the kidneys. All these sympathetic structures are visible on the ventral aspect of the aorta (Fig. H3.13B.)

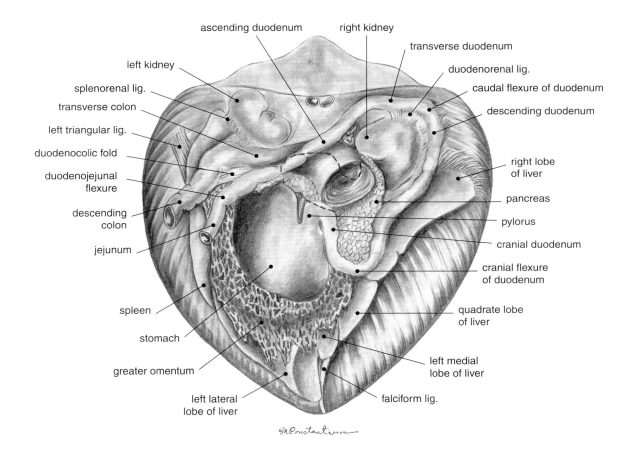

Fig. H3.11. Viscera within the cranial compartment of abdominal cavity in situ, horse, caudal view. Broken line indicates the boundaries of the pancreas.

## The Second Technique

Leaving the triangular ligg. of the liver attached to the diaphragm, carefully remove the rest of the diaphragm from the costal insertions. Leave the crura of the diaphragm in place and retain a strip of diaphragm approximately 10 cm wide, corresponding to the aortic hiatus (dorsally) and the foramen of caudal vena cava (ventrally), up to the sternal attachment of the diaphragm.

Double ligate the esophagus in the thoracic cavity close to the esophageal hiatus and transect it between the two ligatures. Free the esophagus from the diaphragm and the **esophageal impression of the liver** by pulling the stomach backward. At the same time the gastrophrenic lig. will be broken.

Transect the left crus of the diaphragm at the level of the phrenicosplenic lig. Transect the diaphragm around the aortic hiatus, leaving the abdominal aorta in place. Transect the two triangular ligg. after examining their relationship to the diaphragm. Complete the technique on the right side.

Transect the lesser omentum between the liver and the stomach (the hepatogastric lig.) and between the liver and the cranial part of the duodenum (the hepatoduodenal lig.). Transect the hepatorenal lig. (between the caudate lobe of the liver and the right kidney), and at this level transect the **right crus of the diaphragm**. Palpate the caudal vena cava, which travels toward the dorsal border of the liver, and transect it at this level. Palpate the visceral aspect of the liver and identify the **hilus,** the portal V., **hepatic A.,** and **common hepatic duct** (the distal dilated part of which is called **common bile duct** or **choledochus**). Transect the vessels and the duct as far as possible from the liver. Remove the liver with the median strip of the diaphragm from the abdominal cavity and place it on a tray.

Transect the splenorenal and the phrenicosplenic ligg. Double ligate the duodenum between the cranial flexure and the descending part and transect it between the two ligatures. Free the stomach and the attached duodenum from the pancreas and the right dorsal colon. Transect the celiac A. far enough from the aorta to preserve the celiac ggl., so that the stomach, cranial part of the duodenum, and spleen are free and easy to remove.

Free the duodenum from all its attachments up to the duodenojejunal flexure. The **ileum** can be identified by the **ileocecal fold** attached to its greater curvature, whereas the **mesoileum** (part of the mesentery) is attached to the lesser curvature. Transect the small intestine at the end of the ileocecal fold and between two ligatures. *Notice* that the mesoileum is the continuation of the mesojejunum. To remove the jejunoileum, it is necessary to palpate the root of the mesentery and transect it far enough from the aorta to preserve the cranial mesenteric ggl. Remove and place the small intestine on the table.

Identify the transverse colon and the junction with the descending colon. Double ligate the descending colon and transect it between the ligatures. Follow the course of the descending colon toward the pelvic inlet, double ligate and transect it as described above. Identify the dorsal attachment of the **descending mesocolon** and transect it there. Remove the descending colon and compare it to the small intestine.

The last viscera to be removed are the cecum, the ascending colon with its four segments, and the transverse colon. Isolate them from their attachments, remove them, and place them on a low table or on the floor.

Regardless of which technique is used, all the viscera removed from the abdominal cavity are subject to external and internal examination. The blood supply to the viscera is illustrated below in Figures H3.18 and H3.19 and described in the related text (pages 71–72). The sympathetic ggl. and plexuses are dissected with the kidneys and the adrenal glands.

Start with the liver. Dissect the portal V., the hepatic A., and the common hepatic duct. Identify the major branches of the common hepatic duct (choledochus). *Notice* that the common hepatic duct is still connected to the duodenum, if the first technique of exenteration was used *(exenteration is removal of viscera by excision from the abdominal cavity)*. The common hepatic duct merges with the pancreatic duct before opening inside the **hepatopancreatic ampulla** within the **major duodenal papilla**. Make an incision along the greater curvature of the cranial part of the duodenum close to the **pylorus** to identify the major and the **minor duodenal papillae** (Fig. H3.14A). Identify the **portal lnn.**, which are scattered along the hilus. Examine the visceral and diaphragmatic aspects of the liver (Fig. H3.14B,C), with the hepatogastric lig. still in place or transected (depending on the technique of exenteration), and *notice* the "impressions" of other viscera on the embalmed liver. Try to discern the relationship between the liver and those viscera. Look at the fissures and at the limits between the lobes. *Notice* that the horse is the only domestic species that does not have a gall bladder. The number of liver lobes is similar to that in the rabbit (**left lateral, left medial, quadrate, right,** and **caudate**). Examine the diaphragmatic aspect of the liver and identify the caudal vena cava, the coronary lig. (dorsal to the vein), the falciform lig. (ventral to the vein), and the **esophageal impression**.

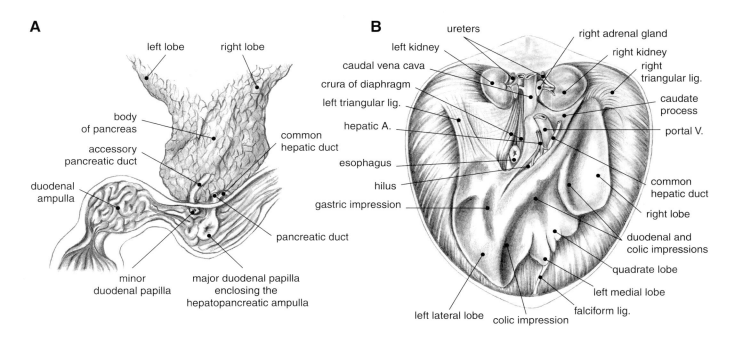

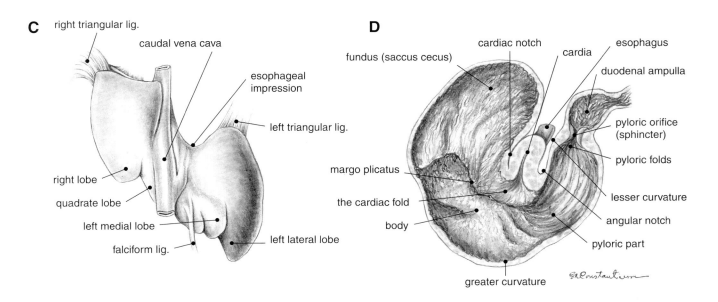

Fig. H3.14. Pancreas, liver, and stomach, horse. **A.** Bile and pancreatic ducts **B.** Liver in situ, visceral aspect, with ligaments. **C.** Liver, diaphragmatic aspect, with ligaments. **D.** Longitudinal section of the stomach.

*Remember!* The **round lig. of the liver** lies in the free edge of the falciform lig.

*Notice* the branches of the celiac A., which supplies the stomach, spleen, and liver. Do not transect them if the first technique of exenteration was used. If the second technique was used, the hepatic A. was previously transected. Examine the **gastric lnn.** located on the lesser curvature of the stomach.

Unfold and spread out the jejunum to examine the **jejunal lnn.** (close to the root of the mesentery) and the arterial and venous arcades, which are 2–4 cm away from the lesser curvature of the jejunum. Compare the arteries supplying the jejunum (the **jejunal Aa.**) and the arteries of the descending colon (the **left colic A.**), whose arcades are very close to the lesser curvature of the colon. Also, *notice* the smooth surface of the jejunum in comparison to the **sacculations** and **bands** of the descending colon (**haustrae** and **teniae**, respectively).

Examine the cecum and its four longitudinal bands (Figs. H3.15, H3.16A,B). Make an incision in the base of the cecum along the greater curvature. Reflect the lateral slip and look at the **ileocecal ostium** and **cecocolic ostium**. The former is provided with the **ileal papilla** and the **ileal sphincter**. The latter is provided with the **cecocolic valve** and **cecal sphincter** (Fig. H3.16C).

As stated earlier, the ascending colon in the horse consists of four "colons." The **right ventral colon** starts with

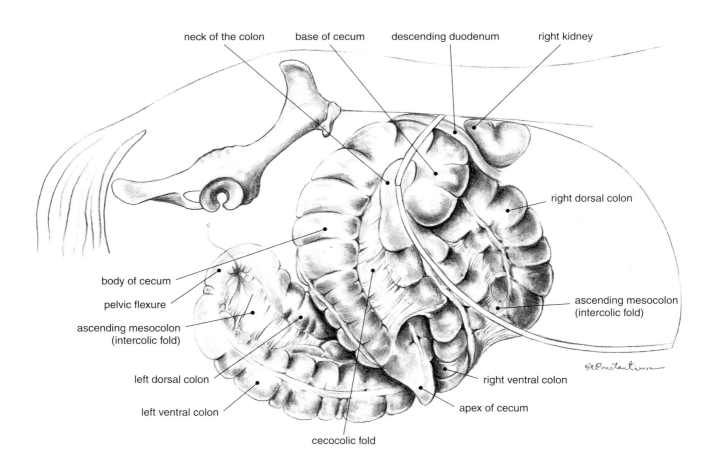

neck of the colon    base of cecum    descending duodenum    right kidney

right dorsal colon

body of cecum

pelvic flexure

ascending mesocolon (intercolic fold)

ascending mesocolon (intercolic fold)

left dorsal colon

right ventral colon

left ventral colon

apex of cecum

cecocolic fold

Fig. H3.15. Cecum and ascending colon, horse, right aspect.

a narrow part, the **neck of the colon**, and runs on the floor of the abdominal cavity in a caudocranial direction, up to the xyphoid cartilage. Here it makes a turn from right to left, horizontally, the **sternal flexure**. From the sternal flexure the ascending colon continues on the floor of the abdominal cavity with the **left ventral colon**, in a craniocaudal direction, up to the pelvic inlet. At this point it makes a turn ventrodorsally, in a vertical position, the **pelvic flexure**. The **left dorsal colon**, parallel to the left ventral colon, has a caudocranial direction and runs to the sternal flexure. It makes a horizontal turn from left to

right, the **diaphragmatic flexure**, and continues in a craniocaudal direction as the **right dorsal colon**, parallel and dorsal to the right ventral colon.

Examine the four longitudinal bands and sacculations of the ventral colon. The left dorsal colon has only one band on the lesser curvature and no sacculations, whereas the right dorsal colon has three longitudinal bands and sacculations. The right dorsal colon is the largest colon, almost double the size of the lumen in comparison with the other three segments of the ascending colon. Examine the sternal, diaphragmatic, and pelvic flexures. The **cecocolic**

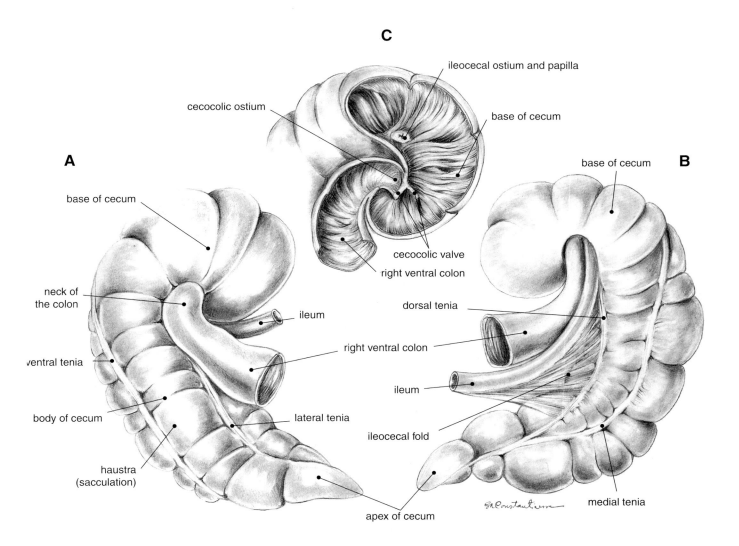

Fig. H3.16. Cecum, horse. **A.** Right aspect. **B.** Left aspect. **C.** The communications of the cecum.

**fold** was previously examined. Look at the **cecal** and **colic lnn.** (Fig. H3.17).

The ileocecal fold (dorsal band of the cecum) and the cecocolic fold (lateral band of the cecum) are important landmarks during exploratory celiotomy surgery. The ileocecal fold is identified on the cecum and used as a landmark to locate the ileum during exploratory surgery. The cecocolic fold is identified on the cecum and traced to the right ventral colon to confirm proper orientation of the large intestine and cecum after correction of a large intestinal displacement or volvulus.

A sudden reduction in lumen size of the right dorsal colon is observed at the medial aspect of the base of the cecum. This is the origin of the **transverse colon**, a short segment of the large intestine with one band and no sac-

culations. It passes from the right to the left, cranial to the cranial mesenteric A.

The reduction in size and change of direction from the cecum to the right ventral colon (the neck of the colon), from the left ventral colon to the left dorsal colon through the pelvic flexure, and from the right dorsal colon to the transverse colon create sites that are susceptible to impaction of ingesta; they are called impaction sites.

Unfold and spread the descending colon, also known as the small colon in comparison to the large (ascending) colon. It has sacculations and two bands. Identify the colic lnn.

The jejunoileum, the cecum, and the colon are illustrated in Figure H3.17.

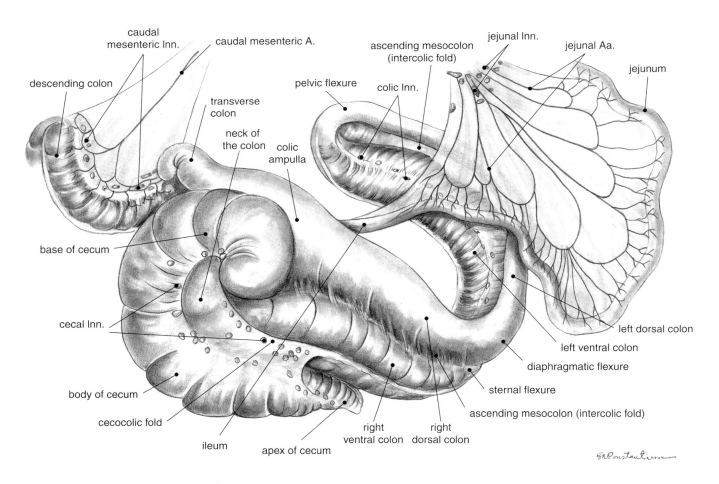

Fig. H3.17. Intestine of the horse.

Examine the spleen with the base, the two borders, and the apex. Inspect the medial aspect with the hilus, splenic A.V., and the **splenic lnn**.

Dissect the celiac A. and its branches and ***notice*** the anastomoses that are indicated in Figure H3.18 by circles.

Make an incision along the greater curvature of the stomach from the **cardia** to the **pylorus** and identify the **cardiac notch** and the **angular notch**. Examine the **margo plicatus**, the **cardiac** and the **pyloric sphincters**, and especially the mucosal folds. The **cardiac fold** allows movement of ingesta *only* from the esophagus to the stomach and *never* back, whereas the **pyloric folds** allow transit from the stomach to the duodenum and back to the stomach (see Fig. H3.14D).

From the cranial mesenteric A. originate branches that supply the whole intestine up to the descending colon. Because of the complexity of the intestinal arteries, certain correlations between the viscera and the name of the

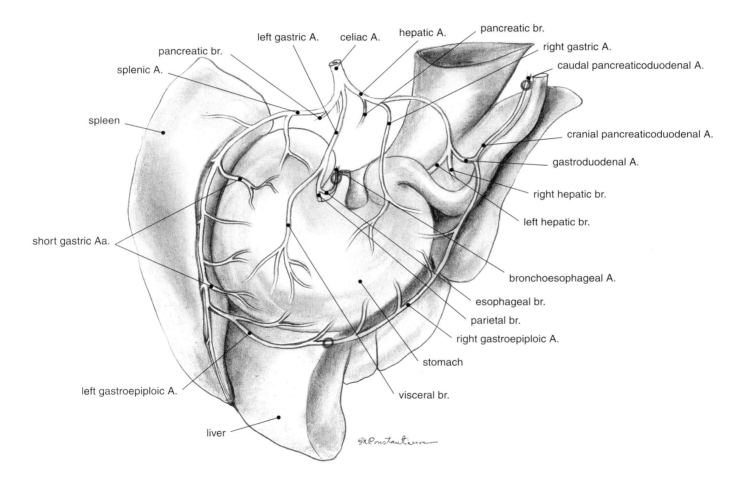

Fig. H3.18. Celiac artery in the horse. The arterial anastomoses are indicated by circles.

arteries are suggested. The **"colic branch"** supplies the first half of the ascending colon (the ventral colon, right and left), whereas the **"right colic A."** supplies the second half of the ascending colon (the dorsal colon, left and right). The middle colic A. supplies the middle portion of the colon, which is the transverse colon.

The first branch of the cranial mesenteric A. is the **caudal pancreaticoduodenal A.**, which anastomoses with the **cranial pancreaticoduodenal A.** (from the gastroduodenal A. of the hepatic A.). The **jejunal Aa.** supply the jejunum, and the **ileal Aa.** supply the ileum. The **ileocolic A.** supplies the cecum (by the **medial** and **lateral cecal Aa.**) and the ventral colon (by the colic branch). The **mesenteric ileal branch** supplies the ileum on its lesser curvature (where the mesentery is attached). The descending colon is supplied by the **left colic A.**, branch of the **caudal mesenteric A.**

The following anastomoses occur: between the caudal and cranial pancreaticoduodenal Aa.; between the last jejunal A. and the ileal Aa.; between the ileal Aa. and the mesenteric ileal A.; between the colic branch and the right colic A. (at the pelvic flexure); between the middle colic A. and the left colic A. The anastomoses are indicated in Figure H3.19 by circles.

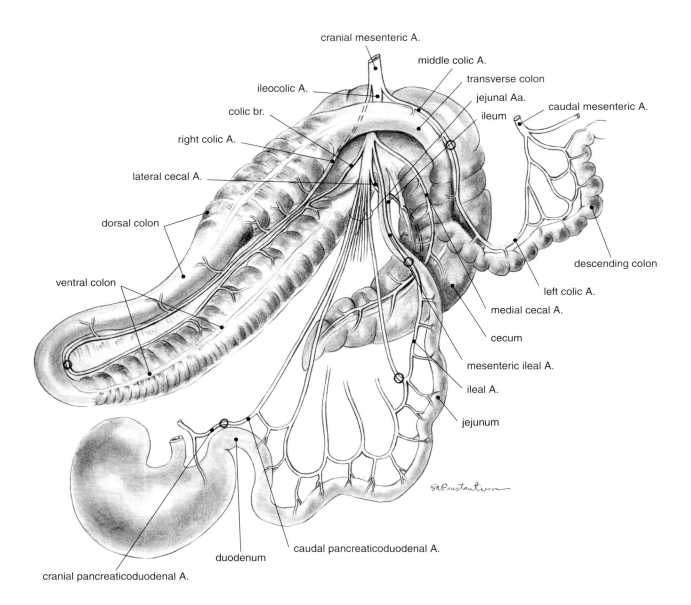

Fig. H3.19. Cranial and caudal mesenteric arteries in the horse. The arterial anastomoses are indicated by circles.

# MODLAB H3

Follow the procedures suggested in the previous modlabs and attempt to first palpate the anatomical structures listed at the beginning of this chapter.

Focus now on the **landmarks** and **approaches** of the most important clinically relevant structures, as follows:

1. **Subiliac ln.** (see Fig. H2.23A)
   A. *Landmarks:* tuber coxae; patella; the cranial border of tensor fasciae latae M.
   B. *Approach*: Press the fingertips of both hands on the cranial border of the tensor fasciae latae M., slightly ventral to the midpoint between the tuber coxae and patella, and roll your fingers deep forward to feel the lymph nodes.
2. **External pudendal A.** (Fig. H3.20A)
   A. *Landmarks*: linea alba; prepubic tendon; superficial inguinal ring
   B. *Approach*: over the caudomedial commissure of the superficial inguinal ring, between the prepubic tendon and the linea alba
   **Caution.** In the male, the external pudendal A. delivers in a cranial direction the superficial caudal epigastric A., which crosses the medial aspect of the spermatic cord; whereas in the female the artery runs 3–4 cm lateral to the linea alba. In both the male and female, the superficial inguinal lnn. (called scrotal in the male and mammary in the female) lie on this artery.
3. **Laparotomy (right-sided approach)** (Fig. H3.20B)
   **Note.** *Laparotomy is the incision of the flank to gain access to the peritoneal cavity.*

*Cecocentesis*
   A. *Landmarks*: right paralumbar fossa
   B. *Approach*: in the middle of the right paralumbar fossa, midway between the last rib and the tensor fasciae latae M., and one hand ventral to the transverse processes of the lumbar vertebrae

*Exploration of the cecum or cecotomy (typhlotomy)*
   A. *Landmarks*: the slope of the right flank; the cranial border of the tensor fasciae latae M.
   B. *Approach*: a vertical incision in the right slope of the flank, one hand cranial to, and parallel with, the cranial border of the tensor fasciae latae M.
4. **Celiotomy (ventrotomy)** (see Fig. H3.20A)
   **Note.** *Celiotomy is the surgical incision into the abdominal cavity at any point to gain access to the peritoneal cavity. Ventral celiotomy, or ventrotomy is the incision into the abdominal cavity through the abdominal wall (there is also a vaginal celiotomy).*
   A. *Landmarks*: umbilicus; linea alba; prepuce or mammary gland; xiphoid cartilage
   B. *Approach*: Length and placement of the incision line depend on the surgical procedure; for example, from the umbilicus toward the xiphoid cartilage on the linea alba in a cesarean section and in most exploratory celiotomies; from the umbilicus toward the prepuce or mammary gland on the linea alba in other interventions, including the approach to the urinary bladder.
5. **Laparotomy for hysterotomy and/or hysterectomy (left-sided approach)** (see Fig. H2.23B)
   A. *Landmarks and Approach*: same as in the exploration of the cecum or cecotomy, but on the left side

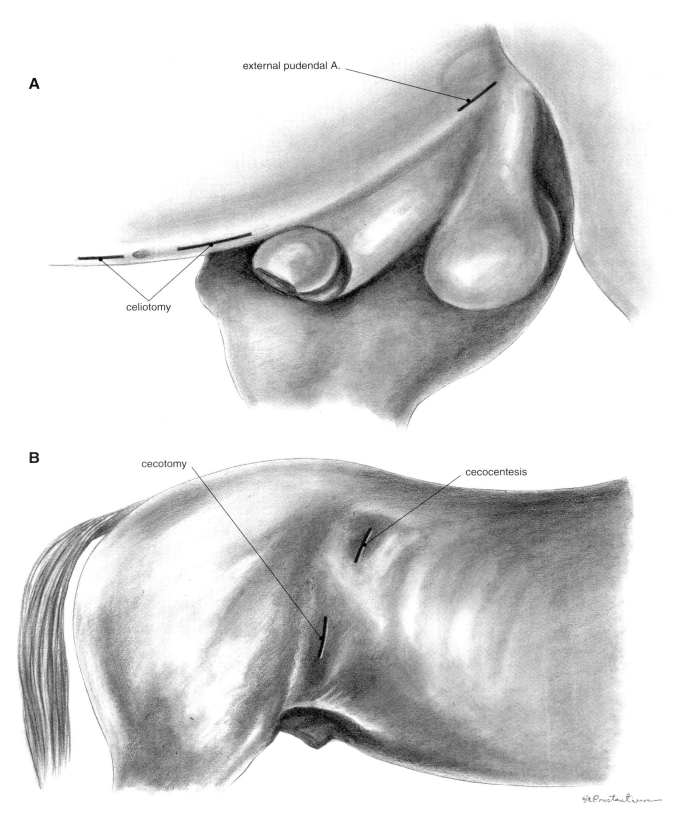

Fig. H3.20. Landmarks and approaches on the abdomen, horse. **A.** Surgical approaches to genital and abdominal structures. **B.** Approaches to cecum.

# H 4

## The Pelvis, Pelvic Viscera, Tail, and External Genitalia

The bones of the pelvis and tail, the **coxal bones**, the **sacrum**, and the **caudal vertebrae**, respectively, are illustrated in Figures H4.1–H4.4. The **obturator membrane** and **canal**, the **sacrosciatic lig.** with the **greater** and **lesser ischiatic foramina**, the **sacroiliac joint** (including the **ventral**, **dorsal**, and **interosseous sacroiliac ligg.**), and the **pelvic symphysis** are illustrated in Fig. H4.5. The hip joint will be exposed in Chapter H5, The Pelvic Limb.

The ventral sacral foramina are valuable landmarks for performing the "subsacral anesthesia," blocking all viscera supplied by the pudendal and caudal rectal Nn. See Landmarks and Approach in item 7 of Modlab H4, the illustration in Figure R4.3, and the technique for large ruminants described on the last page of Chapter R4.

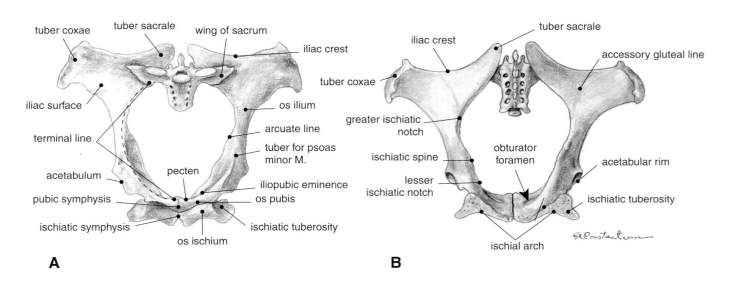

**A**

tuber coxae
tuber sacrale
wing of sacrum
iliac crest
iliac surface
os ilium
terminal line
arcuate line
tuber for psoas minor M.
acetabulum
pecten
iliopubic eminence
pubic symphysis
os pubis
ischiatic symphysis
ischiatic tuberosity
os ischium

**B**

iliac crest
tuber sacrale
tuber coxae
accessory gluteal line
greater ischiatic notch
obturator foramen
ischiatic spine
acetabular rim
lesser ischiatic notch
ischiatic tuberosity
ischial arch

Fig. H4.1. Coxal bones with sacrum, horse. **A.** Cranial aspect. **B.** Caudal aspect.

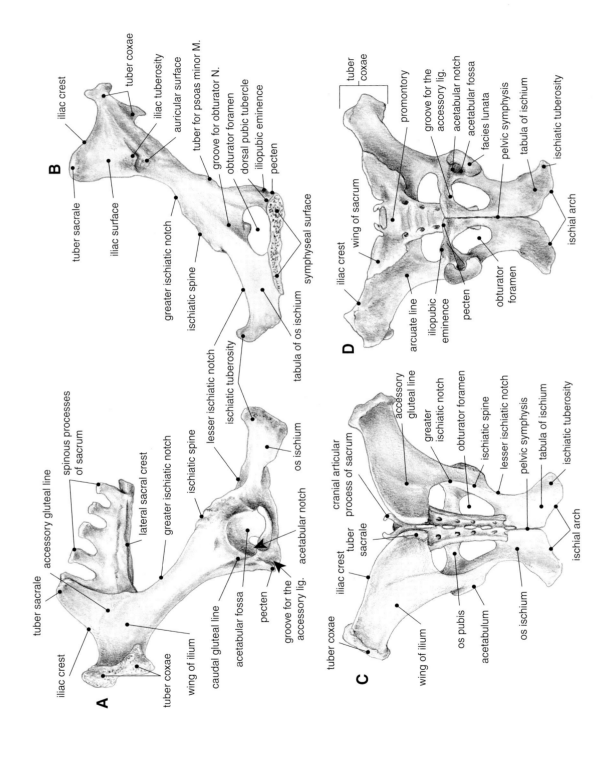

Fig. H4.2. Coxal bones with sacrum, horse. **A.** Left lateral aspect. **B.** Left medial aspect. **C.** Dorsal aspect. **D.** Ventral aspect.

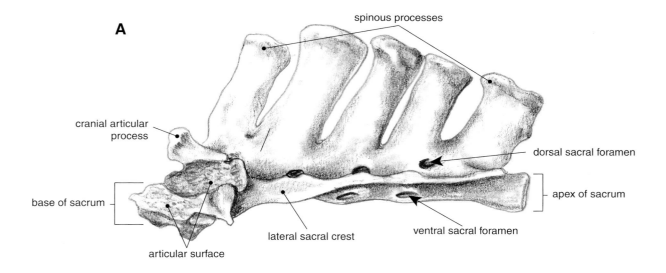

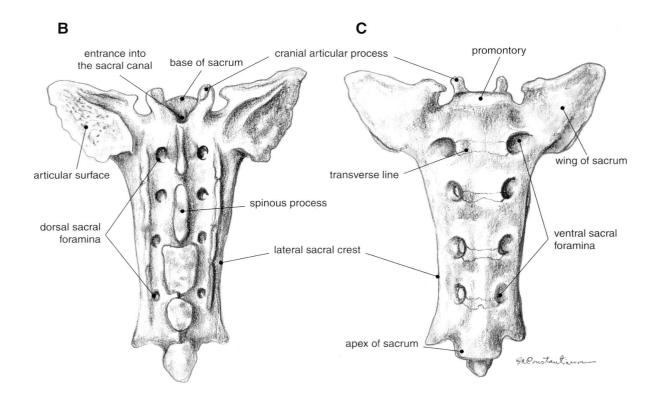

Fig. H4.3. Sacrum, horse. **A.** Left lateral aspect. **B.** Dorsal aspect. **C.** Pelvic aspect.

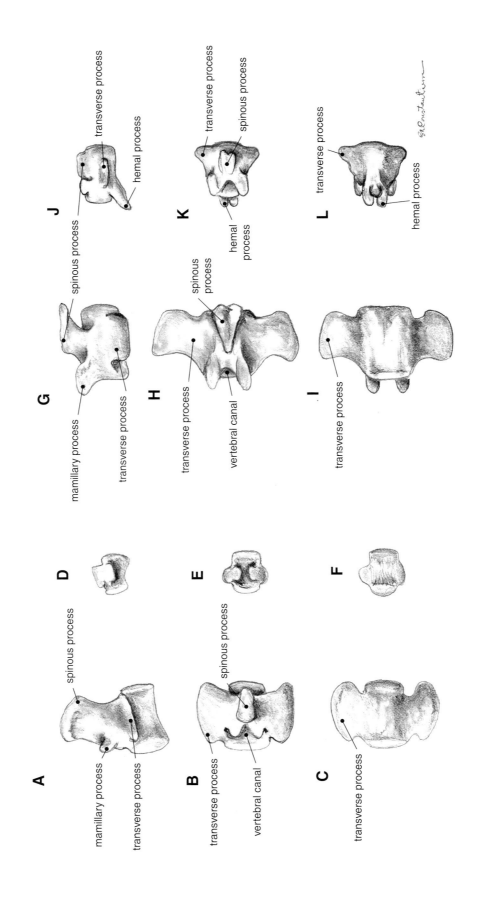

Fig. H4.4. Caudal vertebrae, horse (A–F) and large ruminants (G–L). *First vertebra, horse:* **A.** Left lateral view. **B.** Dorsal view. **C.** Ventral view. *Fourth vertebra, horse:* **D.** Left lateral view. **E.** Dorsal view. **F.** Ventral view. *First vertebra, large ruminants:* **G.** Left lateral view. **H.** Dorsal view. **I.** Ventral view. *Fourth vertebra, large ruminants:* **J.** Left lateral view. **K.** Dorsal view. **L.** Ventral view.

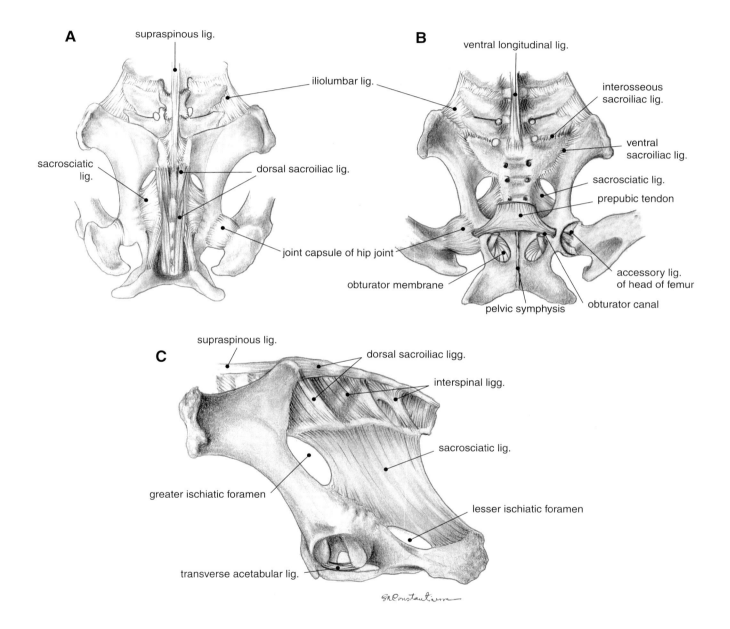

Fig. H4.5. Sacroiliac joint and surrounding articular structures, horse. **A.** Dorsal aspect. **B.** Ventral aspect. **C.** Lateral aspect.

Examine the structures that are common to a male and a female specimen: the symmetrical **rectus abdominis Mm.**, the **linea alba**, the **transversus abdominis Mm.**, the **internal and external abdominal oblique Mm.**, the **rectus sheaths**, **the transverse fascia**, the **parietal peritoneum**, and the arteries and veins.

The rectus abdominis M. is protected by the external and internal laminae of the rectus sheath. The **external lamina** is given by the fusion of aponeuroses of the external and internal abdominal oblique Mm., whereas the **internal lamina** is mostly represented by the aponeurosis of the transversus abdominis M.

Make a longitudinal incision in the parietal peritoneum, transverse fascia, and internal lamina of the rectus sheath parallel and 5 cm lateral to the linea alba and reflect them. The specific fibrous intersections of the rectus abdominis M. are visible. The lateral border of the rectus abdominis is paralleled by the **caudal epigastric A.** Identify the **psoas major** and the **psoas minor Mm.** and the **genitofemoral N.** exiting from between those two muscles.

*Notice* that the psoas minor is located medial to the psoas major, both against the roof of the abdominal cavity, protected and bound down by the **iliac fascia**.

In both male and female, the **descending colon,** suspended by the **descending mesocolon** and supplied by the **left colic A.**, is fully exposed. Close to the **aorta** and around the origin of the **caudal mesenteric A.**, find and dissect the **caudal mesenteric ggl.** and the **hypogastric Nn.**, which are the sympathetic contribution to the **pelvic plexus** (parasympathetic). The **urinary bladder**, lying on the floor of the pelvic cavity is attached to the lateral walls by the symmetrical **lateral vesical ligg.** and to the floor by the **median vesical lig. (median lig. of the bladder)** (see Fig. H4.7). The lateral ligg. enclose the symmetrical **umbilical Aa.**, whereas the median lig. extends up to the **umbilicus** and encloses the **urachus**, a structure from the developmental life. The umbilical Aa. are usually nonpatent; they are transformed into two fibrous cords, the **round ligg.** of the urinary bladder. Before becoming nonfunctional, they supply the **apex of the urinary bladder** by the **cranial vesical Aa.**

Follow the most caudal extent of the aorta and identify first the symmetrical **external iliac Aa.**, then the two **internal iliac Aa.** The external iliac A. takes a caudoventral direction on the lateral side of the pelvic inlet, branching into the **deep circumflex iliac A.** ventral to the tuber coxae. Identify the **cremasteric** or **uterine A.**, which is a branch of the external iliac A., a feature unique to the horse.

Identify the following lymph nodes: aortic lumbar, medial and lateral iliac, and sacral. The **lumbar lnn.** are scattered along the ventral aspect of the aorta and the caudal vena cava, the **medial iliac lnn.** are located along the terminal segment of the aorta and the initial segment of the external iliac A., the **lateral iliac lnn.** are found around the bifurcation of the deep circumflex iliac A., and the **sacral lnn.** are between the two internal iliac Aa.

In the stallion (or gelding), execute an incision of the parietal peritoneum and the transverse fascia at the level of the cranial branch of the deep circumflex iliac A. toward its origin. Follow the course of the **external iliac A.** up to the **deep femoral A.**, which indicates the transition between the external iliac A. and the **femoral A.** Through the transparency of the peritoneum and transverse fascia, identify the caudal border of the internal abdominal oblique M. and the **cremaster M.** Caudally and deep to them, the **arcus inguinalis** is exposed.

*Remember!* The internal abdominal oblique M. represents the cranial border of the deep inguinal ring and the cranial wall of the **inguinal canal**, whereas the arcus inguinalis outlines the caudal border of the deep inguinal ring and the caudal wall of the inguinal canal (Fig. H4.8). The **lateral commissure of the deep inguinal ring** is located dorsally and far from the midline, in comparison to the **medial commissure**, which is located ventrally. The **medial commissure of the deep inguinal ring** is close to, and overlaps, the **caudomedial commissure of the superficial inguinal ring**. The distance between the lateral commissure of the deep inguinal ring and the **craniolateral commissure of the superficial inguinal ring** is much longer. The inguinal canal is found between the two inguinal rings.

*Remember!* The superficial inguinal ring is a slit in the aponeurosis of the external abdominal oblique M. before its attachment to the cranial border of the pubic bone. The ring is outlined by two borders (crura) and two commissures (craniolateral and caudomedial). From the caudomedial commissure a strong fibrous structure 8–10 cm wide (the arcus inguinalis, formerly called the inguinal lig.) courses toward, and attaches to, the tuber coxae within the abdominal cavity. Another structure originating from the superficial inguinal ring, the **femoral lamina**, extends distally to cover the medial aspect of the thigh.

*Remember!* The reflection of the parietal peritoneum through the deep inguinal ring is called **vaginal ring** and is much smaller then the deep inguinal ring.

The vaginal ring surrounds the origin of the **spermatic cord**. Before entering the inguinal canal, the parietal peritoneum changes its name to the **parietal lamina of the vaginal tunic**.

*Remember!* The spermatic cord consists of the **ductus deferens,** surrounded by the **mesoductus deferens,** and

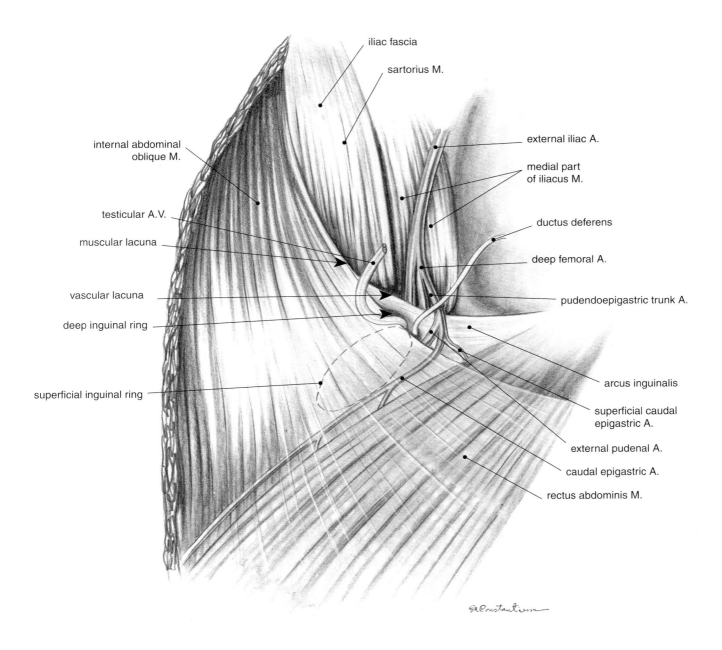

Fig. H4.8. Inguinal rings and associated structures in the stallion, at the pelvic inlet.

the **mesorchium,** which contains the **testicular A.** and the **testicular V. (the pampiniform plexus), autonomic nerves,** and **smooth muscle fibers**. All these structures are surrounded by the **visceral lamina of the vaginal tunic**. The liaison between the parietal and the visceral laminae of the vaginal tunic is the **mesofuniculus** (Fig. H4.9). Between the parietal and visceral laminae of the vaginal tunic the **vaginal canal** is outlined (Fig. H4.10).

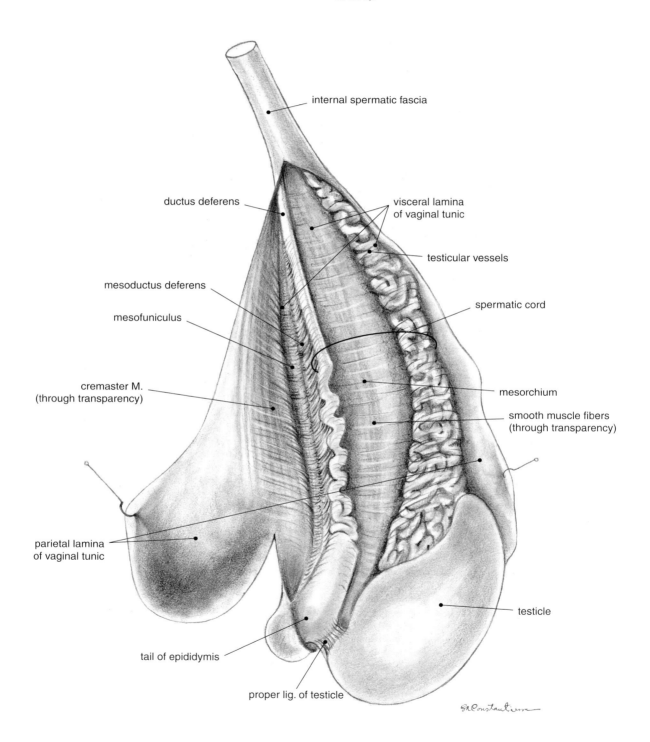

internal spermatic fascia

ductus deferens

visceral lamina of vaginal tunic

testicular vessels

mesoductus deferens

spermatic cord

mesofuniculus

cremaster M. (through transparency)

mesorchium

smooth muscle fibers (through transparency)

parietal lamina of vaginal tunic

testicle

tail of epididymis

proper lig. of testicle

Fig. H4.9. Spermatic cord in the stallion.

*Remember!* The transverse fascia and the peritoneum accompany the **testicle** during its descent through the inguinal canal and finally out of the abdominal cavity. Even though there is a continuation of those structures, their names change as following:

- The transverse fascia becomes the **internal spermatic fascia.**
- The peritoneum becomes the vaginal tunic, with parietal and visceral laminae.
- The peritoneal cavity becomes the vaginal canal within the inguinal canal, and the **vaginal cavity** around the testicle.

Within the inguinal canal, between it and the internal spermatic fascia, the following structures pass:

- The cremaster M., protected by the **cremasteric fascia**
- The **external pudendal A.**
- The **genital branch of the genitofemoral N.**

*Remember!* The cremaster M. originates from the internal abdominal oblique M. and intimately covers the internal spermatic fascia.

The deep femoral A. gives off the **pudendoepigastric trunk** and then continues as the **medial circumflex femoral A.** The external pudendal A. is a branch of the trunk. Before sending the external pudendal A. within the inguinal canal, the trunk sends also the **caudal epigastric A.** The latter runs parallel to and close to the lateral border of the rectus abdominis M., outside of the transverse fascia.

The genitofemoral N. is the ventral branch of the spinal nerves L2 and L3; it branches into the genital and femoral branches. Only the genital branch travels within the inguinal canal, to supply the cremaster M., the **scrotum,** and the **prepuce.**

Make two incisions, one longitudinal and one transverse. Transect the peritoneum, transverse fascia, and internal abdominal oblique M. in a cranial direction from the vaginal ring, parallel to the lateral border of the rectus abdominus M. Transect transversely the caudal tendon of the rectus abdominus M. Reflect all these structures to expose the inguinal canal and the superficial inguinal ring. Make an incision in the longitudinal axis of the internal spermatic fascia; the incision will pass through the parietal lamina of the vaginal tunic at the same time. You are now within the vaginal canal and have exposed the spermatic cord (see Figs. H4.9 and H4.10).

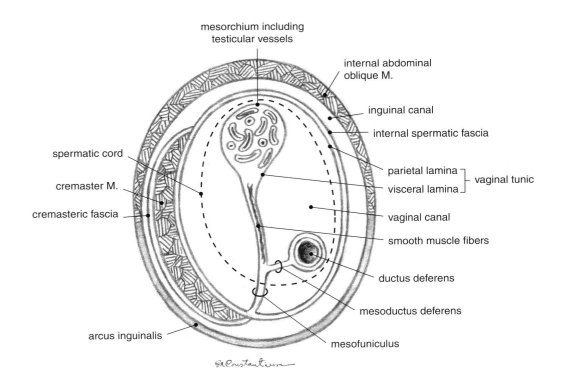

Fig. H4.10. Transverse section through the inguinal canal, horse (schematic).

Following the testicular descent, the testicle is surrounded and protected by two types of tunics: intraabdominal, and extraabdominal. The intraabdominal tunics accompany the testicle during its descent through the inguinal canal. They are the visceral and parietal laminae of the vaginal tunic, and the internal spermatic fascia. The extraabdominal tunic consist of the scrotum, and the continuation of the fascia of the external abdominal oblique M. plus the subcutaneous loose connective tissue. The scrotum has two layers: the **scrotal skin** and the **tunica dartos**. The latter is a layer of smooth muscle, which can be separated from the scrotal skin. The continuation of the fascia of external abdominal oblique M. associated with the subcutaneous loose connective tissue is the **external spermatic fascia**.

Here is the systematization of these tunics:

- Intraabdominal tunics
  - visceral lamina of the vaginal tunic
  - parietal lamina of the vaginal tunic
  - internal spermatic fascia

- Extraabdominal tunics
  - external spermatic fascia
  - tunica dartos (dartos)
  - scrotal skin (scrotum)

There is a **median raphe of scrotum**, separating the two testicles from each other, and also a **scrotal septum**, a median partition formed by the tunica dartos.

The dissection of the extraabdominal testicular tunics and clinical correlations will be explained below, on page 92.

Return to the femoral and the deep femoral Aa. They leave the abdominal cavity to supply muscles of the pelvic limb. The narrow space that they penetrate on their way to the limb is called **lacuna vasorum (vascular lacuna)**. Close to it, identify a similar **lacuna musculorum (muscular lacuna)**, the space allowing the iliopsoas and sartorius Mm. to exit the pelvic limb area toward the abdominal cavity (see Fig. H4.8).

In the mare, the only structures running within the inguinal canal are the external pudendal A., and the genital branch of the genitofemoral N., which supplies the **udder**.

The pelvic inlet shows structures illustrated in Figure H4.11A.

Still looking at the pelvic inlet, in the mare identify the flexuous course of the **ovarian A.**, which (only in the horse, not in ruminants) originates from the aorta, caudal

to the **renal A.** *Remember* that the testicular A. has a similar origin. The ovarian A. runs within the mesovarium.

*Remember!* The **broad lig.**, which suspends the **ovary**, the **uterine tube (or salpinx)**, and the **uterus**, extends from the $L_3$ or $L_4$ vertebra to the level of the $S_4$ vertebra. It is divided into three anatomically nondelineated portions: the **mesovarium**, the **mesosalpinx**, and the **mesometrium**. The mesovarium is divided into proximal and distal segments. The **proximal mesovarium** is considered the portion between the attachment of the broad lig. at the abdominal wall to the origin of mesosalpinx. The **distal mesovarium** is that short portion between the mesosalpinx and the ovary (Fig. H4.11B).

The cranial or free border of the mesovarium is the **suspensory lig. of the ovary**. The cranial border of the mesometrium is delineated by the short **round lig. of the uterus** (Fig. H4.11B).

**The anatomy of the broad ligg. can be clinically relevant in several situations. Exteriorization of the uterine horns or ovaries during surgical procedures is limited by the suspensory lig. The mesovarium is located for écrasement and ligation during ovariectomy, and in standing animals, for local anesthesia. Transrectal palpation of the broad ligg. is necessary for diagnosis of uterine torsion and determination of the direction of torsion.**

There is a duplication of the broad lig. between the ovary and the uterine horn enclosing a cavity called the **ovarian bursa**. The lateral wall of the bursa is represented by the mesosalpinx with the enclosed uterine tube, and the medial wall is the distal mesovarium, which is bordered ventrally by the **proper lig. of the ovary** (see Figs. H4.11B and H4.12).

The ovary, located caudal to the ipsilateral kidney, is reniform in shape and has medial and lateral surfaces, a free border oriented ventrally, a mesovarian border oriented dorsally, a tubal (cranial) end and a uterine (caudal) end, or extremities. The ventral border is concave and indented by the **ovarian (ovulation) fossa**.

*Note.* The ovarian fossa, called by the clinicians "ovulation fossa" and present only in the mare, is the area of the ovary where ovulation occurs.

Examine the **infundibulum** of the uterine tube, its **abdominal opening (ostium),** and the **fimbriae** (see Fig. H4.12). Introduce a finger into the ovarian bursa and palpate the ovarian fossa. The **uterine horns** converge toward the **uterine body**. The body lies on the floor of the pelvic cavity, and the horns are directed toward the dorsal wall of the abdominal cavity, caudal to the kidneys (Fig. H4.11A). Try to identify the **uterine A.V.**

**A**

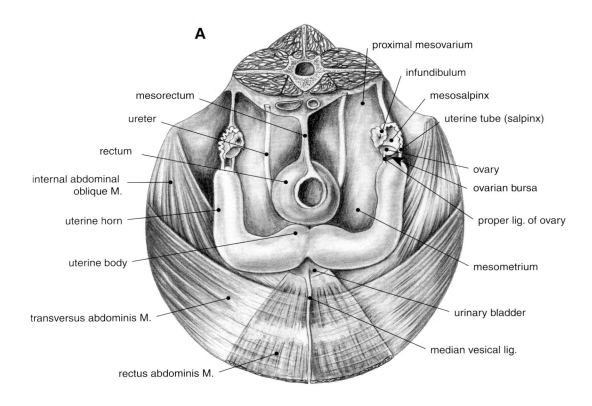

proximal mesovarium

infundibulum

mesorectum

mesosalpinx

ureter

uterine tube (salpinx)

rectum

internal abdominal oblique M.

ovary

ovarian bursa

uterine horn

proper lig. of ovary

uterine body

mesometrium

transversus abdominis M.

urinary bladder

median vesical lig.

rectus abdominis M.

**B**

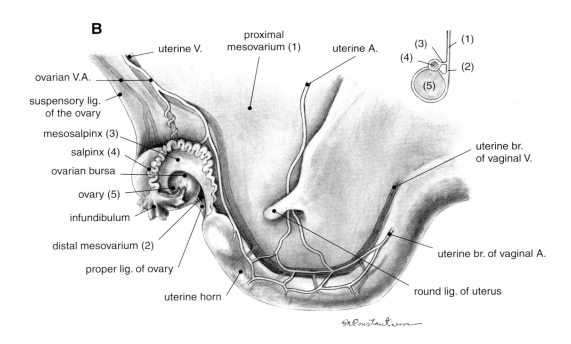

uterine V.

proximal mesovarium (1)

uterine A.

(3)     (1)

ovarian V.A.

(4)          (2)

suspensory lig. of the ovary

(5)

mesosalpinx (3)

salpinx (4)

uterine br. of vaginal V.

ovarian bursa

ovary (5)

infundibulum

distal mesovarium (2)

uterine br. of vaginal A.

proper lig. of ovary

uterine horn

round lig. of uterus

Fig. H4.11. Internal genital organs in the mare. **A.** Cranial view. **B.** Ovary, salpinx, and uterus, mare, left lateral view.

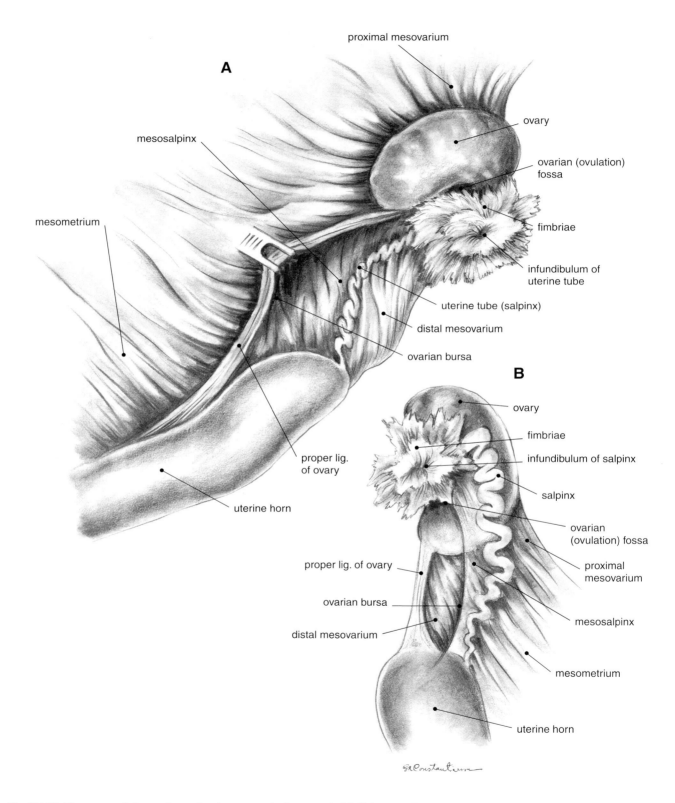

Fig. H4.12. The ovary, salpinx, and associated structures in the mare. **A.** Medial aspect. **B.** Ventral aspect.

Continue to dissect the external pudendal A. outside the inguinal canal, where it branches into cranially and caudally oriented arteries. In the male, identify the cranially oriented branches called the **A. penis cranialis** and the **superficial caudal epigastric A.** (Fig. H4.13). In the female the latter is also called the **cranial mammary A.**, while in the male it gives off **preputial branches**. The caudally oriented branch of the external pudendal A. in the mare is the **ventral labial branch**, also called the **caudal mammary A.** The **ventral scrotal branch** is the terminal branch of the external pudendal A. in the stallion. The arteries are generally accompanied by one or two veins.

The **penis** is protected within the **prepuce**. Examine the **external lamina**, which is the continuation of the skin, and the **internal lamina**, which is attached to the penis at the proximal end of the **free part of the penis**, where it is continuous with the skin of the free end of penis and glans. The internal lamina comes in intimate contact with the fully erect penis. The transition between the external lamina and the internal lamina outlines a circular orifice called **preputial ostium (orifice)**. When the penis is retracted within the prepuce, the internal lamina makes a fold called the **preputial fold**. The preputial fold has a surface facing the internal preputial lamina (**the outer layer**) and another facing the penis (**the inner layer**). The border between the outer and the inner layers has a ring shape and is called the **preputial ring**. On a fully erect penis the ring is shown as a circular prominence. The preputial fold lies within the **preputial cavity** (whose communication with the external environment at the end of the penis is the preputial orifice) (Fig. H4.14A).

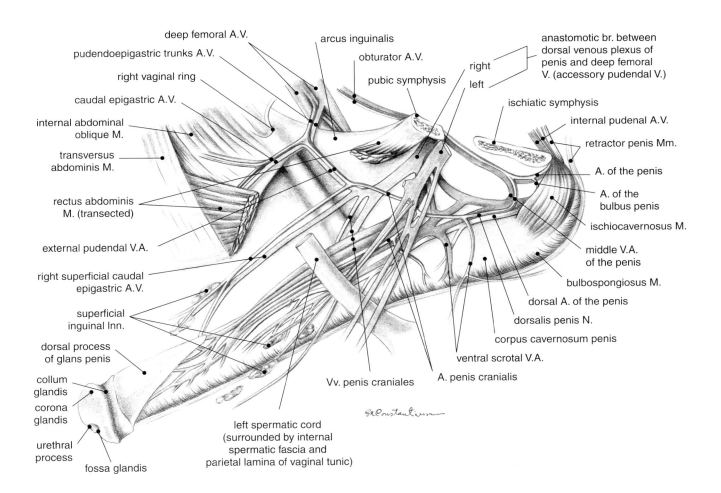

Fig. H4.13. Penis and associated structures in the stallion.

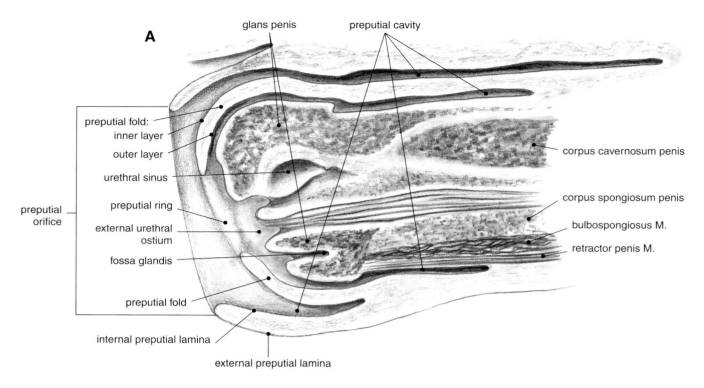

**A**

glans penis

preputial cavity

preputial fold:
inner layer
outer layer

urethral sinus

preputial ring

external urethral
ostium

fossa glandis

preputial fold

internal preputial lamina

external preputial lamina

preputial
orifice

corpus cavernosum penis

corpus spongiosum penis

bulbospongiosus M.

retractor penis M.

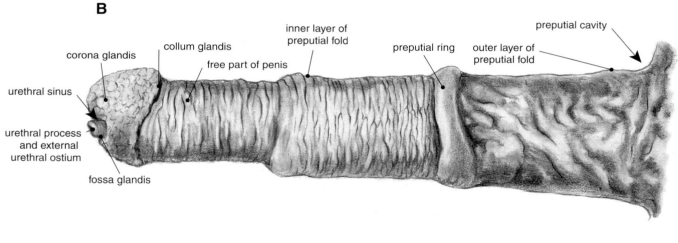

**B**

corona glandis

urethral sinus

urethral process
and external
urethral ostium

fossa glandis

collum glandis

free part of penis

inner layer of
preputial fold

preputial ring

preputial cavity

outer layer of
preputial fold

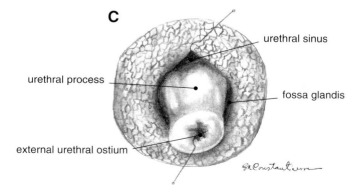

**C**

urethral process

external urethral ostium

urethral sinus

fossa glandis

Fig. H4.14. The penis of the horse. **A.** Median section. **B.** Lateral aspect. **C.** Frontal view of glans penis.

Pull the penis out of the prepuce and identify the preputial ring. Examine the **glans penis** with the **corona glandis** and the **collum glandis** (the neck of the glans penis), the **urethral process** with the **external urethral ostium (orifice)** surrounded by the **fossa glandis**, and dorsal to it the **urethral sinus** (Fig. H4.14B,C).

**The urethral process, the urethra, and the preputial folds are clinically important because they may carry the microorganism *Taylorella equigenitalis*, responsible for contagious equine metritis (CEM).**

Make a midlongitudinal incision on the dorsal aspect of the free part of the penis. Reflect the two borders of the incision and expose the **cranial Aa.** and **Vv. of the penis**, the **dorsal venous plexuses**, and the **dorsal Nn. of the penis**. Follow the cranial A. and V. of the penis caudally, including the dorsal venous plexus and *notice* that the main vein draining the blood from the penis is an anastomotic branch of the dorsal venous plexus to the **deep femoral V.** This branch perforates the origin of the **gracilis M.** through a fibrous ring close to the **pelvic symphysis** and is also called the accessory pudendal V. (see Fig. H4.13).

Transect the penis transversely to obtain several segments and examine each cross surface (Fig. H4.15). The common structures of all sections are the following: the **corpus cavernosum penis** surrounded by the **tunica albuginea** and the **trabeculae** sent by the tunica albuginea to divide the corpus cavernosum into **cavernae** (chambers); **the penile part of the urethra** surrounded by the **corpus spongiosum penis** and lying in the **urethral groove** of the corpus cavernosum; the **corpus spongiosum glandis** is the cranial continuation of the corpus spongiosum penis; the **bulbospongiosus M.** suspending the urethra like a hinge; and the **retractor penis M.**, which is the most ventral structure of the penis. In the most cranial sections, the **dorsal process of the glans penis** overlaps the corpus cavernosum (Fig. H4.15B,C).

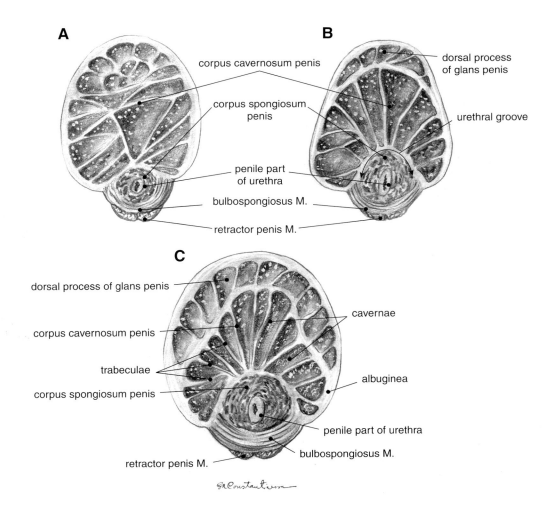

Fig. H4.15. Cross sections through the penis, horse. **A.** Caudal third of penis. **B.** Middle third of penis. **C.** Glans penis.

*Remember!* The glans penis consists of the **corona glandis**, the **collum glandis**, and the **dorsal process of glans penis.**

Next, in the testicular area examine the scrotum and the median raphe. Pull one testicle down into the scrotum, keeping your fingers clamped around the internal spermatic fascia (already exposed) until the scrotum becomes tense. Make a 2 cm sagittal incision in the scrotum, lateral and parallel to the raphe. Bluntly dissect (dilacerate) the external spermatic fascia from the internal spermatic fascia and break the **lig. of the tail of the epididymis.** This ligament attaches to the tunica dartos.

*Remember!* The lig. of the tail of the epididymis and the **proper lig. of the testicle** are the remnants of the **gubernaculum testis** from the developmental life.

In "closed castration," the scalpel incises the scrotal skin and the dartos together. Then, the external spermatic fascia is bluntly dissected. In twisting the internal spermatic fascia and the vaginal tunic enclosing the spermatic cord and applying the emasculator, there is minimal risk for any infection to develop in the vaginal tunic and ascend to the peritoneal cavity. However, peritonitis (sterile, usually) does arise when horses are castrated. It is localized and resolves without treatment (usually). With the closed technique, the amount of tissue in the emasculator may preclude effective crushing of the vasculature. Because of this, the closed technique is used only in young or small horses.

In "open castration" the scalpel incision continues through the internal spermatic fascia and parietal lamina of the vaginal tunic and exposes the spermatic cord. The emasculator is applied directly on the spermatic cord. The internal spermatic fascia, the parietal layer of the vaginal tunic, and the cremaster M. are not removed using this technique. With the open technique, there is an increased risk of a potential infection developing within the vaginal canal and ascending to the peritoneal cavity. Because the emasculator is applied directly on the spermatic cord, crushing off the vasculature is more effective, and larger horses are often castrated using this method.

A modified or half-closed technique is commonly used. The initial incision, similar to the closed technique, incises the scrotal skin and dartos together. The external spermatic fascia is then bluntly dilacerated and the testicle is prolapsed through a smaller incision in the internal spermatic fascia and vaginal tunic. The emasculator is applied directly to the spermatic cord. In larger cords, a separation is created in the mesor-

chium, and the spermatic vasculature is emasculated separately from the ductus deferens and the adjacent structures.

Make an incision through the internal spermatic fascia and the parietal lamina of the vaginal tunic to expose the vaginal cavity around the testicle, and the vaginal canal around the spermatic cord. The testicle and the **epididymis** are intimately covered by the visceral lamina of the vaginal tunic. The epididymis has three segments in continuation with each other: the **head**, the **body**, and the **tail**. The tail is continuous with the ductus deferens. Examine the specific location of the branches of the **testicular A.** Reflect the body of the epididymis proximally and examine the **testicular bursa**, the narrow space on the lateral side of the testicle, between the testicle and the body of the epididymis (Fig. H4.16). At the same time the distal mesorchium is exposed.

The **mesorchium** is divided into the **proximal mesorchium** and the **distal mesorchium** by the attachment of the **mesoepididymis.**

*Notice* that the scrotal skin and the tunica dartos, as well as the internal spermatic fascia and the parietal lamina of the vaginal tunic, are very close to each other. It is difficult, yet possible, to separate them from one another.

In the mare, examine the two **mammary glands** (the udder) (Fig. H4.17A) and the **intermammary groove.** Remove one gland from the midline and the ventral wall of the abdomen. In the removed gland, probe the two or three **papillary openings** of the **papillary ducts** in the tip of the **mammary papilla** (the teat). Make an incision through the papilla and expose the **papillary parts of the lactiferous sinus.** Continue the incision through the body of the gland and expose the **glandular part of the lactiferous sinus**, connected by numerous **lactiferous ducts** with the glandular tissue (Fig. H4.17B).

In both the male and the female, identify the **internal pudendal A.**, as a branch of the **internal iliac A.** The **umbilical A.** branches off close to the origin of the internal pudendal A. and courses toward the **urinary bladder** in the free edge of the lateral lig. of the bladder. The **A. of the ductus deferens** with the **ureteric branch,** and the **cranial vesical Aa.** are branches of the umbilical A. Identify the following structures as landmarks for the dissection of the pelvic walls: the **tuber coxae, tuber sacrale, ischiatic tuberosity, hip joint, greater trochanter,** and **third trochanter.** Skin the croup (or pelvic wall) between the abdominal and perineal areas and the base of the tail, and skin the thigh distal to the stifle joint. Reflect the skin over the crus. The dorsolateral cutaneous branches of the

**A**

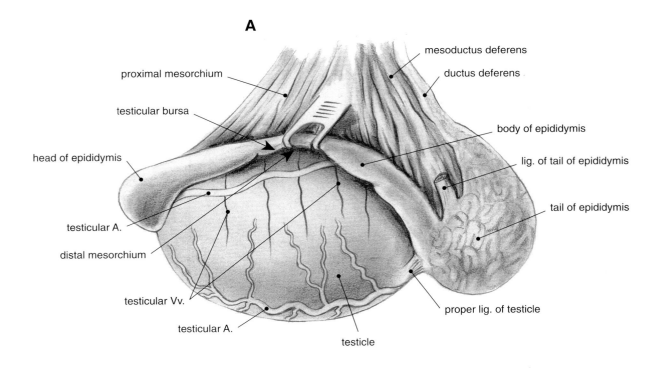

proximal mesorchium

mesoductus deferens

ductus deferens

testicular bursa

head of epididymis

body of epididymis

lig. of tail of epididymis

tail of epididymis

testicular A.

distal mesorchium

testicular Vv.

testicular A.

proper lig. of testicle

testicle

**B**

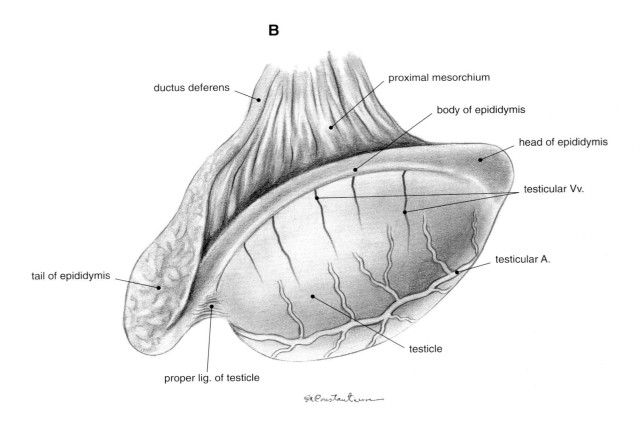

ductus deferens

proximal mesorchium

body of epididymis

head of epididymis

testicular Vv.

testicular A.

tail of epididymis

testicle

proper lig. of testicle

Fig. H4.16. The left testicle, stallion. **A.** Lateral aspect. **B.** Medial aspect.

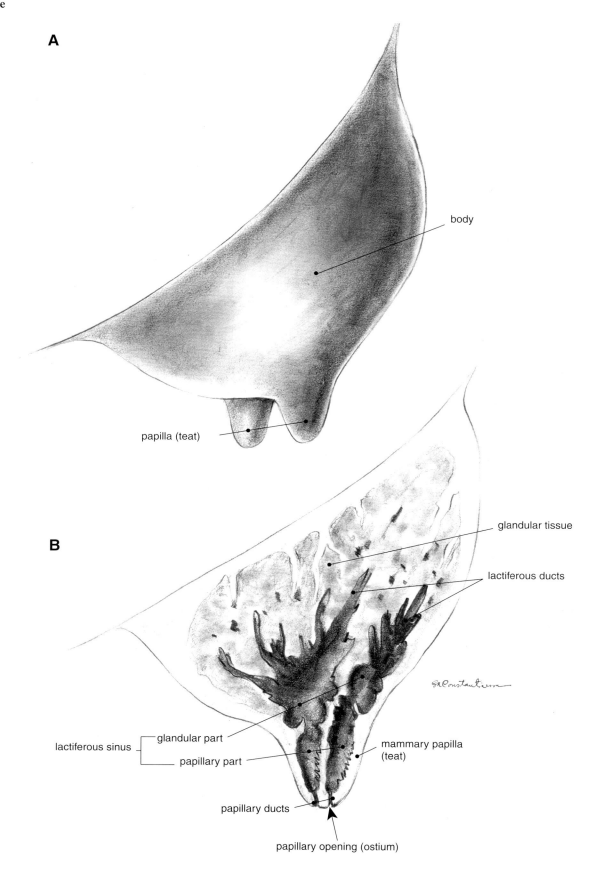

**A**

body

papilla (teat)

**B**

glandular tissue

lactiferous ducts

lactiferous sinus — glandular part
papillary part

mammary papilla
(teat)

papillary ducts

papillary opening (ostium)

Fig. H4.17. Mammary gland of the mare. **A.** Left lateral aspect. **B.** Sagittal section through a mammary gland.

lumbar Nn. (the so-called **cranial clunial Nn.**), the similar branches of the sacral Nn. (the so-called **middle clunial Nn.**), the **caudal cutaneous femoral N.** (the **caudal clunial Nn.**), and the **caudal Nn.** are now exposed (Fig. H4.18).

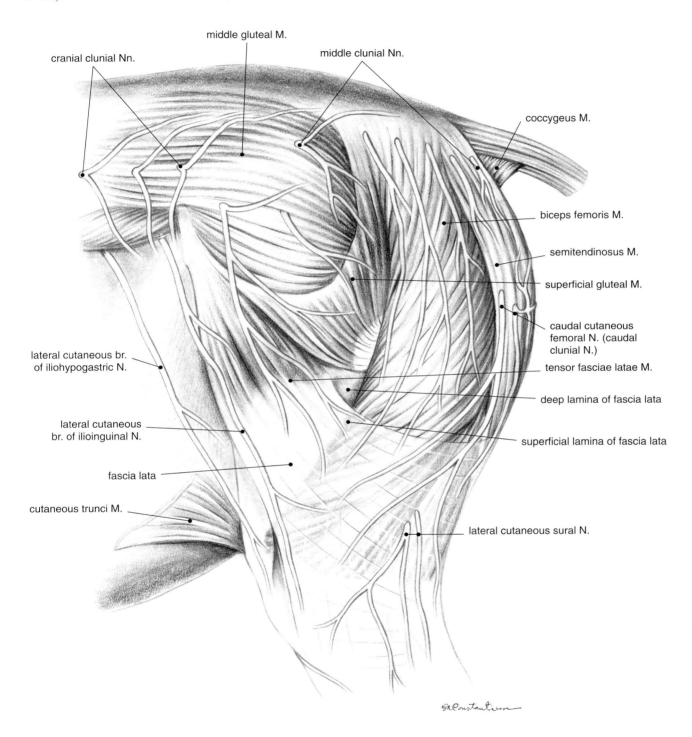

Fig. H4.18. Pelvic wall and thigh, horse, left lateral aspect.

The systematization of the pelvic muscles and the muscles of the tail is shown in Table H4.1.

Between the tuber coxae and the third trochanter, identify (through the **gluteal fascia**) a light white-yellow line separating the **tensor fasciae latae M.** from the **cranial part of the superficial gluteal M.** Make an incision along this line and separate the two muscles. From the third trochanter toward the **sacral spine** try to identify (through the gluteal fascia also) the light-colored line separating the caudal border of the **caudal part of the superficial gluteal M.** from the **biceps femoris M.**, and make an incision along this line. At a distance of three fingers cranial to the last line of separation and parallel to it is the cranial border of the caudal part of the superficial gluteal M. Incise the gluteal fascia on this line up to the tuber sacrale, and separate the superficial gluteal from the **middle gluteal M.**

*Notice* that the superficial gluteal M. is attached to the tuber sacrale by the gluteal fascia and not by its muscular portion. The cranial part of this muscle gets smaller and thinner from the third trochanter to the tuber coxae.

Remove the gluteal fascia from the middle gluteal M. as much as possible. The fascia is in intimate relation to the muscle, and even fused with it in the cranial half of the muscle. The fascia lata splits into a **superficial lamina** and a **deep lamina**, at the cranial border of the **biceps femoris M.** Incise the superficial lamina of the fascia lata parallel to, and 2 cm caudal to, the cranial border of the biceps femoris M. between the third trochanter and the **patella**. Reflect the fascia cranially up to the cranial bor-

der of the muscle. The deep lamina lies deep to the muscle in a caudal direction. The superficial and deep laminae originate from the fascia lata at the cranial border of the biceps femoris M. (see Fig. H4.18). Examine the duplication of the superficial lamina toward the patella.

Return to the croup, carefully separate the superficial gluteal M. from the biceps femoris M., and identify the aponeurosis of the superficial gluteal M., which lies deep to the biceps femoris M. and **semitendinosus M.** and attaches to the ischiatic tuberosity.

*Notice* that the gluteal fascia continues caudally with the **caudal fascia** over the tail, and with the fascia lata over the biceps femoris and semitendinosus Mm.

Free the biceps femoris M. from its **attachments** on the sacrum and the ischiatic tuberosity and reflect it ventrally.

*Caution.* The biceps femoris M. has an attachment on the caudal aspect of the femur (the **tuberosity of biceps M.**). Do not transect it yet.

Transect the proximal attachment of the semitendinosus M., isolate it from the origin of the **sacrocaudales Mm.** (sing. sacrocaudalis) and from the **sacrosciatic lig.** and reflect the semitendinosus M. ventrally. Observe the **ischiatic bursa** of this muscle, between it and the ischiatic tuberosity. Transect the origin of the superficial gluteal M. at the tuber sacrale, free its caudal border from the aponeurosis, and reflect the muscle ventrally.

Identify the caudal part of the **greater trochanter**, where the middle gluteal M. attaches, after gliding on the bone, protected by a **trochanteric bursa**. At a point one-hand cranial to the greater trochanter, make a transverse incision through the middle gluteal M. Five cm deep, the **accessory gluteal M.** will be exposed.

*Notice* the glittery tendon of the accessory gluteal M., which differentiates it from the middle gluteal M.

Identify the cranial part of the greater trochanter and its lateral crest, where the accessory gluteal M. inserts. Between the tendon and the cranial part of the trochanter, probe the **trochanteric bursa** of accessory gluteal M. Reflect the stumps of the middle gluteal M. Toward its caudal attachment, another muscle will be exposed: the **deep gluteal M.**, extending between the **ischiatic spine** and the medial aspect of the cranial part of the greater trochanter. Probe the trochanteric bursa of the middle gluteal M. and identify the **piriformis M.**, which is part of the middle gluteal M. The piriformis M. is attached to the **intertrochanteric crest**. Reflect the cranial stump of the middle gluteal M. over the accessory gluteal M. and up to the cranial border of the **wing of the ilium**. The **accessory gluteal line** separates the territory of attachments of the middle and accessory gluteal Mm. (the middle, medially, and the accessory, laterally) (Fig. H4.19).

Table H4.1. Muscles of the Pelvis and Tail, Horse

**Muscles of the Pelvis**

*Lateral/external aspect*
– superficial gluteus (superficial gluteal M.)
– middle gluteus (middle gluteal M.)
– piriformis
– accessory gluteus (accessory gluteal M.)
– deep gluteus (deep gluteal M.)

*Internal aspect*
– internal obturator
– gemelli
– quadratus femoris
– external obturator

**Muscles of the Tail**
– coccygeus
– sacrocaudalis dorsalis medialis
– sacrocaudalis dorsalis lateralis
– intertransversarii dorsales
– intertransversarii ventrales
– sacrocaudalis ventralis lateralis
– sacrocaudalis ventralis medialis

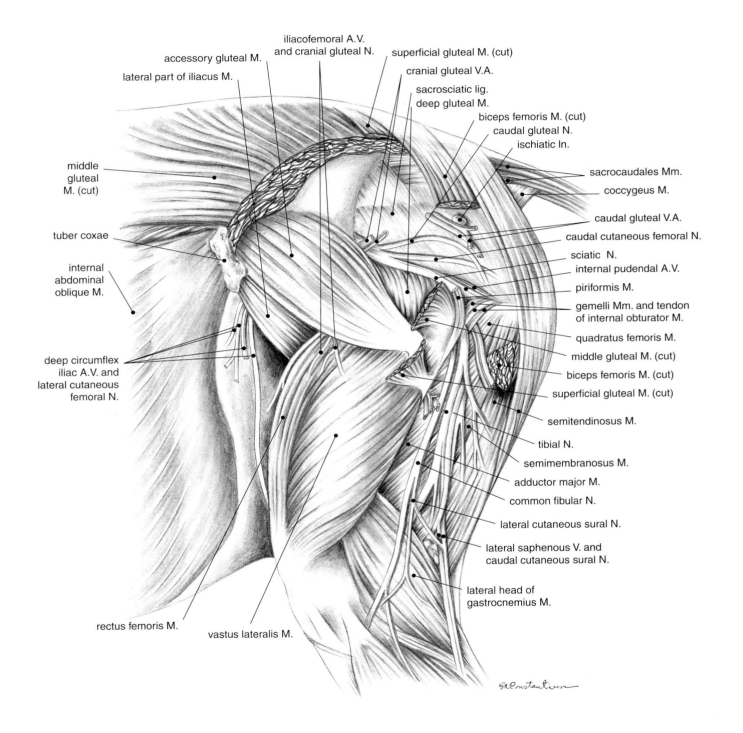

Fig. H4.19. Deep structures of left lateral pelvis and thigh, horse.

Identify the **greater ischiatic foramen**, where the **sciatic N.** becomes apparent. The nerve passes over the deep gluteal M. and surrounds the hip joint on its way toward the thigh. At the caudal aspect of the hip joint, the nerve overlaps the terminal tendon of the **internal obturator M.** accompanied by the **gemelli Mm.** (the twin muscles). The cranial part of the gemelli lies caudal and close to the deep gluteal M. The caudal part of the gemelli lies side by side with the **quadratus femoris M.** The latter comes in contact with the **adductor major M.** (see Fig. H4.19). Reflect the caudal part of the gemelli and the quadratus femoris M. to expose the **external obturator M.**

Transect the tensor fasciae latae M. at a point 5 cm ventral to its attachment on tuber coxae. Close to it, the **iliolumbar A.** and the **ventral branch of spinal nerve L4** are visible after surrounding the lateral border of the wing of the ilium in a mediolateral direction. The **deep circumflex iliac A.** and **V.** and the **lateral cutaneous femoral N.** will be found between the lateral part of the **iliacus M.** and the internal abdominal oblique M. The two parts of the **dorsal sacroiliac lig.** will be found between the wing of the ilium and the lateral border of the sacrum, and between the tuber sacrale and the spinous processes of the sacrum. From between these two parts of the ligament, the **sacrocaudales dorsales Mm.** emerge. The sacrosciatic lig. is widely exposed deep to the middle gluteal, biceps femoris, and semitendinosus Mm. Identify the two **ischiatic foramina:** the greater and the **lesser.** Identify and dissect the nerves and vessels passing through the greater ischiatic foramen from the pelvic cavity to the croup: the cranial gluteal vessels, and the cranial gluteal, sciatic, **caudal gluteal,** and **caudal cutaneous femoral Nn.** (see Fig. H4.19). Identify the **caudal gluteal** and **caudal Aa.** and **Vv.**

Transect the vertebral attachment of the **semimembranosus M.,** isolate it from the **sacrocaudales Mm.,** free its attachments from the sacrosciatic lig. and ischiatic tuberosity and reflect it ventrally. Either transect the sacrosciatic lig. from the proximal attachments and reflect it ventrally, or transect the ligament horizontally and keep a 5 cm wide strap attached dorsally and discard the rest of it (Fig. H4.20).

*Caution.* Some nerves and vessels may travel either on the lateral or the medial side of the sacrosciatic lig. and may perforate it to change sides; they may even travel within the thickness of the ligament. To avoid damaging the nerves or vessels, identify the origin of the nerves as they issue from the **ventral sacral foramina,** and the main arteries and veins before proceeding with the dissection.

On the medial aspect of the sacrosciatic lig. (Fig. H4.21), the following vessels and nerves are exposed: the caudal gluteal A. and V.; the cranial gluteal A., V., and N.; the **obturator A., V., and N.;** the **internal pudendal A.** and **V.,** with the **umbilical, prostatic/vaginal Aa.** and **Vv.** and their corresponding branches; the **pudendal N.;** the **caudal rectal N. (or Nn.);** and the **pelvic Nn.** (parasympathetic). The pelvic Nn. contribute to build up the **pelvic plexus,** which is reached by the symmetrical **hypogastric N.** from the **caudal mesenteric ggl.** (sympathetic). The plexus lies on the lateral aspect of the rectum and sends autonomic fibers, both sympathetic and parasympathetic to the intra- and extrapelvic viscera.

Identify the **coccygeus M.** in an oblique position cranioventrally and separate it from the **levator ani M.,** which runs parallel with and deep to it. *Notice* that the levator ani M. has three portions (**coccygeal, anal,** and **perineal**) (Fig. H4.20).

Carefully transect the coccygeus M. to allow the dissection of the vessels and nerves toward the anogenital area and to fully expose the **peritoneal reflections,** the **retroperitoneal space,** and the **pelvic diaphragm.**

The retroperitoneal space is filled with connective tissue and fat, between the peritoneum and the body wall, and is located just caudal to the peritoneal reflections. The peritoneal reflections mark the end of the peritoneum and are represented by recesses or pouches: the **rectogenital pouch** (between the rectum and the **genital fold** [in the male] or the **broad lig.** [in the female]); the **vesicogenital pouch** (between the urinary bladder and the corresponding genital organs); the **pubovesical pouch** (between the pubis and the urinary bladder). On each side of the **mesorectum** (the peritoneal fold suspending the rectum), two **pararectal fossae** can be identified. Although a **sacrorectal pouch** is not listed in the *N.A.V.,* it is present and is illustrated with the other pouches in the large ruminants (see Fig. R4.21). Those pouches and fossae can be palpated by introducing the hand between the sacrum and the rectum, between the rectum and the genital organs, between the genital organs and the urinary bladder, and between the uninary bladder and the pubis.

The pelvic diaphragm consists of the coccygeus and levator ani Mm. and internal and external fasciae.

Identify and dissect the **retractor penis/retractor clitoridis M.,** partially overlapped by the levator ani M. Some longitudinal muscle fibers from the rectum leave it toward the first few caudal vertebrae as the **rectococcygeus M.**

Continue the dissection of the vessels and the nerves, different in the male and female specimens.

*In the male* identify the following structures: the **prostatic A.** with the **branch to the ductus deferens** (giving off the **caudal vesical A.**), with the **ureteric** and **urethral branches** and the **middle rectal A.;** the **ventral perineal A.** with the **caudal rectal A.;** and the **A. of the penis** with the **A. of the bulbus penis,** the **deep A. of the penis,** and

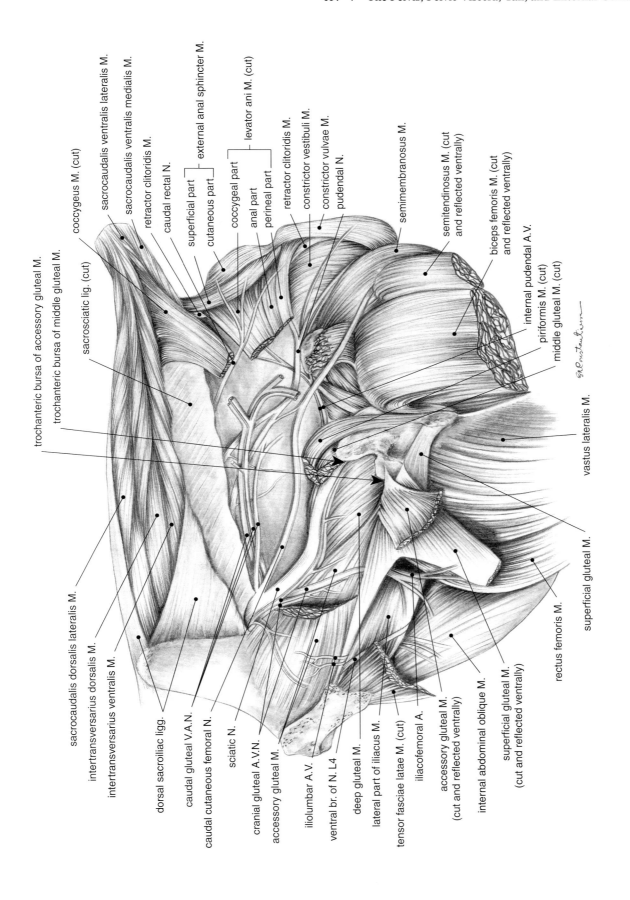

trochanteric bursa of accessory gluteal M.

trochanteric bursa of middle gluteal M.

coccygeus M. (cut)

sacrocaudalis ventralis lateralis M.

sacrocaudalis ventralis medialis M.

retractor clitoridis M.

caudal rectal N.

superficial part

cutaneous part

external anal sphincter M.

coccygeal part

anal part

perineal part

levator ani M. (cut)

retractor clitoridis M.

constrictor vestibuli M.

constrictor vulvae M.

pudendal N.

semimembranosus M.

semitendinosus M. (cut and reflected ventrally)

biceps femoris M. (cut and reflected ventrally)

internal pudendal A.V.

piriformis M. (cut)

middle gluteal M. (cut)

sacrosciatic lig. (cut)

vastus lateralis M.

sacrocaudalis dorsalis lateralis M.

intertransversarius dorsalis M.

intertransversarius ventralis M.

dorsal sacroiliac ligg.

caudal gluteal V.A.N.

caudal cutaneous femoral N.

sciatic N.

cranial gluteal A.V.N.

accessory gluteal M.

iliolumbar A.V.

ventral br. of N. L4

deep gluteal M.

lateral part of iliacus M.

tensor fasciae latae M. (cut)

iliacofemoral A.

accessory gluteal M. (cut and reflected ventrally)

superficial gluteal M.

internal abdominal oblique M.

superficial gluteal M. (cut and reflected ventrally)

rectus femoris M.

Fig. H4.20. Deepest structures of left lateral pelvis, tail, anus, and vulva of the mare.

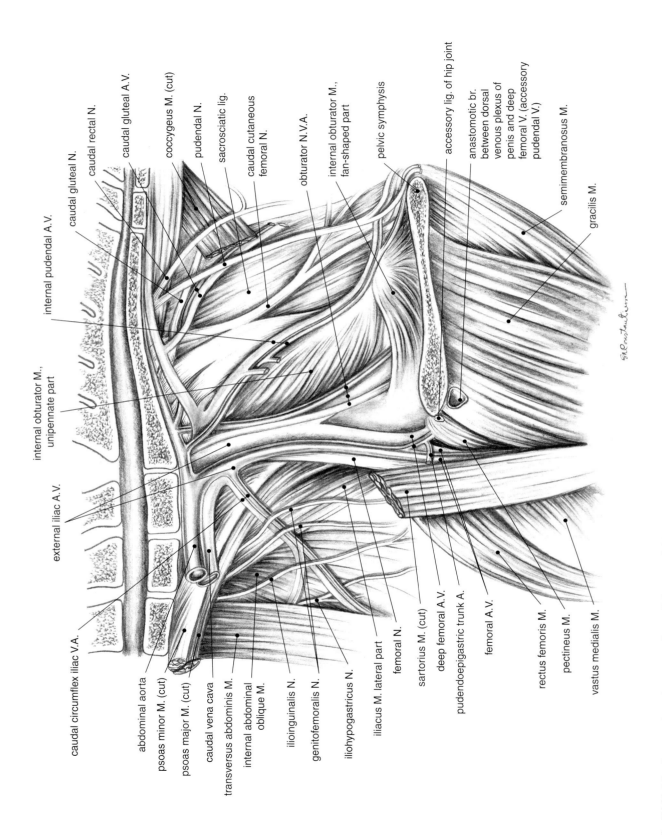

caudal gluteal A.V.

caudal rectal N.

caudal gluteal N.

coccygeus M. (cut)

pudendal N.

internal pudendal A.V.

sacrosciatic lig.

caudal cutaneous femoral N.

obturator N.V.A.

internal obturator M., fan-shaped part

pelvic symphysis

accessory lig. of hip joint

anastomotic br. between dorsal venous plexus of penis and deep femoral V. (accessory pudendal V.)

semimembranosus M.

gracilis M.

internal obturator M., unipennate part

external iliac A.V.

caudal circumflex iliac V.A.

abdominal aorta

psoas minor M. (cut)

psoas major M. (cut)

caudal vena cava

transversus abdominis M.

internal abdominal oblique M.

ilioinguinalis N.

genitofemoralis N.

iliohypogastricus N.

iliacus M. lateral part

femoral N.

sartorius M. (cut)

deep femoral A.V.

pudendoepigastric trunk A.

femoral A.V.

rectus femoris M.

pectineus M.

vastus medialis M.

Fig. H4.21. Muscles, vessels, and nerves on the medial aspect of right pelvis, horse, after removal of the sacrosciatic ligament.

the **dorsal A. of the penis**. *Notice* that the **middle A. of the penis** is a branch of the **obturator A.** in the horse.

*In the female* identify the following arteries: the **vaginal A.** with the **uterine branch** (giving off the **caudal vesical A.**) with the **ureteric** and **urethral** branches and the **middle rectal A.**; the **vestibular branch**; the **ventral perineal A.** with the **caudal rectal A.** and the **dorsal labial branch**; and the **A. of the bulbus vestibuli**. *Notice* that the **middle A. of the clitoris** (with the **deep A. of the clitoris** and the **dorsal A. of the clitoris**) are branches of the **obturator A.** in the mare.

See the systematization of the branches of the internal iliac A. in Table H4.2, on page 105.

In both male and female, dissect the pudendal, caudal rectal, caudal, and pelvic Nn. *Notice* that the pudendal N. branches into the following nerves: the **deep perineal N.**; the **superficial perineal N.** giving off the **dorsal scrotal Nn.** in the male, and the **labial Nn.** in the female; the

**preputial branch** versus the **mammary branch**; the **dorsal N. of the penis** versus the **dorsal N. of the clitoris**.

Palpate the transverse processes of the **caudal vertebrae** as landmarks for dissecting the **sacrocaudales** and **intertransversarii Mm.** (see Fig. H4.20).

Figure H4.21 shows the medial aspect of the muscles, vessels, and nerves after removal of the sacrosciatic lig.

Dissect the **perineal region** in the male (Fig. H4.22) and in the female (Fig.H 4.23). In addition to the muscles dissected from the lateral perspective, *notice*, in the male, the **ischiocavernosus M.**, the **superficial transverse perineal M.**, the **urethralis M.**, and the **external anal sphincter**, with its **cutaneous**, **superficial,** and **deep parts**. In the female pay attention to the **constrictor vaginae M.**, the **constrictor vulvae M.**, the levator ani M. and the external anal sphincter M., as well as to the **perineal septum**. In the horse only, the perineal septum is a fascia between the vestibule, the constrictor vulvae M., the retractor clitoridis M., and the rectum.

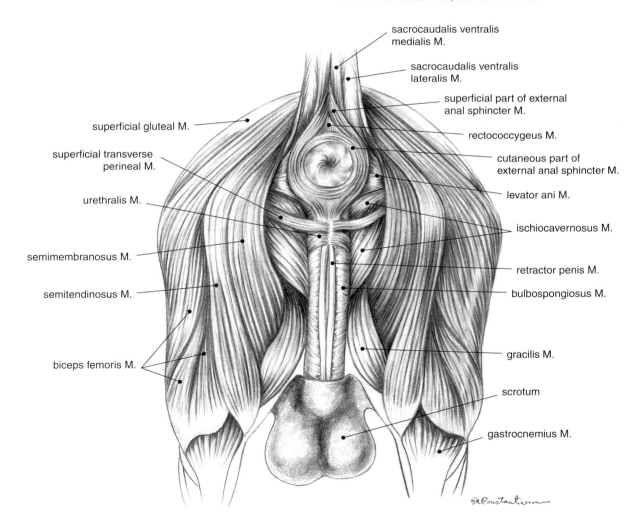

Fig. H4.22. Perineal region in the stallion.

Be prepared to remove the male genital tract from the pelvic cavity. Cut the mesorectum and free the rectum from the roof of the pelvic cavity. Transect all the attachments of the pelvic diaphragm and free the internal male genitalia with their blood and nerve supply already dissected. Transect the three ligaments of the urinary bladder, and the genital fold. Free the ureters and the urethra. Transect the paired ischiocavernosus Mm. with the **crura of the penis** (sing. crus) and free the penis up to the cross section that you have already performed.

*Notice* that the genital fold is a continuous peritoneal structure that surrounds the paired **vesicular glands (seminal vesicles)** laterally, the **ampullae of the ductus deferens** medially, and ventral to them, the ureters. In the middle of the genital fold a rudimentary **masculine uterus** can be seen as a constant structure in the horse (Fig. H4.24).

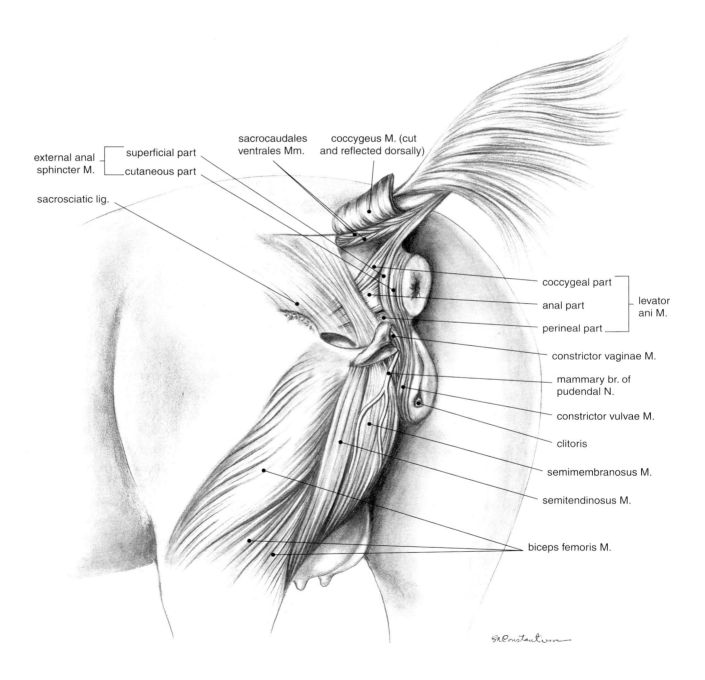

Fig. H4.23. Perineal region in the mare.

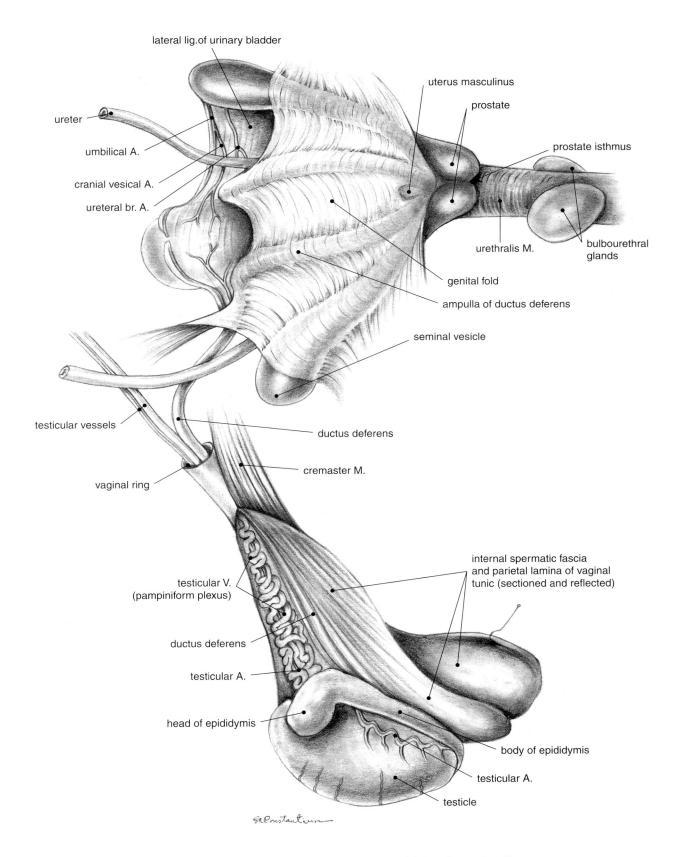

Fig. H4.24. Accessory genital glands (dorsal aspect) and testicle and spermatic cord (left lateral aspect), stallion.

On the dorsal aspect of the **pelvic urethra**, just caudal to the **neck of the urinary bladder,** identify the two right and left lobes of the **prostate gland** united by the **prostate isthmus**. The prostate isthmus overlaps the terminal parts of the seminal vesicles and the ampullae of the ductus deferens. Caudal to the prostate gland, the urethra is surrounded by the **urethralis M.** up to the transition between the pelvic and the **penile urethra**. Close to this transition find the **bulbourethral glands** surrounded by the **bulbourethralis M.;** this muscle is the continuation of the urethralis M.

Make a longitudinal incision on the ventral aspect of the urinary bladder and the urethra. Open up the bladder and examine on the roof the **ureteric columns, orifices,** and **folds**. *Notice* that between the ureteric orifices and folds and the **internal urethral ostium** there is a triangular area called the **vesical trigone**. Caudal to it, identify the **urethral-crest**, a dorsal longitudinal mucosal ridge from the junction of the ureteric folds to the **colliculus seminalis** (a prominence onto which the prostate and the two **ejaculatory ducts** open; Fig. H4.25). *Notice* that the ejaculatory duct is a common secretory passage for the ductus deferens and the seminal vesicle. At the level of the bulbourethral glands, examine the openings of their ducts.

Continue the incision of the urethra through the **urethral isthmus** into the penile urethra and *notice* that the

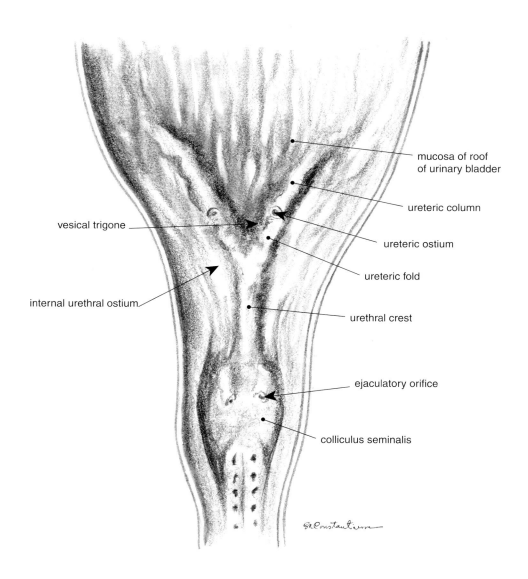

mucosa of roof
of urinary bladder

ureteric column

vesical trigone

ureteric ostium

ureteric fold

internal urethral ostium

urethral crest

ejaculatory orifice

colliculus seminalis

Fig. H4.25. Internal aspect of roof of urinary bladder and male urethra, horse.

lumen of the penile urethra is smaller than that of the pelvic urethra. From its origin, the penile urethra is surrounded by the corpus spongiosum penis, which starts with an expansion called **bulbus penis**.

*Notice* that the two crura of the penis (the attachments of the corpora cavernosa penis [sing. corpus cavernosum penis] on the **ischial arch**) and the bulbus penis make together the **root of the penis**.

Remove the whole genital tract from the pelvic cavity through the pelvic inlet and transfer it to a tray.

In a similar manner, remove the female genital tract, up to and including the vulva. Transect the pudendal A. close to its origin. Free the rectum from the subsacral area. Free the urinary bladder and the genital tract from their peritoneal folds (the broad ligg.) and from the pelvic diaphragm. Transect the **crura of the clitoris** from the **ischial arch**. Free the **vagina**, the **vestibulum,** and the **vulva**, and remove all these structures through the pelvic inlet.

Review the arteries, the veins, and the nerves that supply the genital apparatus.

The systematization of the major branches of the internal iliac A. in the male and in the female horse, according to the *N.A.V.,* is shown in Table H4.2.

Examine the relationship between the terminal portion of the urethra and the **external urethral orifice**, which separates the **vagina** (cranially), from the **vestibule** (caudally). Identify the **constrictor vestibuli M.**, transect it, and expose the **bulbus vestibuli**, an erectile tissue in the lateral wall of the vestibule.

Place the female genitalia in a natural position and make a longitudinal incision through the dorsal commissure of the vulva and the dorsal walls of the vestibule, vagina, cervix, body of the uterus, and one of the uterine horns (Fig. H4.26A).

Examine the vulva with the two **labia** (sing. labium), the two **commissures (dorsal and ventral)** (Fig. H4.26B), and the **clitoris** within the **fossa of the clitoris**, on the floor of the **vestibule** (Fig. H4.26C). Carefully examine the clitoris and adjacent structures, such as the **glans**, the **fossa**, and the **prepuce of the clitoris** (a transverse frenular fold). *Notice* that the fossa of the clitoris is discontinued at the attachment of the glans to the prepuce, called the **frenulum of clitoris. A lateral** and a **ventral recess** can be identified within the fossa of the clitoris (Fig. H4.27A). Pull up the prepuce, and three additional sinuses will be shown: the **median sinus** and two **lateral sinuses** (Fig. H4.27B).

Table H4.2. Major Branches of Internal Iliac A., Male and Female Horse

| Male | Female |
|---|---|
| Caudal gluteal A. | |
| Cranial gluteal A. | |
| Iliolumbar A. | |
| Obturator A. | |
| Iliacofemoral A. | |
| Middle A. of penis | Middle A. of clitoris |
| | Deep A. of clitoris |
| | Dorsal A. of clitoris |
| Median caudal A. | |
| Ventrolateral caudal A. | |
| Dorsolateral caudal A. | |
| Internal pudendal A. | |
| Umbilical A. | |
| A. of ductus deferens | |
| Cranial vesical Aa. | |
| Prostatic A. | Vaginal A. |
| Br. of ductus deferens | Uterine br. |
| Caudal vesical A. | |
| Ureteric br. | |
| Urethral br. | |
| Middle rectal A. | |
| A. of penis | Vestibular br. |
| A. of bulbus penis | Ventral perineal A. |
| Deep A. of penis | Caudal rectal A. |
| Dorsal A. of penis | Dorsal labial br. |
| Ventral perineal A. | A. of bulbus vestibuli |
| Caudal rectal A. | |

**The recesses and especially the sinuses around the glans of the clitoris have a major clinical importance because they may harbor *Taylorella equigenitalis* organisms. Even though the microorganism is also located in the endometrium (the mucosa of the uterus), including the cervix, the three sinuses are often removed to eliminate the infection.** *The removal of the sinuses is called sinusectomy.*

Cranial to the external urethral orifice, examine the transverse fold, which is comparable to the **hymen**. The vagina ends around the **vaginal part of the cervix** as the **vaginal fornix** (see Fig. H4.26A). The aspects of the vaginal part of cervix and of the vaginal fornix are different during the animal's reproductive cycle (**diestrus, estrus,** and **pregnancy**); they are shown in a caudal view and a median section in Figure H4.28. The vaginal part of cervix is anchored to the roof and the floor of the vagina by a **dorsal frenulum** and a **ventral frenulum,** respectively, not listed in the *N.A.V.*

Estrus, or the estrous cycle, is the recurrent, restricted period of sexual receptivity in female species. Diestrus is a short period of sexual quiescence between metestrus (the end of an estrous cycle) and proestrus (the beginning of the following and new estrous cycle).

*Notice* that the horse is the only species in which the uterine body is not (partially) divided. Therefore, its most cranial extent is called the **uterine fundus** (see Fig. H4.26).

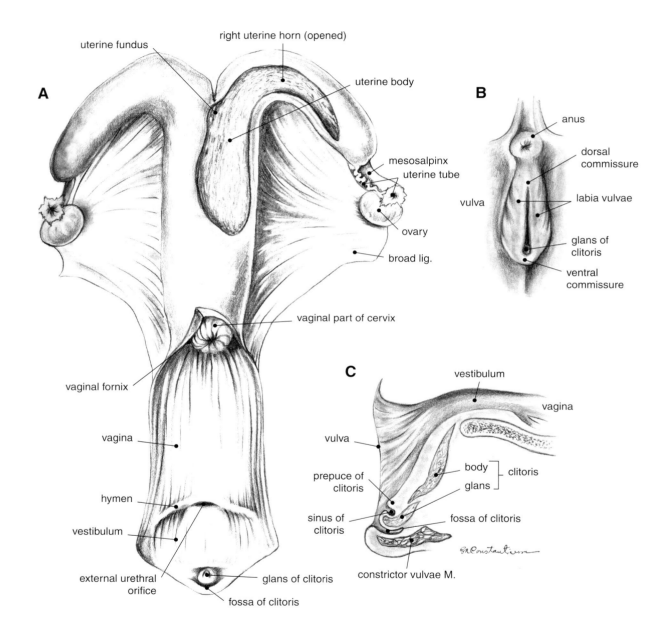

Fig. H4.26. Genital tract, mare. **A.** Dorsal aspect. **B.** Vulva. **C.** Mediosagittal section through the vulva and clitoris.

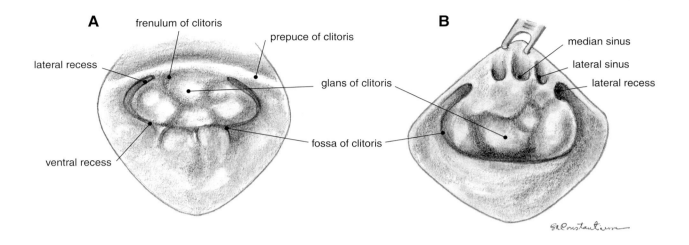

Fig. H4.27. Clitoris of the mare. **A.** Clitoris in situ. **B.** Prepuce reflected.

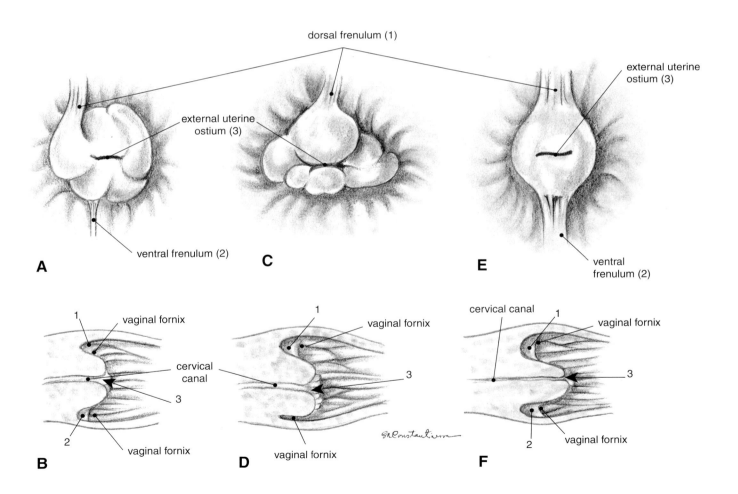

Fig. H4.28. Vaginal part of cervix in the mare, during the diestrus, estrus, and pregnancy. *Diestrus:* **A.** Cervix, caudal view. **B.** Vaginal portion cervix, median section. *Estrus:* **C.** Cervix, caudal view. **D.** Vaginal portion cervix, median section. *Pregnancy:* **E.** Cervix, caudal view. **F.** Vaginal portion cervix, median section.

# MODLAB H4

Attempt to palpate on a live horse the structures with clinical importance listed at the beginning of this chapter.

Anatomical structures of the pelvis, pelvic viscera, tail, and external genitalia that are prone to clinical interventions, with their *landmarks* and *approaches*, as well as the *rectal examination of abdominopelvic viscera (transrectal palpation, or exploration per rectum)* follow.

1. **Superficial perineal N.** (Fig. H4.29A,B)
   A. *Landmarks*: ischiatic tuberosity, ischial arch, root of the penis or vulva
   B. *Approach*: between the ischiatic tuberosity and root of the penis or vulva, on the ischial arch
2. **Median caudal A.V.** (Fig. H4.29C)
   A. *Landmarks*: the midventral line of the base of the tail
   B. *Approach*: on the midventral line of the base of the tail, between the symmetrical sacrocaudalis ventralis medialis Mm., and covered partially by the rectococcygeus M.
3. **Dorsolateral caudal A.V. and dorsal branches of the caudal Nn.** (Fig. H4.29D)
   A. *Landmarks*: transverse processes of the caudal vertebrae
   B. *Approach*: dorsal to the transverse processes and deep, through the skin and caudal fascia, and between the sacrocaudalis dorsalis lateralis and intertransversarii dorsales caudae Mm.
4. **Ventrolateral caudal A.V. and ventral branches of the caudal Nn.** (Fig. H4.29D)
   A. *Landmarks*: transverse processes of the caudal vertebrae
   B. *Approach*: ventral to the transverse processes and deep, through the skin and caudal fascia, and between the sacrocaudalis ventralis lateralis and intertransversarii ventrales caudae Mm.
   *Caution.* Dorsal to the anus and corresponding to the level of the third and fourth caudal vertebrae, the coccygeus M. lies superficially in a subcutaneous and subfascial position, between the two above-mentioned muscles, and overlapping the vessels and the nerves.
5. **Lumbosacral site for collection of cerebrospinal fluid** (see Fig. H4.6)
   A. *Landmarks*: the spinous process of the last lumbar vertebra, the spinous process of the first sacral vertebra, the symmetrical sacral tuberosity and tuber coxae (pl. sacral tuberosities and tubera coxarum)

   B. *Approach*: deep in the middle of the intersection of two perpendicular lines: the line between the symmetrical tuber coxae passing through the symmetrical tuber sacrale and the line that unites the tip of the spinous process of the last lumbar vertebra with the tip of the first spinous process of the sacrum
6. **Epidural anesthesia** (Fig. H4.30A)
   A. *Landmarks*: the spinous process of the last sacral vertebra and the spinous processes of the first and second caudal vertebrae
   B. *Approach*: on the middorsal line either between the sacrum and the first caudal vertebra or between the first and second caudal vertebrae, through the skin and caudal fascia to the vertebral canal
   *Caution.* To easily palpate the intervertebral spaces, raise the tail and move it to the right and to the left, as well as dorsally and ventrally.
7. **Subsacral anesthesia (for the pudendal N. and the caudal rectal N.)** (Fig. H4.30B)
   A. *Landmarks*: the base of tail, anus, ventral aspect of sacrum, promontory, ventral sacral foramina
   B. *Approach*: keep the tail raised, introduce a hand with the palmar aspect oriented dorsally into rectum, and palpate the ventral aspect of the sacrum with the promontory and the paired ventral sacral foramina. Count the foramina and stop your finger on the third (for the pudendal N.), and then on the fourth (for the caudal rectal N.), as the two places for anesthesia. With the other hand, introduce an 18 or 20 gauge, 8 inch, needle with a short beveled point through the skin and the pelvic diaphragm, in the center of the space outlined by the two cutaneous folds between the base of the tail and the anus. Guide the tip of the needle with the hand still in the rectum.
8. **Spermatic cord** (Fig. H4.30C)
   A. *Landmarks*: superficial inguinal ring, testicle, prepuce
   B. *Approach*: between the superficial inguinal ring and the corresponding testicle, lateral to the prepuce
9. **Inguinal approach for stallion castration** (Fig. H4.30C)
   A. *Landmarks*: superficial inguinal ring, testicle, scrotum
   B. *Approach*: through the scrotum and external spermatic fascia, at the level of the superficial inguinal ring

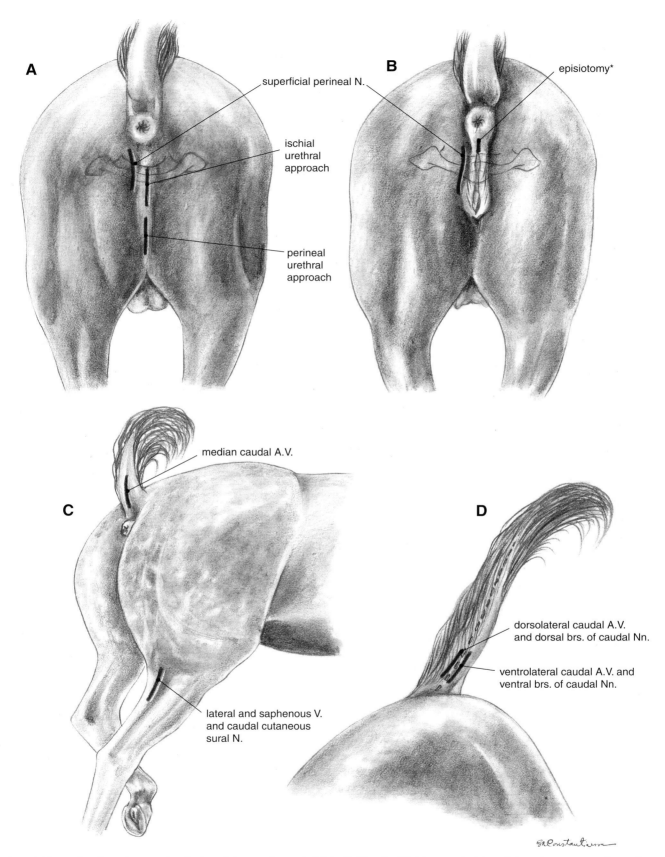

Fig. H4.29. Landmarks and approaches in the pelvic area, horse. **A.** Male. **B.** Female. *Episiotomy: incision of the vulva to prevent laceration during delivery or to facilitate vaginal surgery. **C.** Structures in the popliteal region and tail. **D.** Structures on the tail.

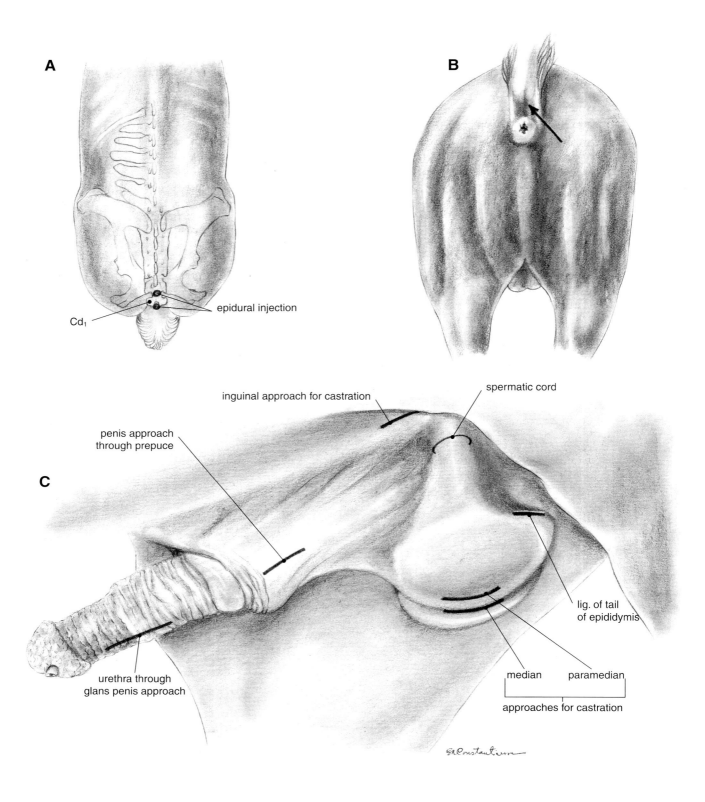

**A**

Cd₁

epidural injection

**B**

**C**

inguinal approach for castration

spermatic cord

penis approach
through prepuce

lig. of tail
of epididymis

urethra through
glans penis approach

median    paramedian

approaches for castration

Fig. H4.30. Landmarks and approaches in the perineal area and external genital organs, stallion. **A.** Epidural anesthesia. **B.** Subsacral anesthesia. **C.** Approaches to male external genitalia.

10. **Paramedian approach for stallion castration** (Fig. H4.30C)
    A. *Landmarks*: spermatic cord, testicle, scrotal raphe
    B. *Approach*: parallel and 2–3 cm lateral to scrotal raphe, through scrotum, dartos, and external spermatic fascia
11. **Median approach for stallion castration** (Fig. H4.30C)
    A. *Landmarks*: scrotal raphe
    B. *Approach*: the middle third of the scrotal raphe
12. **Spongy part of urethra**
    *Ischial approach* (Fig. H4.29A)
    A. *Landmarks*: ischial arch, anus
    B. *Approach*: ventral to the anus, at the level of the ischial arch, through the skin, the superficial perineal fascia, the retractor penis and bulbospongiosus Mm., and the corpus spongiosum penis

    *Perineal approach* (Fig. H4.29A)
    A. *Landmarks*: ischial arch, perineum
    B. *Approach*: same as above, ventral to the ischial arch

    *Glans penis approach* (Fig. H4.30C)
    A. *Landmarks*: prepuce, glans penis

    B. *Approach*: remove the glans penis from the prepuce, turn the glans penis with the ventral aspect up, and pass through the internal preputial lamina, the retractor penis and bulbospongiosus Mm., and the corpus spongiosum penis
13. **Penis** (Fig. H4.30C)
    A. *Landmarks*: prepuce
    B. *Approach*: the penis within the prepuce is located inside the preputial cavity, intimately surrounded by the preputial fold
14. **Perineal body of the mare by episiotomy** (see Fig. H4.29B)
    A. *Landmarks*: anus, vulva
    B. *Approach*: between the anus and the dorsal commissure of the vulva and through skin, the superficial perineal fascia, the communication between the external anal sphincter and the constrictor vulvae, and the perineal septum
15. **Rectal examination of abdominopelvic viscera and other structures**
    **Before starting a rectal exploration you should know that the horse rectum is very fragile and susceptible to injuries, even breakages followed by hemorrhage. If your hand cannot advance, wait until the wave of peristalsis passes over your hand and then continue the examination.**
    A. *Landmarks* (in a caudocranial order) (Fig. H4.31)

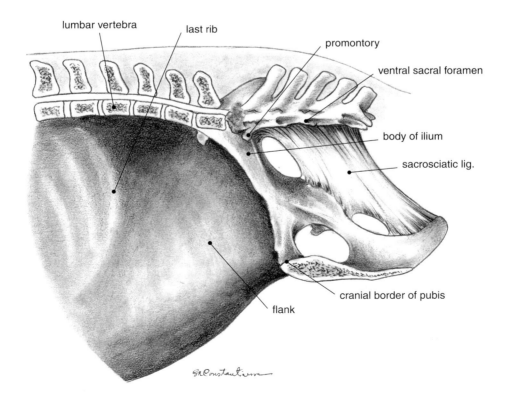

Fig. H4.31. Landmarks for rectal exploration, horse, right side.

*The hand with the palmar aspect oriented dorsally*
a. On midline
   1. The pelvic surface of sacrum with the ventral sacral foramina
   2. The promontory (of sacrum)
   3. The bodies of lumbar vertebrae covered by the aorta (on the left) and the caudal vena cava (on the right)
b. On both lateral sides
   1. The sacrosciatic lig.
   2. The body of the ilium with the internal obturator M.
   3. The flank
   4. The last rib

*The hand with the palmar aspect oriented ventrally*
a. On midline
   1. The internal obturator M.
   2. The cranial border of the pubis
B. *Palpable structures within the pelvic cavity* (on the floor, in a caudocranial order)

*In the male* (Fig. H4.32A)
a. The urethral isthmus
b. The accessory genital glands
   1. The bulbourethral glands (difficult to identify in the horse)
   2. The prostate gland (difficult to identify in the horse)
   3. The seminal vesicles
c. The pelvic part of the urethra
d. The genital fold with the corresponding ductus deferens
e. The urinary bladder (the apex is sometimes dropped into the abdominal cavity depending on the plenitude of the bladder)

*In the female* (Fig. 4.32B)
a. The vestibule and the vagina
b. The cervix
c. The body and horns of the uterus (in older, multiparous mares and pregnant mares, they are usually within the abdominal cavity; in young, nongravid females, these structures may still be within the pelvic cavity)
d. The urinary bladder (see above; in addition, during pregnancy the urinary bladder is compressed by the pregnant uterus and pushed into the abdominal cavity).

C. *Palpable structures within the abdominal cavity*
*In the male*
a. Both ductus deferens continue to course from the pelvic cavity to the pelvic inlet, where they enter the vaginal rings in a craniolateroventral position

*In the female*
a. The uterine horns are convex ventrally and extend in a lateral and dorsal direction toward the roof of the abdominal cavity
b. The uterine tubes can be identified only if enlarged
c. The two ovaries are located dorsal, lateral, and slightly cranial to the respective tips of the uterine horn. They lie in a caudoventral position to the corresponding kidneys.

*In both male and female* (caudocranially) (Figs. H4.32C,D, H4.33, H4.34)
a. On the left side
   1. The descending colon (dorsal in the paralumbar fossa and with sacculations and bands)
   2. The jejunum (medial or lateral, and cranial to the descending colon, smooth and without sacculations and bands)
   3. The left kidney and left renal A. (Only operators with a long reach can palpate the entire left kidney; the caudal pole is frequently palpable.)
   4. The spleen (The caudal border of the spleen can usually be palpated against the left abdominal wall, lateral to the left colons along the last rib.)
   5. The pelvic flexure of the ascending colon (in the pelvic inlet ventrally, but movable; may be located in general area of pelvic inlet)
   6. The left dorsal and ventral colons (continue cranially from the pelvic flexure), just medial to the spleen and the left body wall
   7. The ascending mesocolon (intercolic fold), between the left dorsal and left ventral colons
   8. The left ureter on the left side of abdominal aorta (difficult, but not impossible to palpate, unless abnormal)

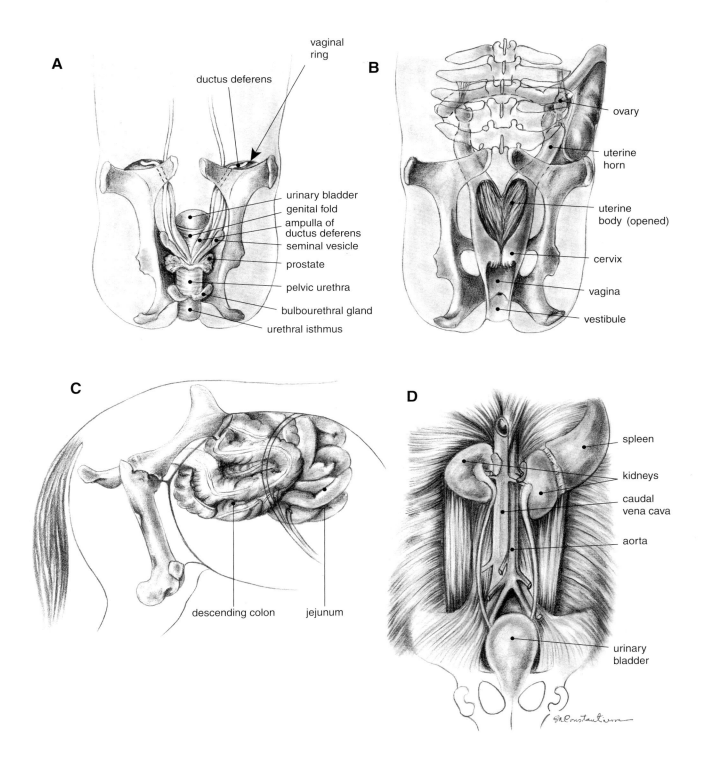

Fig. H4.32. Palpable structures during rectal exploration, horse. **A.** Viscera of pelvic cavity in the male. **B.** In female. **C.** Jejunum and descending colon (right view). **D.** Dorsal wall of abdominal cavity (ventrodorsal view).

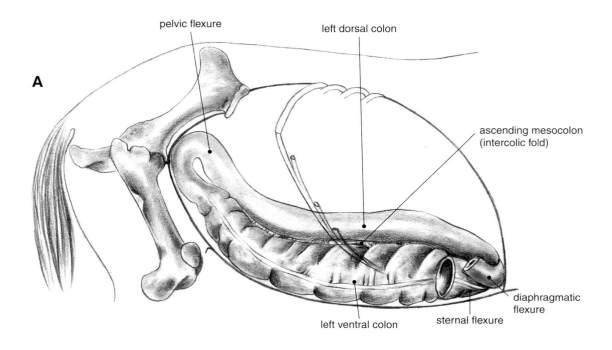

A

pelvic flexure

left dorsal colon

ascending mesocolon
(intercolic fold)

diaphragmatic
flexure

left ventral colon

sternal flexure

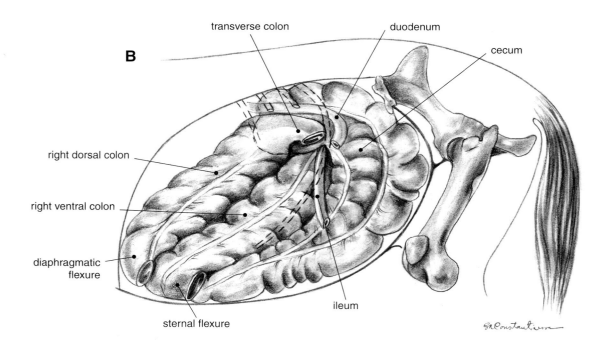

B

transverse colon

duodenum

cecum

right dorsal colon

right ventral colon

diaphragmatic
flexure

ileum

sternal flexure

Fig. H4.33. Large intestine in situ, horse. **A.** Left colon (right view). **B.** Cecum and right colon (left view).

b. On the right side
1. The base of cecum and the proximal part of its body, with the corresponding sacculations and bands
2. The transverse colon (on the medial aspect of the base of cecum), often too far cranial to palpate
3. The right dorsal colon, often too far cranial to palpate
4. The right ureter on the right side of caudal vena cava (difficult, but not impossible to palpate, unless abnormal)
5. The caudal flexure of the duodenum as it passes around the root of the mesentery, smooth and without sacculations and bands

D. *Palpation of the arteries and lymph nodes in the pelvic and abdominal cavities* (in a caudocranial order)
a. Caudal gluteal A. with the sacral branches
b. Obturator A. (on the body of the ilium)
c. Lateral vesical ligg. with the umbilical Aa.
d. Internal iliac A. with the sacral lnn. (on the lateral side of $L_6$ and $S_1$)
e. External iliac A. with the medial iliac lnn.(cranial to the internal iliac A.)
f. The quadrifurcation of the aorta (ventral to $L_5$)
g. Caudal mesenteric A. (can frequently be palpated)
h. Cranial mesenteric A. with the mesenteric lnn. (can occasionally be palpated in association with the root of the cranial mesentery as it branches from the aorta; located too far cranially to be palpated)

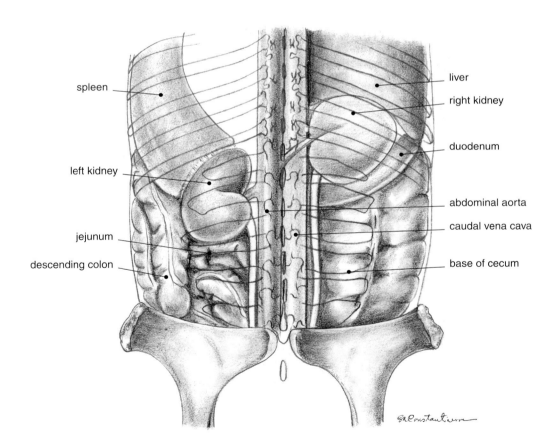

Fig. H4.34. Dorsal view of structures within abdomen, horse.

# H 5

## The Pelvic Limb

The bones of the pelvic limb as a whole, then the **femur and patella**, **tibia** and **fibula**, and **tarsal** and **metatarsal bones** are illustrated in Figures H5.1–H5.5. The phalanges will be illustrated in Chapter 6, the Thoracic Limb, because they look very similar.

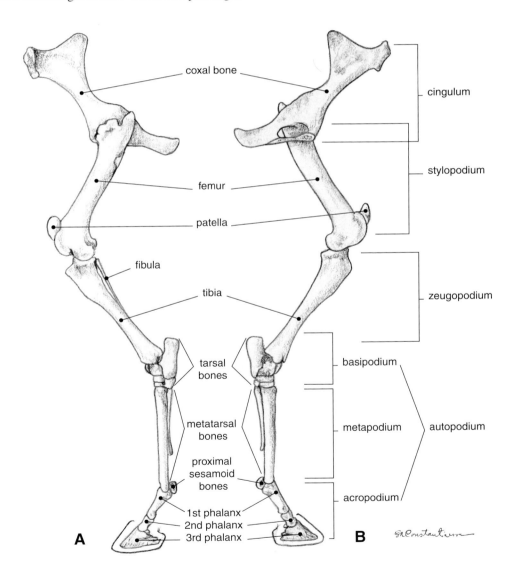

coxal bone

femur

patella

fibula

tibia

tarsal bones

metatarsal bones

proximal sesamoid bones

1st phalanx
2nd phalanx
3rd phalanx

**A**

cingulum

stylopodium

zeugopodium

basipodium

metapodium

acropodium

autopodium

**B**

Fig. H5.1. Skeleton of pelvic limb, horse. **A.** Lateral aspect. **B.** Medial aspect.

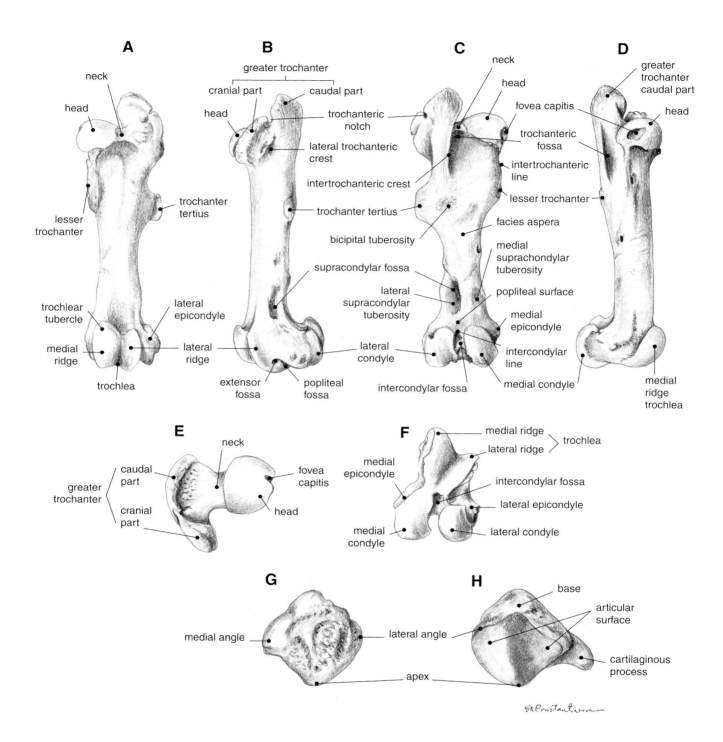

**A**

neck

head

lesser
trochanter

trochanter
tertius

trochlear
tubercle

medial
ridge

lateral
epicondyle

lateral
ridge

trochlea

**B**

greater trochanter

cranial part          caudal part

head

trochanteric
notch

lateral trochanteric
crest

intertrochanteric crest

trochanter tertius

supracondylar fossa

extensor
fossa

popliteal
fossa

**C**

neck

head

fovea capitis

trochanteric
fossa

intertrochanteric
line

lesser trochanter

facies aspera

medial
suprachondylar
tuberosity

popliteal surface

medial
epicondyle

intercondylar
line

medial condyle

bicipital tuberosity

lateral
supracondylar
tuberosity

lateral
condyle

intercondylar fossa

**D**

greater
trochanter
caudal part

head

medial
ridge
trochlea

**E**

neck

greater
trochanter

caudal
part

cranial
part

fovea
capitis

head

**F**

medial
epicondyle

medial
condyle

medial ridge

lateral ridge

trochlea

intercondylar fossa

lateral epicondyle

lateral condyle

**G**

medial angle

lateral angle

apex

**H**

base

articular
surface

cartilaginous
process

apex

Fig. H5.2. Femur and patella, horse, left limb. **A.** Cranial aspect. **B.** Lateral aspect. **C.** Caudal aspect. **D.** Medial aspect. **E.** Proximal extremity of femur, dorsal view. **F.** Distal extremity of femur, ventral view. **G.** Patella, cranial aspect. **H.** Patella, caudal aspect.

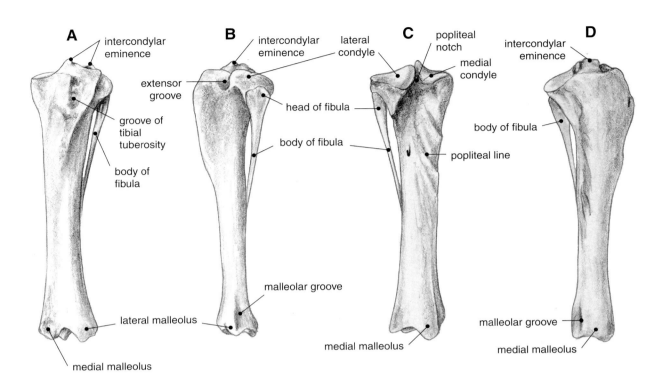

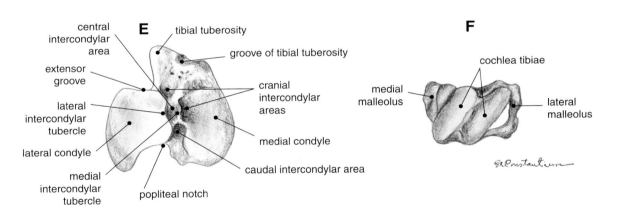

Fig. H5.3. Tibia and fibula, horse, left limb. **A.** Cranial aspect. **B.** Lateral aspect. **C.** Caudal aspect. **D.** Medial aspect. **E.** Proximal articular surface. **F.** Distal articular surface.

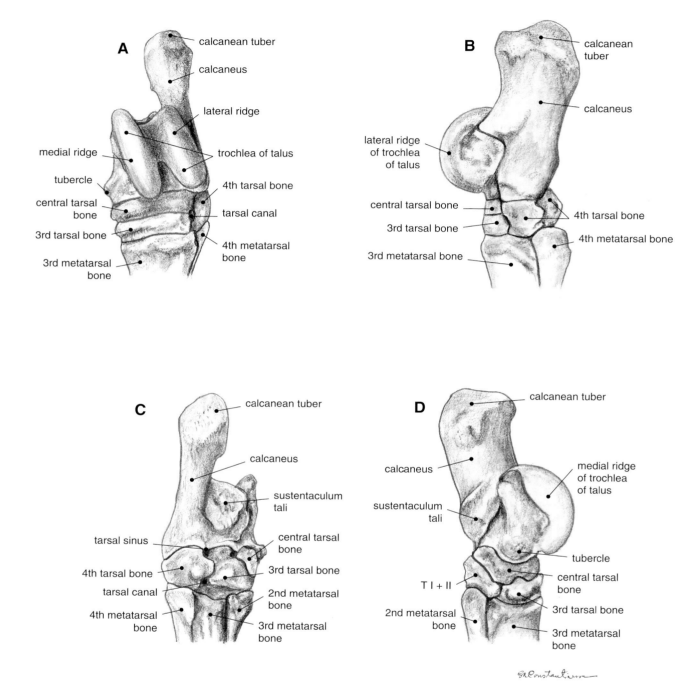

Fig. H5.4. Tarsal bones, horse, left limb. **A.** Dorsal aspect. **B.** Lateral aspect. **C.** Plantar aspect. **D.** Medial aspect.

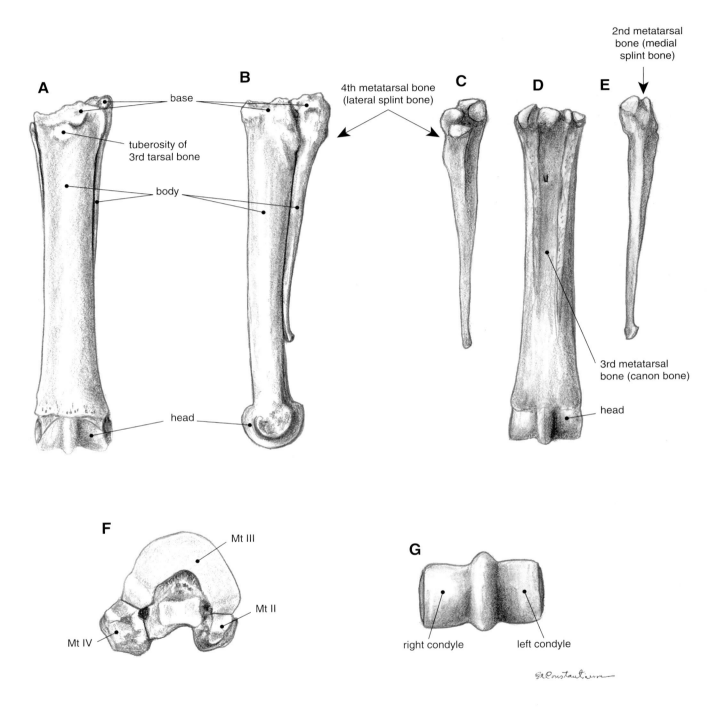

**A**

base

tuberosity of
3rd tarsal bone

body

head

**B**

base

body

head

4th metatarsal bone
(lateral splint bone)

**C**

**D**

**E**

2nd metatarsal
bone (medial
splint bone)

3rd metatarsal
bone (canon bone)

head

**F**

Mt III

Mt IV

Mt II

**G**

right condyle

left condyle

Fig. H5.5. Metatarsal bones, horse, left limb. **A.** Dorsal aspect. **B.** Lateral aspect. **C., D.,** and **E.** Plantar aspect. **F.** Tarsal articular surface.
**G.** Head.

The **hip joint**, the **stifle joint**, and the **tarsal joint** are illustrated in Figures H5.6–H5.10.

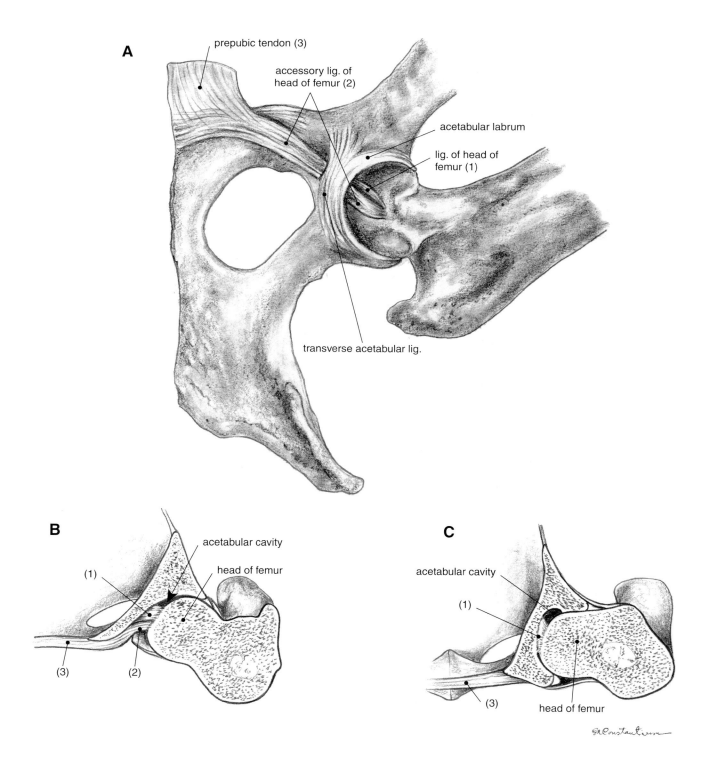

Fig. H5.6. The hip joint in large animals. **A.** Right hip joint, horse, ventral aspect. **B.** Right hip joint, horse, transverse section. **C.** Right hip join, large ruminants, transverse section.

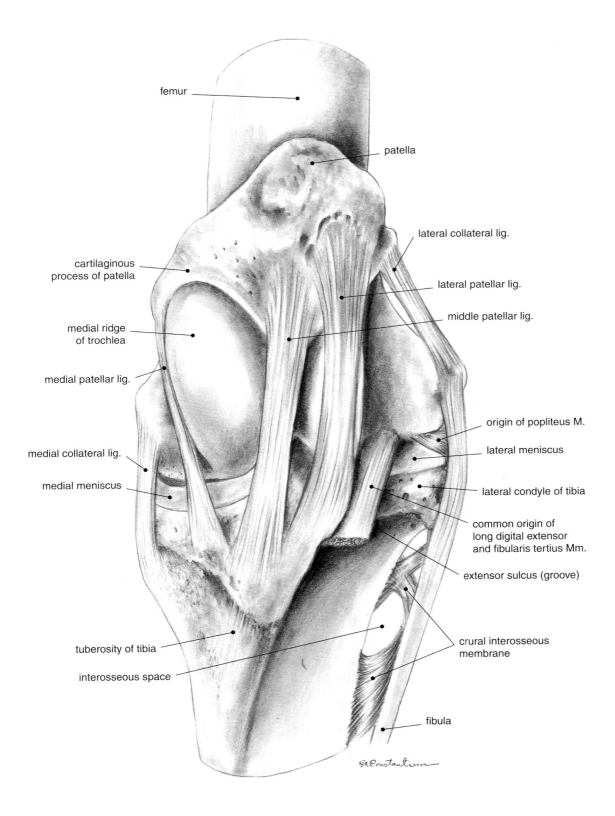

Fig. H5.7. Stifle joint of left pelvic limb, horse, cranial aspect.

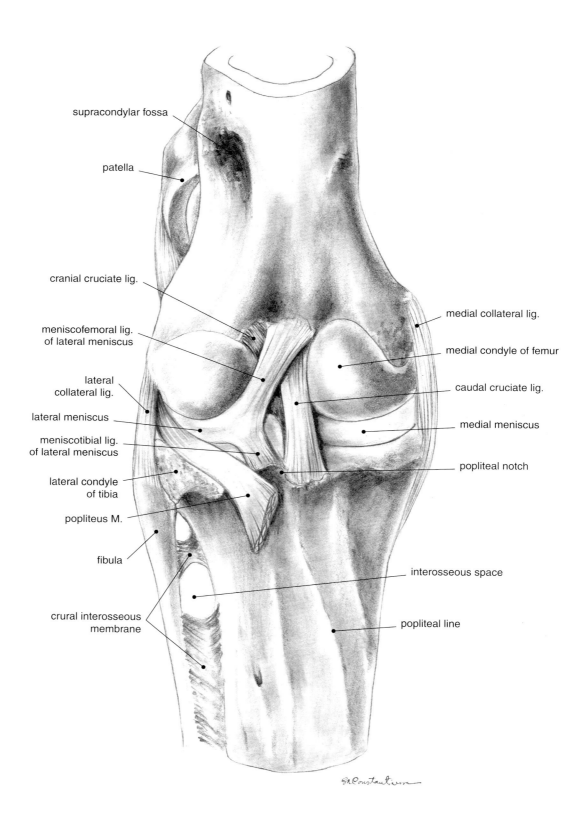

supracondylar fossa

patella

cranial cruciate lig.

meniscofemoral lig.
of lateral meniscus

lateral
collateral lig.

lateral meniscus

meniscotibial lig.
of lateral meniscus

lateral condyle
of tibia

popliteus M.

fibula

crural interosseous
membrane

medial collateral lig.

medial condyle of femur

caudal cruciate lig.

medial meniscus

popliteal notch

interosseous space

popliteal line

Fig. H5.8. Stifle joint of left pelvic limb, horse, caudal aspect.

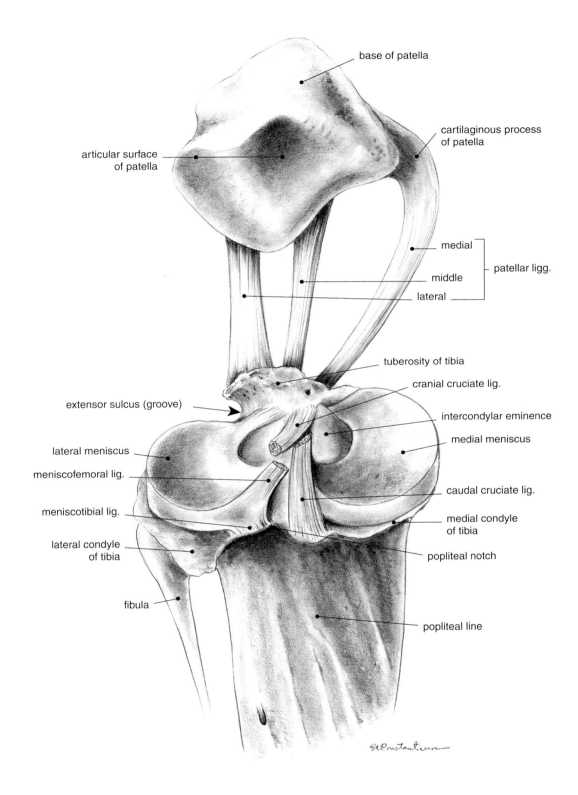

base of patella

cartilaginous process
of patella

articular surface
of patella

medial

middle ⎤ patellar ligg.

lateral

tuberosity of tibia

cranial cruciate lig.

extensor sulcus (groove)

intercondylar eminence

lateral meniscus

medial meniscus

meniscofemoral lig.

caudal cruciate lig.

meniscotibial lig.

medial condyle
of tibia

lateral condyle
of tibia

popliteal notch

fibula

popliteal line

Fig. H5.9. Patella and proximal tibia of left pelvic limb, horse, caudodorsal aspect.

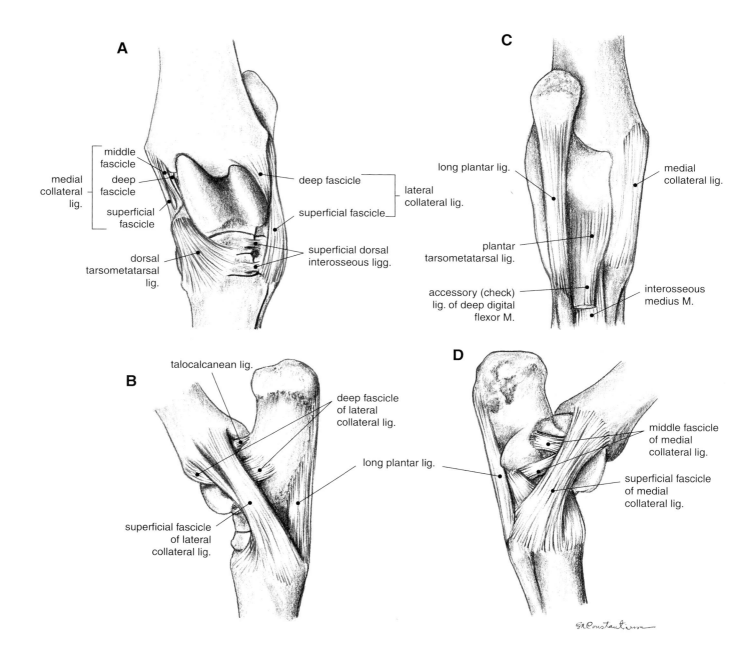

**A**

medial
collateral
lig.

middle
fascicle

deep
fascicle

superficial
fascicle

dorsal
tarsometatarsal
lig.

deep fascicle

superficial fascicle

lateral
collateral
lig.

superficial dorsal
interosseous ligg.

**C**

long plantar lig.

medial
collateral lig.

plantar
tarsometatarsal lig.

accessory (check)
lig. of deep digital
flexor M.

interosseous
medius M.

**B**

talocalcanean lig.

deep fascicle
of lateral
collateral lig.

long plantar lig.

superficial fascicle
of lateral
collateral lig.

**D**

middle fascicle
of medial
collateral lig.

superficial fascicle
of medial
collateral lig.

Fig. H5.10. Left tarsal joint, horse. **A.** Dorsal aspect. **B.** Lateral aspect. **C.** Plantar aspect. **D.** Medial aspect.

*Before starting the dissection, identify the following structures that serve as landmarks for physical examination and/or clinical approach: the greater trochanter with cranial and caudal parts separated by the trochanteric notch, the third trochanter, the lateral and medial epicondyles of the femur, the trochlea of the femur, the patella, the three patellar ligaments, the lateral and medial condyles of tibia, the tibial tuberosity, the craniomedial surface of tibia, the common calcanean tendon, the calcaneus and the calcanean tuber (point of the hock), the distal end of the lateral ridge of the trochlea of the talus, the third metatarsal bone (canon bone), the second and fourth metatarsal bones (splint bones), the tendons of the interosseous medius, deep digital flexor, and superficial digital flexor Mm., the ergot, the proximal sesamoid bones, the metatarsophalangeal joint (fetlock joint), the first phalanx (pastern), the coronet (the narrow area along the proxi-*mal border of the hoof), and the hoof (the wall with the toe, quarters, and heels, and the sole and the frog).

The exenteration (the evisceration or removal) of the urogenital tract and rectum with the anus from the pelvic cavity has already been completed.

With a knife, make an incision along the **linea alba** up to the **pubic symphysis**. With a saw, separate the two pelvic limbs through the lumbosacral and coccygeal midline and the pelvic symphysis. Examine the **vertebral canal** and the **spinal cord** with the **meninges**. *Notice* that in the horse the **conus medullaris** ends at the level of $S_2$ and continues as the **filum terminale** surrounded by the spinal nerves (Fig. H5.11).

*Remember!* The filum terminale and the last sacral and caudal spinal nerves are called the **cauda equina**.

The systematization of the muscles of the pelvic limb are shown in Table H5.1, and the nerve supply to the muscles of the pelvic limb is shown in Table H5.2.

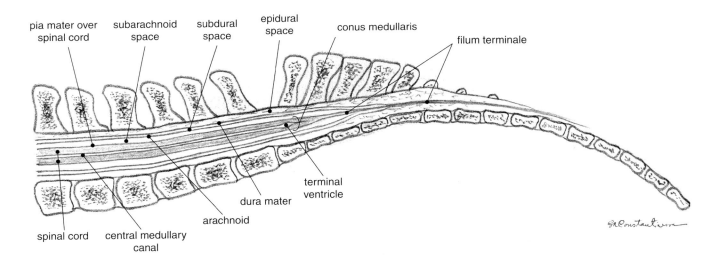

Fig. H5.11. Conus medullaris and associated structures in the horse, median section (schematic) (modified from Nickel, Schummer, and Seiferle, vol. 4).

a- femoral N.
b- saphenous N.
c- obturator N.
d- cranial gluteal N.
e- sciatic N.
f- common fibular N.
g- lateral cutaneous sural N.
h- superficial fibular N.
i- deep fibular N.
j- tibial N.
k- caudal cutaneous sural N.
l- medial plantar N.
m- lateral plantar N.
n- deep branch
o- caudal gluteal N.
p- caudal curtaneous femoral N.
q- pudendal N.
r- caudal rectal N.

1- iliopsoas M.
2- iliacus M.
3- psoas major M.
4- psoas minor M.
5- articularis coxae M.
6- sartorius M.
7- pectineus M.
8- gracilis M.
9- quadriceps femoris M.
10- external obturator M.
11- adductor minor M.
12- adductor major M.
13- middle gluteal M.
14- accessory gluteal M.
15- deep gluteal m.
16- tensor fasciae latae M.
17- superficial gluteal M. – cranial part
18- superficial gluteal M. – caudal part
19- biceps femoris M. – pelvic part
20- semitendinosus M. – pelvic part
21- internal obturator M.
22- gemelli Mm.

23- quadratus femoris M.
24- biceps femoris M.
25- semitendinosus M.
26- semimembranosus M.
27- lateral digital extensor M.
28- long digital extensor M.
29- cranial tibial M.
30- fibularis tertius M.
31- popliteus M.
32- medial digital flexor M.
33- lateral digital flexor m.
34- caudal tibial M.
35- gastrocnemius M. – lateral head
36- gastrocnemius M. – medial head
37- soleus M.
38- superficial digital flexor M.
39- interosseous medius M.

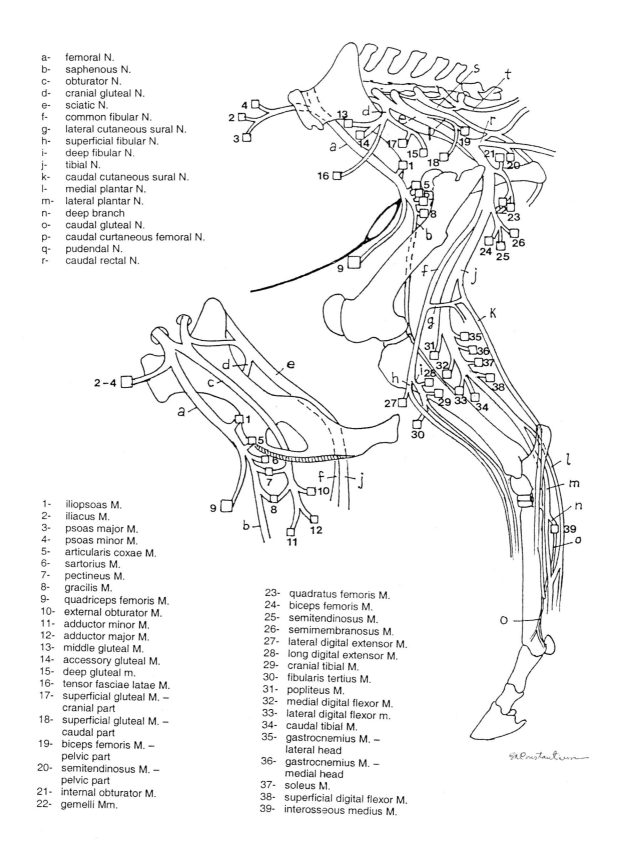

Fig. H5.12. Nerve supply to the muscles of the left pelvic limb, horse. The muscles are represented as little squares.

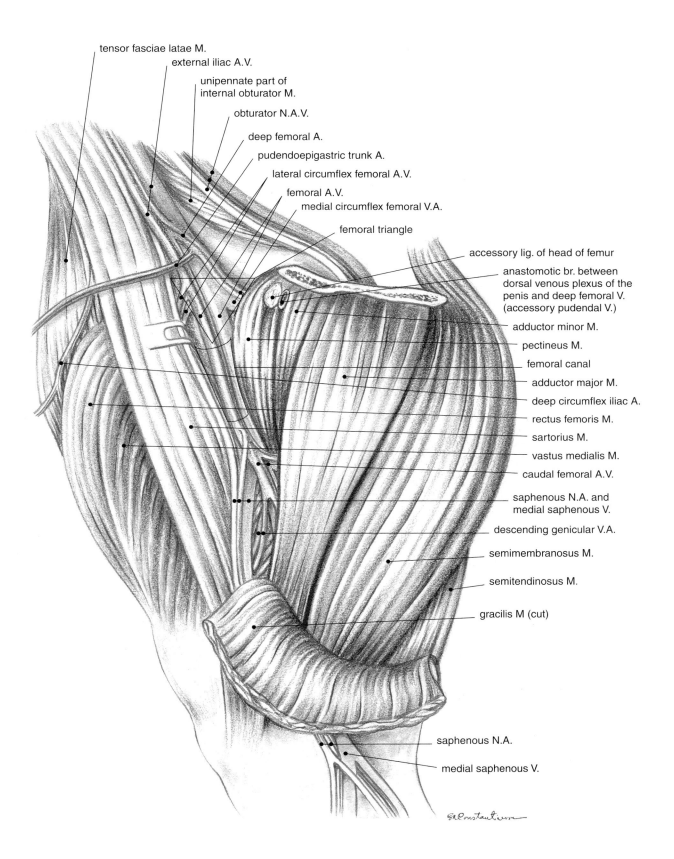

tensor fasciae latae M.

external iliac A.V.

unipennate part of
internal obturator M.

obturator N.A.V.

deep femoral A.

pudendoepigastric trunk A.

lateral circumflex femoral A.V.

femoral A.V.

medial circumflex femoral V.A.

femoral triangle

accessory lig. of head of femur

anastomotic br. between
dorsal venous plexus of the
penis and deep femoral V.
(accessory pudendal V.)

adductor minor M.

pectineus M.

femoral canal

adductor major M.

deep circumflex iliac A.

rectus femoris M.

sartorius M.

vastus medialis M.

caudal femoral A.V.

saphenous N.A. and
medial saphenous V.

descending genicular V.A.

semimembranosus M.

semitendinosus M.

gracilis M (cut)

saphenous N.A.

medial saphenous V.

Fig. H5.13. Medial aspect of right thigh, horse, superficial structures.

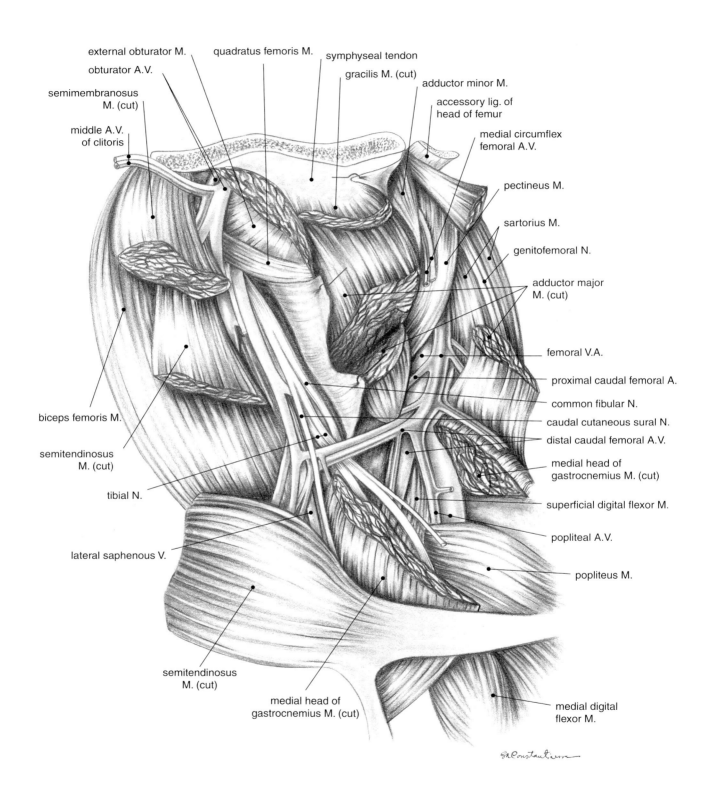

external obturator M.

quadratus femoris M.

symphyseal tendon

obturator A.V.

gracilis M. (cut)

adductor minor M.

semimembranosus M. (cut)

accessory lig. of head of femur

middle A.V. of clitoris

medial circumflex femoral A.V.

pectineus M.

sartorius M.

genitofemoral N.

adductor major M. (cut)

femoral V.A.

proximal caudal femoral A.

common fibular N.

biceps femoris M.

caudal cutaneous sural N.

distal caudal femoral A.V.

semitendinosus M. (cut)

medial head of gastrocnemius M. (cut)

superficial digital flexor M.

tibial N.

popliteal A.V.

lateral saphenous V.

popliteus M.

semitendinosus M. (cut)

medial head of gastrocnemius M. (cut)

medial digital flexor M.

Fig. H5.14. Medial aspect of left thigh, horse, deep structures.

Transect the semimembranosus M., the semitendinosus M., and the medial head of the gastrocnemius M. to widely expose the femoral and the popliteal Aa. (see Fig. H5.14). Transect the **iliopsoas M.** from the **lesser trochanter**, the sartorius M. from the **iliac fascia**, and the pectineus and adductor minor Mm. from their origin to better expose the deepest structures of the medial aspect of the thigh. The **rectus femoris** and **vastus medialis Mm.** are also exposed (Fig. H5.15).

Turn the limb lateral side up. Carefully reflect the ventral stumps of the biceps femoris and semitendinosus Mm. as far as possible without breaking any vessels or nerves.

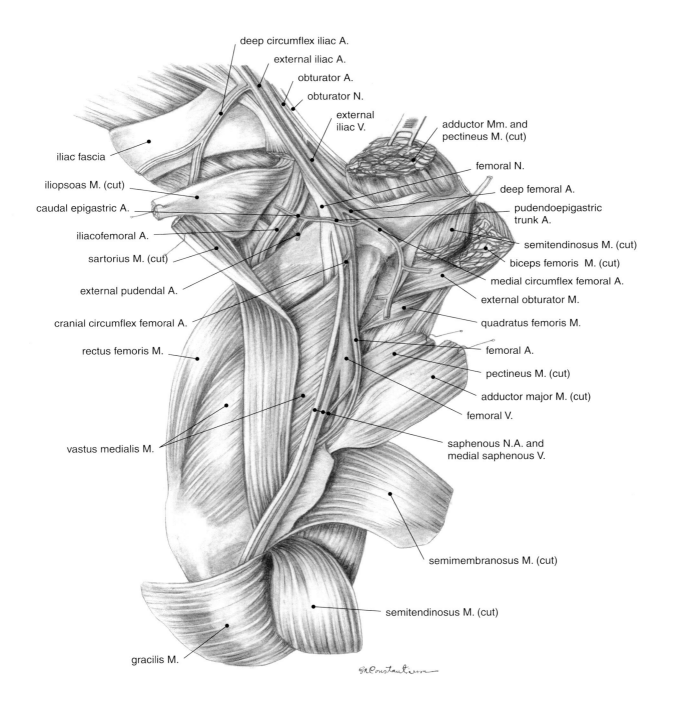

Fig. H5.15. The deepest structures of the medial aspect of the right thigh, horse.

After rounding the hip joint, the **sciatic N.** gives off muscular branches, and then it splits into the **common fibular (peroneal)** and the **tibial Nn.** The common fibular N. runs toward the lateral aspect of the crus, overlapping the lateral head of the gastrocnemius M., whereas the tibial N. penetrates between the two heads of the gastrocnemius M. Identify the **lateral cutaneous sural N.**, a branch of the common fibular N., and the **caudal cutaneous sural N.**, a branch of the tibial N. The caudal cutaneous sural N. is accompanied by the **lateral saphenous V.** all the way to the hock joint, on the lateral aspect of the **calcanean tendon** (Fig. H5.16; see Fig. H4.19). Identify the **deep popliteal lnn.** at the origin of the popliteal A. and V.

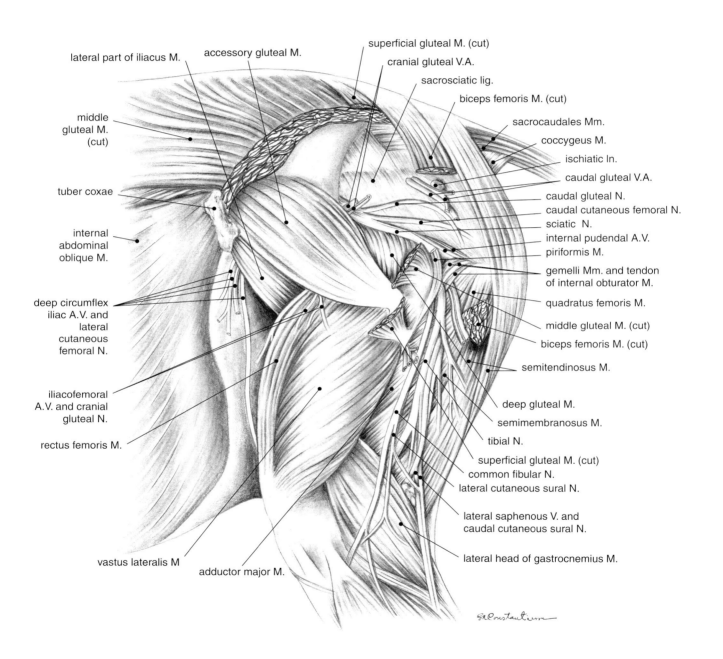

Fig. H5.16. Deep structures of lateral pelvis and thigh, horse, left limb.

Palpate the origin of the rectus femoris M. and the hip joint. Lateral to the origin of the rectus femoris M. and close to the joint capsule of the hip joint, expose the **articularis coxae M.** Transect the **quadriceps femoris M.** in the proximal third and separate the four muscles that compose it from one another. At a certain point of the dissection, transect the quadriceps femoris M. in the middle and look at the relationship of the four muscles.

For a better understanding of the dissection of the crus, first follow the **superficial lamina of the fascia lata** in the crus.

*Remember!* Proximal to the **patella**, this lamina splits into a deep and a superficial layer.

*Notice* that the deep layer is inserted on the patella, whereas the superficial layer continues toward the hock only on the cranial aspect of the crus. It is called the **superficial crural fascia,** and it overlaps the **proper (middle) crural fascia.** The superficial crural fascia becomes loose connective tissue in the metatarsal area.

The entire crus is surrounded and protected by the proper crural fascia. The aponeuroses of the gracilis, sartorius, semitendinosus, and biceps femoris Mm. fuse with one another and with the proper crural fascia. They are considered to be the tensors of this fascia. The proper crural fascia fuses with the **calcanean tendons** of the biceps femoris and semitendinosus Mm. in the **intermediate tendon.** (The intermediate tendon is a major component of the **common calcanean tendon**). In addition, the proper crural fascia builds up three **extensor retinacula** on the dorsal aspect of the hock, and the **flexor retinaculum** on the plantar aspect of the hock. This fascia sends septa that separate the muscles, and fuses with the periosteum on the medial aspect of the tibia. It continues only on the plantar aspect of the metatarsal region with the **plantar fascia.** The deepest fascia is the **deep crural fascia,** the continuation of the **deep lamina of the fascia lata.** This fascia surrounds only the deep caudal muscles of the crus and will not continue in the autopodium region. Figure H5.17 shows these fasciae in a cross section.

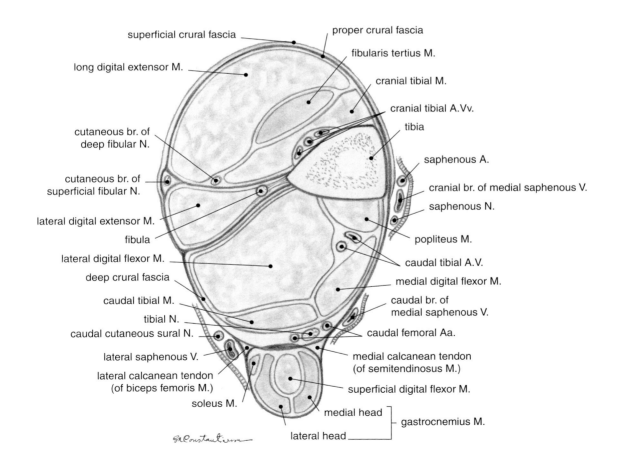

Fig. H5.17. Cross section of left crus, horse (schematic).

Carefully remove the superficial crural fascia and expose the proper crural fascia. Through the transparency of this fascia, outline the **crural (proximal)**, **tarsal (middle)**, and **metatarsal (distal) extensor retinacula**. Identify the **long digital extensor** and the **lateral digital extensor Mm.** (Fig. H5.18).

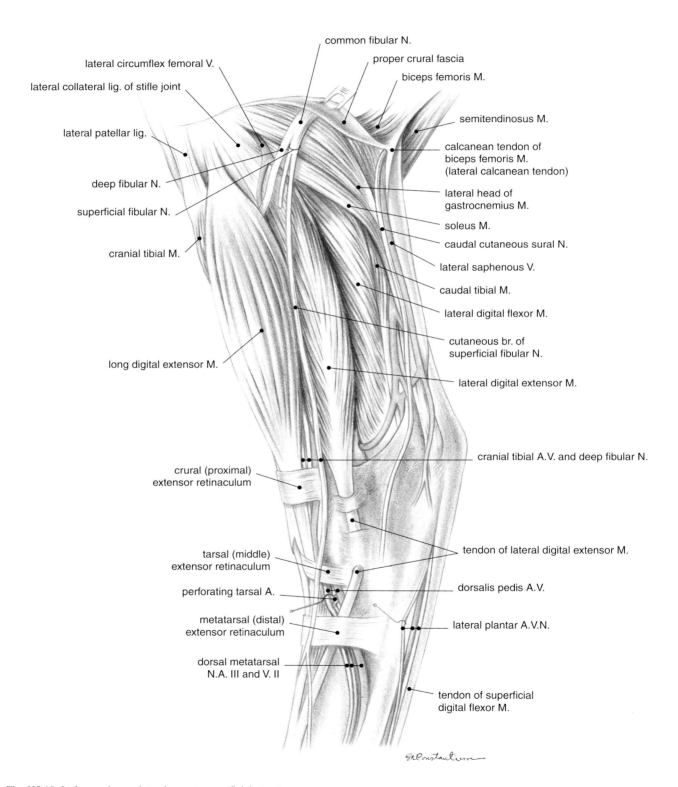

common fibular N.

lateral circumflex femoral V.

proper crural fascia

biceps femoris M.

lateral collateral lig. of stifle joint

semitendinosus M.

lateral patellar lig.

calcanean tendon of
biceps femoris M.
(lateral calcanean tendon)

deep fibular N.

lateral head of
gastrocnemius M.

superficial fibular N.

soleus M.

cranial tibial M.

caudal cutaneous sural N.

lateral saphenous V.

caudal tibial M.

lateral digital flexor M.

cutaneous br. of
superficial fibular N.

long digital extensor M.

lateral digital extensor M.

cranial tibial A.V. and deep fibular N.

crural (proximal)
extensor retinaculum

tendon of lateral digital extensor M.

tarsal (middle)
extensor retinaculum

perforating tarsal A.

dorsalis pedis A.V.

metatarsal (distal)
extensor retinaculum

lateral plantar A.V.N.

dorsal metatarsal
N.A. III and V. II

tendon of superficial
digital flexor M.

Fig. H5.18. Left crus, horse, lateral aspect, superficial structures.

To free the muscles from their individual fascial covers, make a long incision within the proper crural fascia in the long axis of each tendon of these muscles. Introduce the blade of the scalpel through the incision line under the fascia in a position parallel to the muscle, continue the incision to the end of the muscle, and remove the fascia.

Be aware that the **cutaneous branch of the superficial fibular N.** runs between the two extensor muscles. The entire common fibular N. passes over the proximal attachment of the lateral digital extensor M. This nerve becomes apparent from under the proper crural fascia, running in a cranioventral direction, crossing the **lateral condyle of the tibia**, the lateral head of the gastrocnemius M. and the **soleus M.** (see Fig. H5.18).

Either reflect or transect the long digital extensor M. to expose the **fibularis tertius** and the **cranial tibial Mm.** (Fig. H5.19).

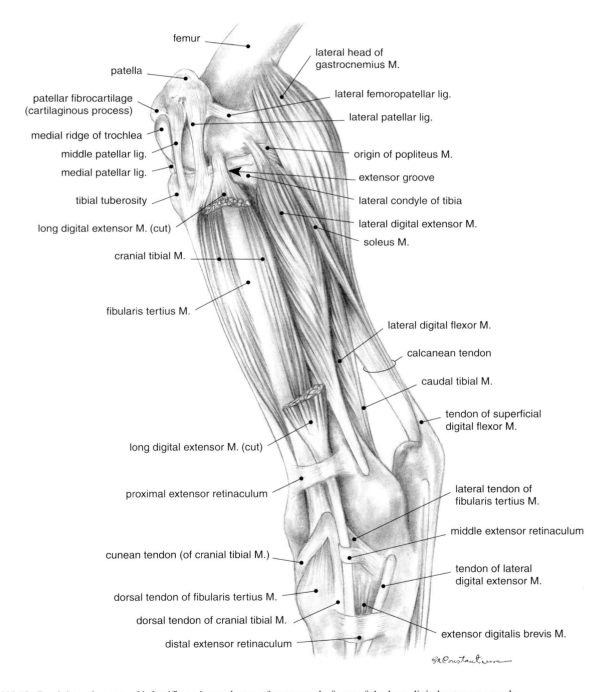

Fig. H5.19. Craniolateral aspect of left stifle and crus, horse, after removal of part of the long digital extensor muscle.

*Caution.* Deep to the long digital extensor, find and protect the **deep fibular N.** Reflect the cranial tibial M. and find the **cranial tibial A.** This artery and the deep fibular N. pass together through the crural extensor retinaculum (see Fig. H5.18).

Once the three extensor retinacula are outlined, carefully remove the proper crural fascia between them and fully expose the tendons running on the dorsal aspect of the hock. Dissect them according to Figures H5.19 and H5.20.

*Notice* that the long digital extensor M. passes through, and is bound down by, all three retinacula; its tendon is surrounded by a tendon sheath.

The fibularis tertius protects and guides the passage of the cranial tibial tendon by a fibrous ring. After passing through this ring, the cranial tibial tendon splits into a **dorsal (metatarsal) tendon** and a **medial (cunean) ten-**

don. The fibularis tertius also has two distal tendons: the **dorsal (metatarsal) tendon** and the **lateral tendon.** *Notice* that the tarsal (middle) retinaculum attaches to the lateral tendon of the fibularis tertius (see Figs. H5.19 and H5.20). Each of these two tendons is surrounded by a tendon sheath.

**Extension of the tarsus while the stifle is flexed is prevented by the fibularis tertius. The ability to extend the tarsus while the stifle is flexed is characteristic of a ruptured fibularis tertius.**

The metatarsal (distal) retinaculum binds down the tendons of the long and lateral digital extensor Mm. and the rudimentary **short digital extensor M. (extensor digitalis brevis M.)** (Fig. H5.20).

*Notice* that the tendon of the lateral digital extensor M. joins the tendon of the long digital extensor M. in the middle third of the dorsal aspect of the metatarsus, in contrast

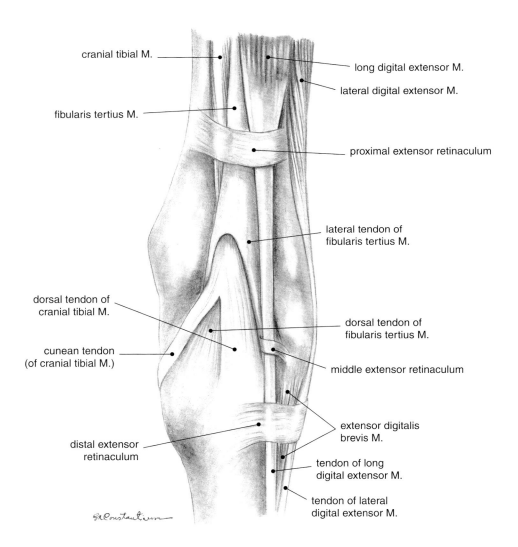

Fig. H5.20. Tarsus, horse, dorsal aspect of left hindlimb.

to the thoracic limb, in which similar tendons run and insert in separate ways. The lateral digital extensor tendon is also protected by a tendon sheath.

**Removal of the lateral digital extensor tendon and the distal portion of the muscle is sometimes performed in the treatment of stringhalt, a neurological and mechanical abnormality of the hind limb.**

Between the tarsal and metatarsal retinacula, carefully dissect the **dorsalis pedis A.** and **V.**, the **perforating tarsal A.** and **V.**, and the **dorsal metatarsal A. III** and **N. III**. The dorsal metatarsal A. and N. and the **dorsal**

metatarsal V. II run distally in the metatarsal area (see Fig. H5.18).

Continue the dissection of the **saphenous A.**, **medial saphenous V.**, and **saphenous N.** on the medial aspect of the crus, from the thigh toward the hock (Fig. H5.21).

*Notice* that the vessels and the nerve cross the aponeurotic attachment of the semitendinosus M. on the **cranial border of tibia** (the former tibial crest), and that the vessels and the nerves usually have two or more branches each (Fig. H5.21).

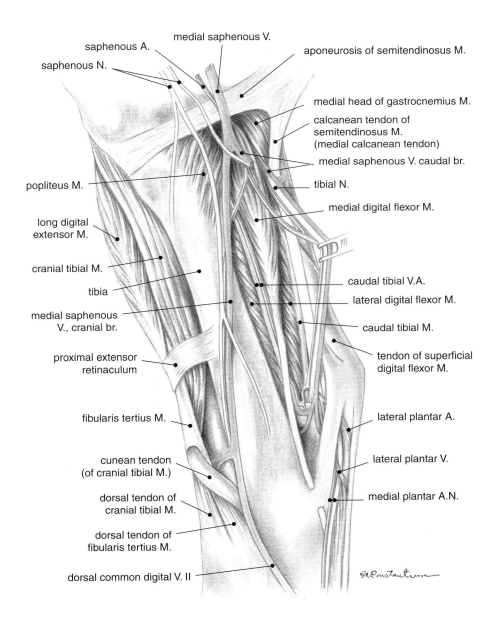

Fig. H5.21. Right crus, horse, medial aspect.

Free the muscles of the medial aspect of the crus from their individual fascial covers and, paying close attention, dissect and protect the following structures: the **caudal tibial A.** and **V.**, passing under the **medial digital flexor (medial head of the deep digital flexor M., flexor pedis longus M.)** and over the **lateral digital flexor (lateral head of the deep digital flexor M., flexor hallucis longus M.)**; the **caudal tibial M. (caudal head of the deep digital flexor M.)** is easy to separate from the lateral head in the distal third of it; the tibial N. lies between the caudal tibial M. and the common calcanean tendon (see Fig. H5.21).

*Note.* The *common calcanean tendon* consists of two groups of structures: the *calcanean tendon* and the *intermediate tendon*. The calcanean tendon is composed of the tendon of the two heads of the gastrocnemius M., the soleus M. (together known as the **triceps surae M.**), and the **superficial digital flexor M.** The intermediate tendon is made up of the calcanean tendons of the biceps femoris and semitendinosus Mm. and the proper crural fascia.

Observe the tendon of the superficial digital flexor M. surrounding the triceps surae tendon from the medial to the lateral side.

Carefully dissect the area at the medial aspect of the crus, distally, between the **tibia** and the **calcaneus**. The caudal branches of both the saphenous A. and the medial saphenous V. anastomose with the corresponding caudal tibial A. and V. and, occasionally, with the distal branches of the caudal femoral A. and V. in an S-shaped artery and vein. The **medial** and **lateral plantar A.** and **V.** originate from this anastomosis. Dorsal to the hock, the tibial N. branches into the **medial** and **lateral plantar Nn.** (Fig. H5.21 and H5.22).

The lateral plantar N. gives off the **deep plantar N.**, which supplies the interosseous medius M. and then continues as the **medial** and **lateral plantar metatarsal Nn.** At the most distal end of the splint bones, the plantar metatarsal Nn. become apparent and supply the dorsal aspect of the fetlock.

On the medioplantar aspect of the hock identify the flexor retinaculum, the continuation of the proper crural fascia. It binds down two of the three heads of the deep digital flexor M., namely the lateral and the caudal heads, surrounded by one common tendon sheath. The tendon of the medial head runs separately, surrounded by its own tendon sheath, and joins the other tendons distal to the hock. From this point, the tendon of the deep digital flexor M. runs as a single structure.

*Remember!* The deep digital flexor M. consists of three heads: lateral, medial, and caudal, also called muscles (see above).

Reflect the deep digital flexor tendon and examine the **check** or **accessory lig.** that fuses with the tendon, as a continuation of the **plantar tarsometatarsal lig.** Examine the **long plantar lig.,** closely attached to the plantar border of the calcaneus (see Fig. H5.10); the tendon of the superficial digital flexor M. intimately passes over this ligament.

**Desmitis (*inflammation of a ligament*) of the long plantar ligament results in a condition called "curb."**

Identify the plantar fascia (in the metatarsal area) and its strong attachments to the splint bones. Remove it carefully to expose the tendons of the superficial and deep digital flexor and interosseous medius Mm., and the vessels and the nerves of the region. The two plantar Nn. run parallel with and between the tendons of the superficial and deep digital flexors. A **communicating branch** is observed between the plantar Nn. in the middle of the metatarsus over the superficial digital flexor tendon (in an oblique position ventrolaterally). The nerves are accompanied by the **superficial branches of Aa.** and **Vv.** and by the **dorsal common digital V. II.** (on the medial side) (Fig. H5.22). The dorsal metatarsal A. III is the major contributor to the **medial** and **lateral digital Aa.**

Do *not* attempt to dissect the digit. It will be described in detail with the thoracic limb (see Chapter 6, The Thoracic Limb). At the end of the dissection of the pelvic limb, cut the metatarsal bones in the middle, store the digit, and dissect it with the thoracic limb. The structures are very similar, and saving the pelvic digits will provide additional specimens for dissection.

After the dissection of the muscles, vessels, and nerves is finished, focus on the joint structures, starting with the hip joint.

Disarticulate the **hip joint** and examine all the components that are specific for the horse, such as the accessory lig. of the femoral head and the articularis coxae M. Also examine the **lig. of the femoral head**, the **transverse acetabular lig.**, the **acetabulum**, and the **femoral head** with the **fovea capitis**, where the two ligaments of the femoral head originate (see Fig. H5.6). Also look at the differences between the horse and the ox.

Return to the **stifle joint** (see Figs. H5.7–H5.9); dissect the three **patellar ligg. (medial, middle, and lateral)** and identify the **infrapatellar fat pad**, between the fibrous and synovial joint capsules. Reflect the common tendon of the quadriceps femoris M. and examine its attachment to the femoropatellar joint capsule, acting as a tensor. Examine the **cartilaginous process** on the medial angle of the patella and try to understand the locking mechanism of the stifle, which will be explained later in this chapter. On both sides of the patella, dissect the **medial** and the **lateral**

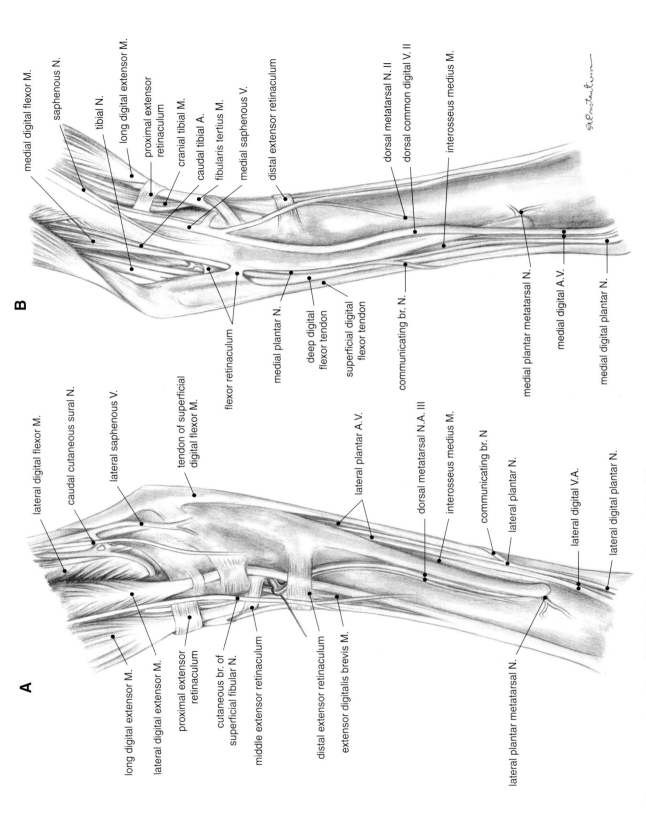

**B**

medial digital flexor M.

saphenous N.

tibial N.

long digital extensor M.

proximal extensor retinaculum

cranial tibial M.

caudal tibial A.

fibularis tertius M.

medial saphenous V.

distal extensor retinaculum

dorsal metatarsal N. II

dorsal common digital V. II

interosseus medius M.

flexor retinaculum

medial plantar N.

deep digital flexor tendon

superficial digital flexor tendon

communicating br. N.

medial plantar metatarsal N.

medial digital A.V.

medial digital plantar N.

**A**

lateral digital flexor M.

caudal cutaneous sural N.

lateral saphenous V.

tendon of superficial digital flexor M.

long digital extensor M.

lateral digital extensor M.

proximal extensor retinaculum

cutaneous br. of superficial fibular N.

middle extensor retinaculum

distal extensor retinaculum

extensor digitalis brevis M.

lateral plantar metatarsal N.

lateral plantar A.V.

dorsal metatarsal N.A. III

interosseus medius M.

communicating br. N

lateral plantar N.

lateral digital V.A.

lateral digital plantar N.

Fig. H5.22. Tarsometatarsal area, horse, left hindlimb. **A.** Lateral aspect. **B.** Medial aspect.

**femoropatellar ligg.** Examine the attachment of the biceps femoris tendon on the lateral femoropatellar lig. and on the lateral patellar lig. Also examine the attachment of the aponeuroses of the gracilis and sartorius Mm. on the medial patellar lig. Transect and reflect the semimembranosus, semitendinosus, and adductor major Mm. and the medial head of the gastrocnemius M. to fully expose the structures shown in Fig. H5.23.

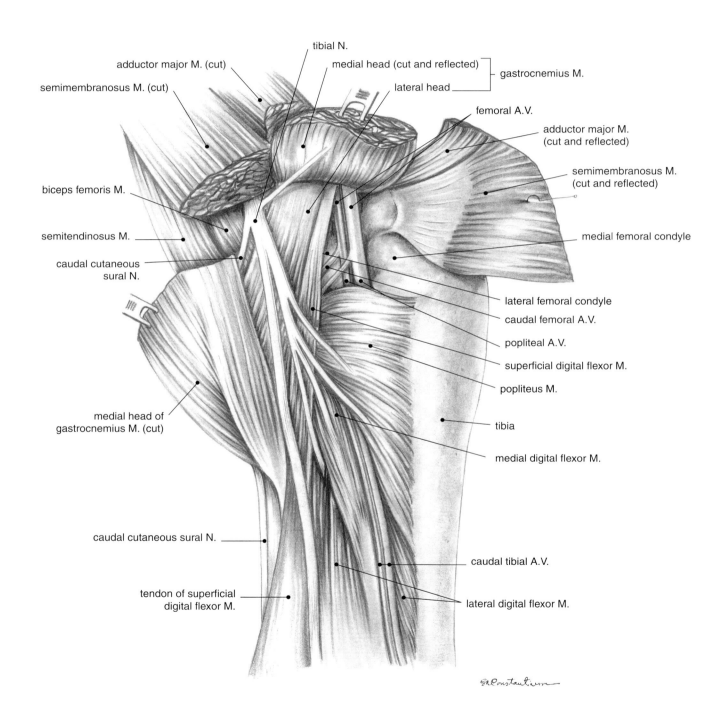

Fig. H5.23. Stifle and proximal crus of left pelvic limb, horse, deep mediocaudal aspect.

Expose the common origin of the long digital extensor and fibularis tertius tendons in the **extensor fossa**, and the origin of the popliteus tendon in the **popliteal fossa**, all of them at the distal end of the femur. Examine the **extensor groove** and the **popliteal notch**, structures of the tibia that are related to these three tendons (see Fig. H5.3).

Follow the route of the popliteus M. and *notice* that it is separated from the lateral head of the deep digital flexor M. by the **popliteal line**, on the caudal aspect of tibia (see Fig. H5.3).

Following the direction of the popliteal A. and V. make an incision within the popliteus M. and expose the caudal tibial A. (superficial) and the origin of the cranial tibial A. (deep), according to Figure H5.24. Remove the caudal joint capsule and explore the two **femorotibial menisci**, the **meniscofemoral lig.**, the unofficially called **meniscotibial lig.** (the caudal attachment of the lateral meniscus on the proximal extremity of the tibia), and the **cranial** and **caudal cruciate ligg.** (see Figs. H5.8 and H5.9).

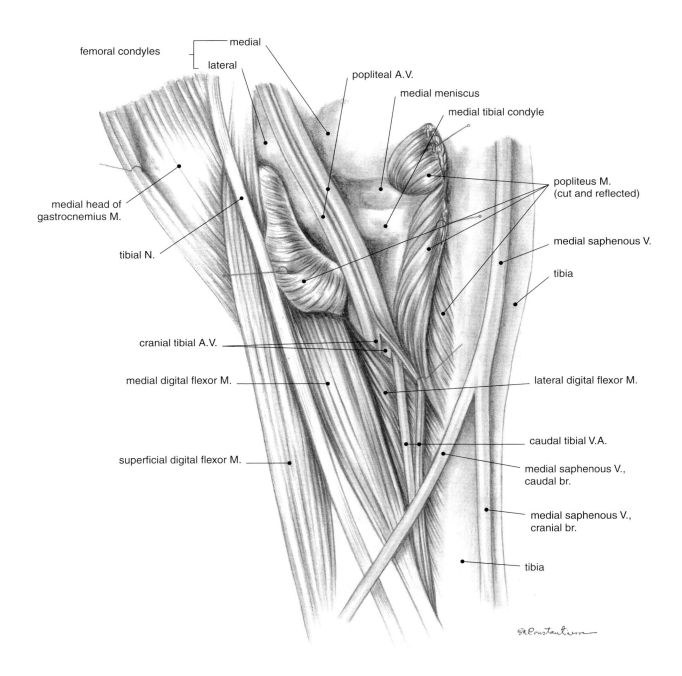

Fig. H5.24. Deep structures of left stifle and crus, horse, mediocaudal aspect.

On the **hock** (see Fig. H5.10), remove the dorsal joint capsule and explore each joint, identifying the bones and the ligaments and attempt to understand the springlike mechanism of the **talocrural joint**, based on the twisted fibers of the **collateral ligg.**, proving that this joint is a **trochlearthrosis (a hinge joint).**

Identify the distal intermediate ridge of the tibia (on the dorsal side of the distal end, between the two malleoli), the most common site of osteochondrosis in the horse.

*The locking mechanism of the stifle* (Fig. H5.25), known also as the patellar locking mechanism, is that action that inhibits flexion of the stifle while in the resting position, to allow for muscles to relax and recuperate. To understand this mechanism, it is necessary to examine the bones involved in the process: the **femoral trochlea** and the patella (see Fig. H5.2). There is a **trochlear tubercle** on the top of the medial trochlear ridge, allowing the loop formed by the cartilaginous process of the patella and the medial and middle patellar ligg. to hang over the trochlear tubercle. When the animal stands with the weight distributed equally on both pelvic limbs, the loop hangs over the trochlear tubercle, and the patella is "locked" in position and can't slip over the gliding surface of the femoral trochlea. Minimal effort is required to keep the trochlea in this position, due to the contraction of the biceps femoris M. on the lateral patellar lig., and the gracilis and sartorius Mm. on the patellar fibrocartilage and medial patellar lig. At the same time the quadriceps femoris M. is relaxed. The horse frequently "rests" on one pelvic limb by partially flexing the hip, stifle, hock, and fetlock so that the limb rests on the toe. The contralateral limb, which becomes the weight-bearing limb, becomes slightly flexed. The patella of the weight-bearing limb rotates slightly medial and slides caudally over the femoral tubercle to essentially "lock" the patella over the medial trochlear ridge and prevent flexion of the stifle. Changing the body weight from one limb to the other requires that the horse unlock the patella, by the contraction of the quadriceps femoris M.

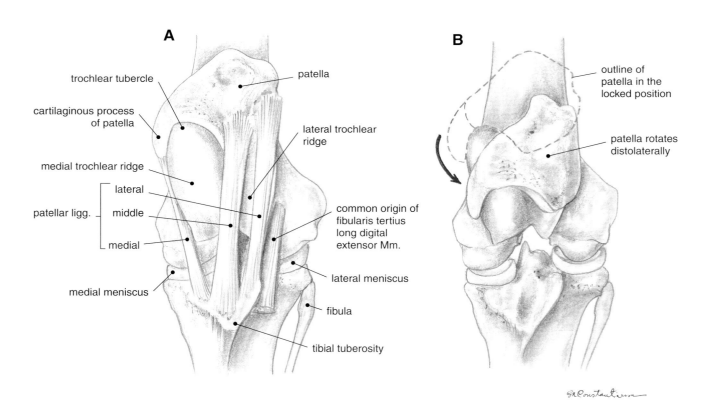

Fig. H5.25. Patellar locking mechanism in the horse, left pelvic limb. **A.** Patella is locked. **B.** Patella is unlocked.

**Transection of the medial patellar lig. disrupts the patellar locking mechanism.**

*The passive stay apparatus* (Fig. H5.26) enables the horse to rest in a standing position with minimal muscular effort. The *passive* stay apparatus is made up of fibrous, inextensible structures that do not get tired (*passive* versus active structures, tendons and ligaments versus muscles).

The locking mechanism is part of the passive stay apparatus. In the pelvic limb, the hip joint is not provided with enough fibrous structures to permanently support the body weight. The structures involved in the stay apparatus are the fibularis tertius, superficial and deep digital flexor, and interosseous medius Mm., and the **distal sesamoidean ligg.**

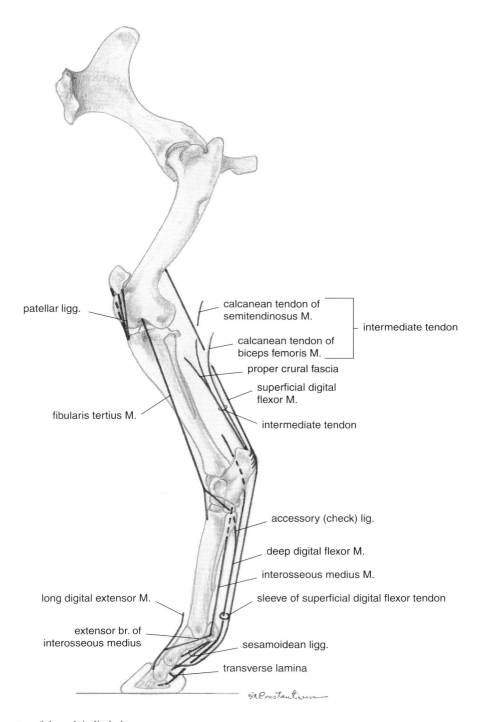

Fig. H5.26. Stay apparatus of the pelvic limb, horse.

When the stifle joint is locked, the hock joint will oppose flexion under pressure of the body weight. The fibularis tertius M. on the cranial aspect of the crus and the superficial digital flexor M. on the caudal aspect act as synergistic structures.

The passive stay apparatus of the fetlock, pastern, and coffin joints will be described in Chapter H6, The Thoracic Limb.

## MODLAB H5

Attempt to palpate on a live horse the structures mentioned at the beginning of this chapter.

The following are *landmarks* and *approaches* for subcutaneous, subfascial, tendinous, subtendinous, and articular bursae, tendons and tendon sheaths, vessels, lymph nodes, and especially nerves for nerve block anesthesia.

1. **Femoral A.V.N. and deep inguinal lnn.** (Fig. H5.27A)
   A. *Landmarks*: cranial border of pubis, caudal border of sartorius M., cranial border of gracilis M.
   B. *Approach*: in the femoral triangle, through the skin and femoral lamina, between the sartorius, gracilis, and pectineus Mm.

2. **Saphenous A.N., and medial saphenous V.** *(in the thigh)* (Fig. H5.27A)
   A. *Landmarks*: cranial border of pubis, intermuscular space between sartorius and gracilis Mm., medial femoral condyle
   B. *Approach*: in the above mentioned intermuscular space, in the distal half of a line between the cranial border of the pubis and the medial femoral condyle

3. **Saphenous A.N., and medial saphenous V.** *(in the crus)* (Fig. H5.27A)
   A. *Landmarks*: the cranial and caudal borders of the tibia, on the medial aspect of the crus
   B. *Approach*: in the middle of the crus, on both borders of the tibia, through the skin and the superficial and proper crural fasciae

4. **Caudal cutaneous sural N. and lateral saphenous V.** (Fig. H5.27B)
   A. *Landmarks*: the common calcanean tendon, the intermuscular space between the biceps femoris and semitendinosus Mm.
   B. *Approach*: between the distal end of the intermuscular space between the biceps femoris and semitendinosus Mm. and along the lateral aspect of the common calcanean tendon, under the skin and the proper crural fascia

5. **Tibial N.** (Fig. H5.27A)
   A. *Landmarks*: the medial groove of the crus separating the common calcanean tendon from the rest of the crus, the calcanean tuber
   B. *Approach*: With the pelvic limb held in flexion, the medial groove of the crus is widely exposed and allows for easy palpation of the nerve; the approach to the nerve is one hand proximal to the calcanean tuber, under the skin and the proper crural fascia.

6. **Cranial tibial A.** (Fig. H5.27A)
   A. *Landmarks*: the medial groove of the crus between the cranial border of the tibia and the long digital extensor M.
   B. *Approach*: deep between the two landmarks, through the skin and the superficial and proper crural fasciae, in the distal third of the crus

7. **Common fibular (peroneal) N.** (Fig. H5.27B)
   A. *Landmarks*: lateral tibial condyle
   B. *Approach*: The nerve is palpable on the lateral condyle of the tibia in an oblique direction cranioventrally, by rolling the fingers firmly back and forth, pressing the skin and the superficial and proper crural fasciae.

8. **Superficial and deep fibular (peroneal) Nn. (sensory branches)** (Fig. H5.27B)
   A. *Landmarks*: the lateral groove of the crus between the long and lateral digital extensor Mm., the calcanean tuber
   B. *Approach*: at a point 10 cm proximal to the calcanean tuber, through the skin and the superficial and proper crural fasciae, in the lateral groove mentioned above (the nerves are parallel to each other, one superficial and one deep)

9. **Dorsal metatarsal A. III** (Fig. H5.27B)
   A. *Landmarks*: the dorsal groove between metatarsal bones III and IV (lateral)
   B. *Approach*: subcutaneous, in the dorsal groove (this is one of the sites for taking the arterial pulse or obtaining arterial blood samples)

10. **Dorsal common digital V. II** (Fig. H5.27A)
    A. *Landmarks*: proximal end of metatarsal bones III and II (medial)
    B. *Approach*: an oblique line crossing the proximal end of metatarsal bones III and II in a distoplantar direction, under the skin

11. **Medial (and lateral) plantar Nn.** (Fig. H5.27C)
    A. *Landmarks*: the tendons of the superficial and deep digital flexor Mm. in the metatarsal area
    B. *Approach*: through the skin and plantar fascia, on both sides of the limb, along the tendons

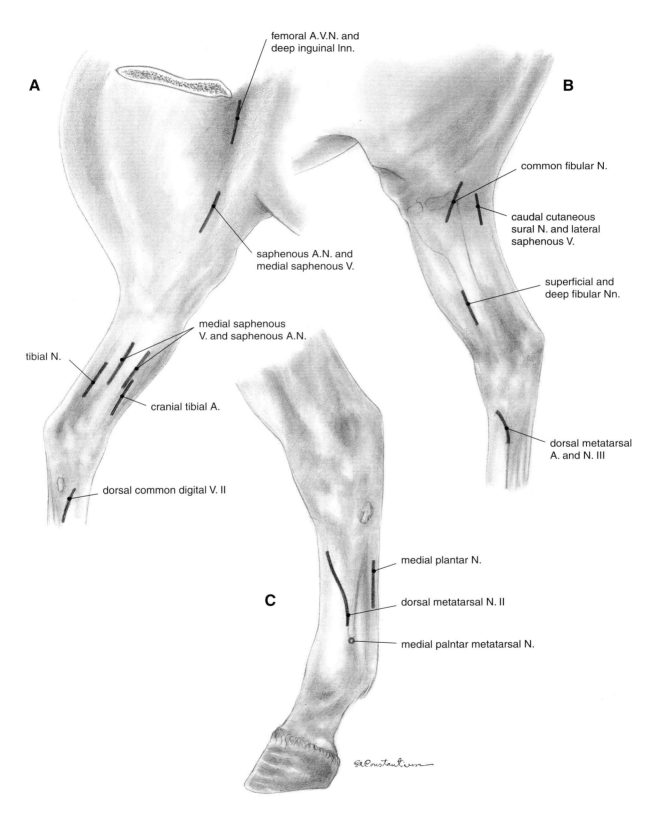

**A**

femoral A.V.N. and deep inguinal lnn.

saphenous A.N. and medial saphenous V.

medial saphenous V. and saphenous A.N.

tibial N.

cranial tibial A.

dorsal common digital V. II

**B**

common fibular N.

caudal cutaneous sural N. and lateral saphenous V.

superficial and deep fibular Nn.

dorsal metatarsal A. and N. III

**C**

medial plantar N.

dorsal metatarsal N. II

medial palntar metatarsal N.

Fig. H5.27. Landmarks and approaches for the pelvic limb, horse. **A.** Medial aspect. **B.** Lateral aspect. **C.** Medial aspect of autopodium.

***Remember!*** There is a communicating branch in the middle of the metatarsal area between the lateral and medial plantar Nn. Choose the right site while blocking one or both nerves, depending on your needs.

12. **Medial (and lateral) plantar metatarsal Nn.** (Fig. H5.27C)

    A. *Landmarks*: the distal ends of metatarsal bones II and IV (the splint bones)

    B. *Approach*: subcutaneous, at the distal end of the palpable splint bones

13. **Dorsal metatarsal Nn.**

    Dorsal metatarsal N. III (Fig. H5.27B)

    A. *Landmarks*: same for dorsal metatarsal A. III

    B. *Approach*: same as for dorsal metatarsal A. III, but continues distally to the lateral aspect of the fetlock

    Dorsal metatarsal N. II (Fig. H5.27C)

    A. *Landmarks*: tendon of the long digital extensor M., metatarsal bone II

    B. *Approach*: In the tarsal area, the nerve parallels the medial border of the tendon of the long digital extensor M., then obliquely crosses metatarsal bone III distoplantarly, running parallel to and between metatarsal bones III and II under the skin.

14. **Subcutaneous bursae**

    *Trochanteric bursa* (Fig. H5.28)

    A. *Landmark and approach*: third trochanter

    *Iliac bursa* (Fig. H5.28)

    A. *Landmark and approach*: tuber coxae

    *Ischiatic bursa* (Fig. H5.28)

    A. *Landmark and approach*: ischiatic tuberosity

    *Prepatellar bursa* (Fig. H5.29A)

    A. *Landmark and approach*: cranial aspect of patella

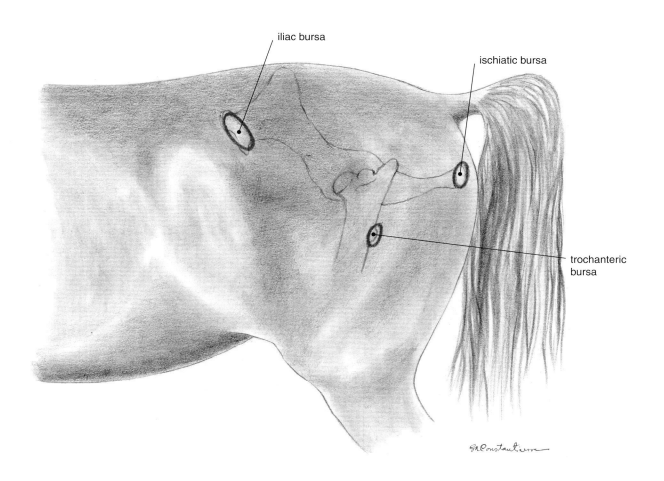

Fig. H5.28. Subcutaneous bursae of proximal left pelvic limb, horse, lateral aspect.

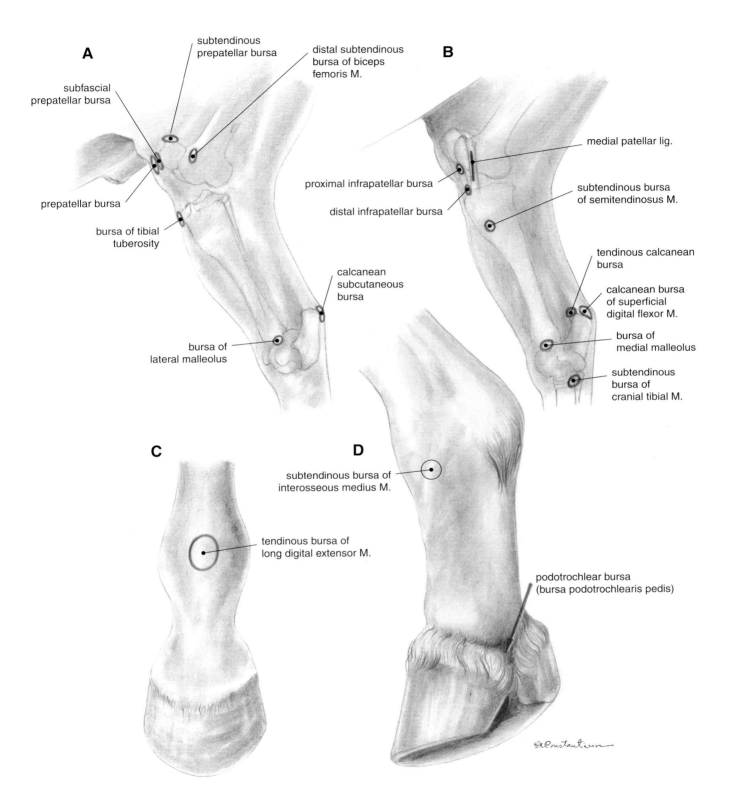

**A**

subfascial
prepatellar bursa

subtendinous
prepatellar bursa

distal subtendinous
bursa of biceps
femoris M.

prepatellar bursa

bursa of tibial
tuberosity

calcanean
subcutaneous
bursa

bursa of
lateral malleolus

**B**

medial patellar lig.

proximal infrapatellar bursa

distal infrapatellar bursa

subtendinous bursa
of semitendinosus M.

tendinous calcanean
bursa

calcanean bursa
of superficial
digital flexor M.

bursa of
medial malleolus

subtendinous
bursa of
cranial tibial M.

**C**

tendinous bursa of
long digital extensor M.

**D**

subtendinous bursa of
interosseous medius M.

podotrochlear bursa
(bursa podotrochlearis pedis)

Fig. H5.29. Tendinous, subtendinous, and subfascial bursae of pelvic limb, horse. **A.** Lateral aspect. **B.** Medial aspect. **C.** Dorsal aspect of the digit. **D.** Plantar aspect of the digit.

*Bursa of tibial tuberosity* (Fig. H5.29A)
A. *Landmark and approach:* tibial tuberosity

*Bursae of lateral and medial malleoli* (Fig. H5.29A,B)
A. *Landmarks and approach*: lateral and medial malleoli (sing. malleolus)

*Calcanean bursa* (Fig. H5.29A)
A. *Landmark and approach*: calcanean tuber

15. **Subfascial, subtendinous, and articular bursae**
*Subfascial prepatellar bursa* (Fig. H5.29A)
A. *Landmark*: cranial aspect of patella
B. *Approach*: through the skin and the superficial layer of the superficial lamina of fascia lata

*Subtendinous prepatellar bursa* (Fig. H5.29A)
A. *Landmark*: patella
B. *Approach*: deep between the base of the patella and the insertion of the quadriceps femoris M.

*Proximal infrapatellar bursa* (Fig. H5.29B)
A. *Landmarks*: patella, middle patellar lig.
B. *Approach*: between the apex of the patella and the patellar attachment of the middle patellar lig.

*Distal infrapatellar bursa* (Fig. H5.29B)
A. *Landmarks*: tibial tuberosity, middle patellar lig.
B. *Approach*: between the tibial tuberosity and the tibial attachment of the middle patellar lig.

*Distal subtendinous bursa of biceps femoris M.* (Fig. H5.29A)
A. *Landmarks*: patella, stifle joint, lateral femoral condyle
B. *Approach*: deep on the lateral aspect of the stifle joint, 5–10 cm caudal to patella and between the aponeurosis of the biceps femoris M. and the lateral femoral condyle

*Subtendinous bursa of semitendinosus M.* (Fig. H5.29B)
A. *Landmark*: cranial border of tibia
B. *Approach*: between the tendon of semitendinosus M. and the cranial border of tibia through the skin, superficial and proper crural fasciae

*Subtendinous bursa of cranial tibial M.* (Fig. H5.29B)
A. *Landmarks*: medial aspect of the hock, proximal end of metatarsal bones III and II
B. *Approach*: through the skin, between the cunean tendon (of the cranial tibial M.) and tarsal bones I

and II, 2–3 cm above the proximal ends of metatarsal bones II and III on the medial aspect of the hock

*Calcanean bursa of superficial digital flexor M.* (Fig. H5.29B)
A. *Landmarks*: calcanean tuber and the attachment of the common calcanean tendon on it
B. *Approach*: between the attachment of the superficial digital flexor tendon and the tendon of the triceps surae M. over the calcanean tuber

*Tendinous calcanean bursa* (Fig. H5.29B)
A. *Landmarks*: same as for the calcanean bursa of superficial digital flexor M. (see above)
B. *Approach*: deep between the attachment of the common calcanean tendon and the calcanean tuber

*Note.* The two calcanean bursae are often fused.

*Tendinous bursa of the long digital extensor M.* (Fig. H5.29C)
A. *Landmarks*: dorsal aspect of the fetlock, the tendon of the long digital extensor M.
B. *Approach*: between the tendon of the long digital extensor M. and the dorsal aspect of the fetlock, over the distal end of metatarsal bone III

*Subtendinous bursa of the interosseous medius M.* (Fig. H5.29D)
A. *Landmarks*: the extensor branches of the interosseous medius M.
B. *Approach*: under the extensor branches of the interosseous medius M. as they obliquely cross the first phalanx

*Podotrochlear bursa* (Fig. H5.29D)
A. *Landmarks*: the navicular bone and the terminal tendon of the deep digital flexor within the hoof
B. *Approach*: on the plantar aspect of the digit, deep within the hoof, between the flexor surface of the navicular bone and the tendon of the deep digital flexor, between the two bulbs of the heels

16. **Medial patellar lig.** (Fig. H5.29B)
A. *Landmarks*: patella, medial ridge of femoral trochlea, tibial tuberosity
B. *Approach*: deep between the patellar cartilaginous process and the tibial tuberosity, along the medial aspect of the medial ridge of femoral trochlea

17. **Intraarticular approach for arthroscopy, arthrocentesis, and intraarticular analgesia**

*Coxofemoral (hip) joint* (Fig. H5.30A)

A. *Landmarks*: the cranial and caudal parts of the greater trochanter

B. *Approach*: A needle is introduced into the joint between the cranial and caudal parts of the greater trochanter through the trochanteric notch, along the femoral neck, and at a 45 degree angle with the sagittal plane.

*Femorotibiopatellar (stifle) joint*

α—Femoropatellar synovial sac (Fig. H5.30A,B)

A. *Landmarks*: patella, medial ridge of femoral trochlea, middle patellar lig.

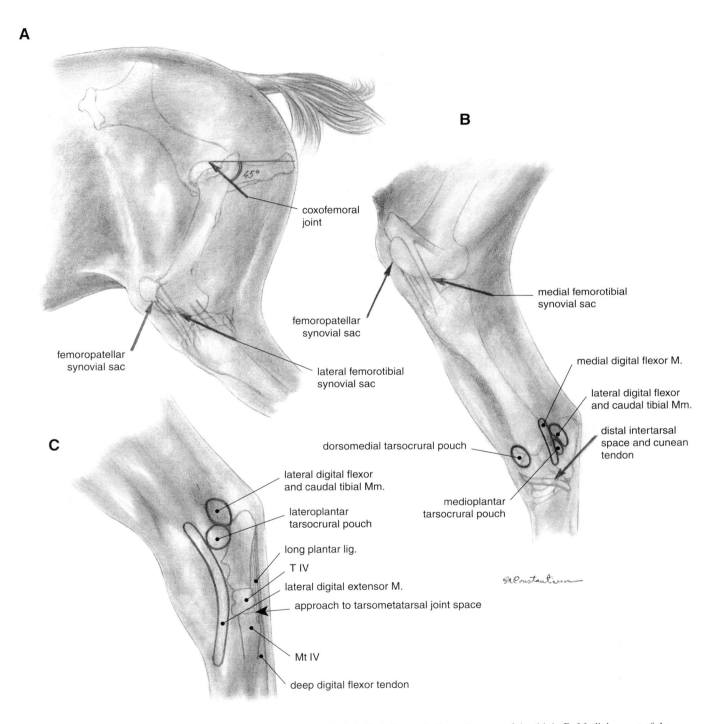

**A**

coxofemoral joint

femoropatellar synovial sac

femoropatellar synovial sac

lateral femorotibial synovial sac

**B**

medial femorotibial synovial sac

medial digital flexor M.

lateral digital flexor and caudal tibial Mm.

distal intertarsal space and cunean tendon

dorsomedial tarsocrural pouch

medioplantar tarsocrural pouch

**C**

lateral digital flexor and caudal tibial Mm.

lateroplantar tarsocrural pouch

long plantar lig.

T IV

lateral digital extensor M.

approach to tarsometatarsal joint space

Mt IV

deep digital flexor tendon

Fig. H5.30. Tendon sheaths, synovial and tendon sheath pouches of pelvic limb, horse. **A.** Lateral aspect of the thigh. **B.** Medial aspect of the crus and hock. **C.** Lateral aspect of the hock.

B. *Approach*: in the angle between the patellar apex, the patellar attachment of the middle patellar lig., and the medial ridge of the femoral trochlea

β—Lateral femorotibial synovial sac (Fig. H5.30A)
A. *Landmarks*: tibial tuberosity, patella, lateral patellar lig., lateral tibial condyle, extensor groove, lateral collateral lig. of stifle joint
B. *Approach*: between the lateral collateral lig. of the stifle and the lateral patellar lig., midway between the patella and the extensor groove (bordered by the tibial tuberosity and the lateral tibial condyle)

γ—Medial femorotibial synovial sac (Fig. H5.30B)
A. *Landmarks*: medial patellar lig., medial condyle of tibia
B. *Approach*: just proximal to the medial condyle of the tibia and the caudal border of the medial patellar lig.

*Tarsal (hock) joint*
α—Distal intertarsal joint space (Fig. H5.30B)
A. *Landmarks*: cunean tendon (of cranial tibial M.) on the medial aspect of the hock; the second, third, and central tarsal bones
B. *Approach*: dorsal to the cunean tendon, on the medial aspect of the hock, at the palpable intersection of the second, third, and central tarsal bones

β—Tarsocrural joint (dorsomedial pouch) (Fig. H5.30B)
A. *Landmarks*: medial malleolus of tibia, medial ridge of trochlea of talus
B. *Approach*: in the dorsal angle between the two landmarks

γ—Tarsocrural joint (medioplantar pouch) (Fig. H5.30B)
A. *Landmarks*: distal extremity of tibia, sustentaculum tali, tendons of the lateral digital flexor and caudal tibial Mm., tendon of the medial digital flexor M.
B. *Approach*: among the four landmarks

δ—Tarsocrural joint (lateroplantar pouch) (Fig. H5.30C)
A. *Landmarks*: lateral malleolus of tibia, calcaneus, tendon of lateral digital extensor M., tendon of lateral digital flexor M.
B. *Approach*: in the angle between the lateral malleolus of tibia and the calcaneus, in the space

between the tendons of the lateral digital extensor and lateral digital flexor Mm.

ε—Tarsometatarsal joint space (Fig. H5.30C)
A. *Landmarks*: the base (proximal end) of the fourth metatarsal bone, tarsal bone IV, long plantar lig., deep digital flexor tendon
B. *Approach*: immediately proximal and slightly dorsal to the base of the fourth metatarsal bone, on the lateral aspect of the hock, in the palpable depression between the landmarks

18. **Muscular bursae** (Fig. H5.31)
*Trochanteric bursa of superficial gluteal M.*
A. *Landmark*: third trochanter
B. *Approach*: through the skin and fascia lata, and deep between the third trochanter and the insertion of superficial gluteal M. on the third trochanter

*Trochanteric bursa of middle gluteal M.*
A. *Landmark*: the caudal part of the greater trochanter
B. *Approach*: through skin and gluteal fascia, deep and in a cranial position between the caudal part of the greater trochanter and the attachment of the middle gluteal M. on the greater trochanter

*Trochanteric bursa of accessory gluteal M.*
A. *Landmark*: the cranial part of the greater trochanter
B. *Approach*: through the skin and the gluteal fascia, deep between the tendon of accessory gluteal M. and the lateral aspect of the cranial part of the greater trochanter

*Trochanteric bursa of biceps femoris M.*
A. *Landmarks*: the caudal part of the greater trochanter, the cranial border of biceps femoris M.
B. *Approach*: through the skin and superficial lamina of fascia lata, deep between the caudal border of the caudal part of greater trochanter, and the cranial border of biceps femoris M.

*Ischiatic bursa of semitendinosus M.*
A. *Landmark*: ischiatic tuberosity
B. *Approach*: through the skin and superficial lamina of the fascia lata, deep between the semitendinosus M. and the ischiatic tuberosity

19. **Vaginal (synovial) tendon sheaths**
*Sheath of the cranial tibial M.* (Fig. H5.32)

A. *Landmarks*: dorsal aspect of the hock, the tendon of long digital extensor M. just above the tarsal area

B. *Approach*: through the skin, around the tendon of cranial tibial M. (deep to the fibularis tertius M.), on the distal third of the dorsal aspect of the crus, medial to and parallel with the tendon of the long digital extensor M.

*Sheath of the long digital extensor M.* (Fig. H5.32)
A. *Landmarks*: same as for the sheath of the cranial tibial M.
B. *Approach*: through the skin and the proper crural fascia, on the dorsal aspect of the hock, around

the tendon between the crural and tarsal retinacula

*Sheath of the lateral digital extensor M.* (Fig. H5.30C)
A. *Landmarks*: lateral aspect of the hock, tendon of lateral digital extensor M., lateral collateral lig. of hock joint, lateral malleolus
B. *Approach*: through the skin and tarsal fascia, around the tendon of the lateral digital extensor M., from the level of the lateral malleolus along the lateral collateral lig. of the hock joint, and to the junction between the tendons of the long and lateral digital extensor Mm.

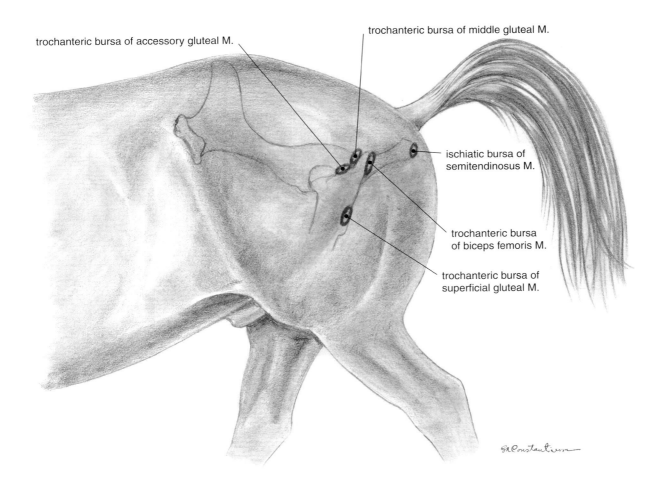

trochanteric bursa of accessory gluteal M.

trochanteric bursa of middle gluteal M.

ischiatic bursa of semitendinosus M.

trochanteric bursa of biceps femoris M.

trochanteric bursa of superficial gluteal M.

Fig. H5.31. Muscular bursae of proximal pelvic limb, horse, lateral aspect.

*Sheath of the lateral digital flexor and caudal tibial Mm.* (Fig. H5.30B,C)

A. *Landmarks*: sustentaculum tali, calcanean tuber, proximal medioplantar aspect of the hock, caudal border of the calcaneus covered by the long plantar lig., the deep group of caudal crural Mm.

B. *Approach*:

   a. Through the skin and flexor retinaculum on the medioplantar aspect of the hock, around the tendons of the lateral digital flexor and caudal tibial Mm., and close to the sustentaculum tali (dorsally) and calcanean tuber (laterally)

   b. On the lateroplantar aspect of the hock, around the same tendons and between the cranial (dorsal) border of the calcanean tuber and the deep group of caudal crural Mm.

*Sheath of the medial digital flexor M.* (Fig. H5.30B)

A. *Landmarks*: medial collateral lig. of the hock joint

B. *Approach*: through skin and tarsal fascia and around the tendon, caudal to and parallel with the medial collateral lig. of the hock joint

20. **Accessory (check) lig. of deep digital flexor M.** (see the similar structure in The Thoracic Limb, page 205). It is significantly smaller than its counterpart on the forelimb.

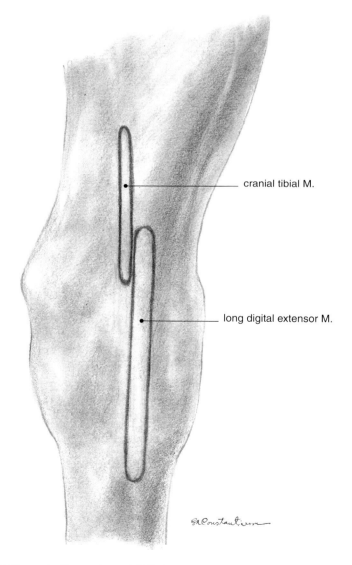

cranial tibial M.

long digital extensor M.

Fig. H5.32. Tendon sheaths on the dorsal aspect of tarsus, horse, left limb.

# H 6

## The Thoracic Limb

The bones of the thoracic limb as a whole, and the separate bones starting with the **scapula** and continuing with the **humerus**, **radius and ulna**, **carpal bones**, **metacarpal bones**, and the **phalanges** are illustrated in Figures H6.1–H6.7.

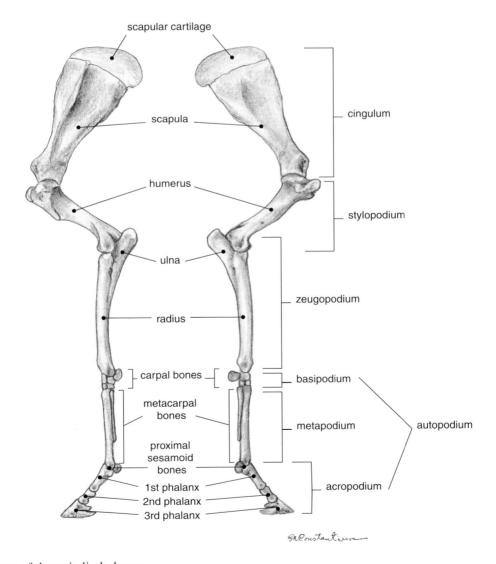

Fig. H6.1. Skeleton of thoracic limb, horse.

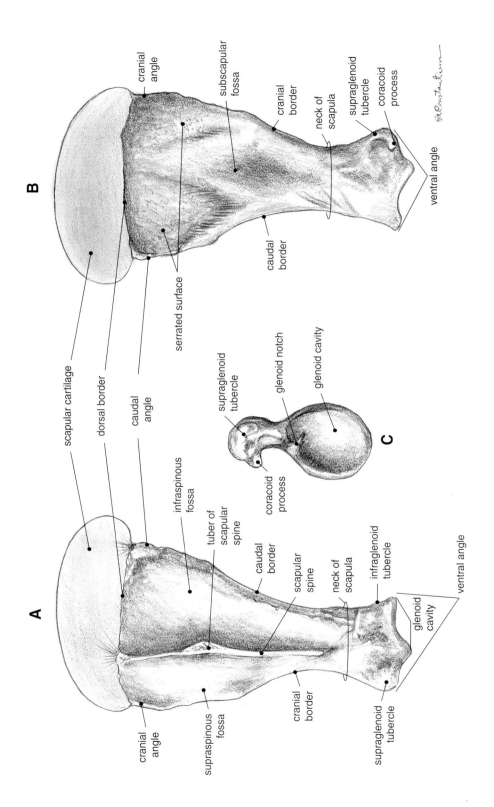

cranial angle

subscapular fossa

cranial border

neck of scapula

supraglenoid tubercle

coracoid process

ventral angle

caudal border

serrated surface

**B**

scapular cartilage

dorsal border

caudal angle

glenoid notch

glenoid cavity

supraglenoid tubercle

coracoid process

**C**

infraspinous fossa

tuber of scapular spine

caudal border

scapular spine

neck of scapula

infraglenoid tubercle

ventral angle

cranial angle

supraspinous fossa

cranial border

glenoid cavity

supraglenoid tubercle

**A**

Fig. H6.2. Left scapula, horse. **A.** Lateral aspect. **B.** Medial aspect (costal surface). **C.** Ventral angle.

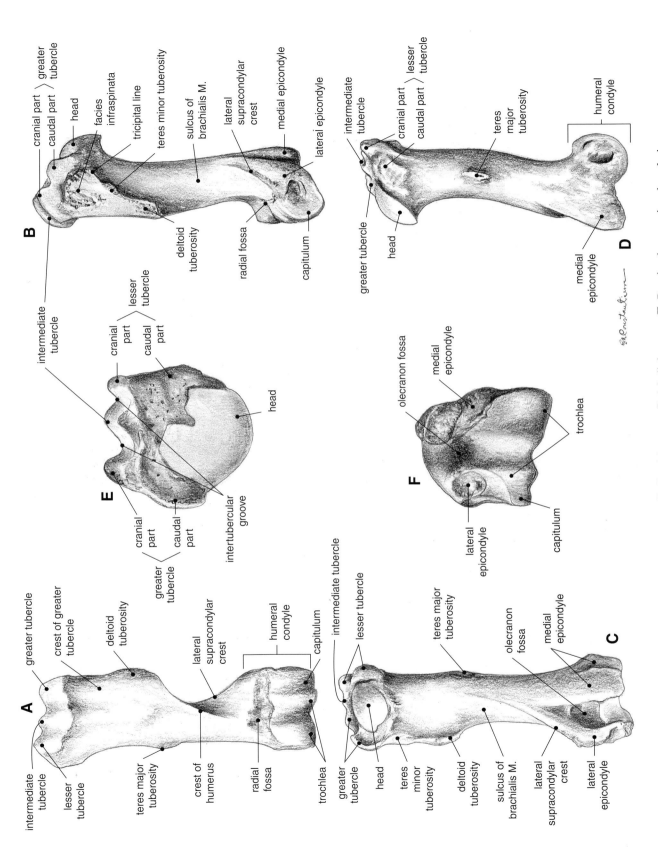

Fig. H6.3. Left humerus, horse. **A.** Cranial aspect. **B.** Lateral aspect. **C.** Caudal aspect. **D.** Medial aspect. **E.** Proximal extremity, dorsal *view.* **F.** Distal extremity, ventral *view.*

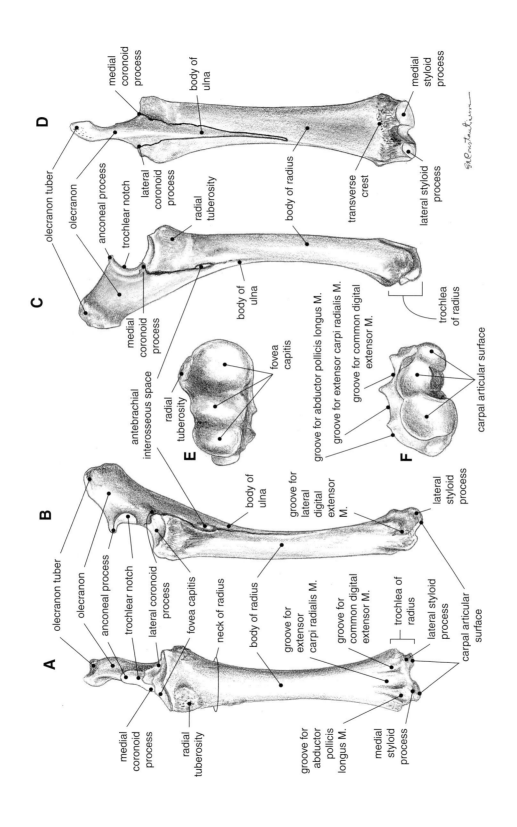

Fig. H6.4. Left radius and ulna, horse. **A.** Cranial aspect. **B.** Lateral aspect. **C.** Medial aspect. **D.** Caudal aspect. **E.** Proximal extremity, dorsal view. **F.** Distal extremity, ventral view.

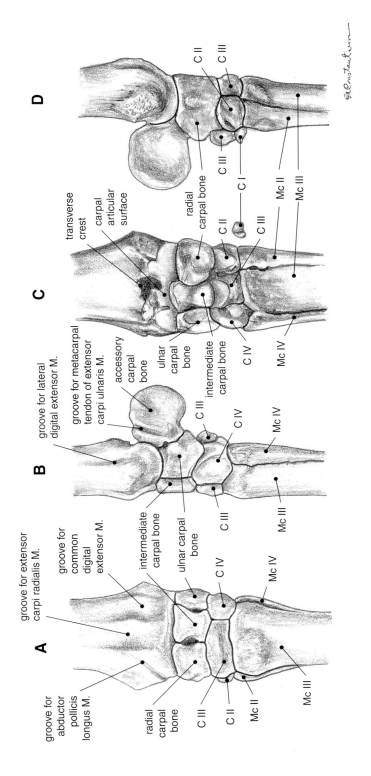

Fig. H6.5. Left carpal bones, horse. **A.** Dorsal aspect. **B.** Lateral aspect. **C.** Palmar aspect (the accessory carpal bone has been removed). **D.** Medial aspect.

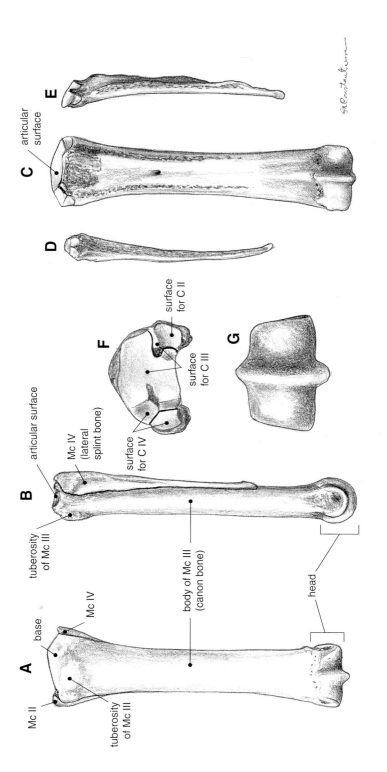

Fig. H6.6. Left metacarpal bones, horse. **A.** Dorsal aspect. **B.** Lateral aspect. **C.** Mc III, plantar aspect. **D.** Lateral splint bone. **E.** Medial splint bone. **F.** Articular surface of Mc III (dorsal view). **G.** Head of Mc III (ventral view).

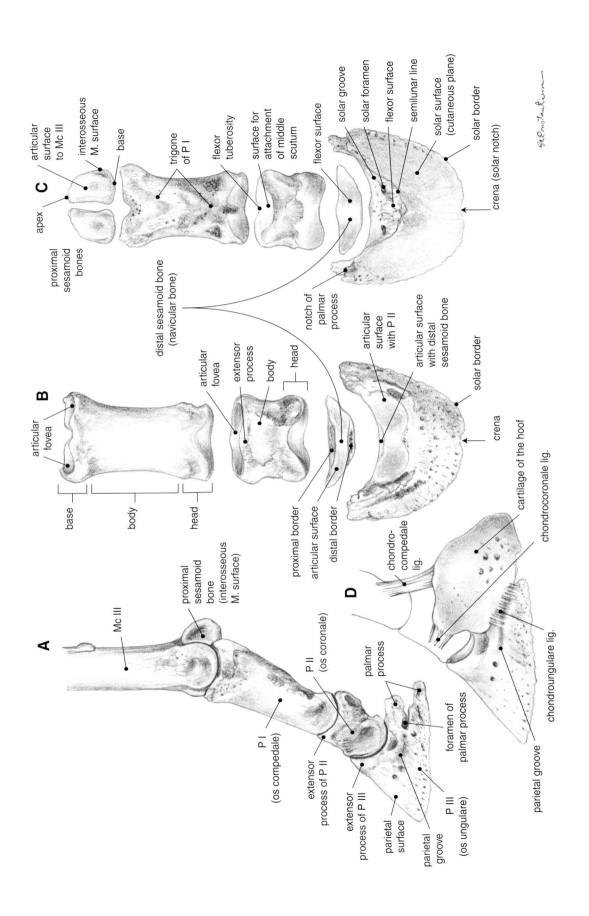

Fig. H6.7. The phalanges and sesamoid bones, horse, thoracic limb. **A.** Lateral/medial aspect. **B.** Dorsal aspect. **C.** Palmar aspect. **D.** Cartilage of the hoof with ligaments (abaxial aspect).

The **scapulohumeral (shoulder) joint**, the **humerora-dioulnar (elbow) joint**, the **carpal joint**, the **metacar-pophalangeal (fetlock) joint**, the **first interphalangeal** (pastern) joint, and the **second interphalangeal (coffin or navicular) joint** are illustrated in Figures H6.8–H6.11.

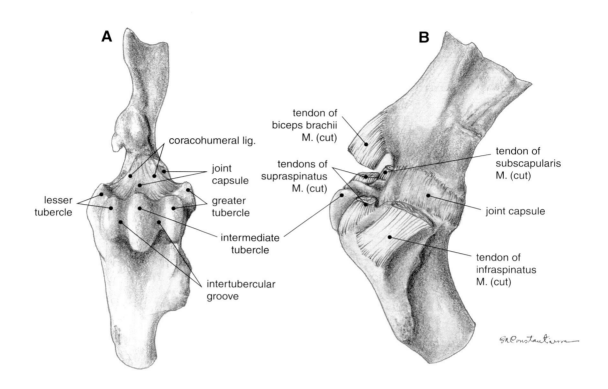

Fig. H6.8. Left scapulohumeral (shoulder) joint in the horse. **A.** Cranial aspect. **B.** Lateral aspect.

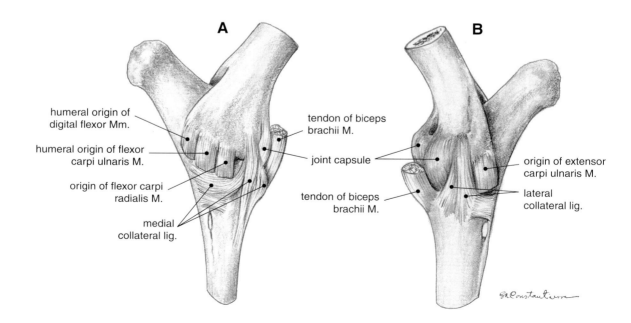

Fig. H6.9. Left humeroradioulnar (elbow) joint in the horse. **A.** Medial aspect. **B.** Lateral aspect.

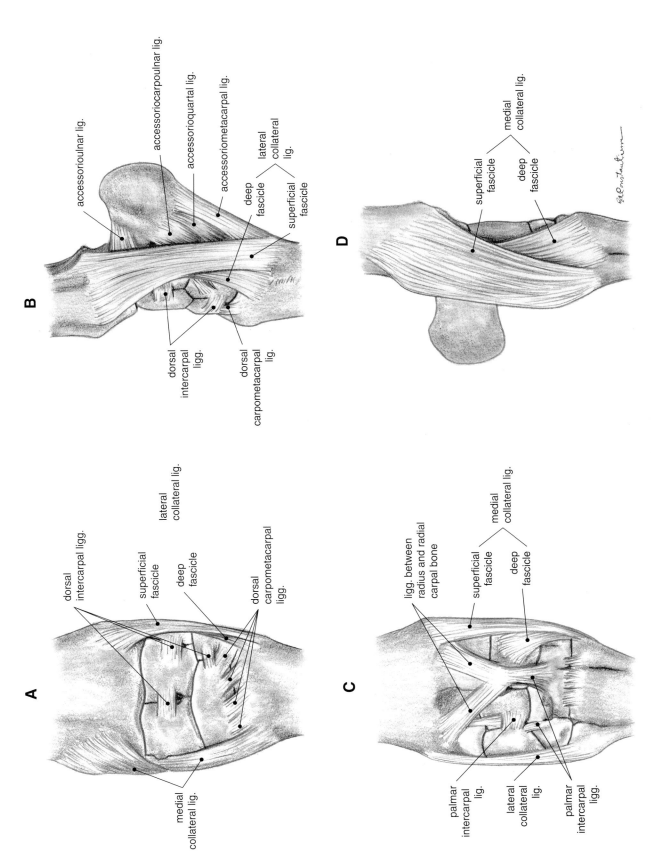

Fig. H6.10. Left carpal joints, horse. **A.** Dorsal aspect. **B.** Lateral aspect. **C.** Palmar aspect. **D.** Medial aspect.

A

dorsal
intercarpal ligg.

lateral
collateral lig.

superficial
fascicle

deep
fascicle

dorsal
carpometacarpal
ligg.

medial
collateral lig.

B

accessorioulnar lig.

accessoriocarpoulnar lig.

accessorioquartal lig.

accessoriometacarpal lig.

deep
fascicle

lateral
collateral
lig.

superficial
fascicle

dorsal
intercarpal
ligg.

dorsal
carpometacarpal
lig.

C

ligg. between
radius and radial
carpal bone

medial
collateral lig.

superficial
fascicle

deep
fascicle

palmar
intercarpal
lig.

lateral
collateral
lig.

palmar
intercarpal
ligg.

D

medial
collateral lig.

superficial
fascicle

deep
fascicle

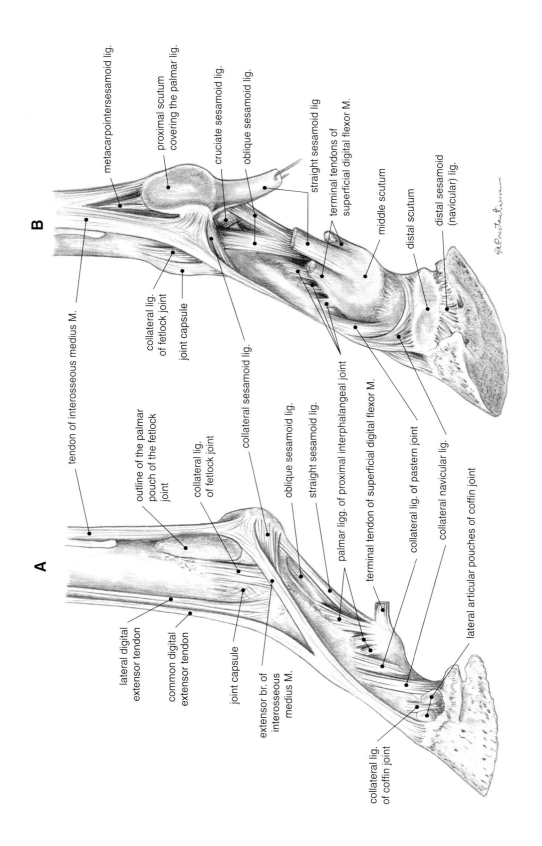

lateral digital
extensor tendon

common digital
extensor tendon

joint capsule

extensor br. of
interosseous
medius M.

collateral lig.
of coffin joint

tendon of interosseous medius M.

outline of the palmar
pouch of the fetlock
joint

collateral lig.
of fetlock joint

collateral sesamoid lig.

oblique sesamoid lig.

straight sesamoid lig.

palmar ligg. of proximal interphalangeal joint

terminal tendon of superficial digital flexor M.

collateral lig. of pastern joint

collateral navicular lig.

lateral articular pouches of coffin joint

A

B

metacarpointersesamoid lig.

proximal scutum
covering the palmar lig.

cruciate sesamoid lig.

oblique sesamoid lig.

straight sesamoid lig

terminal tendons of
superficial digital flexor M.

middle scutum

distal scutum

distal sesamoid
(navicular) lig.

collateral lig.
of fetlock joint

joint capsule

Fig. H6.11. The metacarpophalangeal and interphalangeal joints in the horse. **A.** Lateral/medial aspect. **B.** Palmar aspect.

As in the dissection of the pelvic limb, some important landmarks for physical examination and/or clinical approach should first be identified. Check them with the skeleton.

*Turn the thoracic limb so that the lateral aspect is up and identify by palpation the following landmarks: the caudal angle of the scapula, the tuber of the scapular spine, the supraglenoid tubercle, the greater tubercle of the humerus, the tendon of the infraspinatus M., the deltoid tuberosity, the humeral crest, the olecranon, the elbow, the lateral epicondyle of the humerus, the accessory carpal bone, the carpus, the lateral styloid process of the radius, the accessoriometacarpal lig., the third metacarpal bone (canon bone), the fourth metacarpal bone (the lateral splint bone), the tendons of the interosseous medius, deep digital flexor (DDF), and superficial digital flexor (SDF) Mm., the ergot, the proximal sesamoid bones, the metacarpophalangeal joint (fetlock joint), the first phalanx (pastern), the coronet (the narrow area along the dorsal border of the hoof), and the hoof (the wall, with the toe, quarters, heels, and the bulbs of the heels; the sole; and the frog).*

*In the forearm (antebrachium), identify the two longitudinal grooves: the craniolateral groove, which separates the extensor carpi radialis M. from the common digital extensor M., and the caudolateral groove, which separates the common digital extensor M. from the extensor carpi ulnaris M. Notice that the lateral digital extensor M. lies in the caudolateral groove.*

*Turn the limb medial side up and identify by palpation the following structures: the coracoid process of the scapula, the lesser tubercle of the humerus, the teres major tuberosity, the elbow, the radial and olecranon fossae, the medial epicondyle of the humerus, the radial tuberosity, the interosseous space between radius and the ulna, the body (shaft) of the radius, the medial styloid process of the radius, the carpal joint, the second metacarpal bone (the medial splint bone), and the tendons, bones, and joints that were already identified on the lateral side of the limb.*

*In the antebrachium, palpate the chestnut one hand proximal to the carpus. A vertical line passing through the chestnut separates the flexor carpi radialis M. (cranially) from the flexor carpi ulnaris M. (caudally). Also palpate the medial aspect of the radius and the two vertical grooves between it and the extensor carpi radialis M. (cranially) and flexor carpi radialis M. (caudally).*

The tendon of the supraspinatus M. and the greater tubercle of the humerus are landmarks for scapulohumeral arthroscopy.

The supraglenoid tubercle and the greater tubercle of the humerus are prone to fractures.

The scapular spine is a landmark during the surgical treatment of suprascapular nerve injury (sweeny).

The olecranon and the ulna are commonly susceptible to fractures.

The diagnosis of osteochondral fractures of the carpal bones (carpal chips), accessory carpal bone fractures, carpal hygroma (an inflammation on the dorsal aspect of carpus), and other pathological conditions of the carpus are based on knowledge of the bones, joints, and tendons running over the carpus.

The metacarpal bones, the phalanges, and the proximal sesamoid bones are susceptible to various forms of fractures. Even though the distal sesamoid (navicular) bone is not palpable, it is involved in the so-called "navicular syndrome or navicular disease."

It is important to know all the landmarks listed above that are used to identify injection sites for the regional anesthesia of different nerves, and the approaches to bones, joints, bursae, and other structures.

Skin the limb up to the fetlock and proceed with removal of the hoof. Here is the technique: While one student holds the limb firmly in contact with the table and a second holds the fetlock and the pastern, a third student sections the hoof through the quarters with a saw. If the pastern is fixed in a vice, only one person is needed to perform the sectioning of the hoof. The line of section should be parallel to the long axis of the digit. The use of a wide-bladed saw is suggested. In addition, the thumb of the free hand should make contact with the side of the blade to avoid cutting the fingers. Section the hoof as deep as the third phalanx (the sound is different when the saw is penetrating the bone). With large pliers, first remove the heel, then the rest of the wall, the frog, and the sole. Skin the digit.

*Caution!* Do not skin the digit before removing the hoof.

The hoof might also be removed by boiling the digit for at least one hour. With the limb tied in a vice, the hoof can then be easily pulled out.

Before the dissection of the limb begins, look at the systematization of the muscles listed in Table H6.1.

Begin the dissection of the medial aspect of the thoracic limb by examining the pectoral muscles that were transected while removing the limb. Separate them from each other and at the same time save the vessels and nerves. Identify the **lateral pectoral groove**, between the medial

Table H6.1. Muscles of the Thoracic Limb, Horse

**Shoulder**

*Lateral aspect*
– deltoideus
– supraspinatus
– infraspinatus
– teres minor

*Medial aspect*
– teres major
– subscapularis
– coracobrachialis
– articularis humeri

**Arm**

*Cranial aspect*
- biceps brachii
  • lacertus fibrosus
- brachialis

*Caudal aspect*
– triceps brachii
  • long head
  • lateral head
  • medial head
– anconeus
– tensor fasciae antebrachii

**Forearm**

*Craniolateral aspect*
– extensor carpi radialis
– abductor pollicis longus } muscles with proximal action (to the carpus)
– extensor carpi ulnaris (ulnaris lateralis)
– common digital extensor } muscles with distal action (to the digit)
– lateral digital extensor
– accessory muscles of the common and lateral digital extensors

*Caudomedial aspect*
– flexor carpi ulnaris [with proximal action (to the carpus)]
  • humeral head
  • ulnar head
– flexor carpi radialis [with proximal action (to the carpus)]
– pronator teres (atrophied) [with proximal action (to the carpus)]
– superficial digital flexor [with distal action (to the digit)]
  • sleeve at the level of metacarpophalangeal joint
  • proximal check lig.
– deep digital flexor [with distal action (to the digit)]
  • humeral head
  • ulnar head
  • radial head
  • digital check lig.
  • transverse lamina

*Autopodium*
– lumbricales Mm.
– interosseus medius (III)
– interossei lateralis (IV) and medialis (II) Mm.

border of the **brachiocephalicus M.** and the lateral border of the **descending pectoral M.**

*Remember.* The brachial segment of the **cephalic V.** and the **deltoid branch of the superficial cervical A.** lie in the lateral pectoral groove (Fig. H6.12).

Identify the remnants of the **rhomboideus cervicis** and **thoracis Mm.** and the **serratus ventralis cervicis** and **thoracis Mm.** at the junction where the limb was totally removed from the body wall.

*Notice* the **median pectoral groove**, which separates the two symmetrical descending pectoral Mm.

Deep to the lateral pectoral groove, identify the **subclavius M.**

Separate the descending pectoral M. from the **transverse pectoral M.** The descending pectoral M. is attached to the **humeral crest**, whereas the transverse pectoral M. exceeds the **elbow** and fuses with the **superficial antebrachial fascia** (located only on the medial aspect of the forearm), acting as the tensor of that fascia.

*Remember.* The descending and transverse pectoral Mm. are collectively called the **superficial pectoral Mm.**

Identify and dissect the **external thoracic A.** and **V.**, which are accompanied by a branch of the **lateral thoracic N.** (Fig. H6.12).

Remove the **ascending (deep) pectoral M.** saving only its attachments on both the **greater** and **lesser tubercles of the humerus.** Reflect the superficial pectoral Mm. ventrally to expose the medial aspect of the arm. The **medial brachial fascia** covers and protects all the structures, sending separate sheets around the **coracobrachialis**, **brachialis**, and **biceps brachii Mm.** and around the vessels and nerves. Make a longitudinal incision in that fascia, reflect it, and dissect the muscles (Fig. H6.13) and the vessels and nerves (Fig. H6.14).

Table H6.2 shows the muscles and nerve supply of the thoracic limb in the horse.

Figure H6.15 shows a schematic representation of the **brachial plexus** and the muscles supplied by the nerves of this plexus.

For an easy dissection of the brachial plexus, build a wire or wood Y-shaped device and try to hang the plexus on top of it; then fix the "Y" in the **subscapularis M.** All the nerves of the plexus will be tensed and isolated from the adjacent structures of the limb, easy to identify and dissect.

For a better identification of the nerves, here is the systematization of the two categories of nerves originating from the brachial plexus.

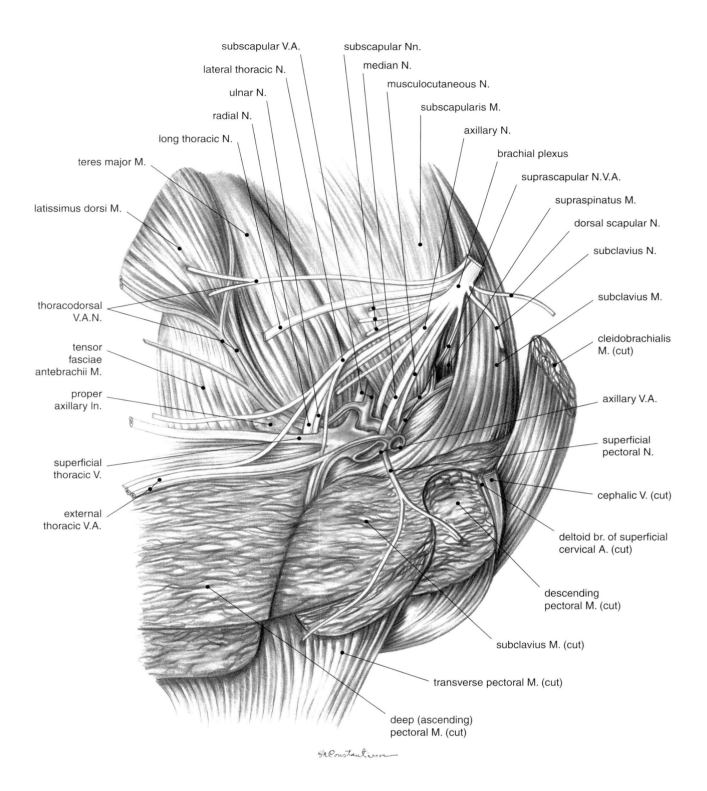

subscapular V.A.

subscapular Nn.

lateral thoracic N.

median N.

ulnar N.

musculocutaneous N.

radial N.

subscapularis M.

long thoracic N.

axillary N.

teres major M.

brachial plexus

latissimus dorsi M.

suprascapular N.V.A.

supraspinatus M.

dorsal scapular N.

subclavius N.

thoracodorsal V.A.N.

subclavius M.

cleidobrachialis M. (cut)

tensor fasciae antebrachii M.

proper axillary ln.

axillary V.A.

superficial pectoral N.

superficial thoracic V.

cephalic V. (cut)

external thoracic V.A.

deltoid br. of superficial cervical A. (cut)

descending pectoral M. (cut)

subclavius M. (cut)

transverse pectoral M. (cut)

deep (ascending) pectoral M. (cut)

Fig. H6.12. Structures of the medial aspect of the shoulder and pectoral region, horse, left thoracic limb.

*Nerves supplying the intrinsic muscles of the forelimb:*

- suprascapular N.
- subscapular N.
- axillary N.
- musculocutaneous N.
- median N.
- ulnar N.
- radial N.

*Nerves supplying the extrinsic muscles of the forelimb:*

- cranial to the axis of the limb
  - dorsal scapular N. (for the rhomboideus cervicis and serratus ventralis cervicis Mm.)
  - subclavius N. (for the subclavius M.)
  - cranial pectoral Nn. (for the superficial pectoral Mm.)
- caudal to the axis of the limb
  - thoracodorsal N. (for the latissimus dorsi M.)
  - long thoracic N. (for the serratus ventralis thoracis M.)
  - lateral thoracic N. (for the cutaneous trunci M.)
  - caudal pectoral Nn. (for the ascending pectoral M.)

Follow the course of the **suprascapular N.**, which penetrates the space between the **supraspinatus** and **subscapularis Mm.**, accompanied by the **suprascapular A.** and **V.** The nerve passes over the **neck of the scapula** at the distal end of the **scapular spine**.

**Damage to the suprascapular nerve results in instability of the shoulder, a condition called "sweeney" (shoulder atrophy, slipped shoulder). This is a neurogenic atrophy due to damage to the suprascapular N., which supplies the supraspinatus and infraspinatus Mm.** *Remember!* **The supraspinatus M. is the only extensor of the shoulder.**

Dissect the **subscapular N.**, which divides into many branches. The **axillary N.** penetrates between the subscapularis and **teres major Mm.** crossing the **subscapular A.** and **V.** on the caudal aspect of the **shoulder joint**. Trace the subscapular A. and identify its branches, the **caudal circumflex humeral**, **circumflex scapular**, and **thoracodorsal Aa.**; the thoracodorsal A. parallels the **thoracodorsal N.** Identify and dissect the **superficial thoracic V. (the spur V.)**, specific to the horse, a branch of the **thoracodorsal V.** without an arterial satellite (Figs. H6.12, H6.14). The **proper axillary lnn.** are found in the angle between the axillary and subscapular arteries.

Dissect the nerves and vessels that travel in the brachial area. Several landmarks are suggested to ease the identification of the structures, as follows. The **musculocutaneous** and **median Nn.** travel cranial to the **brachial A.**, whereas the **ulnar** and **radial Nn.** pass caudal to the artery. The musculocutaneous N. crosses the lateral aspect of the **axillary A.**, while the median N. crosses its medial aspect; they communicate with each other, making a loop that resembles a hinge, or sling, around the artery, which is called the **axillary loop** (see Fig. H6.14).

*Notice* that the **cranial pectoral Nn.** originate from the axillary loop.

Carefully dissect the **proximal muscular branch** of the musculocutaneous N., which penetrates, with the **cranial circumflex humeral A.** and **V.**, between the two parts of the coracobrachialis M. This nerve supplies the coracobrachialis and biceps brachii Mm.

Trace the brachial A. distally and identify the **bicipital** and **transverse cubital Aa.**, in a cranial direction, and the **deep brachial** and **collateral ulnar Aa.**, in a caudal direction. Identify the **cubital lnn.**, specific to the horse, at the origin of the collateral ulnar A. (see Fig. H6.14).

*Notice* that the deep brachial A. accompanies the radial N., passing with it between the coracobrachialis and the **triceps brachii Mm.**, whereas the collateral ulnar A. accompanies the ulnar N.

*Note.* The arteries and veins accompanying nerves are called "collateral."

Pull out the **latissimus dorsi M.** and gently separate it from the **tensor fasciae antebrachii M.** by introducing the hand between the tensor fasciae antebrachii M. and the **long head of the triceps brachii M.** The aponeurosis of the tensor fasciae antebrachii M. fuses with that of the latissimus dorsi M. (see Fig. H6.14), forming a fibrous sulcus for guiding the terminal tendon of the **teres major M.**, on its way to the teres tuberosity.

At approximately the same level with the bicipital A., the musculocutaneous N. separates from the median N. and distributes its **distal muscular branch** (to the **brachialis M.**) and the **medial cutaneous antebrachial N.** (see Fig. H6.14).

Turn the limb lateral side up.

*Caution.* When dissecting the muscles of the lateral scapular area, do not remove the **axillary fascia**. For aesthetic purposes leave it intact, because the fascia is almost fused with the muscles, and the separation is quite impossible.

Dissect the lateral muscles of the shoulder (Fig. H6.16) and reflect the **deltoid M.** caudally to expose the insertions of the infraspinatus and **teres minor Mm.** (Fig. H6.17).

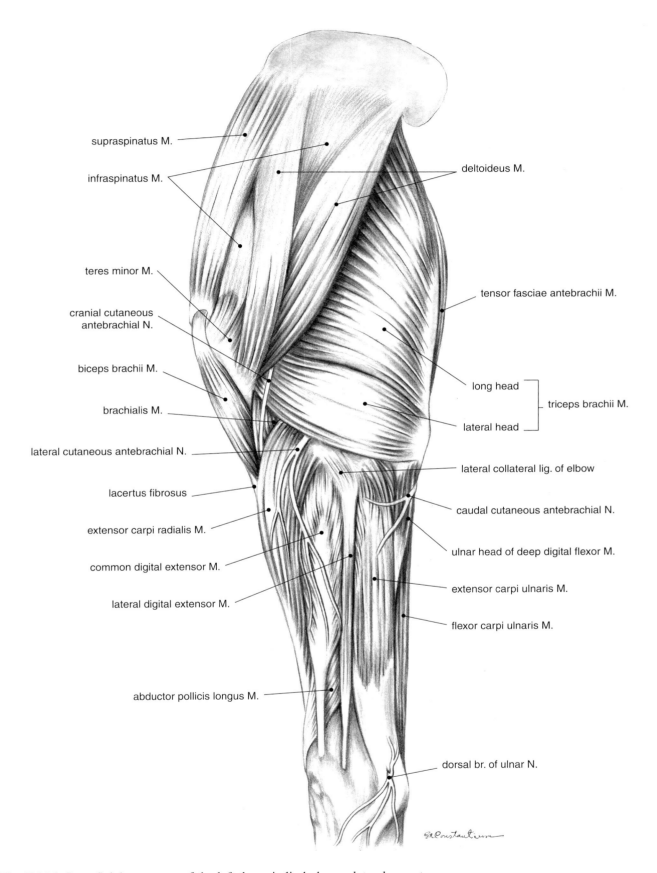

supraspinatus M.

infraspinatus M.

deltoideus M.

teres minor M.

tensor fasciae antebrachii M.

cranial cutaneous
antebrachial N.

biceps brachii M.

long head

brachialis M.

lateral head

triceps brachii M.

lateral cutaneous antebrachial N.

lateral collateral lig. of elbow

lacertus fibrosus

caudal cutaneous antebrachial N.

extensor carpi radialis M.

ulnar head of deep digital flexor M.

common digital extensor M.

extensor carpi ulnaris M.

lateral digital extensor M.

flexor carpi ulnaris M.

abductor pollicis longus M.

dorsal br. of ulnar N.

Fig. H6.16. Superficial structures of the left thoracic limb, horse, lateral aspect.

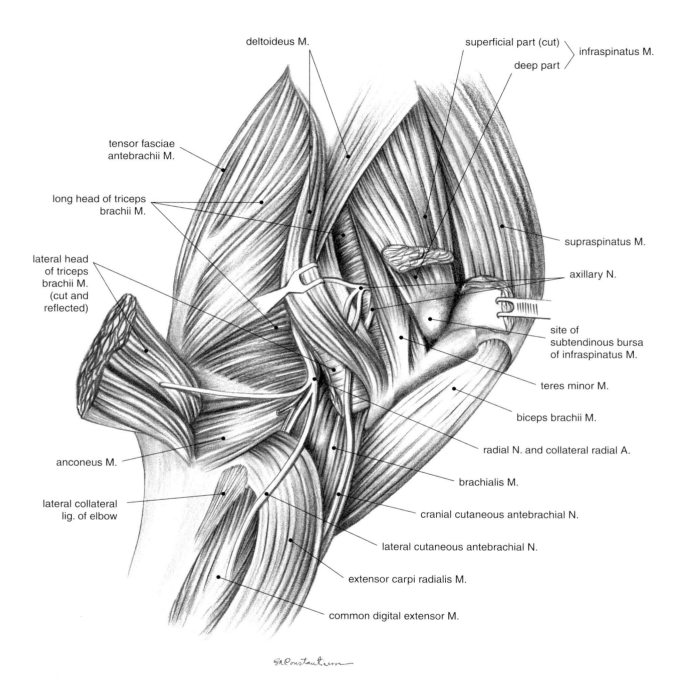

deltoideus M.

superficial part (cut)

deep part

infraspinatus M.

tensor fasciae antebrachii M.

long head of triceps brachii M.

lateral head of triceps brachii M. (cut and reflected)

supraspinatus M.

axillary N.

site of subtendinous bursa of infraspinatus M.

teres minor M.

biceps brachii M.

radial N. and collateral radial A.

anconeus M.

lateral collateral lig. of elbow

brachialis M.

cranial cutaneous antebrachial N.

lateral cutaneous antebrachial N.

extensor carpi radialis M.

common digital extensor M.

Fig. H6.17. Deep structures of the right thoracic limb, horse, lateral aspect.

*Notice* that the infraspinatus M. has two portions close to its insertion, one superficial, and one deep (see Fig. H6.17). Transect the superficial to expose the deep portion.

The **subtendinous bursa of the infraspinatus M.** is located between the superficial part of the tendon and the caudal part of the greater tubercle of humerus. Transect the distal end of the supraspinatus M. distal to the route of the suprascapular N. and expose it fully. (Trace the nerve from the point of entry between the subscapularis and the supraspinatus Mm. and estimate the level of transection of the supraspinatus M.)

Caudal to the teres minor M., the **axillary N.** and the **caudal circumflex humeral A.** and **V.** are visible. One of the branches of the axillary N. exceeds the deltoid M. caudal to the **deltoid tuberosity** and becomes the **cranial cutaneous antebrachial N.** (see Fig. H6.17).

Dissect the **long** and **lateral heads of the triceps brachii M.** Transect the lateral head in the middle, reflect the stumps, and expose the radial N., accompanied by the **collateral radial A.** and **V.** At the ventral border of this muscle, the radial N. sends the **lateral cutaneous antebrachial N.** deep to the lateral head. Identify a portion of the long head, the **anconeus M.**, and a portion of the brachialis M. (see Fig. H6.17).

Stay on the lateral aspect of the limb and continue to dissect the structures of the forearm (see Fig. H6.16). Start the dissection proximal to the carpus, where the tendons of the extensors are detectable under the fascia (the **extensor carpi radialis**, the **common** and **lateral digital extensors**, the **abductor pollicis longus**, and the **extensor carpi ulnaris Mm.**). Make an incision in the long axis of each tendon and introduce the blade of the scalpel under the fascia with the blade parallel to the tendon. Continue the incision of the fascia proximally, up to the origin of each muscle. Reflect and remove the fascia, freeing the muscles one by one. All tendons running over the dorsal aspect of the carpus are accompanied by tendon sheaths. Here the tendons are bound down by the **extensor retinaculum**, which is the continuation of the **proper antebrachial fascia** over the carpus. Between the extensor retinaculum and the **dorsal joint capsule** several septa that completely separate the tendons from each other are formed. The tendon sheaths extend proximal and distal to the extensor retinaculum.

During this procedure protect the cutaneous antebrachial nerves (in addition to those listed above, dissect the **caudal cutaneous antebrachial N.** and the **dorsal branch of the ulnar N.**) and the superficial vein (the cephalic V.). *Notice* that the dorsal branch of the ulnar N. exits between the two distal tendons of the extensor carpi ulnaris. The lateral extensor M. is very thin and is located between the common digital extensor and the extensor carpi ulnaris Mm.

Transect the common digital extensor M. in the middle and reflect it to expose the radial N., the **collateral radial A.**, the **cranial interosseous A.**, and the **accessory M. of the common digital extensor M.** (the muscle of Thiernesse, not listed in the *N.A.V.*). Also, at the caudal border of the common digital extensor M., find a very thin tendon, which will join the lateral digital extensor tendon in the middle third of the metacarpus; this is the **accessory M. of the lateral digital extensor M.** (the muscle of Phillips, also not mentioned in the *N.A.V.*) (see Fig. H6.18). *Note.* The muscles of Thiernesse and Phillips are rudimentary, not important, but they are there.

Turn the limb medial side up and first focus on the **elbow.** Dissect the **lacertus fibrosus**, a connecting fibrous structure between the tendons of the biceps brachii and the extensor carpi radialis Mm., which is a landmark for the apparent origin of the **medial cutaneous antebrachial N.** (Fig. H6.19) and for regional anesthesia (see Modlab R2).

Make an incision in the transverse pectoral M. and the superficial antebrachial fascia in the longitudinal axis of the forearm, and reflect the fascia protecting the antebrachial segment of the cephalic V., the **accessory cephalic V.**, the medial cutaneous antebrachial N., and the **median cubital V.** The latter connects the cephalic V. to the **brachial V.** (see Fig. H6.19). The proper antebrachial fascia is now exposed.

*Note.* There are two layers of the **antebrachial fascia**: superficial and deep (or proper). The deep antebrachial fascia surrounds the entire forearm, whereas the **superficial antebrachial fascia** overlaps the deep fascia only on the medial aspect of the forearm. The tensor of the deep fascia is the tensor fasciae antebrachii, whereas the tensor of the superficial fascia is the transverse pectoral M.

Using same technique described for the lateral aspect of the forearm, dissect the superficial muscles of the medial aspect, the **flexor carpi radialis** and the **flexor carpi ulnaris Mm.**, and on the proximal third of the region, the muscular part of the **ulnar head of the DDF M.** *Notice* that the flexor carpi ulnaris M. has two heads, the **humeral head** (the main one) and the **ulnar head.** The distal end of the brachialis M. and the **medial collateral lig. of the elbow joint** will also be exposed proximally. Distally, only part of the **humeral head of the DDF M.** is shown, between the other two muscles (see Fig. H6.19).

*Note.* The deep digital flexor M. (DDF) has three heads: humeral, ulnar, and radial.

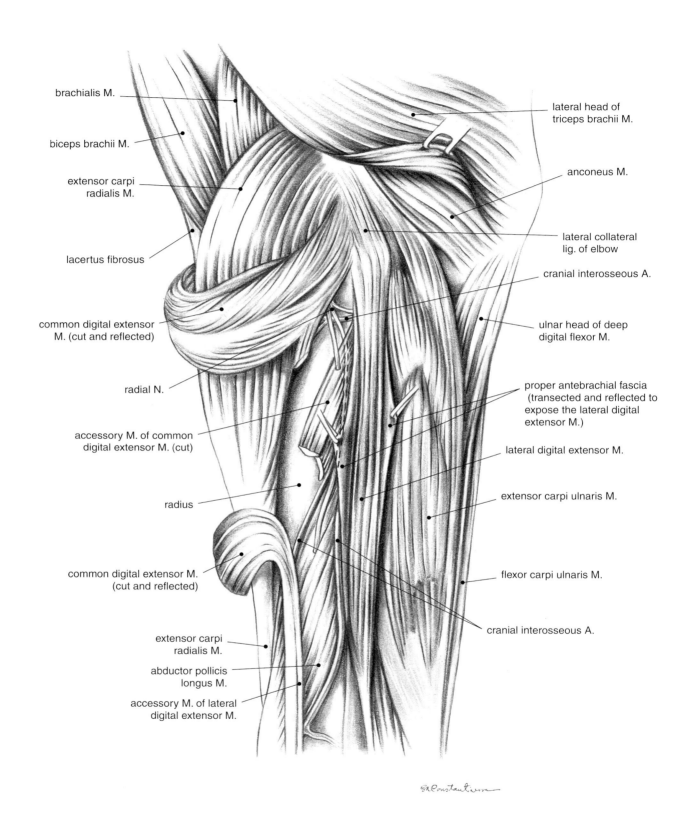

brachialis M.

biceps brachii M.

extensor carpi
radialis M.

lacertus fibrosus

common digital extensor
M. (cut and reflected)

radial N.

accessory M. of common
digital extensor M. (cut)

radius

common digital extensor M.
(cut and reflected)

extensor carpi
radialis M.

abductor pollicis
longus M.

accessory M. of lateral
digital extensor M.

lateral head of
triceps brachii M.

anconeus M.

lateral collateral
lig. of elbow

cranial interosseous A.

ulnar head of deep
digital flexor M.

proper antebrachial fascia
(transected and reflected to
expose the lateral digital
extensor M.)

lateral digital extensor M.

extensor carpi ulnaris M.

flexor carpi ulnaris M.

cranial interosseous A.

Fig. H6.18. Deep structures of the left forearm, horse, lateral aspect.

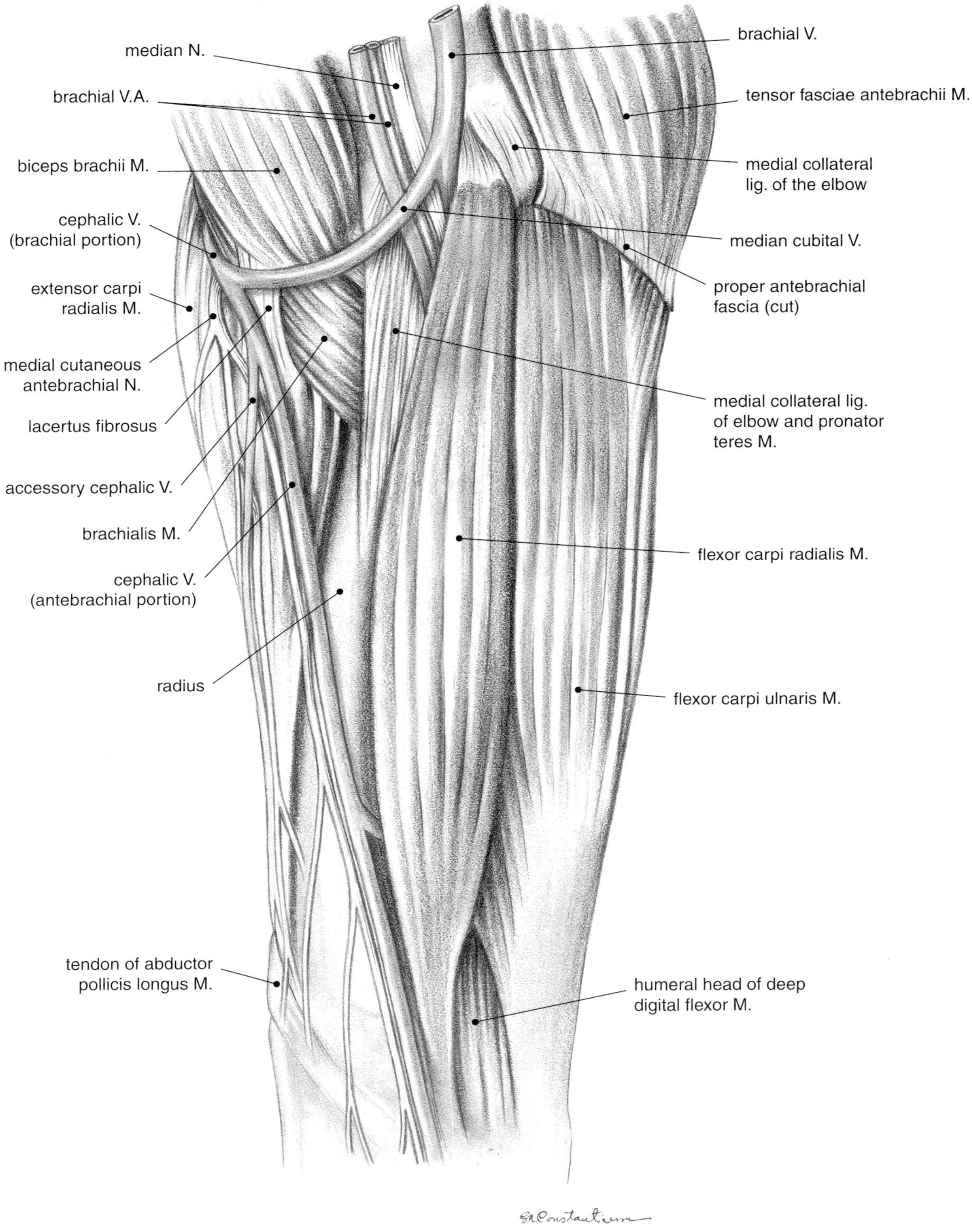

median N.

brachial V.A.

biceps brachii M.

cephalic V.
(brachial portion)

extensor carpi
radialis M.

medial cutaneous
antebrachial N.

lacertus fibrosus

accessory cephalic V.

brachialis M.

cephalic V.
(antebrachial portion)

radius

tendon of abductor
pollicis longus M.

brachial V.

tensor fasciae antebrachii M.

medial collateral
lig. of the elbow

median cubital V.

proper antebrachial
fascia (cut)

medial collateral lig.
of elbow and pronator
teres M.

flexor carpi radialis M.

flexor carpi ulnaris M.

humeral head of deep
digital flexor M.

SRConstantine

Fig. H6.19. Superficial structures of the right forearm, horse, medial aspect.

*Notice* that the medial and lateral collateral ligg. have twisted fibers, to minimize the muscular contraction during the flexion and extension of the elbow. Also *notice* that sometimes the **pronator teres M.** is present (usually not), attached to the medial collateral lig.

Leaving 2–3 cm of the proper antebrachial fascia attached to the tensor fasciae antebrachii M., reflect this muscle caudally. Expose the **medial head of the triceps brachii M.** and dissect the ulnar N. and the collateral ulnar A. and V. Continue to dissect the brachial A. and V. (Vv.) and the median N., obliquely crossing the elbow. Transect the flexor carpi radialis and the flexor carpi ulnaris Mm. in the middle and reflect the stumps to allow for deep dissection. The **common interosseous A.** and the **cranial** and the **caudal interosseous Aa.** represent the limit between the brachial A. and the **median A.** (Fig. H6.20). Dissect the median A. and its major branches, the **deep antebrachial**, **proximal radial**, and **radial Aa.** Dissect the humeral head and the **radial head of the DDF M.** *Caution.* The humeral head of the DDF M. is made up of three portions that should stay together. Do not attempt to separate them from each other.

To isolate the **superficial digital flexor M. (SDF)** from the humeral head, flex the carpus as much as possible and feel the space between these two muscles 5–10 cm proximal to the carpus. With the scalpel and the fingers separate the SDF from the DDF. Continue the separation manually up to the elbow and feel the triangular shape of the SDF and the corresponding triangular groove of the humeral head of the DDF. Once the SDF is separated, pull it caudally and expose (on the caudal aspect of the radius distally) its tendinous attachment, called the **accessory lig. of the superficial digital flexor**, or the **proximal check lig.** (Fig. H6.20), an important contribution to the passive-stay apparatus of the thoracic limb.

Still on the medial aspect of the limb, identify the **flexor retinaculum**, which is the continuation of the proper antebrachial fascia over the mediopalmar aspect of the carpus. It is attached to the medial aspect of the carpus and the accessory carpal bone and covers the **carpal canal**. The carpal canal is the triangular space between the palmar joint capsule that overlaps the palmar aspect of the radial and intermediate carpal bones, the medial aspect of the accessory carpal bone, and the flexor retinaculum. The tendons of the SDF and the DDF, surrounded by a **common tendon sheath** and accompanied by an artery and a nerve, pass within the carpal canal.

Before dissecting those vessels and nerves, review the branches of the arteries and of the nerves, as follows:

The main artery in the region is the median A. It passes through the carpal canal with the **medial palmar N.**, surrounded by the common tendon sheath. Proximal to the carpus, the median A. (and the **median V.**) deliver the **radial A. and V.** and the **palmar branch A. and V.** The radial vessels perforate the flexor retinaculum close to its medial attachment; distal to the carpus, they will anastomose with the palmar branches, forming the **deep palmar arch A.V.** The palmar branches cross the palmar aspect of the carpus in an oblique direction laterodistally to anastomose with the **collateral ulnar A. and V.**, then perforate the flexor retinaculum close to the accessory carpal bone. Distal to the carpus they divide into a **deep branch**, which ends in the deep palmar arch, and a **superficial branch.**

*Note.* The palmar branches are located on the deep aspect of the tendon of the flexor carpi ulnaris M.

The median and ulnar Nn. accompany the median and collateral ulnar Aa., respectively. The median N. splits proximal to the carpus into the **medial palmar N.** and the **lateral palmar N.** The medial palmar N. accompanies the median A. through the carpal canal, whereas the lateral palmar N. fuses with the **palmar branch of the ulnar N.** and accompanies the palmar branch of the median A.V.

The ulnar N. splits proximal to the carpus into a **dorsal branch** and a palmar branch. The dorsal branch passes between the two tendons of the extensor carpi ulnaris M. and becomes cutaneous for the laterodorsal aspect of the carpus and metacarpus.

For a better exposure, transect the flexor carpi ulnaris and flexor carpi radialis Mm. close to their insertions, carefully reflect the distal stumps, and dissect all the structures shown in Figure H6.21.

Make a vertical incision within the flexor retinaculum to expose the carpal canal. Identify all the structures passing through it. *Notice* that the flexor retinaculum looks like it has a superficial and a deep sheet. Then trace the radial A. and V. through the flexor retinaculum, between the two sheets. Do the same thing with the palmar branches (A.V.) and the lateral palmar N. and identify on your specimen all the structures included in Figure H6.22.

Continue the dissection of the palmar aspect of the metacarpus. The flexor retinaculum continues as the **palmar fascia**, which is attached to the splint bones. Transect and remove it from the most superficial structures in the area, namely the SDF tendon, the medial and lateral palmar Nn., the median A. and V. (medially), and the superficial branch of the palmar branch A. and V. (laterally).

*Caution.* In the middle third of the SDF tendon, the palmar Nn. are connected by an obliquely lateroventrally oriented **communicating branch** (see Fig. H6.22). Also, the two superficial arteries anastomose with each other via the slender **superficial palmar arch.**

From the superficial palmar arch distally, the median A. becomes the **palmar common digital A. II**, whereas the

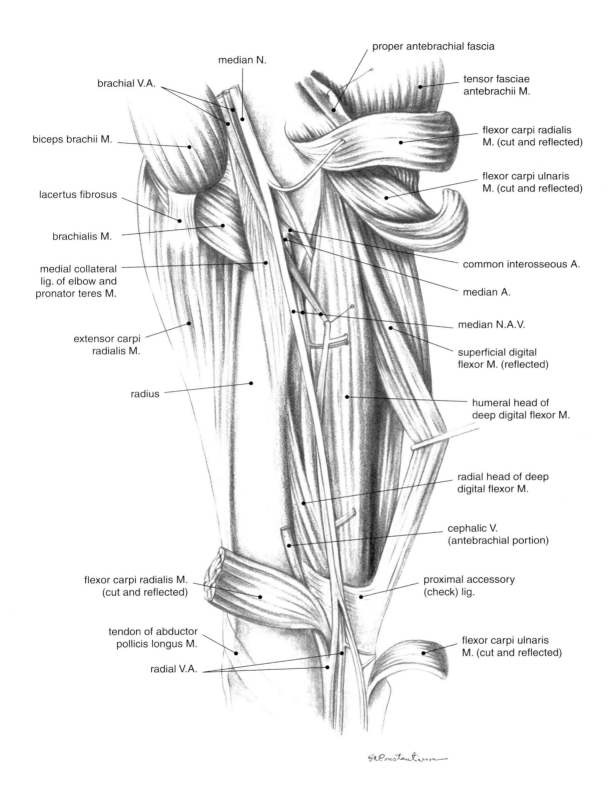

proper antebrachial fascia

median N.

brachial V.A.

tensor fasciae
antebrachii M.

biceps brachii M.

flexor carpi radialis
M. (cut and reflected)

flexor carpi ulnaris
M. (cut and reflected)

lacertus fibrosus

brachialis M.

common interosseous A.

medial collateral
lig. of elbow and
pronator teres M.

median A.

extensor carpi
radialis M.

median N.A.V.

superficial digital
flexor M. (reflected)

radius

humeral head of
deep digital flexor M.

radial head of deep
digital flexor M.

cephalic V.
(antebrachial portion)

flexor carpi radialis M.
(cut and reflected)

proximal accessory
(check) lig.

tendon of abductor
pollicis longus M.

flexor carpi ulnaris
M. (cut and reflected)

radial V.A.

Fig. H6.20. Deep structures of the right forearm, horse, medial aspect.

superficial branch of the palmar branch becomes the **palmar common digital A. III.**

Dissect and transversely transect at different levels the tendons of the SDF and DDF and reflect them proximally. On the deep aspect of the DDF tendon identify, dissect and isolate the **accessory lig. of the DDF, or distal check lig.**

**Surgical transection of the accessory ligament of the DDF is sometimes performed in the treatment of "club foot" (deep digital flexure contracture).**

Reflect the DDF proximally and dissect the vessels and nerves deep to it (see Fig. H6.23). Focus your attention on the lateral palmar N. It sends a **superficial branch** and a **deep branch.** The superficial branch continues within the lateral palmar N., while the latter supplies the interosseous medius M. and continues as the **lateral** and **medial palmar metacarpal Nn.**

**The accessoriometacarpal lig. is a landmark for nerve block anesthesia of the deep branch, when anesthesia of the interosseous medius M. is required.**

The palmar metacarpal nerves accompany the borders of the interosseous medius M., between the palmar aspect of metacarpal bone III and the splint bones. In their course, they are paralleled by the corresponding **palmar metacarpal Aa.** and **Vv.** (see Fig. H6.24). At the free end of the splint bones, the palmar metacarpal Nn. become cutaneous and supply the dorsolateral and dorsomedial aspects of the fetlock.

Continue to dissect the structures on the palmar aspect of the metacarpus. Before that, identify the **ergot** and the ligaments attaching it to the free ends of the splint bones and to the **cartilages of the hoof.** These are called the **ligg. of the ergot.**

**The lig. of the ergot is a landmark for nerve block anesthesia of the palmar branch of the lateral/medial digital Nn.**

The palmar Nn. continue as **lateral** and **medial (palmar) digital Nn.** *Note.* Since in the horse there are no dorsal digital nerves, the term "palmar" may be omitted.

The palmar common digital Aa. and Vv. anastomose with the palmar metacarpal Aa. and Vv. proximal to the fetlock (see Fig. H6.24). From this point, dissect the **lateral** and **medial digital Aa.** and **Vv.**

The following technique is suggested for dissecting the digit: use one side of the digit for the tendons, ligaments, and fasciae, and the other side for the vessels and nerves. You will save time and still have all structures dissected.

Start by removing the vessels and nerves from one side of the digit, then separate the **fascia of the digital cushion** (not mentioned in the *N.A.V.*) from the **digital fascia** (see Fig. H6.25). The digital fascia is composed of the **palmar annular lig. (superficial transverse metacarpal lig.)** and the **proximal digital annular lig.** The former

attaches on the abaxial sides of the **proximal sesamoid bones**, whereas the latter attaches on the proximal *and* distal extremities of the first phalanx (P I) (see Fig. H6.26). From the lateral/medial perspective, outline and expose those attachments; between them, identify the tendons of the SDF and DDF Mm.

Identify the **distal digital annular lig.**, outline its attachments on P I, and expose the tendon of the DDF, slipping from under the SDF on its way to the third phalanx.

The **digital cushion** is a pyramidal fibroelastic structure located between the distal digital annular lig. on the dorsal side, the **frog** on the palmar side (see Fig. H6.27A), and the paired **fibrocartilages of the hoof** on the lateral and medial sides. The base of the digital cushion, which is protected by the **bulbs of the heels**, is partly subcutaneous.

*Remember!* From carpus distally, the cranial aspect of all structures is called "dorsal," whereas the caudal aspect is called "palmar."

The fibrocartilages of the hoof are slightly rectangular, with the dorsal half attached to the **palmar processes of P III**, and the palmar half attached to the digital cushion. With the exception of the proximal (convex) borders, which contribute to the anatomical basis of the **coronet** (above the coronary border of the hoof), the cartilages are included within the hoof (see Fig. H6.27B).

Hold the **distal interphalangeal joint** in extension and remove the digital cushion. Identify the ligaments of the cartilages of the hoof on their deep aspect; they attach the cartilages to P I, P II, P III, and the **distal sesamoid (navicular) bone** (see Fig. H6.27C). Remove the cartilage from the side where you are dissecting the tendons, ligaments, and fasciae.

Transect the attachments of the palmar annular lig., proximal digital annular ligg., and the distal tendons of the SDF. Reflect the tendons of both the SDF and DDF and *notice* the presence of the **sleeve of the superficial digital flexor**, which surrounds the tendon of the DDF. *Notice* that the DDF is surrounded by a tendon sheath, and the SDF glides upon it. The SDF is not surrounded by the tendon sheath, because the digital fascia is partially fused with it.

**Involvement of the digital fascia, tendon sheath, SDF, and DDF is common in distal limb lacerations due to their superficial location.**

On the palmar aspect of the proximal sesamoid bones identify the **proximal scutum**, a fibrocartilage that covers the **palmar lig.** (between the two bones), providing a gliding surface for the flexor tendons (see Fig. H6.28). *Notice* the attachment of the bifurcated tendon of the SDF on the **middle scutum**, which provides a gliding surface only for the DDF tendon.

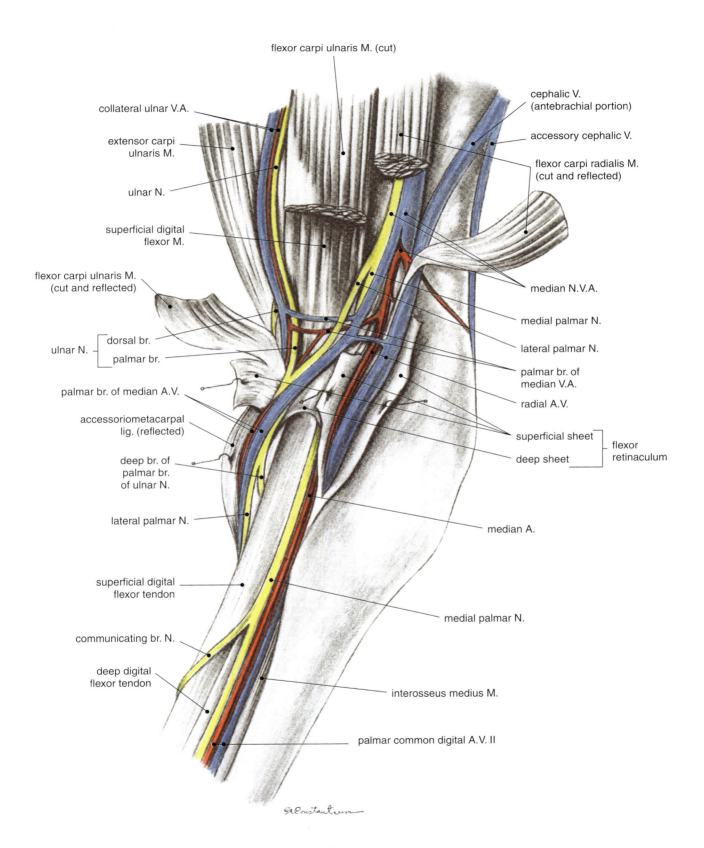

flexor carpi ulnaris M. (cut)

collateral ulnar V.A.

extensor carpi
ulnaris M.

ulnar N.

superficial digital
flexor M.

flexor carpi ulnaris M.
(cut and reflected)

ulnar N. — dorsal br.
— palmar br.

palmar br. of median A.V.

accessoriometacarpal
lig. (reflected)

deep br. of
palmar br.
of ulnar N.

lateral palmar N.

superficial digital
flexor tendon

communicating br. N.

deep digital
flexor tendon

cephalic V.
(antebrachial portion)

accessory cephalic V.

flexor carpi radialis M.
(cut and reflected)

median N.V.A.

medial palmar N.

lateral palmar N.

palmar br. of
median V.A.

radial A.V.

superficial sheet    ⎤ flexor
deep sheet          ⎦ retinaculum

median A.

medial palmar N.

interosseus medius M.

palmar common digital A.V. II

Fig. H6.21. Deep structures of the left carpus, horse, mediopalmar aspect.

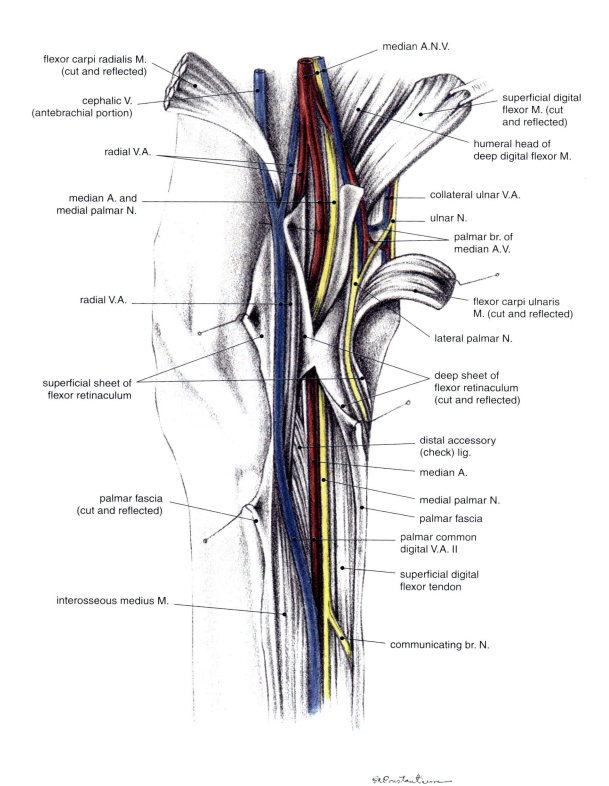

flexor carpi radialis M.
(cut and reflected)

cephalic V.
(antebrachial portion)

radial V.A.

median A. and
medial palmar N.

radial V.A.

superficial sheet of
flexor retinaculum

palmar fascia
(cut and reflected)

interosseous medius M.

median A.N.V.

superficial digital
flexor M. (cut
and reflected)

humeral head of
deep digital flexor M.

collateral ulnar V.A.

ulnar N.

palmar br. of
median A.V.

flexor carpi ulnaris
M. (cut and reflected)

lateral palmar N.

deep sheet of
flexor retinaculum
(cut and reflected)

distal accessory
(check) lig.

median A.

medial palmar N.

palmar fascia

palmar common
digital V.A. II

superficial digital
flexor tendon

communicating br. N.

Fig. H6.22. Deep structures of the right carpus, horse, mediopalmar aspect.

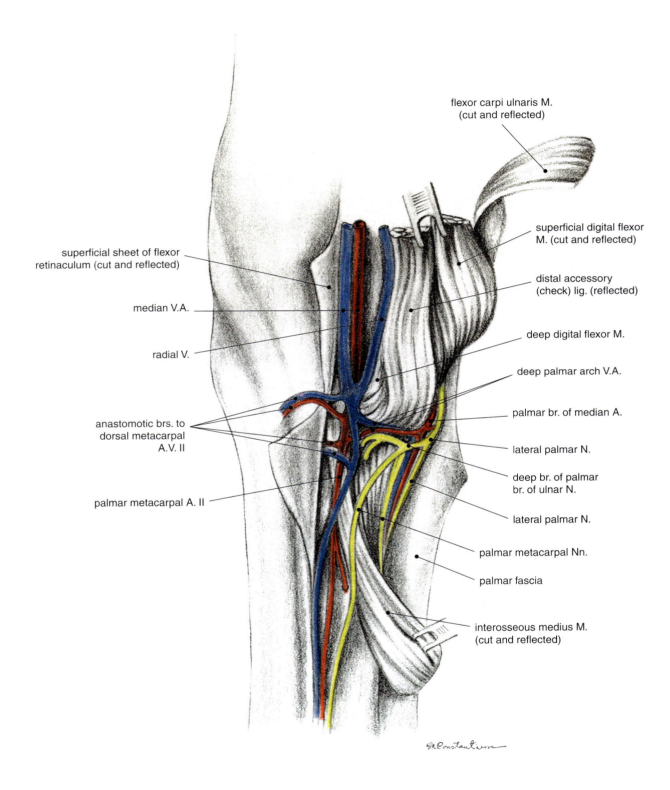

flexor carpi ulnaris M.
(cut and reflected)

superficial digital flexor
M. (cut and reflected)

superficial sheet of flexor
retinaculum (cut and reflected)

distal accessory
(check) lig. (reflected)

median V.A.

deep digital flexor M.

radial V.

deep palmar arch V.A.

palmar br. of median A.

anastomotic brs. to
dorsal metacarpal
A.V. II

lateral palmar N.

deep br. of palmar
br. of ulnar N.

palmar metacarpal A. II

lateral palmar N.

palmar metacarpal Nn.

palmar fascia

interosseous medius M.
(cut and reflected)

Fig. H6.23. Deep structures of the right carpometacarpal area, horse, mediopalmar aspect.

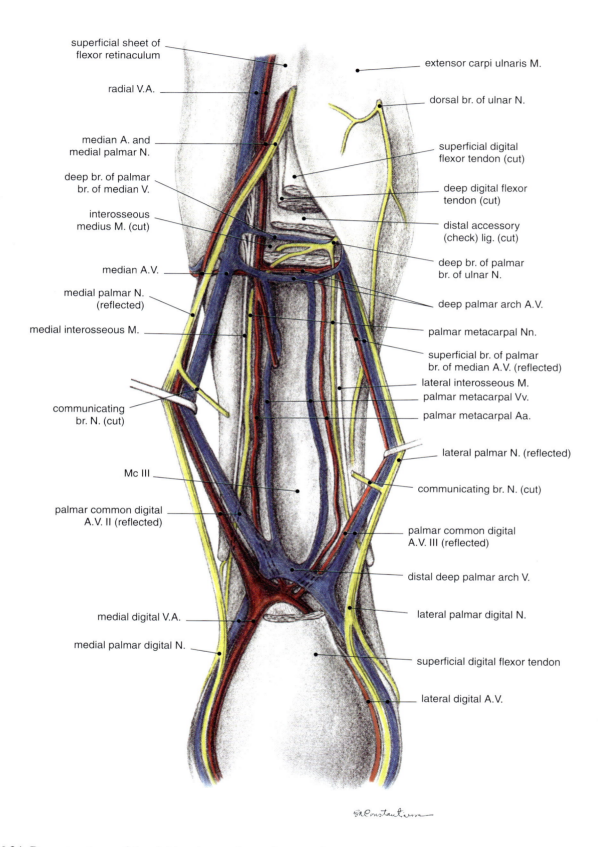

superficial sheet of
flexor retinaculum

radial V.A.

median A. and
medial palmar N.

deep br. of palmar
br. of median V.

interosseous
medius M. (cut)

median A.V.

medial palmar N.
(reflected)

medial interosseous M.

communicating
br. N. (cut)

Mc III

palmar common digital
A.V. II (reflected)

medial digital V.A.

medial palmar digital N.

extensor carpi ulnaris M.

dorsal br. of ulnar N.

superficial digital
flexor tendon (cut)

deep digital flexor
tendon (cut)

distal accessory
(check) lig. (cut)

deep br. of palmar
br. of ulnar N.

deep palmar arch A.V.

palmar metacarpal Nn.

superficial br. of palmar
br. of median A.V. (reflected)

lateral interosseous M.

palmar metacarpal Vv.

palmar metacarpal Aa.

lateral palmar N. (reflected)

communicating br. N. (cut)

palmar common digital
A.V. III (reflected)

distal deep palmar arch V.

lateral palmar digital N.

superficial digital flexor tendon

lateral digital A.V.

Fig. H6.24. Deep structures of the right metacarpal area, horse, palmar aspect.

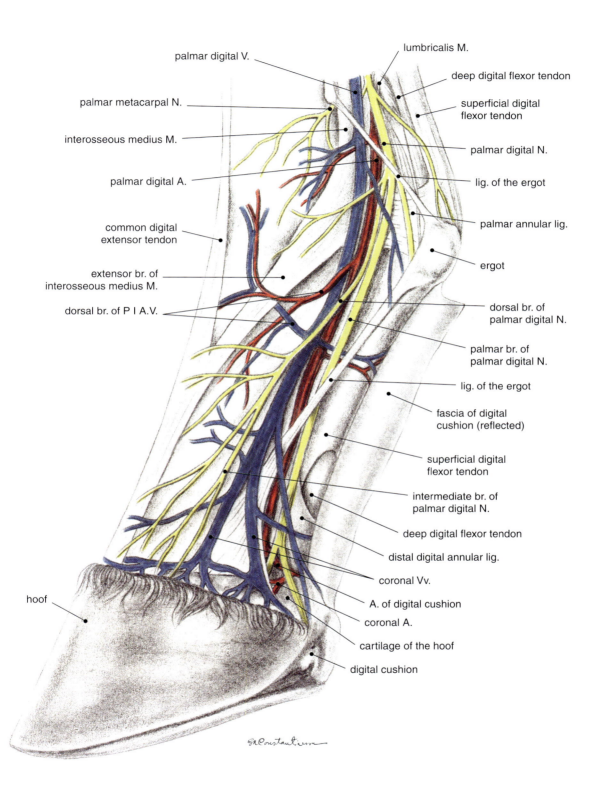

Fig. H6.25. Vessels and nerves of digit of right limb, horse, medial aspect.

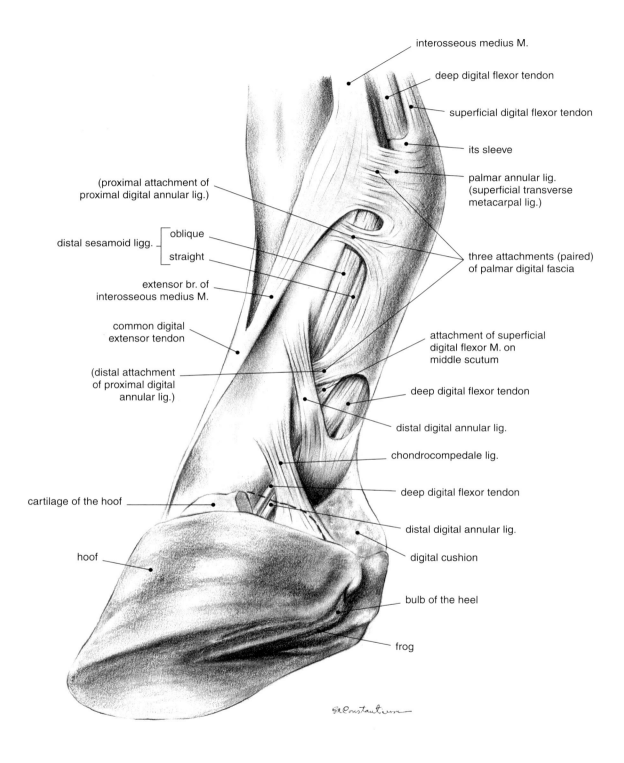

interosseous medius M.

deep digital flexor tendon

superficial digital flexor tendon

its sleeve

palmar annular lig.
(superficial transverse
metacarpal lig.)

(proximal attachment of
proximal digital annular lig.)

distal sesamoid ligg. ⎡ oblique
⎣ straight

three attachments (paired)
of palmar digital fascia

extensor br. of
interosseous medius M.

common digital
extensor tendon

attachment of superficial
digital flexor M. on
middle scutum

(distal attachment
of proximal digital
annular lig.)

deep digital flexor tendon

distal digital annular lig.

chondrocompedale lig.

cartilage of the hoof

deep digital flexor tendon

distal digital annular lig.

digital cushion

hoof

bulb of the heel

frog

Fig. H6.26. Tendons of digit of thoracic limb, horse, mediopalmar aspect, superficial level.

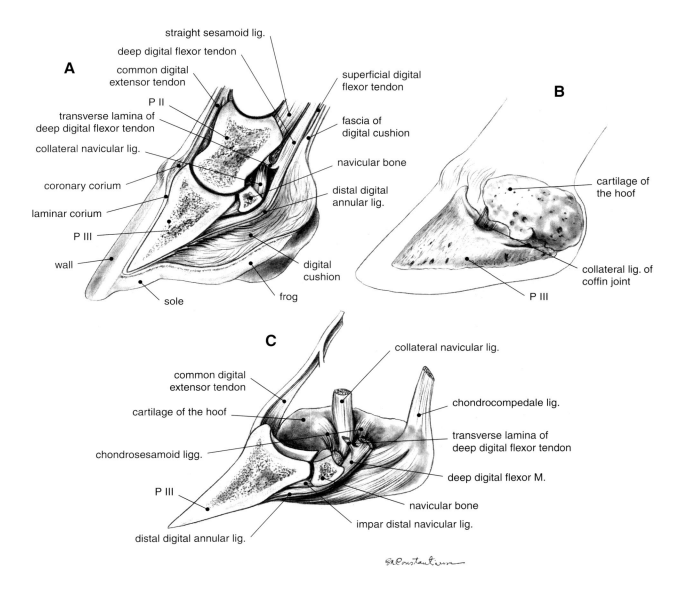

Fig. H6.27. Structures of the digit, horse. **A.** Median section through the digit. **B.** Topography of the cartilage of the hoof (abaxial aspect). **C.** Ligaments of the cartilage of the hoof (axial aspect).

The distal sesamoid ligg. are attached to the base of the proximal sesamoid bones. The **straight (superficial, "Y") lig.** is the only one extending to P II. Transect it and fully expose the **oblique (middle, "V") lig.** Between the two arms of the V-shaped ligament, dissect the **cruciate ("X")** lig. (Fig. H6.28). The **short ligg.** extend from the base of the sesamoid bones to the proximal end of P I, deep to the proximal attachment of the oblique lig.

The areas of attachment of all ligaments and tendons on the distal metacarpal bones, phalanges, and sesamoid bones are shown in Figure H.29.

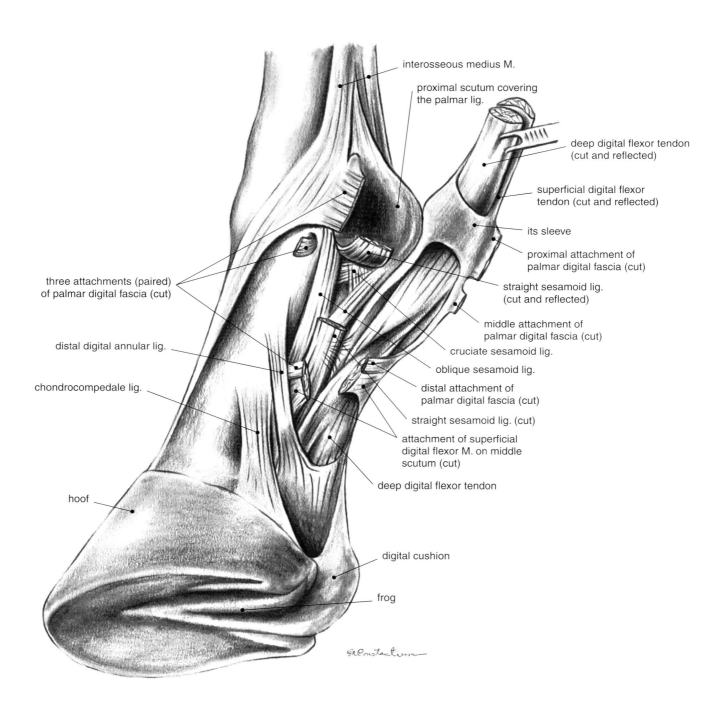

Fig. H6.28. Tendons of digit of thoracic limb, horse, mediopalmar aspect, deep level.

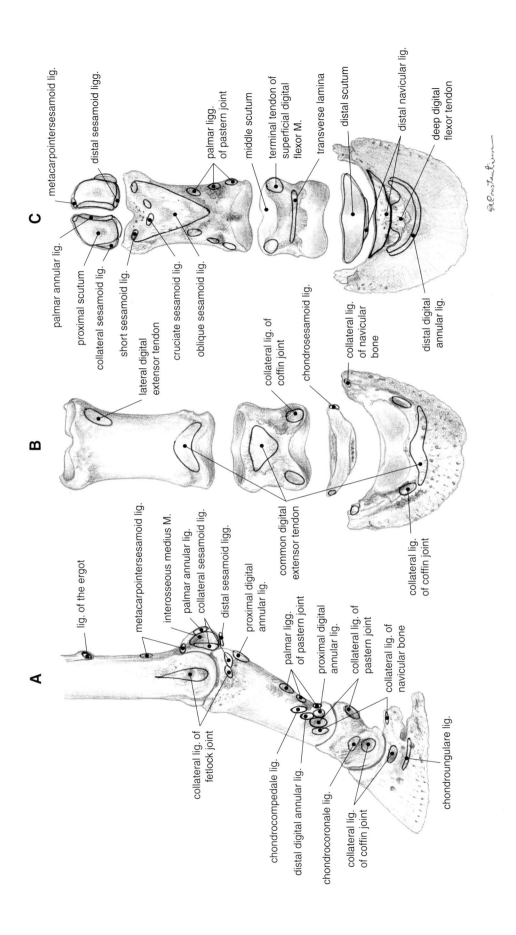

Fig. H6.29. The areas of attachment of ligaments and tendons on the distal metacarpal bones, phalanges, and sesamoid bones in the horse. **A.** Lateral/medial aspect. **B.** Dorsal aspect. **C.** Palmar aspect.

Holding the digit with the palmar side up, make a vertical incision in the middle of the distal digital annular lig. and the DDF tendon, up to the **semilunar line**, where these two structures attach. Remove one-half of those structures to expose the navicular bone, covered by the **distal scutum**, the **impar distal sesamoid (navicular) lig.**, and the **flexor surface of P III** (Fig. H6.30A). While making the section in the DDF tendon, you transected the **transverse lamina** (not mentioned in the *N.A.V.*), an attachment of the DDF on the palmar aspect of P II.

**The clinical importance of the transverse lamina is that it separates the tendon sheath of the DDF from its tendinous navicular (podotrochlear) bursa.**

**In certain circumstances, such as after a long run, or as a consequence of an inflammatory or infectious condition, the tendon sheath forms small, symmetrical, tumor-like expansions (pouches) between the attachments of the digital fascia, and two nonsymmetrical pouches, proximal and distal. The proximal (nonsymmetrical) pouch can be felt between the interosseous medius M. and the tendons of the DDF and the SDF, proximal to the fetlock. The distal (nonsymmetrical) pouch touches the transverse lamina and can be seen on a live horse on the palmar aspect of the digit, proximal to and between the bulbs of the heels (see Fig. H6.37B, Modlab H6).**

**The tendinous bursa fills the space between the DDF tendon and the distal scutum, the impar distal navicular lig., and the flexor surface of P III. It is important to preserve it during surgical interventions on different aspects of navicular syndromes (diseases).**

Turn the digit with the vessels and nerves up and start the dissection.

*Remember* that the lig. of the ergot attached to the free end of the splint bone obliquely crosses all the vessels and nerves.

Dissect the vessels and the nerves while passing over the abaxial aspect of the sesamoid bone. The relationship between the digital vessels and nerve is, in dorsopalmar order: V., A., N. After that, the palmar digital N. gives off a **dorsal branch** and a **middle branch** (not mentioned in the *N.A.V.*), then continues parallel to the long axis of the phalanges and enters the hoof (see Fig. H6.25).

The digital artery gives off **dorsal and palmar branches for P I and P II**, a **branch for the digital cushion**, a **dorsal branch for P III**, a **coronal A.**, and the **terminal arch**. The terminal arch is formed by the anastomosis of the symmetrical digital Aa. inside the **solar canal** (Fig. H6.30C). The digital vein originates from venous plexuses of the dorsal and palmar aspects of P III, the lateral and medial aspects of the cartilages of the hoof, the **V.**

of the digital cushion, the **coronal V.**, and the **terminal arch (venous)** (Fig. H6.30B,C).

**The digital V. is clinically important for performing venograms. In cases of acute "club foot," acute and chronic laminitis, and other conditions, venograms help in correctly diagnosing and treating these conditions.**

The hoof was already removed. Look at the continuation of the dermis (the sensitive tissue) within the hoof. It consists of five adjacent structures (Fig. H6.31A,B), all of them located within the hoof. The hoof represents the epidermis (the nonsensitive tissue).

The dermis, also known as the **corium**, consists of a rich vascular connective tissue. The corium has the same relation to the hoof as the dermis has to the skin. Three out of five structures of the dermis are located in contact with the internal aspect of the wall of the hoof. They are, in a proximodistal order the **perioplic (limbic) corium**, the **coronary corium**, and the **laminar (lamellar) corium**. At the solar aspect of the digit, the **cuneal corium** (the corium of the frog) and the **solar corium** (the corium of the sole) are the main structures; the **laminar corium of the bars** is also present, as a component of the lamellar corium of the solar surface of the digit (see Fig. H6.31).

The perioplic corium (1 mm wide) consists of many fine papillae. It continues as the **bulbar corium** toward the heels and is protected within the **perioplic groove** of the hoof. The coronary corium (1 cm wide) bears papillae that are similar to those of the perioplic corium, and it continues in a manner similar to that of the bulbar corium. It is protected within the **coronary groove** of the hoof and lies on a supportive subcutaneous tissue, called the **coronary cushion**. The lamellae of the laminar corium, which are equal in number to the **horny lamellae of the hoof,** cover the parietal aspect of P III and the corresponding area of the bars (the **horny lamellae of the bars**), between the cuneal corium and the solar corium (Fig. H6.32A,C).

The cuneal corium and the solar corium bear fine papillae and join the laminar corium to form a continuous envelope for the deep structures (see Fig. H6.31).

Identify the three main components of the hoof: the wall (see Fig. H6.32A), the frog (Fig. H6.32B), and the sole (see Fig. H6.32C). These structures represent the continuation of the epidermis.

The wall is conventionally divided externally into a frontal region (the **toe**), the lateral and medial sides (the **quarters**), and the most palmar areas (the **heels**) (see Fig. H6.33).

The proximal parts of the heels, on the palmar borders, are called the **bulbs of the heels.**

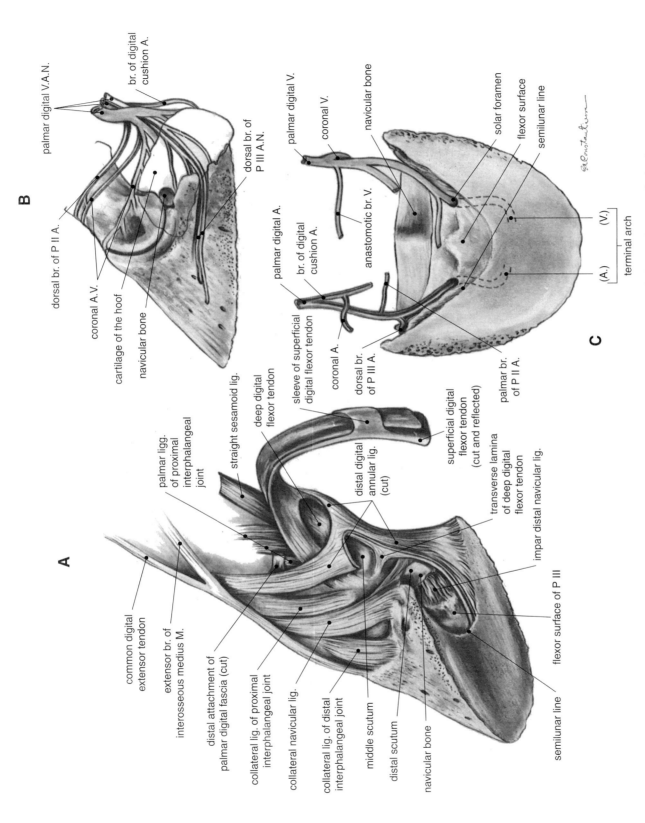

**B**

palmar digital V.A.N.

br. of digital cushion A.

dorsal br. of P II A.

coronal A.V.

cartilage of the hoof

navicular bone

dorsal br. of P III A.N.

palmar digital V.

coronal V.

navicular bone

solar foramen

flexor surface

semilunar line

palmar digital A.

br. of digital cushion A.

anastomotic br. V.

coronal A.

dorsal br. of P III A.

palmar br. of P II A.

(V.)

terminal arch

(A.)

**C**

**A**

common digital extensor tendon

extensor br. of interosseous medius M.

distal attachment of palmar digital fascia (cut)

collateral lig. of proximal interphalangeal joint

collateral navicular lig.

collateral lig. of distal interphalangeal joint

middle scutum

distal scutum

navicular bone

palmar ligg. of proximal interphalangeal joint

straight sesamoid lig.

deep digital flexor tendon

sleeve of superficial digital flexor tendon

distal digital annular lig. (cut)

superficial digital flexor tendon (cut and reflected)

transverse lamina of deep digital flexor tendon

impar distal navicular lig.

flexor surface of P III

semilunar line

Fig. H6.30. Deep structures of the digit, horse. **A.** Lateroventral aspect. **B.** Terminal branches of palmar digital vessels (ventral view). **C.** Terminal branches of palmar digital A.V. N.

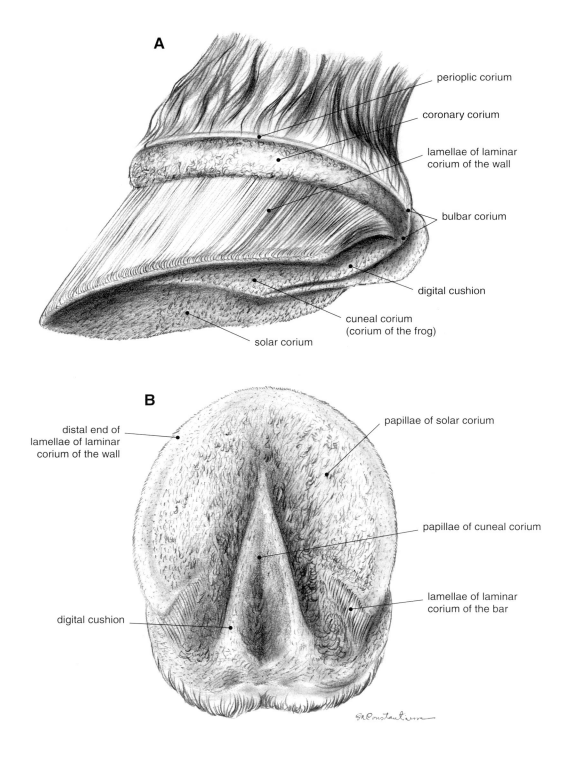

**A**

perioplic corium

coronary corium

lamellae of laminar
corium of the wall

bulbar corium

digital cushion

cuneal corium
(corium of the frog)

solar corium

**B**

distal end of
lamellae of laminar
corium of the wall

papillae of solar corium

papillae of cuneal corium

lamellae of laminar
corium of the bar

digital cushion

Fig. H6.31. Corium of digit, horse, after removal of hoof. **A.** Lateroventral aspect. **B.** Ventral aspect.

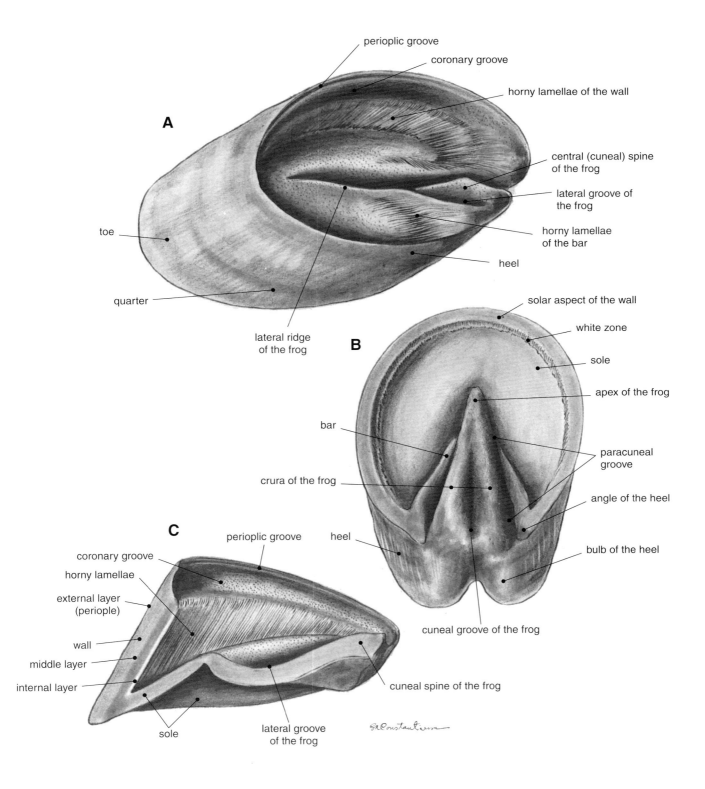

Fig. H6.32. The hoof, horse. **A.** Internal aspect of the hoof. **B.** Solar aspect of the hoof. **C.** Median section through the hoof (internal aspect).

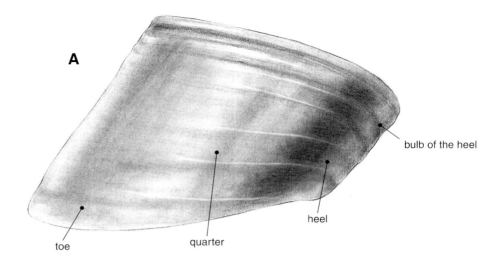

A

bulb of the heel

heel

quarter

toe

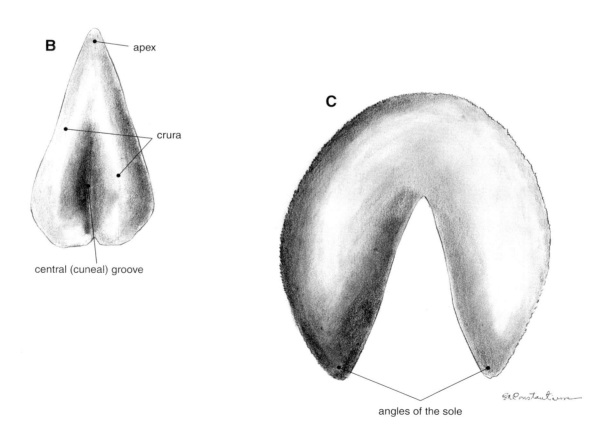

B

apex

crura

central (cuneal) groove

C

angles of the sole

Fig. H6.33. The hoof, horse. **A.** Wall. **B.** Frog. **C.** Sole.

*Notice* that the toe is taller than the heels.

The heels bend themselves (the angles of the heels) and continue forward as two symmetrical, thin, pointed laminae called bars, visible only on the contact surface of the hoof. Between the wall and the bars, the two angles of the sole are visible. The bars parallel the two **crura of the frog** and are separated from the frog by the **paracuneal grooves** (see Fig. H6.32B).

Examine the frog, with the V-shaped crura that meet dorsally in the **apex** and are separated from each other by the **central (cuneal) groove**. The **sole** and the frog are turned toward the ground when the limb is in a resting position. The sole fills the space between the solar surface of the wall, the bars, and the frog. The bars separate the frog (except the apex) from the sole. At the junction of the sole with the wall, regardless of the color of the horn of the hoof, a **white zone** is observed (see Fig. H6.32B). The interdigitations between the nonpigmented horny (insensitive) lamellae and the lamellae of the laminar corium (sensitive, living tissue) are referred to as the white zone, which has a practical importance.

**While nailing the horseshoe, make sure that the nails do not penetrate the sole (inside of the white zone), but only the wall of the hoof. Through the sole, the nail will hit the papillary solar corium, and even P III. Dramatic consequences may occur.**

The internal aspect of the hoof wall consists of the following three structures (starting from the coronary border of the hoof): (1) the **perioplic groove** (1 mm wide), which receives and protects the perioplic corium; (2) the **coronary groove** (1 cm wide), which receives the coronary corium; and (3) the 550–600 **horny lamellae (laminae)**, which interdigitate with the same number of lamellae (laminae) of the laminar corium. The horny lamellae also continue at the level of the bars. The perioplic and coronary grooves are provided with very fine holes for the papillae of the perioplic and coronary coria (plural of corium) (see Fig. H6.32A,C).

The internal aspects of the frog and sole consist of very small holes that perforate the entire surface to receive the papillae of the cuneal and solar coria. The frog has the following characteristics: one **central spine (the cuneal spine)**, which corresponds to the **central (cuneal) groove** (on the external aspect of the frog); two **lateral grooves**, which correspond to the crura of the frog (on the external aspect); and two **lateral ridges**, which correspond to the **paracuneal grooves** (on the external aspect) (see Fig. H6.32A,C).

Make a vertical section through the wall and examine the three layers of the epidermis (the horny wall): the external layer (**stratum externum**), which is represented by the **periople** (a very thin protective layer produced by the perioplic corium); the internal layer (**stratum internum**), which is represented by the horny lamellae (nonpigmented); and the middle layer (**stratum medium**), which is the thickest layer and is represented by pigmented horn (see Fig. H6.32C).

Dissect and examine the collateral ligg. of all the digital joints. Check with a skeleton as many times as necessary.

At the carpal joint, dissect and examine the dorsal and palmar joint capsules, the collateral ligg., and the four ligg. of the accessory carpal bone. Identify the carpal and metacarpal bones on a skeleton and on your specimen.

**Identify the intercarpal lig. on the palmar aspect of the joint, between the proximal aspect of the third carpal bone and the distal aspect of the radial carpal bone. This ligament can be damaged during high-speed exercise.**

Dissect and examine the cranial fibrous joint capsule of the elbow joint, which has no corresponding structure on the caudal aspect. The only structure present both cranially and caudally is the humeroradial synovial membrane.

After the entire thoracic limb is dissected, if you do not plan to save it for other purposes, disarticulate it joint by joint to examine the articular surfaces of the bones.

The passive-stay apparatus of the thoracic limb (Fig. H6.34) is complete, in comparison to that of the pelvic limb, which has no provision for the hip joint. Therefore, all the joints of the thoracic limb are covered and provided with connective tissue structures to keep the angles between bones in a steady position, even during sleep, while the limbs are on the ground.

The *shoulder joint* does not flex under the body weight (see the suspensory apparatus of the body—Fig. H2.22), due to the tendon of the biceps brachii M. that joins the supraglenoid tubercle of scapula to the radial tuberosity.

At the same time, the distal insertion of the muscle pulls the *elbow* proximally and forward and also does not allow it to flex.

The *carpal joint* is balanced between two forces: one on the dorsal aspect and one on the palmar aspect. The distal tendon of the extensor carpi radialis M., joined by the lacertus fibrosus of the biceps brachii tendon, pulls the carpus proximally (on the dorsal aspect). The proximal check lig. (of the SDF) and the distal check lig. (of the DDF) pull the carpus distally (on the palmar aspect).

To understand the action of the structures acting on the palmar aspect of carpus, concentrate your attention on the *fetlock*. This joint has a flexion angle of approximately 220 degrees and is prone to hyperextension under the pressure of the body weight (55–60% of the body weight

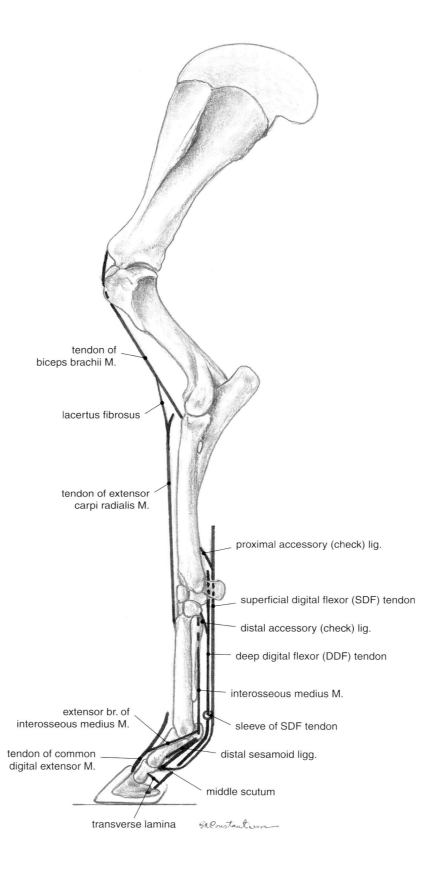

tendon of
biceps brachii M.

lacertus fibrosus

tendon of extensor
carpi radialis M.

proximal accessory (check) lig.

superficial digital flexor (SDF) tendon

distal accessory (check) lig.

deep digital flexor (DDF) tendon

interosseous medius M.

extensor br. of
interosseous medius M.

sleeve of SDF tendon

tendon of common
digital extensor M.

distal sesamoid ligg.

middle scutum

transverse lamina

Fig. H6.34. The passive-stay apparatus of the thoracic limb in the horse.

is supported by the thoracic limbs). The interosseous medius opposes this tendency by pulling the sesamoid bones in a proximal direction. By means of the distal sesamoid ligg., the hyperextension of the fetlock and of the *pastern joint* is prevented. At the same time, the pressure of the fetlock in the palmar direction, against the SDF and DDF tendons, keeps them under continuous tension. This process is translated by pulling the palmar aspect of the carpus distally, and the palmar aspect of the *pastern* and *coffin* proximally, by the two digital flexor muscles. Explanation: the proximal and the distal check ligg. pull the carpus in a distal direction, balancing the action of the extensor carpi radialis tendon on the dorsal aspect of carpus, which pulls the carpus in a proximal direction. The SDF tendon, inserted on the middle scutum (pastern joint), and the DDF tendon, inserted on the semilunar line (coffin joint), pull those joints in a proximal direction, while the extensor branches of the interosseous medius join the tendon of the common digital extensor and balance the flexion-extension action upon the phalangeal joints.

# MODLAB H6

Attempt to palpate on a live horse all the structures listed at the beginning of this chapter.

Check your specimen and adapt to the live horse the following **landmarks** and **approaches** of the most clinically relevant anatomical structures for physical examination and/or clinical interventions (including the nerve block or regional anesthesia).

1. **Median A.V.N.** (Fig. H6.35A)
   *Proximal approach*
   A. *Landmark:* medial aspect of elbow
   B. *Approach:* through the skin, transverse pectoral M., and brachial fascia on the medial aspect of the elbow. The vessels and nerve produce a popping motion when rolled back and forth under a firmly pressing finger.
   *Notice* that the median N. is in a caudal position to the vessels.

   *Distal approach*
   A. *Landmarks:* chestnut on medial aspect of forearm; radius; flexor carpi radialis M.
   B. *Approach:* on the medial aspect of the forearm deep through the skin and superficial and proper antebrachial fasciae, and between the radius and the flexor carpi radialis M., one hand proximal to the chestnut. The median A.V.N. lie on the caudal aspect of the radius.

2. **Ulnar N. and collateral ulnar A.V.** (Fig. H6.35B)
   A. *Landmarks:* accessory carpal bone; olecranon; flexor and extensor carpi ulnaris Mm.
   B. *Approach:* at a point one hand wide, proximal to the accessory carpal bone, between the flexor and extensor carpi ulnaris Mm., on the line between the accessory carpal bone and the olecranon, and through the skin and proper antebrachial fascia

3. **Cranial cutaneous antebrachial N.** (Fig. H6.35C)
   A. *Landmarks:* deltoid tuberosity; deltoid M.
   B. *Approach:* emerging on the lateral aspect of the arm, caudodorsal to the deltoid tuberosity and caudal to the insertion of the deltoideus M., in a dorsoventral direction through the skin, brachial fascia, and cutaneous omobrachialis M.

4. **Lateral cutaneous antebrachial N.** (Fig. H6.35D)
   A. *Landmarks:* the ventral border of the lateral head of the triceps brachii M.; deltoid tuberosity; olecranon; common digital extensor M. (bordered on both sides by two vertical grooves on the lateral aspect of the forearm)
   B. *Approach:* midway between the deltoid tuberosity and the olecranon, emerging from under the ventral border of the lateral head of the triceps brachii M., in a dorsoventral direction, and along the long axis of the common digital extensor M., through the skin and proper antebrachial fascia
   *Caution.* The nerve regularly has two branches close to and parallel to one another.

5. **Caudal cutaneous antebrachial N.** (Fig. H6.35B)
   A. *Landmarks:* olecranon tuberosity; accessory carpal bone; flexor and extensor carpi ulnaris Mm.
   B. *Approach:* subcutaneous and 10 cm ventral to olecranon tuberosity on a line between the olecranon and the accessory carpal bone, and between the flexor and extensor carpi ulnaris Mm.

6. **Medial cutaneous antebrachial N.** (Fig. H6.35A)
   A. *Landmark:* lacertus fibrosus
   B. *Approach:* on the medial aspect of the lacertus fibrosus
   *Caution.* The nerve is accompanied by the accessory cephalic V. and the antebrachial segment of the cephalic V. and is palpable by rolling the fingers upon the lacertus fibrosus.

7. **Dorsal branch of ulnar N.** (Fig. H6.35D)
   A. *Landmarks:* accessory carpal bone; the two distal tendons of the extensor carpi ulnaris M.
   B. *Approach:* through the skin on the lateral aspect of the carpus, just proximal to the accessory carpal bone, between the two distal tendons of the extensor carpi ulnaris M., where a small fingertip-like depression may be palpated

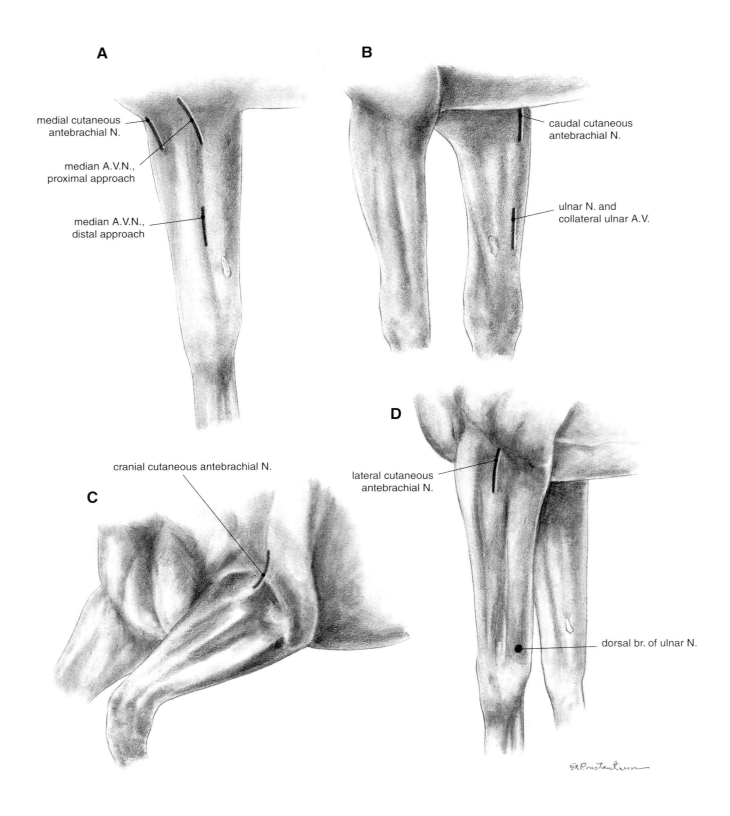

Fig. H6.35. Landmarks and approaches on the thoracic limb for nerve block anesthesia, horse. **A.** Medial aspect. **B.** Caudomedial aspect. **C.** Craniolateral aspect. **D.** Lateral aspect.

8. **Deep branch of radial N.** (Fig. H6.35D)
   A. *Landmarks:* common digital extensor tendon in the forearm; caudal groove of the lateral aspect of forearm; carpus
   B. *Approach:* one hand proximal to the carpus in the caudal groove of the lateral aspect of the forearm, parallel to the common digital extensor tendon, through the skin and proper antebrachial fascia
9. **(Lateral) and medial palmar Nn.** (Fig. H6.36A)
   A. *Landmarks:* interosseous medius M.; the tendons of the SDF and the DDF in the palmar metacarpal area
   B. *Approach:* through the skin and palmar fascia on both sides between the interosseous medius and the two tendons of the digital flexors
   *Caution.* The medial palmar N. is accompanied by the palmar common digital A.V. II, whereas the lateral palmar N. is accompanied by the palmar common digital A.V. III. The relationship between the nerves and vessels is the following: V.A.N. in a dorsopalmar direction.
10. **Lateral and medial sesamoidean Nn.** (not mentioned in *N.A.V.*) (Fig. H6.36A). These nerves were mentioned by Cornelissen (1997), and they are branches of the lateral and medial palmar nerves, respectively.
    A. *Landmarks:* the proximal sesamoid bones; the attachment of the interosseous medius on the abaxial aspects of the proximal sesamoid bones
    B. *Approach:* The needle should be introduced between the attachment of the interosseous medius on the abaxial aspects of the corresponding proximal sesamoid bone and the dorsal side of the abaxial border of the proximal sesamoid bone.
11. **Deep branch of palmar branch of ulnar N.** (Fig. H6.36A)
    A. *Landmarks:* accessory carpal bone; accessoriometacarpal lig.; lateral border of the tendons of the SDF and the DDF on the mediopalmar aspect of the carpus, just distal to flexor retinaculum
    B. *Approach:* A needle can be inserted in a proximodistal direction and deep between the medial aspect of the accessoriometacarpal lig. and the two above mentioned tendons.
    *Caution.* Repeated flexions and extensions of the carpus are suggested.
12. **Lateral and medial palmar metacarpal Nn.**
    A. *Landmarks and approaches:* Similar to those for the lateral and medial plantar metatarsal Nn. (see page 148)

13. **(Lateral) and medial palmar digital Nn.** (Fig. H6.36A)
    A. *Landmarks:* the abaxial aspect of the proximal sesamoid bones, which is the place of insertion of the interosseous medius M.
    B. *Approach:* The nerves, accompanied by the corresponding arteries and veins in a subcutaneous position, produce a popping movement when rolled back and forth under firmly pressing fingers.
    *Caution.* The relationship between the nerves and vessels is as follows: V.A.N. in a dorsopalmar direction.
    **This is the most common peripheral nerve block performed.**
    *Note.* Similar landmarks and approaches should be considered for the plantar digital Nn.
14. **Palmar branch of palmar digital N.** (Fig. H6.36A)
    A. *Landmarks:* pastern, lig. of the ergot, ergot, fibrocartilage of the hoof
    B. *Approach:* with the hoof held in extension, the lig. of the ergot may be exposed and felt under the skin, in a oblique direction from the ergot toward the dorsal end of the fibrocartilage of the hoof. A needle can be inserted in the long axis of the digit in the pastern region, between the middle and palmar thirds of the area, deep to the lig. of the ergot.
15. **Intraarticular approaches**
    *Scapulohumeral (shoulder) joint* (Fig. H6.36B)
    A. *Landmark:* the notch between the cranial and caudal parts of the greater tubercle of the humerus (on the lateral aspect of the shoulder)
    B. *Approach:* A needle is inserted in an approximately horizontal position and directed craniocaudally in a 45-degree angle with the body. It penetrates the skin, the brachial fascia, and the notch separating the two parts of the greater tubercle of the humerus.
    *Note.* The notch is bordered by the supraspinatus M., which attaches to the cranial part, and the infraspinatus M., whose tendon glides over the caudal part of that tubercle.

    *Humeroradial (elbow) joint* (Fig. H6.36B)
    A. *Landmarks:* the lateral prominence of the humeral condyle, the lateral collateral lig. of the elbow, the lateral groove on the lateral aspect of the forearm
    B. *Approach:* Palpate the humeral condyle and the lateral collateral lig. of the elbow while flexing the joint; reflect the caudal border of the common digital extensor M. from the caudal groove (see above) cranially and feel a depression between the

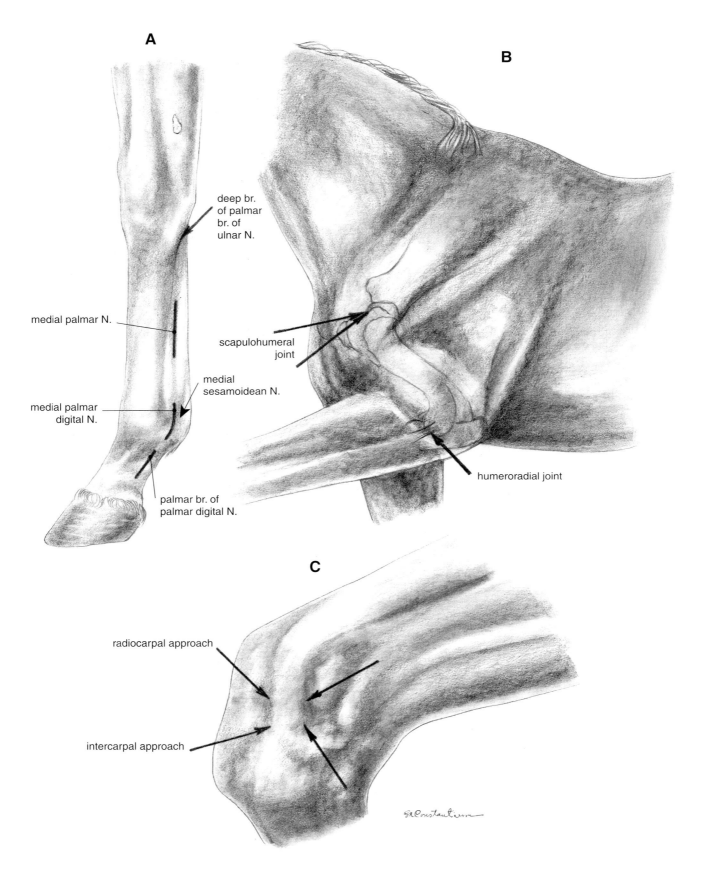

**A**

deep br.
of palmar
br. of
ulnar N.

medial palmar N.

scapulohumeral
joint

medial
sesamoidean N.

medial palmar
digital N.

humeroradial joint

palmar br. of
palmar digital N.

**B**

**C**

radiocarpal approach

intercarpal approach

Fig. H6.36. Landmarks and approaches on the thoracic limb, horse. **A.** Nerve block anesthesia, medial aspect of autopodium. *Intraarticular approaches:* **B.** Lateral aspect. **C.** Dorsal aspect of carpus.

first two landmarks. A needle is inserted in a horizontal position and is directed slightly obliquely craniocaudally and lateromedially through the skin and proper antebrachial fascia.

*Radiocarpometacarpal (carpal) joint* (Fig. H6.36C)

α—Radiocarpal joint

A. *Landmarks:* the dorsal aspect of carpus, the tendon of extensor carpi radialis M.

B. *Approach:* While flexing the carpus, a deep depression can be felt between the radius and the proximal row of carpal bones. Here is the site for the approach through the skin and extensor retinaculum, at either the medial or the lateral border of the tendon of the extensor carpi radialis M.

β—Intercarpal joint

A. *Landmarks:* same as above

B. *Approach:* Proceed in a manner similar to that for the previous approach, and another depression can be felt, between the two rows of carpal bones. Continue in a similar manner as previously.

*Metacarpo/metatarsophalangeal (fetlock) joint* (Fig. H6.37A,B)

A. *Landmarks:* metacarpal (metatarsal) bone III, proximal sesamoid bones, interosseous medius M.

B. *Approach:* through the skin, 1–2 cm proximal to the proximal sesamoid bones, between the bone and the tendon

*Proximal interphalangeal (pastern) joint* (Fig. H6.37A)

A. *Landmarks:* the pastern, the tendon of the common (long in the pelvic limb) digital extensor M.

B. *Approach:* A needle is inserted on either side of the tendon and directed toward the pastern joint through the skin in an oblique direction proximodistally and dorsopalmarly/plantarly.

*Distal interphalangeal (coffin) joint* (see Fig. H6.37A)

A. *Landmarks:* the coronary border of the hoof, the tendon of the common (long in the pelvic limb) digital extensor M.

B. *Approach:* A needle is inserted on either side of the tendon through the skin and toward the distal interphalangeal (coffin) joint at the coronary border of the hoof in a direction similar to that performed for the pastern.

16. **Subcutaneous bursae**

*Prescapular bursa* (see Fig. H6.38A)

A. *Landmark* and *approach:* tuberosity of scapular spine

*Olecranon bursa* (see Fig. H6.38 A)

A. *Landmark* and *approach:* olecranon tuberosity

*Dorsal carpal bursa* (see Fig. H6.38B)

A. *Landmark* and *approach:* dorsal aspect of carpus

17. **Subtendinous bursae**

*Bursa of infraspinatus M.* (see Fig. H6.38A)

A. *Landmarks:* the caudal part of the greater tubercle of humerus, the tendon of the infraspinatus M.

B. *Approach:* through the skin and between the tendon and the bone

*Intertubercular bursa (bursa of biceps brachii M.)* (see Fig. H6.38A)

A. *Landmarks:* deltoid tuberosity of humerus, cranial part of the greater tubercle of the humerus

B. *Approach:* A needle is inserted craniodorsally at the level of the deltoid tuberosity, along the cranial aspect of the humerus toward the cranial part of the greater tubercle, deep through the skin and brachial fascia, and between the humerus and the cleidobrachialis M. Finally, the needle is located between the humerus and the biceps brachii M.

*Bursa of brachialis M.* (see Fig. H6.38C)

A. *Landmarks:* medial aspect of proximal extremity of radius, medial collateral lig. of the elbow

B. *Approach:* through the skin and the superficial and proper antebrachial fascia, at the cranial border of the medial collateral lig. of the elbow, deep between the brachialis M. and the medial aspect of the proximal extremity of the radius

*Bursa of extensor carpi radialis M.* (see Fig. H6.38B)

A. *Landmarks:* the tuberosity of metacarpal bone III, the attachment of the extensor carpi radialis M. on that tuberosity

B. *Approach:* through the skin and between the insertion of the muscle on metacarpal bone III, at the distal end of the extensor retinaculum

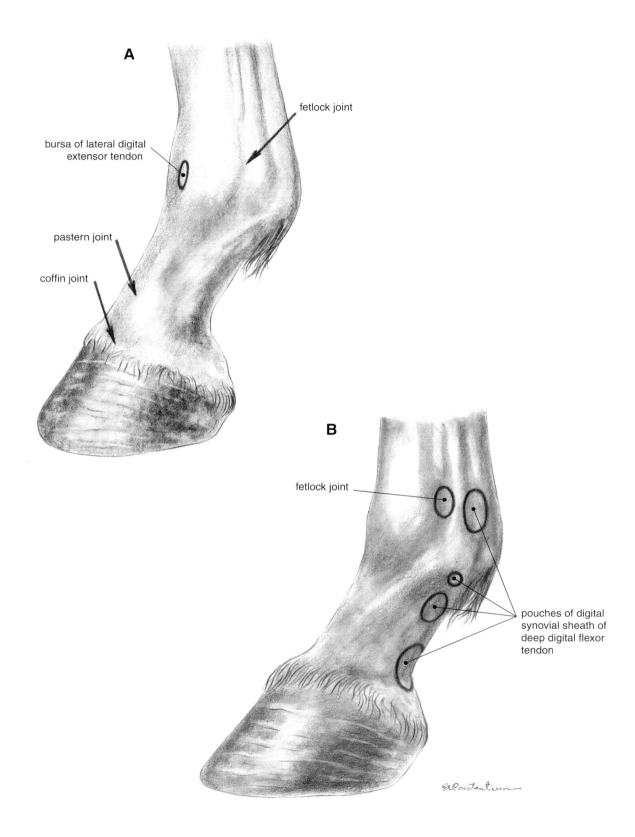

Fig. H6.37. Landmarks and approaches in the digital area, horse. **A.** Intraarticular approaches for the fetlock and interphalangeal joints, horse. **B.** Articular and tendinous pouches of the digit, horse.

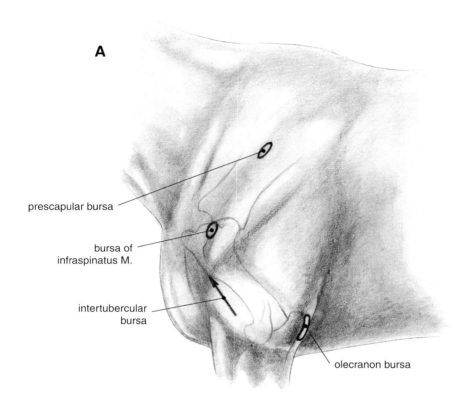

A

prescapular bursa

bursa of
infraspinatus M.

intertubercular
bursa

olecranon bursa

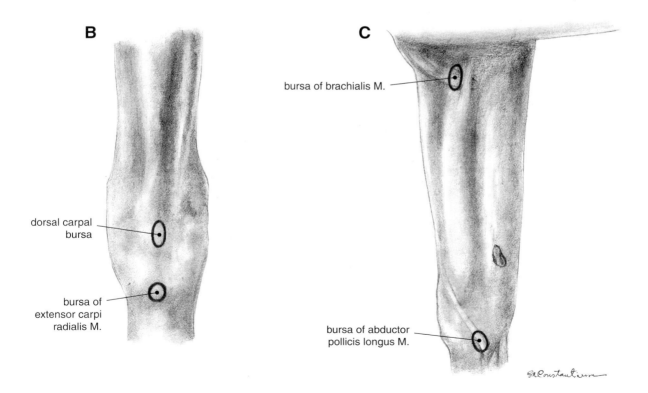

B

dorsal carpal
bursa

bursa of
extensor carpi
radialis M.

C

bursa of brachialis M.

bursa of abductor
pollicis longus M.

Fig. H6.38. Subcutaneous and subtendinous bursae of the thoracic limb, horse. **A.** Lateral aspect of left shoulder. **B.** Dorsal aspect of left carpus. **C.** Medial aspect of right forearm and carpus.

*Bursa of abductor pollicis longus M.* (see Fig. H6.38C)

A. *Landmarks:* the base of metacarpal bone II, the attachment of the abductor pollicis longus M. on that bone

B. *Approach:* through the skin and between the bone and the tendon of abductor pollicis longus M.

*Bursa of common digital extensor M.*

A. *Landmarks* and *approach:* similar to those used for the long digital extensor M. in the pelvic limb (see page 150)

*Bursa of lateral digital extensor M.* (Fig. H6.37A)

A. *Landmarks:* the dorsal aspect of the fetlock, the tendon of the lateral digital extensor M.

B. *Approach:* through the skin and between the tendon and the dorsal aspect of the fetlock

*Podotrochlear bursa*

A. *Landmarks* and *approach:* similar to those used in the pelvic limb (see page 150)

18. **Vaginal (synovial) tendon sheaths**

*Sheath of the extensor carpi radialis M.* (Fig. H6.39A)

A. *Landmarks:* the dorsal aspect of carpus, the tendon of the extensor carpi radialis M.

B. *Approach:* through the skin, around the tendon, proximal to the extensor retinaculum, and between the extensor retinaculum and the dorsal carpal joint capsule

*Sheath of the abductor pollicis longus M.* (Fig. H6.39A)

A. *Landmarks:* tendons of the extensor carpi radialis and abductor pollicis longus Mm. proximal to the carpus

B. *Approach:* through the skin, between the two tendons, and around the tendon of the abductor pollicis longus, in an oblique position ventromedially

*Sheath of the common digital extensor M.* (Fig. H6.39A)

A. *Landmarks:* dorsal aspect of the carpus, the tendon of the common digital extensor M.

B. *Approach:* through the skin around the common digital extensor tendon, between the extensor retinaculum and the dorsal carpal joint capsule, and exceeding the extensor retinaculum by 2–3 cm proximally and distally

*Sheath of the lateral digital extensor M.* (Fig. H6.39A)

A. *Landmarks:* lateral aspect of carpus, the tendon of the lateral digital extensor M.

B. *Approach:* through the skin around the lateral digital extensor tendon, between the superficial and deep fascicles of the lateral collateral lig. of the carpus, and exceeding the extensor retinaculum by 2–3 cm proximally and distally

*Sheath of the flexor carpi radialis M.* (Fig. H6.39B)

A. *Landmarks:* accessory carpal bone, chestnut, distal extent of radius on the medial aspect of the forearm

B. *Approach:* midway between the accessory carpal bone and the chestnut, parallel to the caudal border of the distal third of the radius, and through the skin and the superficial and proper antebrachial fasciae

*Common synovial sheath of SDF and DDF tendons* (Fig. H6.39B)

A. *Landmarks:* lateral and medial aspects of carpus; accessory carpal bone; tendons of lateral digital extensor, extensor carpi ulnaris, flexor carpi ulnaris, and flexor carpi radialis Mm.; metacarpal bones II and IV

B. *Approach:* through the skin, proximal and distal to the limits of the extensor and flexor retinacula. On the lateral aspect, proximal to the extensor retinaculum between the tendons of the lateral digital extensor M. (cranially) and extensor carpi ulnaris (caudally) and distal to the extensor retinaculum, in a palmar position to the metacarpal bone IV. On the medial aspect, proximal to the flexor retinaculum between the tendons of the flexor carpi radialis M. (cranially) and the flexor carpi ulnaris M. (caudally) and distal to the flexor retinaculum, in a palmar position to the metacarpal bone II

*Sheath of the deep digital flexor tendon*

A. *Landmarks:* the fetlock, the pastern, P I, the interosseous medius M., the tendons of the SDF and DDF

*Note.* There are six pouches associated with this sheath (see Fig. H6.37B), visible and palpable after a long run or in pathological conditions related to tenosynovitis. They are located subcutaneously and are described on page 190.

B. *Approach:* on the lateral and medial aspects of the fetlock, between the interosseous medius M. and the tendon of the SDF (the sheath surrounds the

DDF); on the lateral and medial aspects of the pastern, between P I and the tendon of the SDF; on the palmar/plantar aspects of the pastern, between the bifurcation of the tendon of the SDF and the distal digital annular lig.

19. **Accessory (check) lig. of the SDF (proximal check lig.)** (Fig. H6.39B)

    A. *Landmarks:* medial aspect of carpus, radius, flexor carpi radialis and flexor carpi ulnaris Mm.

    B. *Approach:* through the skin and the superficial and proper antebrachial fascia 2–3 cm proximal to the medial aspect of the carpus, in a horizontal or slightly oblique position between the radius and the tendon of the flexor carpi ulnaris M. The tendon of the flexor carpi radialis M. crosses the ligament.

20. **Accessory (check) lig. of the DDF (distal check lig.)** (Fig. H6.39B)

    A. *Landmarks:* lateral and medial palmar aspects of metacarpus/metatarsus, the splint bones, the interosseous medius M., the tendons of the SDF and DDF

    B. *Approach:* distal to the carpus/tarsus, on both sides of the metacarpus/metatarsus, between the splint bones and the corresponding border of the interosseous medius M. and the tendons of the superficial and deep digital flexors, in the proximal third of the area. It is located deep under the skin and palmar/plantar fascia, on the dorsal aspect of the deep digital flexor tendon. It is significantly smaller in the pelvic limb.

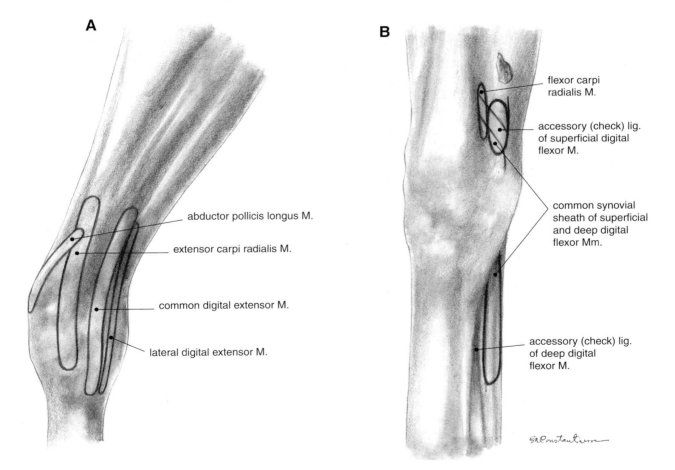

Fig. H6.39. Synovial tendon sheaths around the carpus, horse. **A.** Lateral aspect of carpus. **B.** Medial aspect of carpus.

# H 7

# The Head

The skull is illustrated from the frontal, lateral, and ventral perspectives (Figs. H7.1–H7.3); the orbital area and the cranial cavity are also illustrated (Figs. H7.4 and H7.5); the lateral, dorsal, and ventral aspects of the mandible are shown in Fig. H7.6; and the hyoid apparatus is shown in Fig. H7.7. A thorough study of all of the characteristics and structures of the skull is strongly suggested before trying to identify the head structures, which follow. The structures of the skull are important not only as landmarks for physical examination and/or clinical approach (illustrated in Fig. H7.8), but also because they are related to the muscle attachments, passage of vessels and nerves, and the location of other structures, such as ganglia, glands, paranasal sinuses, and so on. The skull also protects the initial segments of the respiratory and digestive systems.

Before starting the dissection, identify on the head the following landmarks for physical examination and/or clinical approach.

*On the frontal aspect of the head locate the philtrum of the upper lip, the incisive bones, the nasal process, the nasal aperture, the nostrils, the alar cartilages, the nasal diverticula (sing. diverticulum; the false nares), the infraorbital foramina, the orbitae, the supraorbital foramina, the zygomatic arches, the temporal lines, the temporal fossae, the external occipital protuberance, the base of the ear, and the mane.*

*On the lateral aspect, identify the upper and the lower lips, the oral cleft, the commissure of the lips, the nostril, the alar cartilage (at the medial border of the nostril), the nasal process, the nasoincisive notch, the nasal aperture, the chin, the mental foramen, the superior and inferior incisors, premolars and molars, the diastema, the facial tubercle and crest, the infraorbital foramen, the orbita, the supraorbital foramen, the zygomatic arch, the temporal fossa, the ear, the temporomandibular joint, the jugular (paracondylar) process of the occipital bone, the caudal border of the ramus of the mandible and the*

*angle of the mandible, the styloid angle of the stylohyoid bone, the vascular notch of the mandible (the notch for the facial vessels), the rostral border of the masseter M., the linguofacial V., the tendon of the sternomandibularis M., and the occipitomandibular part of the digastricus M.*

*On the ventral aspect, identify the paired bodies of the mandible, with the incisive and molar parts, the mylohyoideus Mm., the basihyoid bone, and the larynx.*

**Passing a gastric tube or exploring the nasal cavity, pharynx, guttural pouches, larynx, esophagus, stomach, trachea, and bronchi endoscopically is accomplished by introducing the tube or the endoscope through the nostrils (then the ventral meatus, the choana, the naso- and laryngopharynx, etc).**

**The temporal line marks the medial and rostral borders of the temporal fossa.**

**The external occipital protuberance is a landmark for collection of cerebrospinal fluid (see Chapter H1, The Neck).**

**The facial tubercle and crest, the medial canthus of the eye (at the medial angle of the orbita), and the infraorbital foramen are landmarks for trepanation/trephination of the paranasal sinuses *(a trepan or trephine is a saw for removing a circular disk of bone, chiefly from the skull, and also an instrument for removing a circular area of cornea, as in corneal transplant operations)*.**

**The caudal border of the ramus of the mandible, the linguofacial V., the tendon of the sternomandibularis M., and the occipitomandibular part of the digastricus M. outline Viborg's triangle, used in several approaches to the guttural pouch.**

**The jugular (paracondylar) process of the occipital bone and the styloid angle of the stylohyoid bone are landmarks for an additional approach to the guttural pouch.**

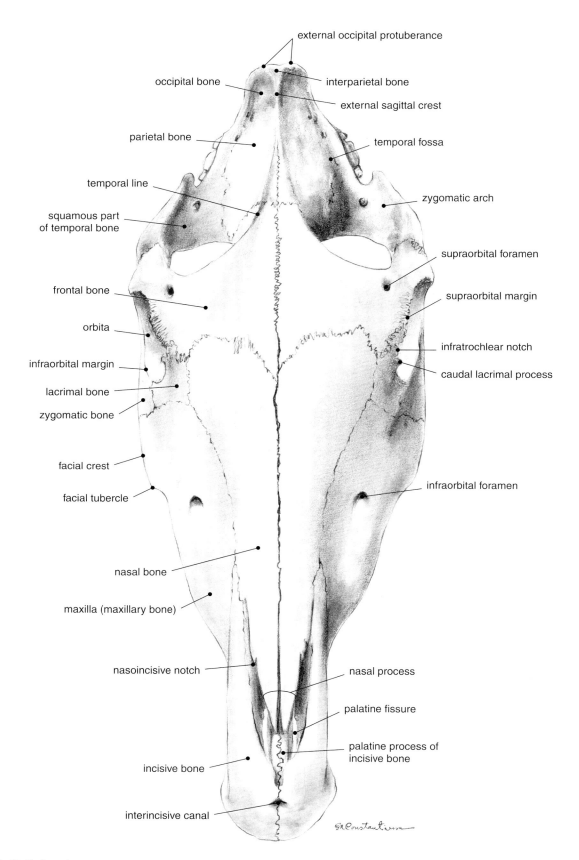

external occipital protuberance

occipital bone

interparietal bone

external sagittal crest

parietal bone

temporal fossa

temporal line

zygomatic arch

squamous part
of temporal bone

supraorbital foramen

frontal bone

supraorbital margin

orbita

infratrochlear notch

infraorbital margin

caudal lacrimal process

lacrimal bone

zygomatic bone

facial crest

infraorbital foramen

facial tubercle

nasal bone

maxilla (maxillary bone)

nasoincisive notch

nasal process

palatine fissure

palatine process of
incisive bone

incisive bone

interincisive canal

Fig. H7.1. Skull, frontal aspect.

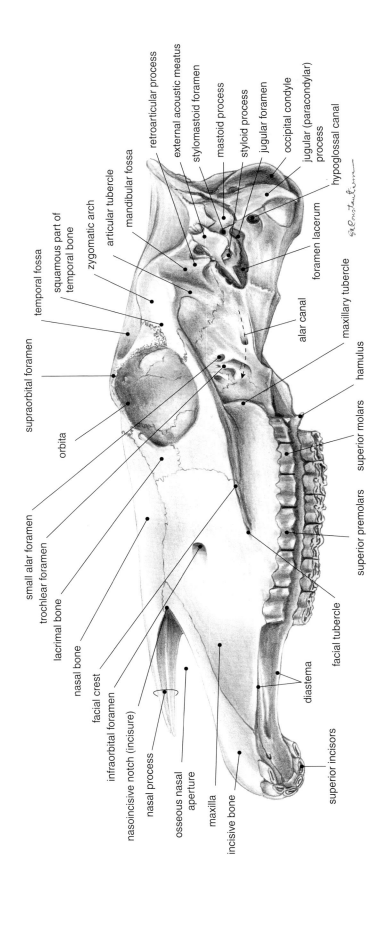

retroarticular process

external acoustic meatus

stylomastoid foramen

mastoid process

styloid process

jugular foramen

occipital condyle

jugular (paracondylar) process

hypoglossal canal

articular tubercle

mandibular fossa

squamous part of temporal bone

zygomatic arch

temporal fossa

foramen lacerum

alar canal

maxillary tubercle

supraorbital foramen

orbita

hamulus

superior molars

superior premolars

small alar foramen

trochlear foramen

lacrimal bone

nasal bone

facial crest

infraorbital foramen

nasoincisive notch (incisure)

nasal process

osseous nasal aperture

maxilla

incisive bone

diastema

facial tubercle

superior incisors

Fig. H7.2. Skull, lateral aspect, without mandible.

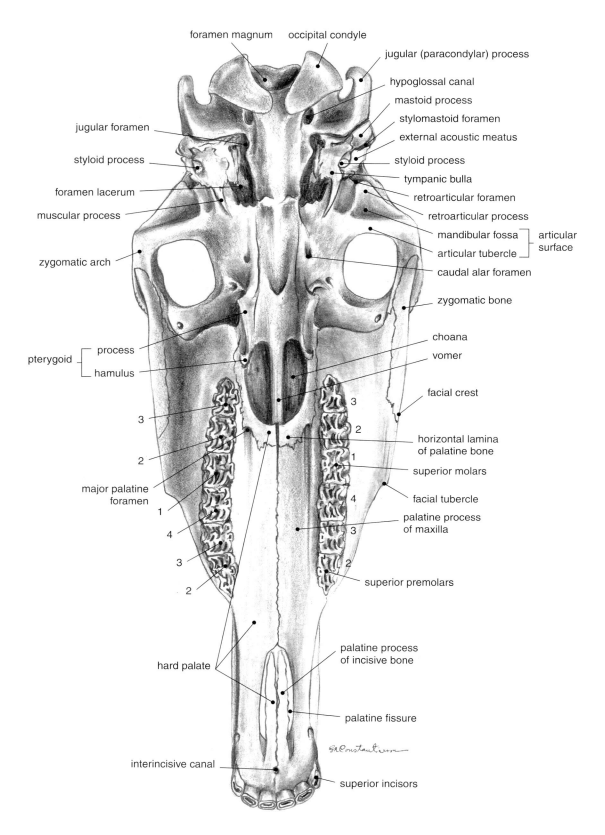

foramen magnum

occipital condyle

jugular (paracondylar) process

hypoglossal canal

mastoid process

stylomastoid foramen

external acoustic meatus

styloid process

tympanic bulla

retroarticular foramen

retroarticular process

mandibular fossa ⎤ articular
articular tubercle ⎦ surface

caudal alar foramen

zygomatic bone

choana

vomer

facial crest

horizontal lamina
of palatine bone

superior molars

facial tubercle

palatine process
of maxilla

superior premolars

palatine process
of incisive bone

palatine fissure

superior incisors

jugular foramen

styloid process

foramen lacerum

muscular process

zygomatic arch

pterygoid ⎡ process
⎣ hamulus

major palatine
foramen

hard palate

interincisive canal

3

2

1

4

3

2

3

2

1

4

3

2

Fig. H7.3. Skull, ventral aspect, without mandible.

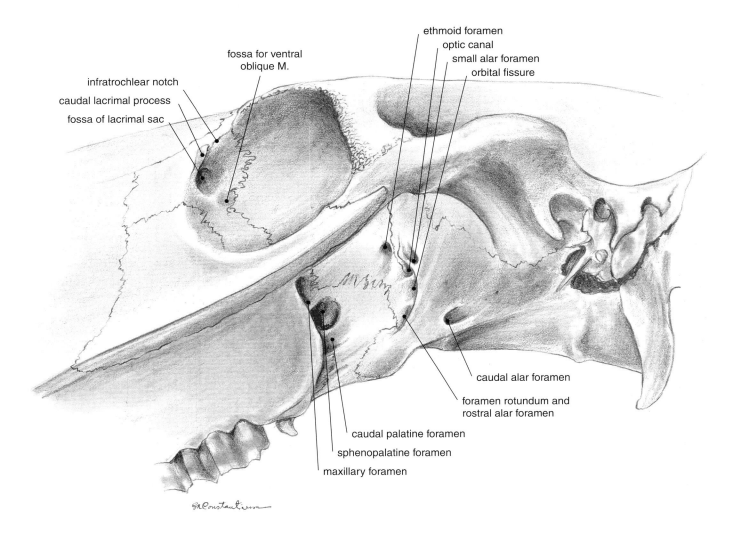

infratrochlear notch

caudal lacrimal process

fossa of lacrimal sac

fossa for ventral
oblique M.

ethmoid foramen

optic canal

small alar foramen

orbital fissure

caudal alar foramen

foramen rotundum and
rostral alar foramen

caudal palatine foramen

sphenopalatine foramen

maxillary foramen

Fig. H7.4. Orbital area on the skull, lateroventral aspect.

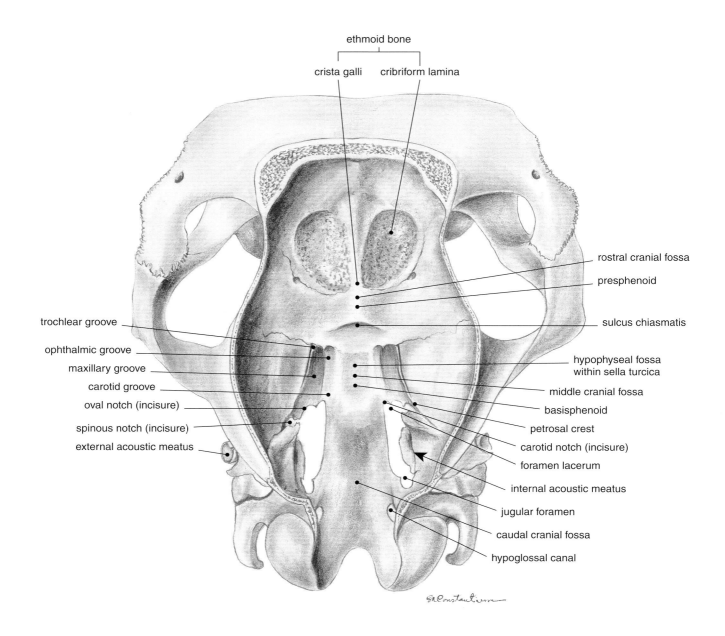

ethmoid bone

crista galli  cribriform lamina

rostral cranial fossa

presphenoid

trochlear groove

sulcus chiasmatis

ophthalmic groove

maxillary groove

hypophyseal fossa
within sella turcica

carotid groove

middle cranial fossa

oval notch (incisure)

basisphenoid

spinous notch (incisure)

petrosal crest

external acoustic meatus

carotid notch (incisure)

foramen lacerum

internal acoustic meatus

jugular foramen

caudal cranial fossa

hypoglossal canal

Fig. H7.5. Cranial cavity, rostral wall and floor.

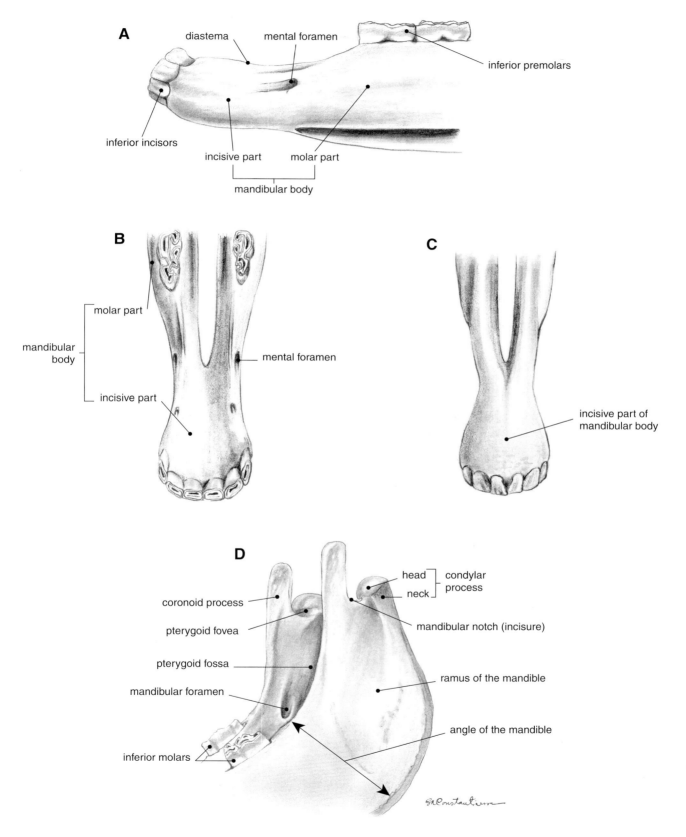

Fig. H7.6. Mandible in the horse. **A.** Rostral end of mandible, lateral aspect. **B.** Rostral end of mandible, dorsal aspect. **C.** Rostral end of mandible, ventral aspect. **D.** Caudal half of mandible, rostrolateral aspect.

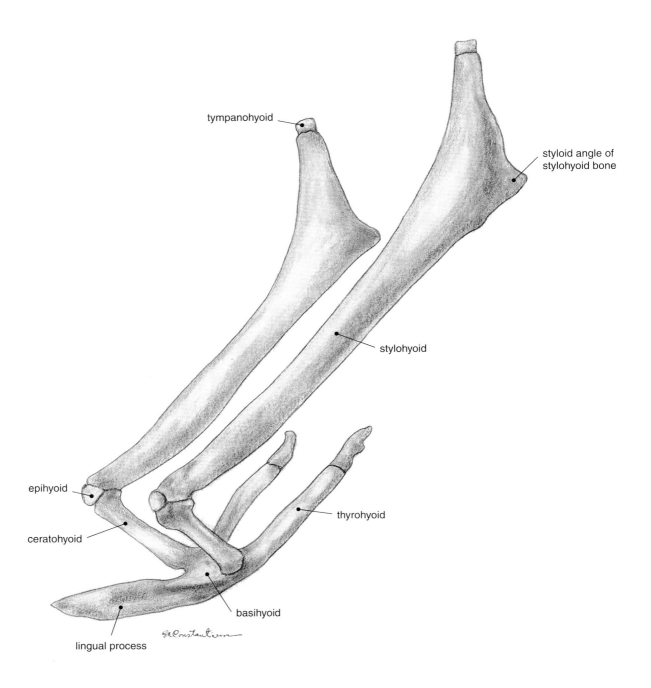

tympanohyoid

styloid angle of
stylohyoid bone

stylohyoid

epihyoid

ceratohyoid

thyrohyoid

basihyoid

lingual process

Fig. H7.7. The hyoid apparatus, horse, left aspect.

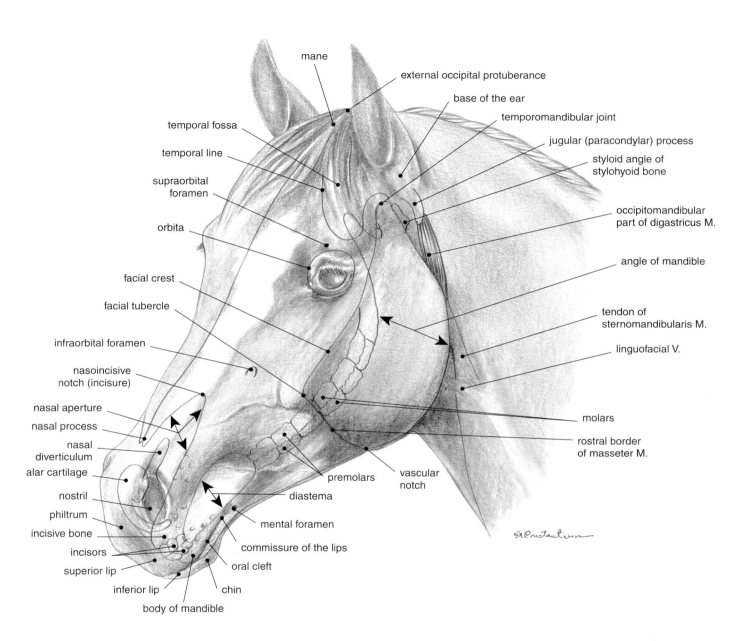

mane

external occipital protuberance

base of the ear

temporomandibular joint

jugular (paracondylar) process

styloid angle of stylohyoid bone

temporal fossa

temporal line

supraorbital foramen

occipitomandibular part of digastricus M.

orbita

angle of mandible

facial crest

facial tubercle

tendon of sternomandibularis M.

linguofacial V.

infraorbital foramen

nasoincisive notch (incisure)

nasal aperture

nasal process

molars

rostral border of masseter M.

nasal diverticulum

alar cartilage

nostril

philtrum

incisive bone

incisors

superior lip

inferior lip

chin

body of mandible

premolars

diastema

mental foramen

commissure of the lips

oral cleft

vascular notch

Fig. H7.8. Landmarks for physical examination and/or clinical approach to the head, horse.

The **mylohyoideus M.**, the **basihyoid bone**, and the notch for the **facial vessels** are landmarks for access to the mandibular lnn.

The other structures, single or combined, are landmarks for nerve block anesthesia.

All structures listed above will be used at the end of this chapter in Modlab H7 for physical examination and/or clinical approach.

Make an incision in the skin, starting from the **chin**, around the **commissure of the lips**, caudal to the **nostrils**, and up to the dorsal midline. Make a 1 cm skin incision around the **eyelids**, and another around the base of the **ear**. Make a last incision in the skin on the midventral line and begin skinning in a ventrodorsal direction.

*Caution*. The more carefully the skin is removed, the better the underlying structures will be exposed. There is only a very small amount of subcutaneous loose connective tissue!

The muscles of the head are presented in a systematic order in Table H7.1.

The muscles of the hyoid apparatus, pharynx, and larynx will be described separately.

The **cutaneous faciei M.**, continuous with the **cutaneous colli M.**, is the most superficial muscle exposed (within the **superficial fascia of the head**). The cutaneous faciei M. is attached to the **orbicularis oris M.**, at the level of the **commissure of the lips**, as the **depressor anguli oris M.** Start removing the cutaneous faciei M. in a rostral direction, from the parotid region to the commissure of the lips. Leave only a few centimeters of the cutaneous faciei M. attached to the commissure of the lips as the depessor anguli oris M. and discard the rest of it. Several nerves, vessels, and muscles are now exposed. Outline and then dissect them carefully as they are illustrated in Figure H7.9.

Parallel with the rostral border of the **masseter M.** identify, in rostrocaudal order, the **facial A.**, the **facial V.**, and the **parotid duct**.

While dissecting the **levator labii superioris M.**, pay attention to the symmetrical tendons (in a rostral direction) that fuse with each other to form an aponeurosis. The aponeurosis overlaps the **dilator naris apicalis M.** and blends its fibers with the orbicularis oris M.

Before dissecting the four parts of the **lateral nasal M.**, introduce a finger through the dorsal commissure of the **nostril** into the **nasal diverticulum (the false naris)**, which is the size and shape of a glove finger. It lies against the membrane that fills the **osseous nasal aperture**. Its secretion, mixed with particles of dust, is emptied by the vibration of the membrane, activated by the lateral nasal M.

Table H7.1. Muscles of the Head, Horse and Large Ruminants

**Facial Muscles**
– frontalis *(except eq)*
– lateralis nasi
– dilatator naris apicalis
– orbicularis oculi
– levator anguli oculi medialis
– retractor anguli oculi lateralis *(except eq)*
– malaris
– incisivus superior
– incisivus inferior
– mentalis
– orbicularis oris
– depressor anguli oris
– zygomaticus
– levator nasolabialis
– levator labii superioris
– caninus
– depressor labii superioris *(except eq)*
– depressor labii inferioris
– buccinator

**Muscles of Mastication**
– masseter
– temporalis
– pterygoideus medialis
– pterygoideus lateralis
– digastricus
  • pars occipitomandibularis *(only in eq)*

**Muscles of the Ear**
– auriculares rostrales
  • scutuloauriculares superficiales
  • scutuloauriculares profundi
  • frontoscutularis
  • zygomaticoscutularis
  • zygomaticoauricularis
– auriculares dorsales
  • interscutularis
  • parietoscutularis
  • parietoauricularis
– auriculares caudales
  • cervicoscutularis
  • cervicoauricularis superficialis
  • cervicoauricularis medius
  • cervicoauricularis profundus
– auriculares ventrales
  • parotidoauricularis
  • styloauricularis

*Note*. The lateral nasal M. consists of four parts. The dorsal, caudal, and ventral parts originate from the osseous nasal aperture. The rostral part is attached to the tip of the **cornu** of the **alar cartilage** and is a dilator of the nostril.

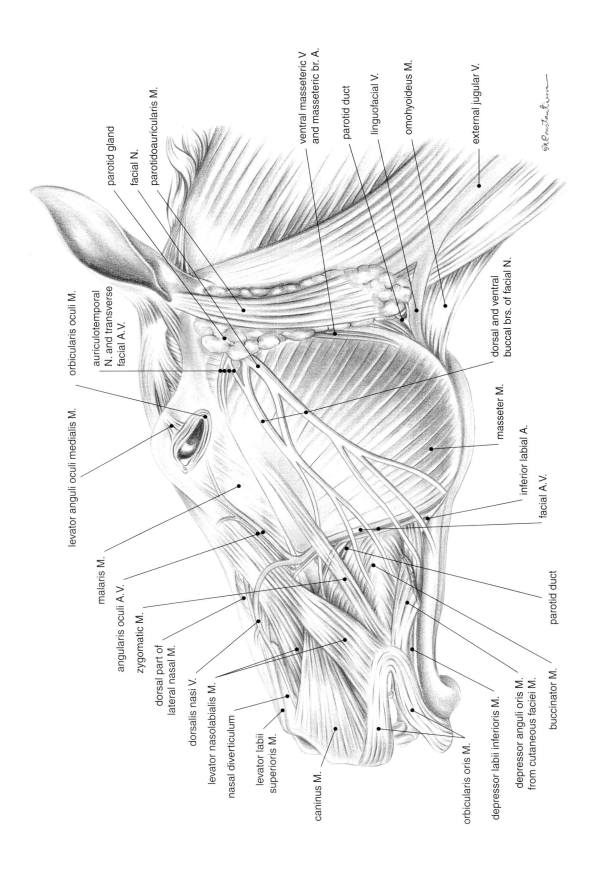

Fig. H7.9. Superficial structures of the head, lateral aspect.

orbicularis oculi M.

parotid gland

facial N.

parotidoauricularis M.

ventral masseteric V
and masseteric br. A.

parotid duct

linguofacial V.

omohyoideus M.

external jugular V.

auriculotemporal
N. and transverse
facial A.V.

dorsal and ventral
buccal brs. of facial N.

levator anguli oculi medialis M.

masseter M.

inferior labial A.

facial A.V.

malaris M.

angularis oculi A.V.

zygomatic M.

dorsal part of
lateral nasal M.

dorsalis nasi V.

levator nasolabialis M.

levator labii
superioris M.

nasal diverticulum

caninus M.

parotid duct

orbicularis oris M.

depressor labii inferioris M.

depressor anguli oris M.
from cutaneous faciei M.

buccinator M.

Focus your attention on the parotid region. Branches of cervical spinal nerves 2 and 3 and the cutaneous colli M. cover the **parotid gland** and the **parotidoauricularis M.** and should be reflected caudally. *Remember* that you already dissected these nerves in the cervical region. Sev-

eral vessels and nerves are seen before reflecting the gland (Fig. H7.10).

Start the removal of the parotid gland from the **facial N.** Pay attention to the small **parotid ln.**, lying on the **transverse facial A.** This artery is accompanied by the **auricu-**

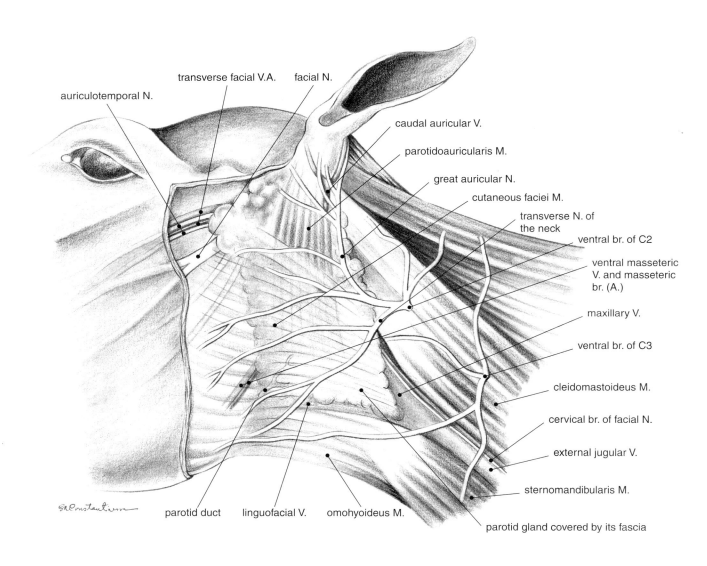

Fig. H7.10. Superficial structures in the parotid region, horse.

lotemporal N., a branch of the **mandibular N.** from the **trigeminal N.** Carefully reflect the rostroventral angle of the gland to protect the parotid duct.

Dissect the facial and auriculotemporal Nn. in a rostral direction and *notice* that they communicate with each other and build up a plexus-like net, the **buccal branches** of the facial N.

The **superficial temporal V.** crosses the facial N. in a position parallel to the caudal border of the ramus of the mandible and very close to it. Dissect the vein dorsally and ventrally and identify the merging point with the **maxillary V.** Dissect the maxillary V. and identify the merging point with the **linguofacial V.**, which is the origin of the **external jugular V.** (Fig. H7.11).

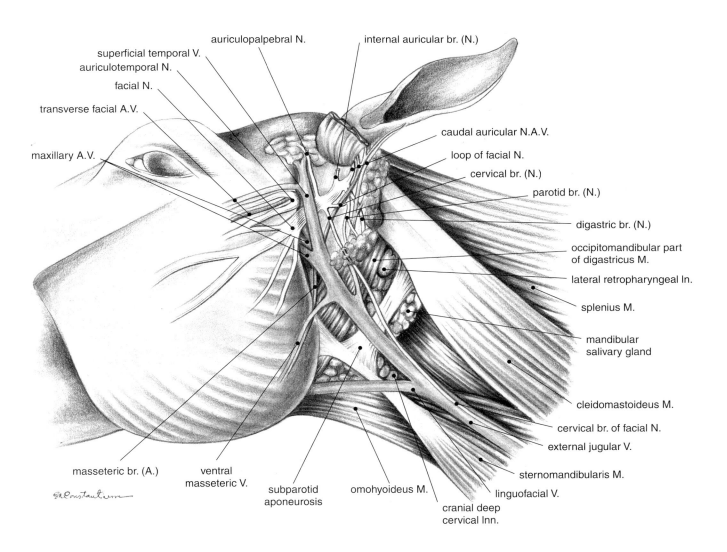

Fig. H7.11. Structures located deep to the parotid gland, horse.

*Caution.* Unless injected with latex, the dissection of these veins should be performed with care because they usually travel within the parotid gland.

Continue to dissect the facial N. and identify its three dorsally oriented branches and three ventrally oriented branches. The dorsal branches are in a rostrocaudal order: the **auriculopalpebral N.** (parallel with and caudal to the superficial temporal V.), the **internal auricular branch,** and the **caudal auricular N.**, accompanied by the **caudal auricular A.V.** The ventral branches are the **cervical branch**, the **parotid branch**, and the muscular branches (**digastric** and **stylohyoid**) (see Fig. H7.11). The cervical branch has an inconstant route with regard to the parotid gland, but it finally accompanies the external jugular V., supplying the parotidoauricularis M. and the cutaneous colli M. In addition, identify a loop of the facial N. surrounding the caudal auricular A.

Between the tendons of the **sternomandibularis** and **cleidomastoideus Mm.,** identify and dissect a fibrous bridge, unofficially called the **subparotid aponeurosis**. It lies deep to the maxillary V. and separates the parotid from the **mandibular salivary gland**. Also deep to the vein, identify the **occipitomandibular part of the digastricus M.** Between it and the subparotid aponeurosis, the **lateral retropharyngeal ln.** is exposed (see Fig. H7.11).

Retract the maxillary V. rostrally and transect the occipitomandibular part of the digastricus M. to expose the **caudal belly of the digastricus M.**, the **occipitohyoideus** and **stylohyoideus Mm.**, the **stylohyoid bone**, the **glossopharyngeal** and **hypoglossal Nn.**, and the **external carotid A.** with two branches and two terminal arteries. The two branches are the **caudal auricular A.** and the **masseteric br.**, while the two terminal arteries are the **maxillary** and the **superficial temporal Aa.** (Fig. H7.12). *Notice* that the glossopharyngeal N. (in a dorsal position) crosses the external carotid A. on the medial (deep) side, whereas the hypoglossal N. (in a ventral position, parallel to the glossopharyngeal N.) crosses the artery on the lateral (superficial) side.

Reflect the digastricus M. caudally and expose the deepest structures of the area covering the **guttural pouch** (Fig. H7.13). The guttural pouch is the **diverticulum of the mucosa of the auditory,** or **pharyngotympanic,** or **Eustachian tube.** To ease the dissection, pull caudally the **common carotid A.**, the **vagosympathetic trunk**, and the **recurrent laryngeal N.** and extend the head on the neck as much as possible.

Prepare to split the head into two halves. With a knife, make a precise midline incision through the **lips**, the **tip of the nose**, and the ventral aspect of the head. Deepen the incision on the ventral aspect through the **tongue, larynx,** **pharynx**, and the **esophagus**. Do the same on the dorsal midline of the neck. Saw the head carefully to obtain two symmetrical halves.

To expose, dissect, and identify the deep structures of the head (Fig. H7.14), it is necessary to *remove the mandible* from one-half of the split head. First, transect the buccal branches of the facial N. Free and reflect them from the **masseter M.** Transect the masseter M. parallel and 1 cm ventral to the **facial crest** and reflect it ventrocaudally, saving the three veins that join the facial V. In dorsoventral order they are the **transverse facial, deep facial**, and **buccal Vv.**

*Notice* that in the horse these three veins form dilations called venous sinuses.

The transverse facial V. connects the facial V. to the superficial temporal V.; the deep facial V. discharges blood from the **orbital** and **pterygopalatine regions**. The buccal V. connects the facial V. to the maxillary V.

Transect the facial A.V. and the parotid duct at the level of the **mandibular notch for the facial vessels** and reflect them. Make an incision in the mucosa of the **vestibule of the oral cavity** following the ventral border of the **depressor labii inferioris M.** all the way through the **mental foramen**. Transect the occipitomandibular part of the digastricus M., the tendon of the sternomandibularis M., and the **masseteric** and transverse facial vessels close to the caudal border of the ramus of the mandible.

Using a chisel and a hammer, make four sections in the skull (Fig. H7.15): (1) a transverse section of the **zygomatic process of the frontal bone**, as close as possible to the base of the process; (2) a transverse section of the **temporal process of the zygomatic bone** rostral to the **medial canthus of the eye**; (3) an oblique section of the **zygomatic arch** caudal to the temporomandibular joint in a caudorostral direction; and (4) a transverse section of the mandible between the **incisive** and the **molar parts**, caudal to the palpable mental foramen.

Turn the head so that the ventral intermandibular aspect is up. Dissect the **mylohyoideus M.** and the **rostral belly of the digastricus M.**, the **mandibular lnn.**, the **omohyoideus** and **sternohyoideus Mm.**, the facial A. and V., and the parotid duct. Reflect the vessels and the parotid duct caudally. Free the mylohyoideus M. and the rostral belly of the digastricus M. from the medial aspect of the mandible. Gently pull the mandible and free it from the mylohyoideus M. to detach the muscle from its insertion. Toward the caudal extent of the mylohyoideus M., remove the periosteum from the medial aspect of the mandible to protect the **mylohyoid N.**

Turn the head lateral side up and remove the zygomatic arch. To accomplish this, it is necessary to free the zygo-

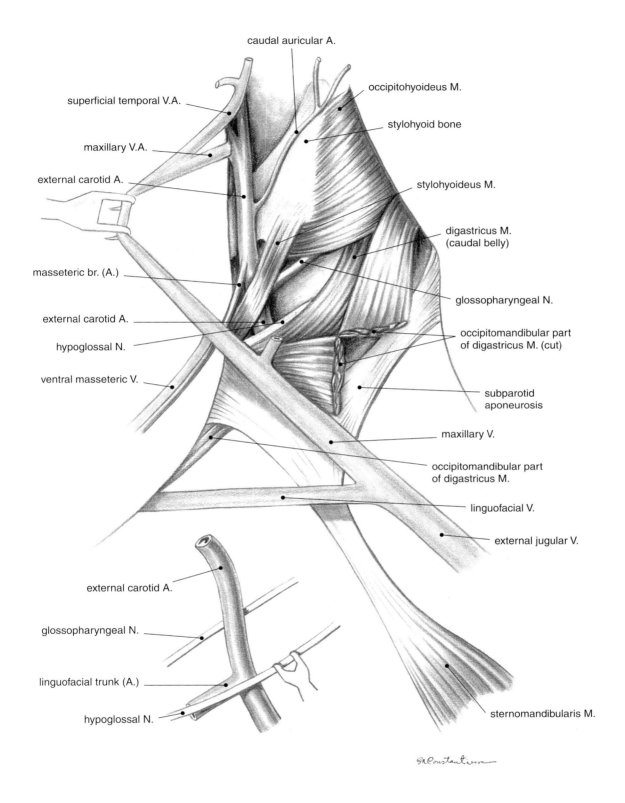

caudal auricular A.

occipitohyoideus M.

superficial temporal V.A.

stylohyoid bone

maxillary V.A.

stylohyoideus M.

external carotid A.

digastricus M. (caudal belly)

masseteric br. (A.)

glossopharyngeal N.

external carotid A.

occipitomandibular part of digastricus M. (cut)

hypoglossal N.

ventral masseteric V.

subparotid aponeurosis

maxillary V.

occipitomandibular part of digastricus M.

linguofacial V.

external jugular V.

external carotid A.

glossopharyngeal N.

linguofacial trunk (A.)

hypoglossal N.

sternomandibularis M.

Fig. H7.12. Deep structures within the left parotid region, horse.

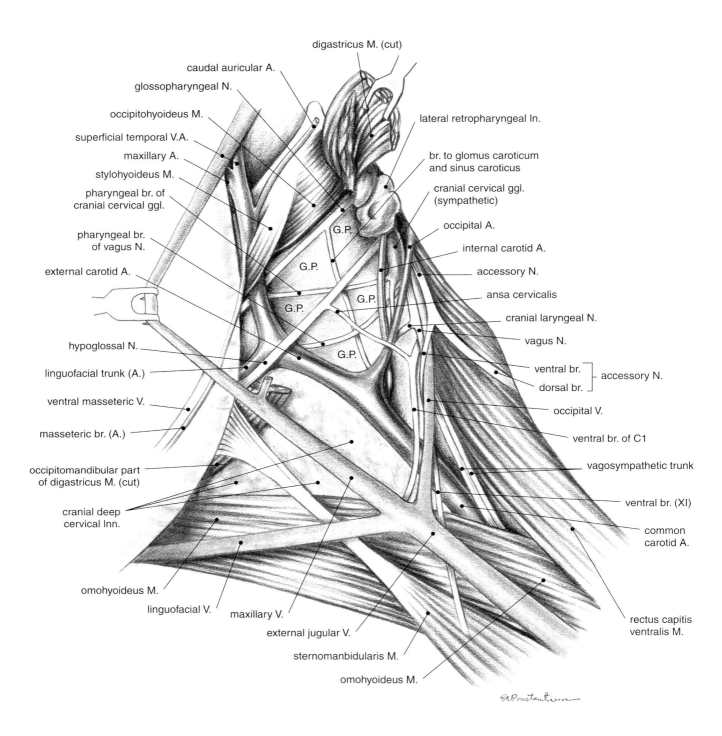

caudal auricular A.

digastricus M. (cut)

glossopharyngeal N.

occipitohyoideus M.

superficial temporal V.A.

maxillary A.

stylohyoideus M.

pharyngeal br. of
cranial cervical ggl.

pharyngeal br.
of vagus N.

external carotid A.

hypoglossal N.

linguofacial trunk (A.)

ventral masseteric V.

masseteric br. (A.)

occipitomandibular part
of digastricus M. (cut)

cranial deep
cervical lnn.

omohyoideus M.

linguofacial V.

maxillary V.

external jugular V.

sternomanbidularis M.

omohyoideus M.

lateral retropharyngeal ln.

br. to glomus caroticum
and sinus caroticus

cranial cervical ggl.
(sympathetic)

occipital A.

internal carotid A.

accessory N.

ansa cervicalis

cranial laryngeal N.

vagus N.

ventral br.
dorsal br.  ] accessory N.

occipital V.

ventral br. of C1

vagosympathetic trunk

ventral br. (XI)

common
carotid A.

rectus capitis
ventralis M.

G.P.

G.P.

G.P.

G.P.

G.P.

Fig. H7.13. The left guttural pouch (G.P.) and adjacent structures, horse.

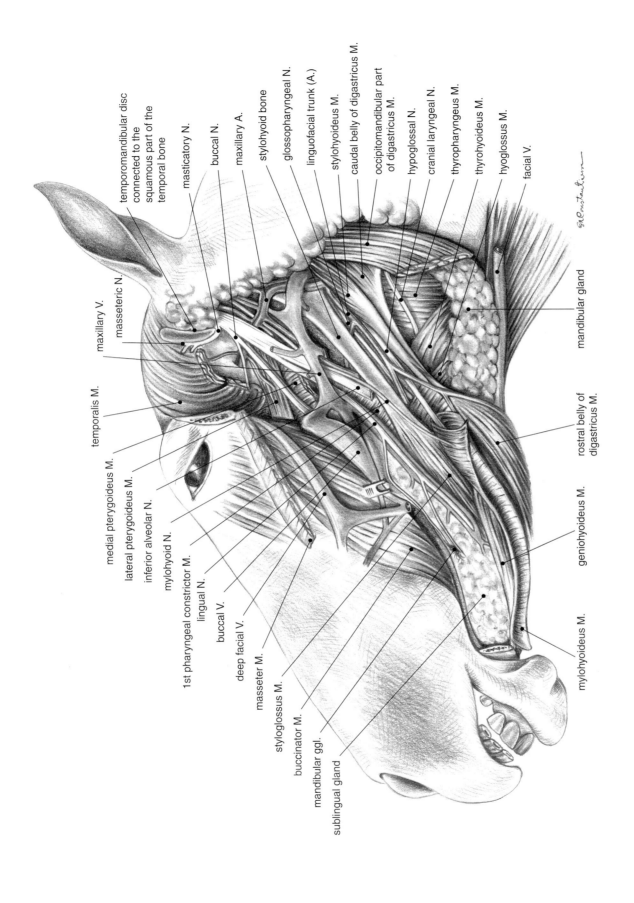

temporomandibular disc connected to the squamous part of the temporal bone

masticatory N.

buccal N.

maxillary A.

stylohyoid bone

glossopharyngeal N.

linguofacial trunk (A.)

stylohyoideus M.

caudal belly of digastricus M.

occipitomandibular part of digastricus M.

hypoglossal N.

cranial laryngeal N.

thyropharyngeus M.

thyrohyoideus M.

hyoglossus M.

facial V.

mandibular gland

maxillary V.

masseteric N.

temporalis M.

medial pterygoideus M.

lateral pterygoideus M.

inferior alveolar N.

mylohyoid N.

1st pharyngeal constrictor M.

lingual N.

buccal V.

deep facial V.

masseter M.

styloglossus M.

buccinator M.

mandibular ggl.

sublingual gland

mylohyoideus M.

geniohyoideus M.

rostral belly of digastricus M.

Fig. H7.14. Deep structures of the head, lateral aspect, horse. (Mandible has been removed.)

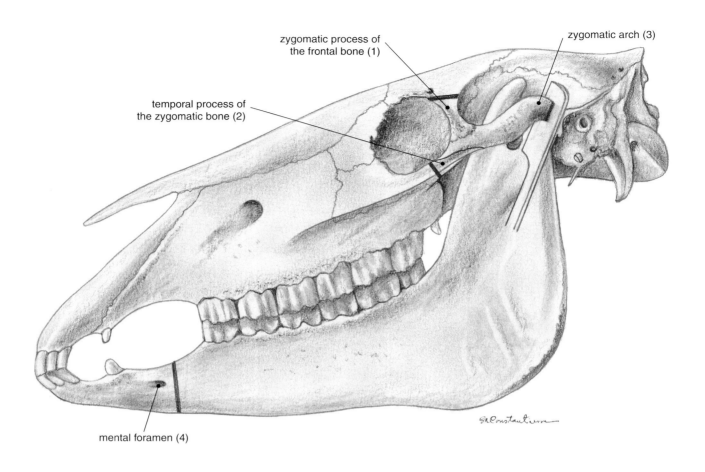

zygomatic process of
the frontal bone (1)

zygomatic arch (3)

temporal process of
the zygomatic bone (2)

mental foramen (4)

Fig. H7.15. Sites for cutting the skull and removing the mandible in the horse.

matic arch from both the **temporalis** and the **masseter Mm.** Leave the **temporomandibular disc** connected to the **squamous part of the temporal bone** after sectioning the joint capsule around the joint (see Fig. H7.14).When the mandible is pulled higher and higher, the following muscles are sectioned: the **medial pterygoideus M.** from the **pterygoid fossa** (on the medial aspect of the ramus of the mandible), the attachment of the temporalis M. from the medial aspect of the **coronoid process of the mandible**, and the attachment of the **lateral pterygoideus M.** from the **pterygoid fovea** (on the medial aspect of the **neck** and **condyle of the mandible**).

Continue to carefully detach the periosteum from the

medial aspect of the mandible up to the **mandibular foramen**.

*Caution*. The slender mylohyoid N., which supplies the mylohyoideus M. and the rostral belly of the digastricus M., runs between the bone and the periosteum.

Transect the **inferior alveolar A., V.,** and **N.** before entering the mandibular foramen.

At the conclusion of the procedure, the mandible is removed.

For a better understanding of the cranial nerves, Table H7.2 shows the foramina through which these nerves pass in and out of the cranial cavity, the quality of the fibers that they carry, and some observations.

Table H7.2. The Cranial Nerves in the Horse and Large Ruminants

| Nerve | Leaves Skull Through | Motor | Sensory | Mixed | Para-sympathetic | Observations |
|---|---|---|---|---|---|---|
| I. Olfactory | Cribriform plate ethmoid | | SVA | | | Terminal ggl. |
| II. Optic | Optic canal | | SSA | | | |
| III. Oculomotor | Foramen orbitorotundum (Ru) Orbital fissure (eq) | GSE | | | GVE | Ciliary ggl. (parasymp.); short ciliary Nn. postggl. fibers |
| IV. Trochlear | Foramen orbitorotundum (Ru) Orbital fissure/Foramen trochleare (eq) | GSE | | | | |
| V. Trigeminal | | | | * | | |
| 1. Ophthalmic | Foramen orbitorotundum (Ru) Orbital fissure (eq) | | GSA | | | |
| 2. Maxillary | Foramen orbitorotundum (Ru) Foramen rotundum (eq) | | GSA | | | Trigeminal ggl. (sens.) |
| 3. Mandibular | Foramen ovale | SVE | GSA | | | |
| VI. Abducent | Foramen orbitorotundum (Ru) Orbital fissure (eq) | GSE | | | | |
| VII. Facial | Enters facial canal Leaves stylomastoid foramen Leaves petrotympanic fissure for chorda tympani N. | SVE | GSA | * | GVE | Geniculate ggl. (sens.) Pterygopalatine ggl. (parasymp.) Greater petrosal N. preggl. fibers Mandibular ggl. (parasymp.) Chorda tympani N. preggl. fibers |
| VIII. Vestibulococh-lear | Enters internal acoustic meatus | | SP | | | Vestibular ggl. |
| | | | SSA | | | Spiral ggl. |
| IX. Glossopharyngeal | Jugular foramen | SVE | | | | Proximal ggl. |
| | | SVA | | * | | Distal ggl. |
| | | GVA | | * | | |
| | | GSA | | * | | |
| | | | | | GVE | Lateropharyngeal ggl. (bo, ov) Otic ggl. (parasymp.) Lesser petrosal N. preggl. fibers |
| X. Vagus | Jugular foramen | SVE | GSA | * | | Proximal ggl. (sens.) |
| | | | | GVA | | Distal ggl. (sens.) |
| | | | | SVA | | |
| XI. Accessory | Jugular foramen | SVE | | | GVE | |
| XII. Hypoglossal | Hypoglossal canal | GSE | | | | |

*Note:* GSE = general somatic efferent; GVE = general visceral efferent; GSA = general somatic afferent; GVA = general visceral afferent; SVA = special visceral afferent; SVE = special visceral efferent; SSA = special somatic afferent; SP = special proprioception.
* = mixed nerves.

Carefully remove the two pterygoid muscles, preserving the vessels and the nerves and, in addition, the delicate and thin wall of the guttural pouch. All the branches of the **mandibular N.** of the **trigeminal N. (V3)** can be dissected. They all cross the lateral aspect of the **maxillary A.** (see Fig. 7.14).

The rostral border of the temporomandibular disc is paralleled by the **masticatory N.**, whose branches are the **masseteric N.** for the masseter M., and the **caudal** and **middle deep temporal Nn.**, which supply the temporalis M. The next branch of the V3 is the **buccal N.**, mixed, supplying part of the temporalis M. by the **rostral deep**

**temporal N.** and then supplying the mucosa of the cheeks. Identify the **otic ggl.** (parasympathetic) at the origin of the buccal N.

*Remember!* The otic ggl. is the site for synapsis between the **minor petrosal N.**, carrying preganglionic parasympathetic fibers from the **glossopharyngeal N.** and the postganglionic fibers supplying the parotid and **buccal** glands.

The **lateral pterygoid N.**, the **medial pterygoid N.**, the **tensor veli palatini N.** and the **tensor tympani N.** supply the muscles with the same names. The **lingual N.** supplies the mucosa of the tongue and at the same time protects the route of the **chorda tympani N.** The latter carries preganglionic parasympathetic fibers from the **intermediate N. (part of the intermediofacial, or facial N.).** These fibers synapse in the **mandibular ggl.**, at the origin of the **sublingual N.** (the sublingual N. is a branch of the lingual N.). The mandibular ggl. supplies the mandibular and **sublingual** glands.

*Note.* In the horse, the sublingual salivary gland is represented only by the **polystomatic sublingual gland**.

*Note.* The chorda tympani joins the lingual N. crossing the medial aspect of the maxillary A.; therefore, it is easily detectable.

The only hard structures within the area following the removal of the mandible are the stylohyoid bone, which is surrounded by the guttural pouch, and the jugular (paracondylar) process of the occipital bone.

The guttural pouch is the protrusion of the mucosa of the auditory tube through a ventral fissure of the cartilaginous part of the tube. The tube has an osseous part and a cartilaginous part, a tympanic opening, and a pharyngeal opening (in the nasopharynx). The pouch has an average capacity of 300–500 ml. The largest capacity ever reported was 5.7 l.

The guttural pouch is divided into two compartments by the stylohyoid bone: a large medial and a small lateral compartment. As a whole, the guttural pouch is located dorsal to the pharynx, coming in contact with the **sphenoid bone**, the **tympanic bulla**, the **temporohyoid joint**, and the **ventral condylar fossa**. The lateral aspect comes in contact with the medial pterygoideus and digastricus Mm. and the parotid and mandibular salivary glands. Medially, they touch each other rostrally and are separated caudally by the **longus capitis** and the **rectus capitis ventralis Mm.** Ventrally, the **medial retropharyngeal lnn.** are located between the guttural pouch and the pharynx.

**Enlargement and rupture of these lymph nodes into the guttural pouch results in a condition called "guttural pouch empyema"** *(accumulation of a large amount of purulent material).*

The guttural pouch extends caudally up to the **atlas**. Figure H7.16 illustrates the muscles, arteries, and the nerves in intimate contact with the right guttural pouch (the cast) (de Lahunta and Habel 1986).

**Endoscopic exploration of the guttural pouches can lead to the diagnosis of several conditions, such as tympany, empyema, mycosis, retropharyngeal lymphadenomegaly, temporohyoid osteoarthropathy, and others.**

**The surgical drainage of the guttural pouch, which is dictated in case of empyema, mycosis, foreign bodies, and other conditions, necessitates a perfect knowledge of the anatomical structures in contact with the guttural pouch. There are different approaches to the drainage of the guttural pouch, such as the hyovertebrotomy, the Chabert-Fromage approach, the Viborg's triangle approach, and the Whitehouse and the modified Whitehouse approaches, using as landmarks the jugular (paracondylar) process of the occipital bone, the angle of the stylohyoid bone, the caudal border of the ramus of the mandible, the tendon of the sternomandibularis M., the occipitomandibular part of the digastricus M., and the linguofacial V.**

Turn the head again with the lateral side up, and focus your attention on the larynx, trachea, and **esophagus**.

On the lateral aspect of the head continue the dissection of the structures exposed by the removal of the mandible, as illustrated in Figure H7.17.

Follow the common carotid A. toward the head and identify the **recurrent laryngeal N.** just ventral to the artery as it courses toward the larynx. At the larynx, it is called the **caudal laryngeal N.** and supplies all but one of the laryngeal muscles (the **cricothyroideus M.**, supplied by the **external branch of the cranial laryngeal N.** from the vagus N.). Both laryngeal nerves supply the mucosa of the larynx and communicate with each other.

Locate the **thyroid fissure** and the **thyroid foramen**, where the **internal branch** of the cranial laryngeal N. penetrates the larynx.

Identify the **thyrohyoideus M.**, the already known **sternothyroideus** and **sternohyoideus Mm.**, and the **thyroid** and **parathyroid glands**.

There are three symmetrical **longitudinal esophageal Mm.** that converge to the so-called **cricoesophageal tendon**.

Identify the **stylohyoideus M.** and its split tendon, which allows for passage of the tendon of the digastricus M. Identify the external carotid A., exiting from the deep aspect of the stylohyoideus M., as it runs over the lateral aspect of the stylohyoid bone (the angle) and terminates by branching into the maxillary and superficial temporal Aa. Between the stylohyoid bone and the stylohyoideus

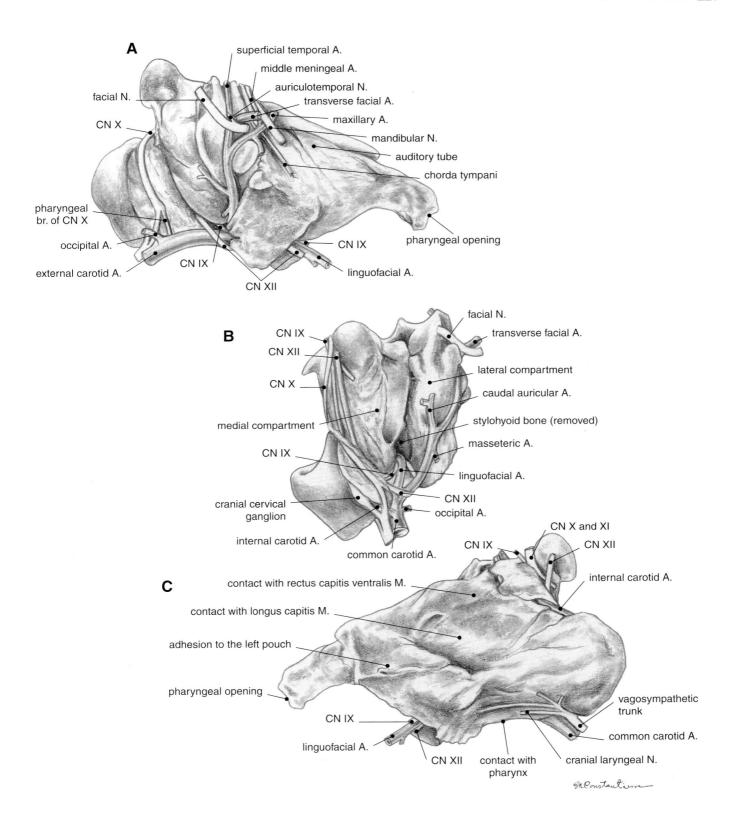

**A**
superficial temporal A.
middle meningeal A.
auriculotemporal N.
facial N.
transverse facial A.
CN X
maxillary A.
mandibular N.
auditory tube
chorda tympani
pharyngeal br. of CN X
pharyngeal opening
occipital A.
CN IX
external carotid A.
CN IX
linguofacial A.
CN XII

**B**
CN IX
facial N.
CN XII
transverse facial A.
CN X
lateral compartment
caudal auricular A.
medial compartment
stylohyoid bone (removed)
masseteric A.
CN IX
linguofacial A.
cranial cervical ganglion
CN XII
occipital A.
internal carotid A.
common carotid A.

**C**
CN X and XI
CN IX
CN XII
contact with rectus capitis ventralis M.
internal carotid A.
contact with longus capitis M.
adhesion to the left pouch
pharyngeal opening
vagosympathetic trunk
CN IX
common carotid A.
linguofacial A.
CN XII
contact with pharynx
cranial laryngeal N.

Fig. H7.16 Cast of the left guttural pouch of the horse and of the vessels and nerves in contact with it. **A.** Lateral aspect. **B.** Caudal aspect. **C.** Medial aspect.

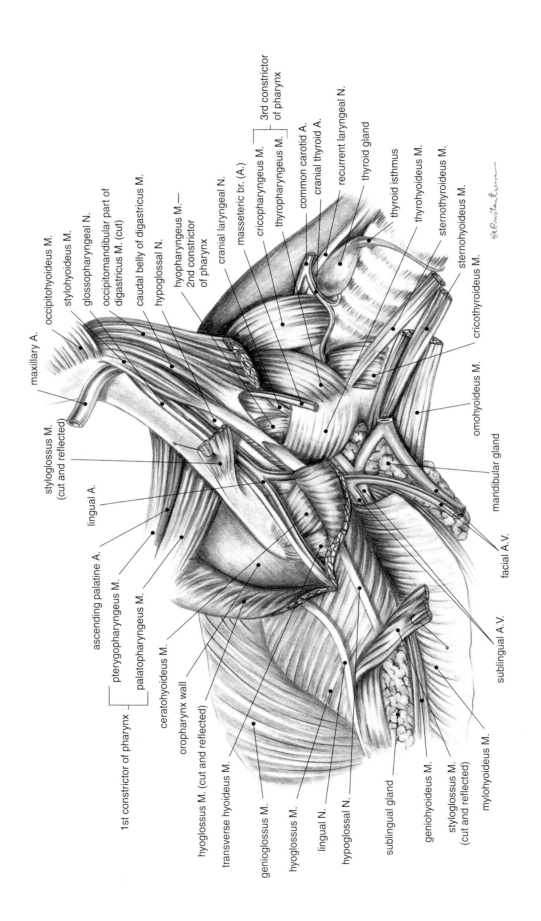

maxillary A.

occipitohyoideus M.

stylohyoideus M.

glossopharyngeal N.

occipitomandibular part of digastricus M. (cut)

caudal belly of digastricus M.

hypoglossal N.

hyopharyngeus M.— 2nd constrictor of pharynx

cranial laryngeal N.

masseteric br. (A.)

cricopharyngeus M.

thyropharyngeus M.

3rd constrictor of pharynx

common carotid A.

cranial thyroid A.

recurrent laryngeal N.

thyroid gland

thyroid isthmus

thyrohyoideus M.

sternothyroideus M.

sternohyoideus M.

cricothyroideus M.

omohyoideus M.

mandibular gland

facial A.V.

sublingual A.V.

styloglossus M. (cut and reflected)

lingual A.

ascending palatine A.

pterygopharyngeus M.

palatopharyngeus M.

1st constrictor of pharynx

ceratohyoideus M.

oropharynx wall

hyoglossus M. (cut and reflected)

transverse hyoideus M.

genioglossus M.

hyoglossus M.

lingual N.

hypoglossal N.

sublingual gland

geniohyoideus M.

styloglossus M. (cut and reflected)

mylohyoideus M.

Fig. H7.17. Structures of tongue, hyoid apparatus, pharynx, and larynx, left lateral aspect, horse.

M. the largest branch of the external carotid A. is exposed: the **linguofacial trunk**. This artery is paralleled by the **glossopharyngeal N.** (rostrally), and by the **hypoglossal N.** (caudally). Identify the **ascending palatine, lingual, facial**, and **sublingual Aa.**

Reflect the lingual mucosa and continue the dissection of those structures that continue into the tongue, such as the lingual N. and Vv., the glossopharyngeal and hypoglossal Nn., the lingual A., and the **styloglossus, hyoglossus, genioglossus**, and **geniohyoideus Mm.** Transect and reflect the styloglossus and hyoglossus Mm. to expose the **ceratohyoideus** and **transverse hyoideus Mm.**

Turn the split head median side up and concentrate on the muscles of the soft palate and pharynx. First dissect the **tensor** and **levator veli palatini Mm.** from this perspective (Fig. H7.18). Palpate the **pterygoid hamulus** close to the caudal extent of the **hard palate** and remove the mucosa of the nasopharynx in a caudal direction, all the way between the roof of the nasopharynx and the soft palate. *Remember:* The roof of the nasopharynx is also called the **fornix**. The **palatinus M.** is a slender symmetrical muscle that shortens and bends the caudal border of the soft palate ventrally. It is located on both sides of the midline.

**The palatinus M. also increases tension to offset dynamic collapse during exercise. Its failure leads to dorsal displacement of the soft palate, exercise intolerance, and noise.**

Between the **soft palate** and the **pterygoid bone** on one side, and the stylohyoid bone on the other side, dissect the **pterygopharyngeus** and the **palatopharyngeus Mm.** (known also as the **first constrictor of the pharynx**). Caudal to the stylohyoid bone, identify the **hyopharyngeus M.** (the **second constrictor of the pharynx**) and the **thyropharyngeus** and **cricopharyngeus Mm.** (known as the **third constrictor of the pharynx**) (see Fig. H7.17).

Leave the median section of the **cerebrum** for a later examination. Remove the entire mucosa of the nasopharynx and the laryngopharynx, and the guttural pouch; transect and reflect the rectus capitis ventralis and longus capitis Mm. The **occipitohyoideus M.** is now exposed. Dissect the structures illustrated in Figure H7.19.

Between the stylohyoid bone and the levator and tensor veli palatini Mm., identify the medial and lateral pterygoid Mm.

**The tensor veli palatini M. plays a role in the dorsal displacement of the soft palate.**

Reflect the roof of the nasopharynx and laryngopharynx. From the medial aspect of the stylohyoid bone, identify the only dilator of the pharynx, the **stylopharyngeus M.** Caudal to the stylohyoid bone identify the stylohy-

oideus M. On the medial aspect of the digastricus M., identify the external carotid A., the linguofacial trunk, and the glossopharyngeal, hypoglossal, vagus, and **accessory Nn.**, as well as the **cranial cervical ggl.**, the **cervical sympathetic trunk**, the branches and communicating branches of these nerves, and the ganglion. The vagus N. and the cervical sympathetic trunk run together as the **vagosympathetic trunk**. The **internal carotid** and **occipital Aa.** branch from the **common carotid A.** caudal to the digastricus M. The internal carotid A. runs toward the **carotid foramen,** parallel to the cranial cervical ggl.

*Remember!* The terminal branches of the common carotid A. are the external carotid, internal carotid, and occipital Aa.

*Note.* The carotid foramen is built between the **carotid notch** of the sphenoid bone and the periosteum covering the **foramen lacerum**.

Identify the **glomus caroticum** and the **carotid sinus** at the origin of the internal carotid A. The glomus is a small nodule containing chemoreceptors, and the sinus is a luminal enlargement of the origin of this artery.

Focus your attention on the ear muscles, systematized into rostral, dorsal, caudal, and ventral groups. They originate from the surrounding bones, the **ligamentum nuchae**, or the **scutiform cartilage** and insert either on the **auricle** or on the scutiform cartilage (this cartilage transmits the action of some muscles to the auricle). There is an additional cartilage to the **external ear**: the **annular cartilage**, interposed between the auricle and the **external acoustic meatus**. The muscles are illustrated in Figure H7.20. To dissect the rostral muscles, pull the ear caudally to tense those muscles. To dissect the caudal muscles, pull the ear rostrally. For the dorsal muscles pull the ear ventrally, and for the ventral muscles pull the ear dorsally.

Concentrate on the **eye**. Examine the following structures: the two **eyelids**; the **palpebral fissure,** which starts and ends in the **lateral/medial angles of the eye** (called by the clinicians **canthi—sing. canthus**); the **lateral and medial palpebral commissures** (the union of upper and lower lids); inside of the medial canthus, identify the **lacrimal caruncle** and the two **lacrimal puncta**, which are located dorsal and ventral to the caruncle, close to the **posterior palpebral limbus** of each eyelid (Fig. H7.21A). (The posterior palpebral limbus is the posterior edge of the free border of the eyelid). There is also an anterior palpebral limbus for each eyelid.

The lacrimal puncta lead the tears into the **lacrimal canaliculi,** which open into the **lacrimal sac**, the origin of the **nasolacrimal duct.**

The lateral and medial palpebral commissures are connected to the lateral and medial borders of the orbita by

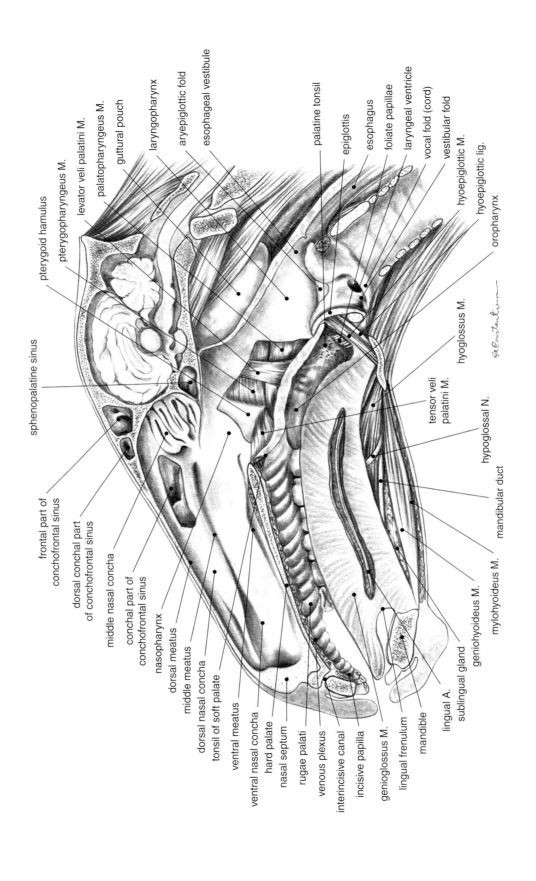

sphenopalatine sinus

frontal part of
conchofrontal sinus

dorsal conchal part
of conchofrontal sinus

middle nasal concha

conchal part of
conchofrontal sinus

nasopharynx

dorsal meatus

middle meatus

dorsal nasal concha

tonsil of soft palate

ventral meatus

ventral nasal concha

hard palate

nasal septum

rugae palati

venous plexus

interincisive canal

incisive papilla

genioglossus M.

lingual frenulum

mandible

lingual A.

sublingual gland

geniohyoideus M.

mylohyoideus M.

mandibular duct

hypoglossal N.

tensor veli
palatini M.

hyoglossus M.

oropharynx

hyoepiglottic lig.

hyoepiglottic M.

vestibular fold

vocal fold (cord)

laryngeal ventricle

foliate papillae

esophagus

epiglottis

palatine tonsil

esophageal vestibule

aryepiglottic fold

laryngopharynx

guttural pouch

palatopharyngeus M.

levator veli palatini M.

pterygopharyngeus M.

pterygoid hamulus

Fig. H7.18. Structures on the median aspect of the head, horse.

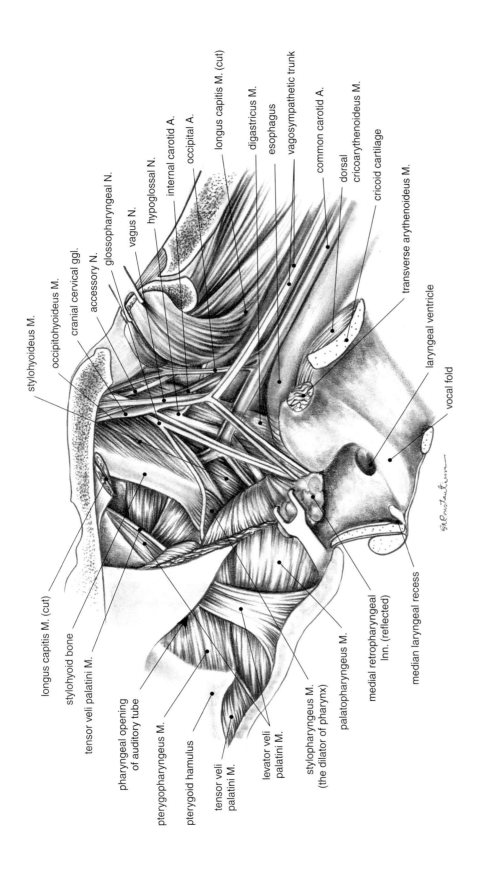

longus capitis M. (cut)

stylohyoid bone

tensor veli palatini M.

pharyngeal opening
of auditory tube

pterygopharyngeus M.

pterygoid hamulus

tensor veli
palatini M.

levator veli
palatini M.

stylopharyngeus M.
(the dilator of pharynx)

palatopharyngeus M.

medial retropharyngeal
Inn. (reflected)

median laryngeal recess

stylohyoideus M.

occipitohyoideus M.

cranial cervical ggl.

accessory N.

glossopharyngeal N.

vagus N.

hypoglossal N.

internal carotid A.

occipital A.

longus capitis M. (cut)

digastricus M.

esophagus

vagosympathetic trunk

common carotid A.

dorsal
cricoarythenoideus M.

cricoid cartilage

transverse arythenoideus M.

laryngeal ventricle

vocal fold

Fig. H7.19. Structures of pharynx, larynx, and hyoid apparatus, medial aspect, horse.

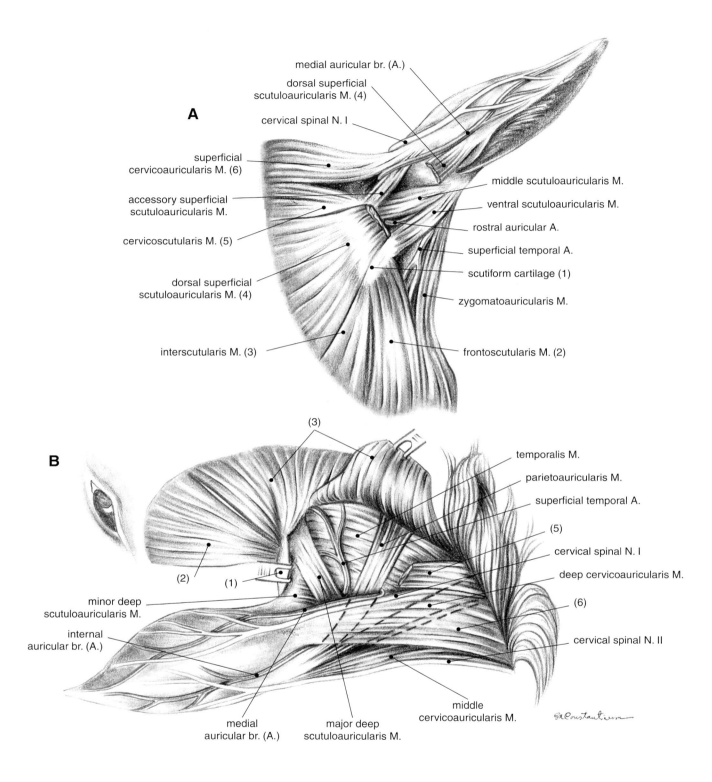

**A**

medial auricular br. (A.)

dorsal superficial
scutuloauricularis M. (4)

cervical spinal N. I

superficial
cervicoauricularis M. (6)

accessory superficial
scutuloauricularis M.

cervicoscutularis M. (5)

dorsal superficial
scutuloauricularis M. (4)

interscutularis M. (3)

middle scutuloauricularis M.

ventral scutuloauricularis M.

rostral auricular A.

superficial temporal A.

scutiform cartilage (1)

zygomatoauricularis M.

frontoscutularis M. (2)

**B**

(3)

temporalis M.

parietoauricularis M.

superficial temporal A.

(5)

cervical spinal N. I

deep cervicoauricularis M.

(6)

cervical spinal N. II

(2)

(1)

minor deep
scutuloauricularis M.

internal
auricular br. (A.)

medial
auricular br. (A.)

major deep
scutuloauricularis M.

middle
cervicoauricularis M.

Fig. H7.20. Muscles, arteries, and nerves of the left external ear, horse. **A.** Auricular structures, dorsal aspect. **B.** Deep auricular structures, dorsal aspect.

**A**

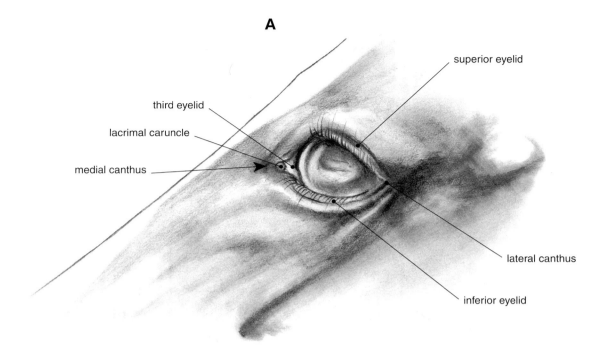

third eyelid

lacrimal caruncle

medial canthus

superior eyelid

lateral canthus

inferior eyelid

**B**

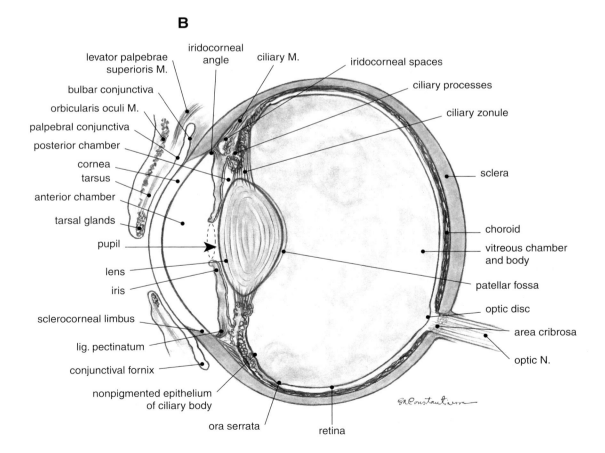

levator palpebrae
superioris M.

iridocorneal
angle

ciliary M.

iridocorneal spaces

ciliary processes

ciliary zonule

bulbar conjunctiva

orbicularis oculi M.

palpebral conjunctiva

posterior chamber

cornea

tarsus

anterior chamber

tarsal glands

pupil

lens

iris

sclerocorneal limbus

lig. pectinatum

conjunctival fornix

nonpigmented epithelium
of ciliary body

ora serrata

retina

sclera

choroid

vitreous chamber
and body

patellar fossa

optic disc

area cribrosa

optic N.

Fig. H7.21. The eye of the horse. **A.** External features. **B.** Vertical section through the eye.

the **lateral and medial palpebral ligg.** They both assure that the palpebral fissure, when narrowed by the orbicularis oculi M., remains elliptical rather than becoming circular.

Evert the eyelids and identify the **palpebral** and **bulbar conjunctivae**, the **superior and inferior conjunctival fornices (sing. fornix)**, and the **conjunctival sac**. (The conjunctival fornix is formed by the reflection of the palpebral conjunctiva onto the bulbar conjunctiva. The conjunctival sac is the space between the palpebral and the bulbar conjunctivae) (see Fig. H7.21B).

Make an incision through one of the eyelids from the free border to the conjunctival fornix. On the cut surface examine the **tarsus**, the **tarsal (Meibomian) glands**, and the cross section of the **orbicularis oculi M.** In the superior eyelid, also identify the **levator palpebrae superioris M.** (see Fig. H7.21B). Examine the tunics and the related structures on Figure H7.21B.

The eyelids are attached to the border of the **orbita (orbital cavity)** by means of the **orbital septum**; the latter is represented by fibrous membranes extending up to the tarsi (pl. for tarsus).

Examine the **semilunar fold (the third eyelid)** at the medial angle of the eye (see Fig. H7.21A).

The zygomatic arch has already been removed. Manually remove the **extraperiorbital fat,** the large amount of fat separating the orbital area from the temporalis M. The **periorbita**, the cone-shaped fibrous membrane enclosing the eyeball and its muscles, vessels, and nerves is now exposed. The periorbita is attached by its base to the bony rim of the orbita, fusing with the periosteum. The vessels and nerves enter the periorbita through its apex.

After the extraperiorbital fat is removed, the branches of the **maxillary A.** and **N.** are exposed.

The maxillary A. enters the **alar canal** through the **caudal alar foramen** and exits from the **rostral alar foramen** (see Fig. H7.4). Before entering the alar canal it branches into the **rostral tympanic**, **middle meningeal**, and **caudal deep temporal Aa.** (in a caudorostral direction, dorsally oriented). The **inferior alveolar A.** and the **pterygoid branches** are ventrally oriented. Within the alar canal, the maxillary A. gives off the **rostral deep temporal A.**, which exits through the **small alar foramen**. After exiting through the rostral alar foramen, the maxillary A. branches into the **external ophthalmic A.** (dorsally oriented), the **infraorbital A.** (rostrally oriented), and the **buccal** and the **minor palatine Aa.** (ventrally oriented), and continues as the **descending palatine A.** The descending palatine A. runs parallel to the infraorbital A. and branches into the **sphenopalatine** and the **major palatine Aa.**

The maxillary N. runs in the **groove for the maxillary N.** on the cerebral surface of the **sphenoid bone** (see Fig.

H7.5), and exits through the **foramen rotundum**, on the medial side of the rostral alar foramen. It gives off the zygomatic N., which enters the periorbita, and then the maxillary N. continues rostrally and divides into the **infraorbital** and the **pterygopalatine Nn.** The pterygopalatine N. branches into the **caudal nasal N.** and the **major palatine N.**, which gives off the **minor** and **accessory palatine Nn.**

The infraorbital A. and N. enter the **maxillary foramen** and exit the **infraorbital foramen**. The sphenopalatine A. and the caudal nasal N. enter the **sphenopalatine foramen** within the nasal cavity. The major palatine A. and N. enter the **caudal palatine foramen** and exit the **major palatine foramen** (see Figs. H7.4 and H7.2).

**Clinically important is the fact that the symmetrical major palatine Aa. anastomose with each other at the level of the second or third palatine ruga (close to the incisive papilla) before entering as a single vessel in the interincisive canal (see Fig. H7.3).**

Return to the periorbita. Between the dorsal and lateral rectus Mm., in the projection area (they are under the periorbita and cannot be seen), a yellow strip is visible through the transparency. Here, make an incision in the long axis of the periorbita, separate it from the orbital septum, and carefully transect it from the attachment on the **pterygoid crest.** *Remember* that the pterygoid crest extends caudal to the optic canal, orbital fissure, foramen rotundum, and the rostral alar foramen (see Fig. H7.4). The yellow strip is part of the **intraperiorbital fat.** Reflect the periorbita as far as possible, saving the **lacrimal gland** that lies in the **lacrimal fossa** of the frontal bone. In dorsoventral order, identify the **frontal, lacrimal,** and **zygomatic Nn.**, running on the surface of the **dorsal rectus** and **lateral rectus Mm.** (Fig. H7.22A).

The frontal N. passes through the **supraorbital foramen** and branches into the **supraorbital N.** (caudally), and the **supratrochlear N.** (rostrally). The zygomatic N. branches into the **zygomaticotemporal**, and the **zygomaticofacial Nn.**, and sometimes sends a communicating branch to the lacrimal N.

Reflect the muscles of the eyeball as far laterally as possible and identify the **dorsal oblique M.,** and the **trochlear N.** lying on it, and the trochlea surrounded by the tendon of this muscle.

Evert the lateral rectus M. and identify the branch of the **abducent N.** supplying it (the nerve also supplies the **retractor bulbi M.**). Reflect the lateral rectus M. dorsally and the **ventral rectus M.** ventrally to expose the **oculomotor N.**, with its dorsal and ventral branches. The dorsal branch supplies the dorsal rectus and the levator palpebrae superioris Mm., whereas the ventral branch supplies the ventral rectus M., the **medial rectus**, and the **ventral oblique Mm.** At the origin of the ventral branch, identify

**A**

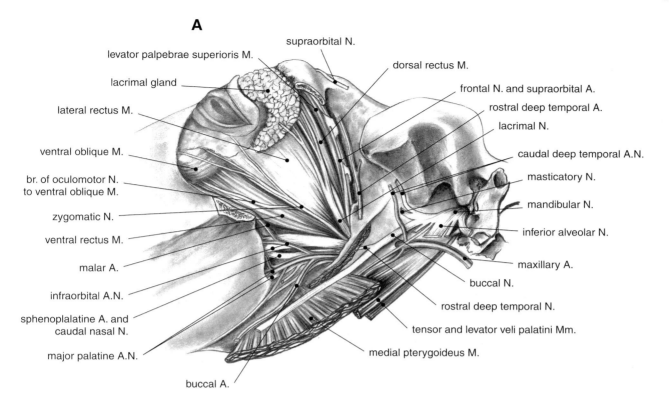

levator palpebrae superioris M.

supraorbital N.

lacrimal gland

dorsal rectus M.

lateral rectus M.

frontal N. and supraorbital A.

rostral deep temporal A.

ventral oblique M.

lacrimal N.

br. of oculomotor N. to ventral oblique M.

caudal deep temporal A.N.

zygomatic N.

masticatory N.

mandibular N.

ventral rectus M.

inferior alveolar N.

malar A.

maxillary A.

infraorbital A.N.

buccal N.

sphenoplalatine A. and caudal nasal N.

rostral deep temporal N.

tensor and levator veli palatini Mm.

major palatine A.N.

medial pterygoideus M.

buccal A.

**B**

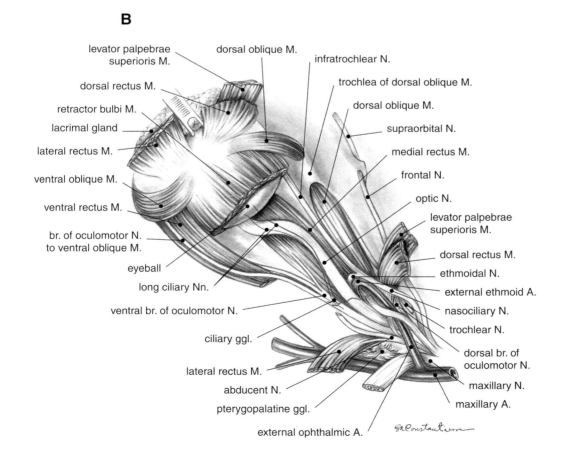

levator palpebrae superioris M.

dorsal oblique M.

infratrochlear N.

dorsal rectus M.

trochlea of dorsal oblique M.

retractor bulbi M.

dorsal oblique M.

lacrimal gland

supraorbital N.

lateral rectus M.

medial rectus M.

ventral oblique M.

frontal N.

ventral rectus M.

optic N.

br. of oculomotor N. to ventral oblique M.

levator palpebrae superioris M.

eyeball

dorsal rectus M.

long ciliary Nn.

ethmoidal N.

ventral br. of oculomotor N.

external ethmoid A.

nasociliary N.

ciliary ggl.

trochlear N.

lateral rectus M.

dorsal br. of oculomotor N.

abducent N.

maxillary N.

pterygopalatine ggl.

maxillary A.

external ophthalmic A.

Fig. H7.22. Structures of the eye, horse. **A.** Structures of the eye and orbital area. **B.** Deep structures of the eye.

the tiny parasympathetic **ciliary ggl.** and the **short ciliary Nn.** (Fig. H7.22B).

Very deep between the dorsal rectus M. and the lateral rectus M., find the **nasociliary N.**, which gives off the **ethmoidal N.** (entering the **ethmoidal foramen**) and the **infratrochlear N.** (continuing forward parallel to the ventral aspect of the dorsal oblique M.) (see Fig. H7.22B). The nasociliary N. also sends the **long ciliary Nn.**

*Note.* The frontal, lacrimal, and nasociliary Nn. are branches of the **ophthalmic N.** (the first major branch of the trigeminal N.).

Take a chisel and a hammer and remove the lateral wall of the alar canal. Carefully transect the maxillary N. and reflect the stumps to expose the **pterygopalatine ggl.** (parasympathetic). This ganglion is the site of synapsis between the **major petrosal N.** of the facial N. and the postganglionic fibers that supply the **lacrimal** and **nasal glands.**

Remove the eye from the orbita by transecting the muscles, nerves, and arteries from the pterygoid crest (see Figs. H7.4 and H7.22A); free the trochlea of the dorsal oblique M. from the medial wall of the orbita; free the ventral oblique M. from the **fossa of the ventral oblique M.** (see Fig. 7.4); free the eyelids from the orbital septum and the palpebral ligaments; transect the zygomatic N. from the foramen rotundum and the **A. malaris** from the infraorbital A.; transect the frontal N. and the **supraorbital A.** below the supraorbital foramen; and transect the ethmoidal N. and the **external ethmoid A.** at the entrance into the **ethmoidal foramen.** Remove the eyeball with the accessory structures and place it on a tray.

*Note.* The malaris A. supplies the eyelids. The supraorbital A. is a branch of the external ophthalmic A. and parallels the frontal N. The external ethmoid A. is a branch of the external ophthalmic A.

Identify the **anterior** and **posterior poles**, the **axis,** and the **equator** of the eyeball. An infinite number of **parallels** and **meridians** can be traced.

Make a vertical incision in the axis of the eyeball through the **tunics of the eyeball (fibrous, vascular,** and **nervous), anterior and posterior chambers**, and **vitreous body** (see Fig. H7.21B).

Examine the fibrous tunic, consisting of **sclera** (opaque) and **cornea** (transparent); identify the **area cribrosa,** where the **optic N.** penetrates.

The vascular tunic is represented by the **choroid,** including the **tapetum lucidum,** the **ciliary body,** and the **iris** perforated by the **pupil.** The ciliary body consists of the **ciliary processes** and the **ciliary M.** Identify the **iridocorneal angle** with the **pectinate lig.** and the **iridocorneal spaces.**

The nervous tunic of the eyeball is represented by the **retina,** a translucent structure easily removable from the

choroid. Identify the **ora serrata**, which separates the retina from the **nonpigmented epithelium of the ciliary body.**

There is still a wrong idea in most anatomy books, including the *Nomina Anatomica Veterinaria,* that the retina is divided in two major parts, the visual and nonvisual, and that the nonvisual part consists of a ciliary part and an iridic part. Albeit this conception is true from an embriological perspective, in postnatal life there is only one retina, which ends at the level of ora serrata.

Identify the **optic disc,** which marks the origin of the optic N. Examine the arborization of the **central A. of the retina**, the design of which is unique for each species.

Examine the **lens,** with the **capsule,** the soft **cortex,** and the hard **nucleus.** The lens is surrounded and supported by the **ciliary zonule (zonule of Zinn, or suspensory apparatus of the lens).** The zonule is attached to the ciliary body. Observe that between the cornea and the lens there are two chambers that communicate via the pupil. They are called the **anterior chamber** (between the cornea and the iris), and the **posterior chamber** (between the iris and the lens). They are filled with the **aqueous humor,** a transparent and waterlike fluid. On the other side of the lens, between it and the retina, there is another space, called **vitreous chamber,** in which the **vitreous body,** a gel-like structure, is located. The **vitreous humor** is the liquid filling the meshes of the vitreous body.

The next section on the dissection of the head is focused on the structures exposed on the median section, as they are shown in Figures H7.18 and H7.23.

Focus your attention on the **nasal cavity.** Remove the **nasal septum,** lying on the groove of the **vomer bone,** and identify the conchae and the meatuses (meatus or meatuses are accepted as the plural of meatus), as follows: the **dorsal nasal concha,** the **ventral nasal concha,** and the small and caudally located **middle nasal concha.** The conchae are separated from each other and from the walls of the nasal cavity: the **dorsal meatus** between the roof of the cavity and the dorsal concha; the **ventral meatus** between the floor and the ventral concha; the **middle meatus** between the dorsal and ventral conchae; and the **common meatus** on each side of the nasal septum. The dorsal, middle, and ventral meatuses communicate with the common meatus. The middle meatus splits into two channels that surround the middle concha. The dorsal and middle meatuses end at the osseous wall separating the nasal cavity from the **cranial cavity.** Only the ventral meatus communicates with the nasopharynx, via the **choana** (pl. **choanae**).

**The ventral meatus is the only passage between the nasal cavity and the nasopharynx. An endoscope or a gastric tube should be introduced only via the ventral meatus for exploring the nasal cavity, the nasophar-**

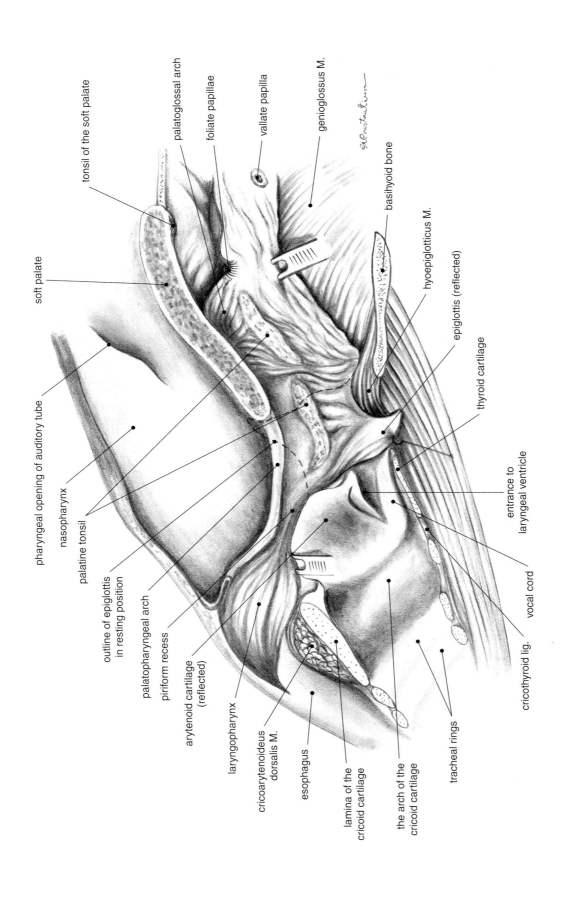

tonsil of the soft palate

palatoglossal arch

foliate papillae

vallate papilla

genioglossus M.

soft palate

basihyoid bone

hyoepiglotticus M.

pharyngeal opening of auditory tube

epiglottis (reflected)

nasopharynx

thyroid cartilage

palatine tonsil

outline of epiglottis
in resting position

palatopharyngeal arch

entrance to
laryngeal ventricle

piriform recess

vocal cord

arytenoid cartilage
(reflected)

cricothyroid lig.

laryngopharynx

cricoarytenoideus
dorsalis M.

esophagus

lamina of the
cricoid cartilage

the arch of the
cricoid cartilage

tracheal rings

Fig. H7.23. Median section of the pharynx and larynx, medial aspect of the left half, horse

ynx, the laryngopharynx, the larynx, trachea, and bronchial tree, and the esophagus, stomach, and duodenum. Sometimes clinicians also explore the middle and dorsal meatuses via endoscopy.

Make one window in the rostral portion and another in the caudal portion within the dorsal and ventral conchae and explore them. The rostral and caudal portions of these two conchae are separated only in the horse by **conchal septa**. In the rostral portion, only the osseous scrolls can be seen, whereas in the caudal portion the **dorsal conchal sinus** and the **ventral conchal sinus** are sculpted. In the horse only, the dorsal conchal sinus communicates with the **frontal sinus**, forming the **conchofrontal sinus**; it communicates with the middle meatus via the **caudal maxillary sinus**. The ventral conchal sinus communicates with the middle meatus via the **rostral maxillary sinus**. Identify the **palatine** and the **sphenoid sinuses** that are continuous only in the horse and are known as the **sphenopalatine sinus**; it communicates with the caudal maxillary sinus (see Fig. H7.18).

Examine the **hard palate**, which consists of the **palatine processes of the incisive bones**, the **palatine processes of the maxillae**, and the **horizontal laminae of the palatine bones**. Examine the soft palate in the resting position: its caudal border comes in intimate contact with the rostral aspect of the epiglottis. This is a specific feature of the horse and is due to the presence of the strong **hyoepiglottic lig.** (see Fig. H7.18).

**One cause of exercise intolerance in horses is intermittent displacement of the soft palate above the epiglottis during intense exercise.**

Identify the **palatoglossal arch**, connecting the soft palate to the base of the tongue; they outline together the **isthmus faucium**, or **aditus pharyngis**, the entrance into the **oropharynx**, and at the same time the communication between the oral cavity and the pharynx (the oropharynx compartment). *Notice* that the oropharynx is also called **fauces**. Now identify the **palatopharyngeal arch**, which connects the caudal border of the soft palate to the lateral wall of the pharynx to form the **intrapharyngeal ostium** (opening), separating the **nasopharynx** from the **laryngopharynx** (see Fig. H7.23).

Properly identify the three compartments of the pharynx: the nasopharynx, the oropharynx, and the laryngopharynx.

The nasopharynx communicates rostrally with the nasal cavity via the two choanae, and caudally with the laryngopharynx via the intrapharyngeal ostium. The roof is also called pharyngeal fornix, while the floor is shared with the roof of the oropharynx. On the lateral wall the slit **pharyngeal opening of the auditory tube** is seen (see Fig. H7.23). Caudodorsal to this opening is a prominence, caused by the cartilage of the auditory tube, called the

**torus tubarius**. Rostroventral from the same opening is another prominence, caused by the levator veli palatini M., called **torus levatorius**. The niche in the caudodorsal angle of the nasopharynx is the **pharyngeal recess**. On the caudodorsal wall of the nasopharynx is the **pharyngeal tonsil**.

The laryngopharynx is positioned dorsal to the larynx. Between the lateral wall of the laryngopharynx and the **aryepiglottic fold** is a narrow and deep groove, the **piriform recess**. It allows passage of a small amount of saliva into the esophagus without closing the laryngeal opening, and also the passage of milk in suckling animals, simultaneous with breathing. The aryepiglottic fold is the mucosal fold between the arytenoid cartilage and the epiglottis. That part of the laryngopharynx between the arytenoid cartilages and the origin of the esophagus is called **esophageal vestibule** (see Figs. H7.18 and H7.23).

Examine the **oropharynx** and identify the **tonsil of the soft palate**, the **palatine tonsil** and the lingual papillae: **filiform**, **fungiform**, **vallate**, and **foliate**. The oropharynx ends at the rostral aspect of the epiglottis, where there are three mucosal folds between the root of the tongue and the epiglottis: the **median glossoepiglottic fold** and the symmetrical **lateral glossoepiglottic folds**. Between these three folds, identify the two **valleculae epiglotticae**, the symmetrical depressions on both sides of the median glossoepiglottic fold.

The median glossoepiglottic fold is due to the presence of the hyoepiglotticus M.

As a whole, the pharynx has seven communications with the surrounding structures: two rostrodorsal communications with the nasal cavity via the choanae; the rostroventral communication with the oral cavity via the isthmus faucium; two lateral communications with the auditory tubes; one caudodorsal communication with the esophagus; and one caudoventral communication with the larynx via the **aditus laryngis** (the entrance into the larynx).

Reflect the tendon of the genioglossus M. to better expose the hyoglossus, geniohyoideus and mylohyoideus Mm., the hypoglossal N., the **mandibular duct**, and the **polystomatic sublingual salivary gland** (the only sublingual salivary gland in the horse).

To study the oral cavity in an organized manner, it is necessary first to distinguish the **oral cavity proper** from the **vestibule**. The oral cavity proper is medial to and surrounded by the teeth; it includes the tongue, mucosa, and some of the salivary glands. The vestibule is the space between the teeth, and the lips and cheeks. In the resting position (with the mouth closed and the masticatory [occlusal] surface of the teeth against each other), communication is possible between the vestibule and the oral cavity proper, caudal to the last molars and through the diastema (see Figs. H7.1, H7.2, and H7.6A,B,C). The diastema is the space between the incisive and premolar teeth on the same dental arcade. Within the vestibule, some of the salivary ducts course and/or open.

Examine the structures of the oral cavity proper. Look at the **palatine rugae** (the transversely oriented crests of the mucosa of the hard palate) and the **palatine raphe** (the median line of junction or separation between the two halves of the mucosa of the hard palate). There is an elevation of the mucosa at the level of the second or third mucosal crest called the **incisive papilla**. Explore the floor of the oral cavity proper and identify the **sublingual caruncles**, on both sides of the **lingual frenulum** (see Fig. H7.18). The sublingual caruncles are mucosal flaps that protect the openings of the mandibular ducts. Examine the **tongue** with the **apex, body**, and **root**. The apex lies on the **body of the mandible**, overlapping the sublingual caruncle. Reflect the tongue medially (toward you). Still within the oral cavity proper, examine the **lateral sublingual recess**, a narrow space under the tongue. The **minor sublingual ducts** (of the polystomatic sublingual salivary gland) open along the **sublingual fold**. This fold is located within the sublingual recess.

*Note.* In the horse, there is no **monostomatic sublingual salivary gland**, as there is in the other species; therefore, no **major sublingual duct** is present in the horse.

Examine the **teeth**. There are three symmetrical **incisors** or **incisive teeth** (upper and lower): I1, **central**; I2, **intermediate**; and I3, **corner**. There is one symmetrical **canine tooth** (upper and lower) in the male, sometimes in the female. There are three symmetrical **premolars** and three symmetrical **molars** (upper and lower), together called **cheek teeth**.

There are two distinct types of teeth in the domestic mammals: brachydont and hypsodont. A **brachydont** tooth consists of a distinct **crown** (the visible part), a **root** (implanted within the **alveolus**), and a **neck** in between (slightly constricted). The horse is a **hypsodont** species, in which crown and neck of the permanent teeth cannot be easily distinguished; therefore, there is only a **body** and a root.

*Notice* that the free part of the body of a permanent tooth, regardless of the category (incisor, canine, premolar, or molar) is called the **clinical crown**. The part of the tooth that is concealed by the gingiva and alveolus is the **clinical root**.

There are also several types of premolars and molars in the domestic animals: tuberculosectorial (carnivores), bunodont (pig), both brachydont species, and selenodont and lophodont (hypsodont) species. In bunodont species the cheek teeth are provided with cusps. In selenodont species (ruminants), the cusps are flat and curved, looking like croissants (crescent moon–shaped; *selena*, in Greek, means *moon*). The horse is a **lophodont** species. In the horse, there are folds and ridges of enamel separated by infundibula (only in the maxillary cheek teeth) on the occlusal surface, and the walls between the cusps have several indentations (*lophos*, in Greek, means *ridge*).

As far as the relationship between the **upper dental arch** and the **lower dental arch** is concerned, the animals are divided into two groups: isognathous and anisognathous. In the **isognathous** species (only the pig), the occlusal surface of the upper dental arch completely covers the occlusal surface of the lower dental arch. In the **anisognathous** species, including the horse, the upper dental arch is wider than the lower dental arch.

A tooth consists of three structures: dentin, enamel, and cement (Fig. H7.24A).

The **dentin**, a calcified collagenous matrix permeated by the processes of odontoblasts, is the main substance of the teeth. The **enamel**, a white substance covering the dentin in the crown or the body of the tooth, is the hardest structure in the body. In the horse and ruminants an **invagination of the enamel** on the occlusal surface of the cheek teeth is observed; this is the **infundibulum** (in the horse, only present on the maxillary arcade). The external (peripheral) enamel and the internal (central) enamel, which lines the infundibulum, are continuous with each other until the tooth becomes worn. The black cavity of the infundibulum is called the **cup**. With the age, the cup narrows and disappears, but the bottom of the infundibulum remains as the **enamel spot**. The **cement** is the bone-like substance that covers the root. In the hypsodont species, the cement of permanent teeth also covers the crown, lines the enamel within the infundibulum, and lines the dental cavity; the latter is called **secondary dentine**. When the cup disappears, the **dental star** appears between the infundibulum and the vestibular surface of the tooth. The dental star is darker in color and represents the secondary dentine (that fills the dental cavity).

In the horse, there are **deciduous teeth** (the so-called **milk dentition**) and **permanent teeth**. The formula for the deciduous teeth is

$$2(Di3/3; Dc0/0; Dp3/3) = 24$$

The formula of the permanent teeth is

$$2(I3/3; C1/1; P3(4)/3; M3/3) = 40 \text{ or } 42$$

*Note.* The first of the four upper premolars (within parentheses) is the wolf tooth (see explanation on page 244.

*Note.* The molars are *not* present in the formula for the deciduous teeth.

As far as the deciduous and permanent teeth are concerned, the animals are either monophyodont, or diphyodont. The **monophyodont** species (the rabbit) have one dentition all life long; there is no separate milk and permanent dentition. The **diphyodont** species (all domestic mammals) have deciduous teeth gradually replaced by permanent teeth.

There are fundamental differences between the deciduous and the permanent incisors. Examine a deciduous incisor (Fig. H7.24B,C,D). Each tooth has a **vestibular surface**, a **lingual surface**, two **contact surfaces** (except the corner incisors), and an **occlusal (masticatory) surface** (which comes in contact with the opposing tooth when the mouth is closed). Each incisor is curved, with the concave surface toward the tongue. A rostral view of an incisor shows a broad **crown**, a narrow **root**, and an obvious transitional area called **neck**. At the **apex** of the root, the **apical foramen of the root canal** leads into the **cavity of the tooth** that contains the **pulp**. The cavity of the tooth within the root is called **root canal**. The pulp supports the vessels and nerves supplying the tooth.

The teeth are implanted within the **alveoli** (sing. alveolus) of the maxillae, incisive bones, and mandibulae. There is a ligament between the tooth and its alveolus, called the **periodontium** (periodontal lig.). The bone of the alveolus is called **lamina dura**. The periodontium attaches the tooth and the **gingiva** (the gum) to the alveolus. The gingiva is the mucosa of the oral cavity surrounding the neck or the transition between the crown and the root of a tooth.

Examine a permanent incisor (Fig. H7.24E,F,G). The body is curved, prismatic, or cylindrical and has no neck. The teeth are worn differently from animal to animal, according to the quality of the food. With age, the shape and other features of the occlusal surface change. For estimating age one looks at the occlusal surface of the lower incisive teeth. In examining the aspects of the occlusal surface at different stages, keep in mind that there are

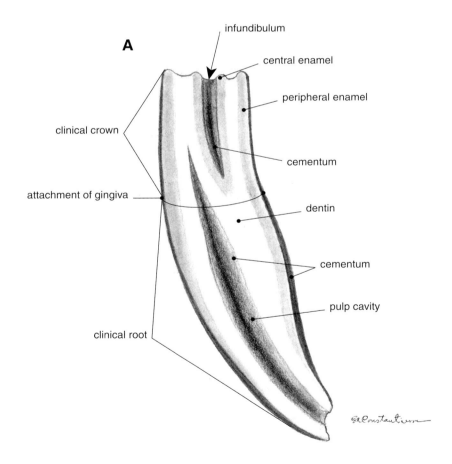

Fig. H7.24. Teeth of the horse. **A.** Vertical section in a permanent incisor, horse. *(continues)*

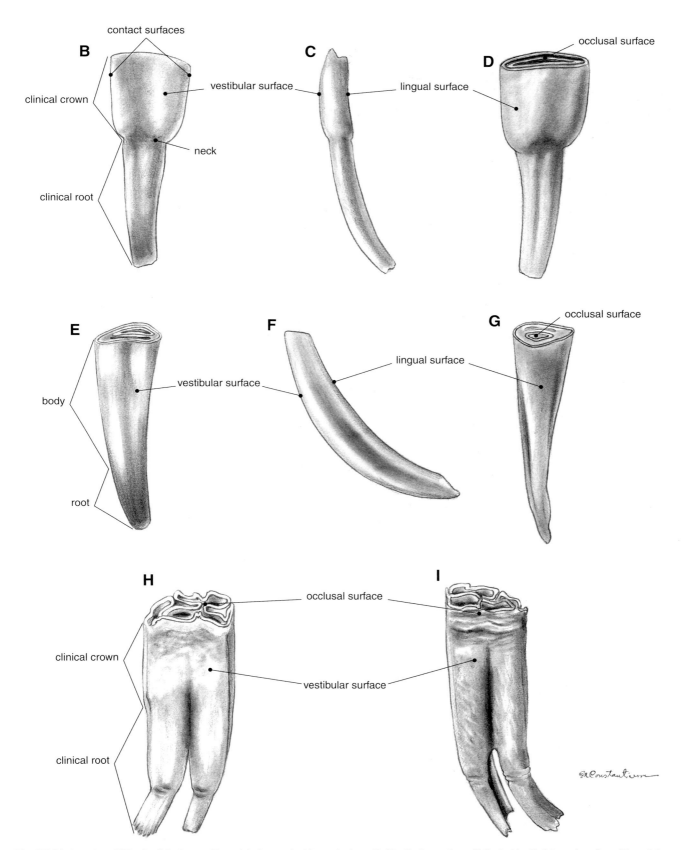

Fig. H7.24. *(continued)* Teeth of the horse. *First right lower deciduous incisor:* **B.** Vestibular surface. **C.** Left side. **D.** Lingual surface. *First right lower permanent incisor:* **E.** Vestibular surface. **F.** Left side **G.** Lingual surface. **H.** *Third right lower permanent premolar,* vestibular surface. **I.** *Second left lower permanent molar,* vestibular surface.

three distinct events in the growing process of a tooth: the eruption, the time the tooth is "in wear," and the time the tooth is "level." **Eruption** is the moment that the tooth breaks the gingiva that covered it from the very beginning of its development. A tooth is **"in wear"** when it reaches its opposing tooth (at the masticatory level) and the

enamel starts to wear. When the peripheral enamel as well as the central enamel are in wear and separated by dentin, the tooth is **"level."**

Figure H7.25 shows the occlusal surface of the lower incisors at different ages.

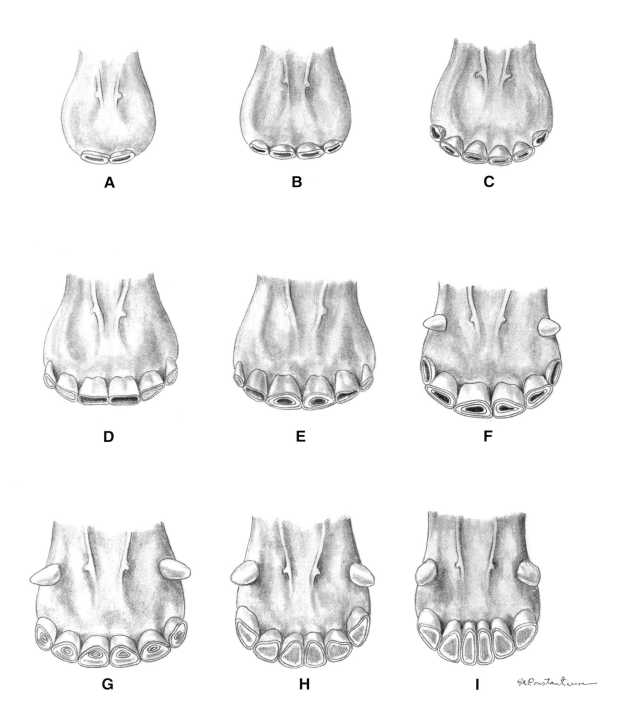

Fig. H7.25. Occlusal surface of lower incisors of the horse at different ages. **A.** 4–7 days old. **B.** 3–5 weeks old. **C.** 7 months old. **D.** 3 years old. **E.** 4 years old. **F.** 5 years old. **G.** 10 years old. **H.** 15 years old. **I.** 20 years old.

Figure H7.26 shows the shape and other features of the horse teeth at different ages. Additional information regarding the aging of a horse by its teeth includes the angle between the upper and lower incisors, the relative dimensions of the vestibular surfaces of the incisors, **Galvayne's groove,** and the **hook of the corner upper incisors.**

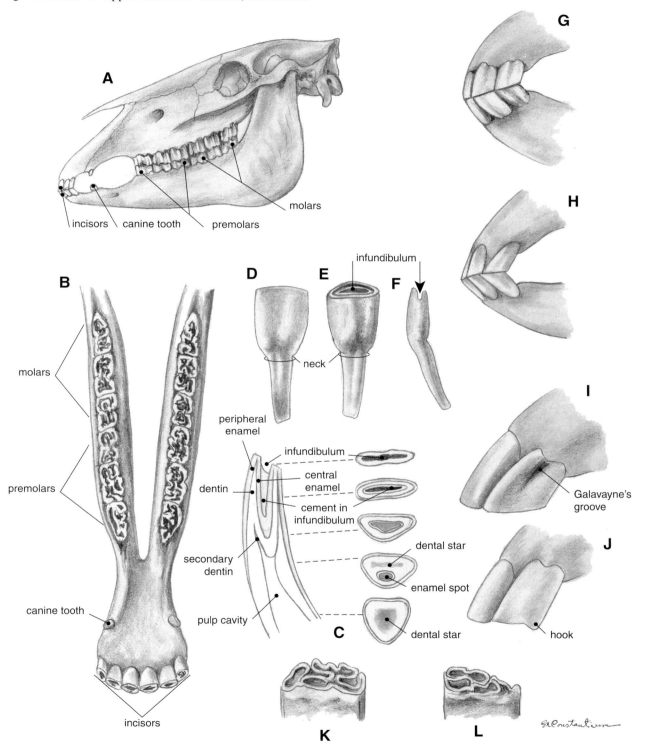

Fig.H7.26. Features of the dentition in the horse. **A.** The teeth of the horse, profile. **B.** The mandibular teeth, dorsal view. **C.** Serial transverse sections through a permanent incisor. **D.** Vestibular aspect of deciduous incisor. **E.** Lingual aspect of deciduous incisor. **F.** Profile of deciduous incisor. **G.** 6 years old. **H.** and **I.** 10 years old. **J.** 7–9 years old. **K.** Lower molar. **L.** Lower premolar.

The following is a brief description of the eruption of the incisors in the horse (after Barone 1976).

- The central incisors (Di1) are sometimes visible at birth; they erupt between four and seven days, are in wear in the second month, and are level at 12 months old.
- The intermediate incisors (Di2) erupt between 25 and 35 days, are in wear in the fourth month, and are level at 15–18 months of age.
- The corner incisors (Di3) erupt between 6 and 8 months, are in wear at 12–15 months, and are level at 24 months of age.

According to the same author (in combination with the shape of the occlusal surface and the disappearance of the cup—the so-called **"cup gone"**):

- The Di1 are replaced by permanent teeth (I1) at 2½ years and are in wear at 3 years.
- The Di2 are replaced by I2 at 3½ years and are in wear at 4 to 4½ years.
- The Di3 are replaced by I3 at 4½ years, and are in wear at 5½ years.
- At 6 years, the I1 are level, the lower I1 cup is gone, and the occlusal surface is elliptical and transversely oriented.
- At 7 years, the I2 are level, the lower I2 cup is gone, and the occlusal surface is elliptical and transversely oriented.
- At 8 years, the I3 are level, the lower I3 cup is gone, the occlusal surface is elliptical and transversely oriented, and the dental star is visible on I1 and I2.
- At 9 years, the lower I1 occlusal surface is round.
- At 10 years, the lower I2 occlusal surface is round, and the dental star is visible.
- At 11 years, the lower I3 occlusal surface is round.
- At 12 years, the cement of the infundibulum dissapears on the lower I1 and I2.
- At 13 years, the cement of the infundibulum disappears on the lower I3, and the dental star is in the middle of the occlusal surface.
- At 14 years, the occlusal surface of the lower I1 is triangular.
- At 15 years, the occlusal surface of the lower I2 is triangular.
- At 16 or 17 years, the occlusal surface of the lower I3 is triangular.
- At 18 years, the occlusal surface of the lower I1 is biangular.
- At 19 years, the occlusal surface of the lower I2 is biangular.
- At 20 years, the occlusal surface of the lower I3 is biangular.

The premolars and molars are similar to one another. They are straight, prismatic teeth with multiple roots and a very discrete neck. The four surfaces (vestibular, lingual, and contact surfaces) border a square-shaped occlusal surface. The upper P1, rudimentary and only occasionally shown, is called **wolf tooth**. It erupts between five and six months, and if it falls out in young individuals it will not be replaced. Also present in the lower jaw, it does not commonly erupt. Wolf teeth hardly ever "fall out," but they must be removed if causing problems.

The permanent premolars on each arch are called P2, P3, and P4.

**The extent of the roots of the upper premolars and molars in the horse (see Fig. H7.37A) is of great clinical importance in two instances: during trepanation of the maxillary sinuses either during treatment of sinusitis or in case of the expulsion of a cheek tooth. The approach to the trepanation should take into consideration the age of the individual. The trepanation is also commonly performed to explore/inspect the sinuses for sinus neoplasia, cysts, and other conditions.**

The eruption and replacement of the cheek teeth differs from author to author. Here is an average:

- The deciduous premolars (Dp2, Dp3, and Dp4) erupt before birth or during the first two weeks.
- Permanent premolar 2 (P2) replaces the Dp2 at 2–2½years.
- Permanent premolar 3 (P3) replaces the Dp3 at 2½–3 years.
- Permanent premolar 4 (P4) replaces the Dp4 at 3½ years.
- The first molar (M1) erupts between 6 and 12 months.
- The second molar (M2) erupts at 2½ years.
- The third molar (M3) erupts at 3½–4½ years.

With the median (split) side of the head up, identify the **basihyoid bone** and the following structures of the larynx (see Fig. H7.27A; see Figs. H7.18, H7.19, and H7.23):
- The **epiglottis**, with the **cuneiform process** (present only in the horse)
- The **hyoepiglottic lig.** and **hyoepiglotticus M.**
- The **arytenoid cartilage**, with the **corniculate** and **vocal processes**
- The median section of the **thyroid cartilage**
- The **cricothyroid lig.** (see Fig. H7.23)
- The median section of the **cricoid cartilage** (both the plate—**lamina**—and the ring—**arcus**)
- The **tracheal cartilages** (see Fig. H7.23)

- The aryepiglottic fold
- The **vestibular** and **vocal folds** separated by the **laryngeal ventricle (saccule)** (see Fig. H7.18)
- The **median laryngeal recess**

Look at the medial aspect of the larynx and identify the following structures:

- The **aditus laryngis** (the entrance into the larynx)
- The **laryngeal vestibule** (between the entrance and the vocal folds)
- The **rima glottidis** (between the vocal folds and the arytenoid cartilages)
- The **infraglottic cavity** (between the **glottis** and the trachea)

The glottis is the vocal apparatus of the larynx and consists of the vocal cords (the vocal lig. and vocalis M. covered by the mucosa—vocal fold), arytenoid cartilages, and rima glottidis. Carefully remove the mucosa of the larynx and expose the two parts of the **thyroarytenoideus M.,** namely the **ventricularis M.** (rostrally) and the **vocalis M.** (caudally), separated by the laryngeal ventricle. The ventricularis M. is accompanied by the **vestibular lig.,** whereas the vocalis M. is paralleled by the **vocal lig.** Cau-

dal to the vocalis M., the **cricoarytenoideus lateralis M.** is exposed. Also identify the **arytenoideus transversus M.,** and the **cricoarytenoideus dorsalis M.** (both transversely sectioned).

**The surgery for correction of idiopathic laryngeal hemiplegia attempts to replace the function of the cricoarytenoideus dorsalis M. (to abduct the corniculate process).**

Reflect the free end of the cricoarytenoideus dorsalis M. to expose its origin on the caudodorsal aspect of the cricoid cartilage and the insertion on the muscular process of the arytenoid cartilage.

Remove the hyoid apparatus with the tongue and larynx attached, as follows. Free the stylohyoid bone from the **styloid process of the temporal bone (the petrosal part)**, by transecting the **tympanohyoid** (the cartilage between the two bones). Section the occipitohyoideus M., and the attachments of the rostral belly of the digastricus, the mylohyoideus, geniohyoideus, and genioglossus Mm. from the mandible. Section the attachment of the lingual mucosa to the oral cavity and oropharynx. Section the attachments of the dorsal walls of the pharynx, transect the cranial laryngeal N., and free the larynx from any other attachments. Remove the hyoid apparatus, tongue, and larynx and place them on a tray.

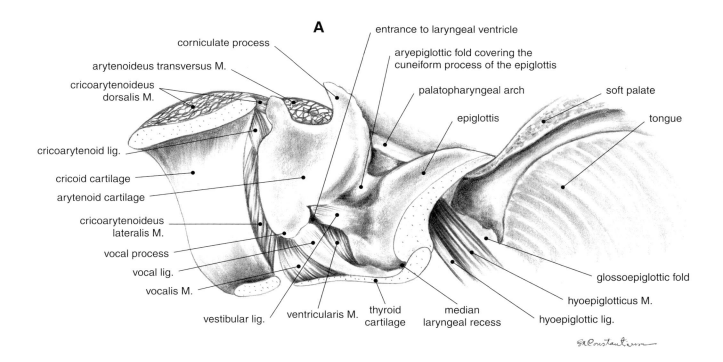

Fig. H7.27. The larynx in the horse. **A.** Larynx after mucosa has been removed, left medial aspect. *(continues)*

**B**

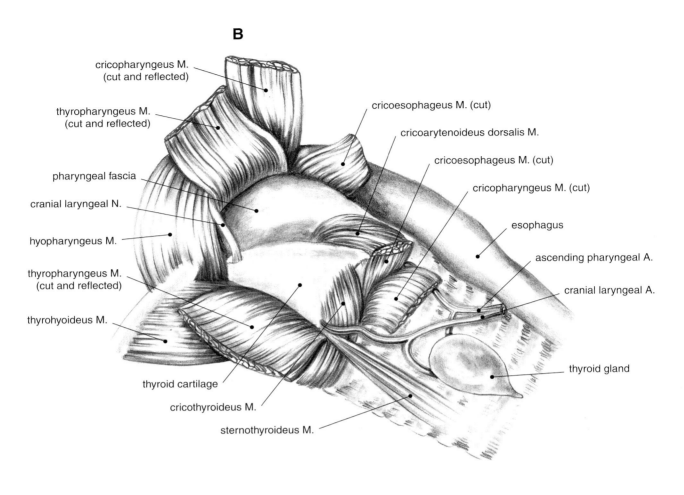

cricopharyngeus M.
(cut and reflected)

thyropharyngeus M.
(cut and reflected)

pharyngeal fascia

cranial laryngeal N.

hyopharyngeus M.

thyropharyngeus M.
(cut and reflected)

thyrohyoideus M.

thyroid cartilage

cricothyroideus M.

sternothyroideus M.

cricoesophageus M. (cut)

cricoarytenoideus dorsalis M.

cricoesophageus M. (cut)

cricopharyngeus M. (cut)

esophagus

ascending pharyngeal A.

cranial laryngeal A.

thyroid gland

**C**

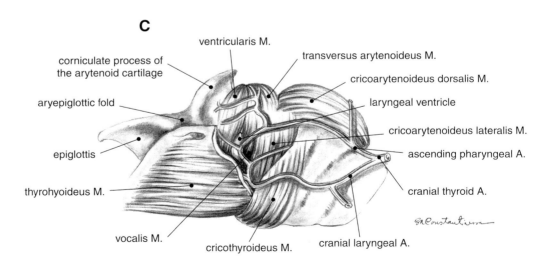

ventricularis M.

corniculate process of
the arytenoid cartilage

aryepiglottic fold

epiglottis

thyrohyoideus M.

vocalis M.

cricothyroideus M.

transversus arytenoideus M.

cricoarytenoideus dorsalis M.

laryngeal ventricle

cricoarytenoideus lateralis M.

ascending pharyngeal A.

cranial thyroid A.

cranial laryngeal A.

Fig. H7.27. *(continued)* The larynx in the horse. **B.** Deep larynx, left laterodorsal aspect. **C.** Arterial supply of the left larynx.

Turn all these structures lateral side up. Transect the thyropharyngeus and cricopharyngeus Mm., reflect the stumps, and expose the **wing (lamina) of the thyroid cartilage** and the **pharyngeal fascia** (Fig. H7.27B). Make a window within the lamina of the thyroid cartilage and expose the cricoarytenoideus lateralis, ventricularis, and vocalis Mm., and the bottom of the laryngeal ventricle (Fig. H7.27C). Dissect the **laryngeal A.,** the **laryngeal branch** of the **cranial thyroid A.,** and the cranial and caudal laryngeal Nn., all the way inside the larynx (see Fig. H7.27C).

Separate the components of the hyoid apparatus and the cartilages of the larynx and examine them one by one.

The **paranasal sinuses** differ from species to species. The following sinuses are present in the horse: the rostral and caudal maxillary sinuses, the conchofrontal sinus (Fig. H7.28), the sphenopalatine sinus, and the ventral and the middle conchal sinuses (see Fig. H7.18).

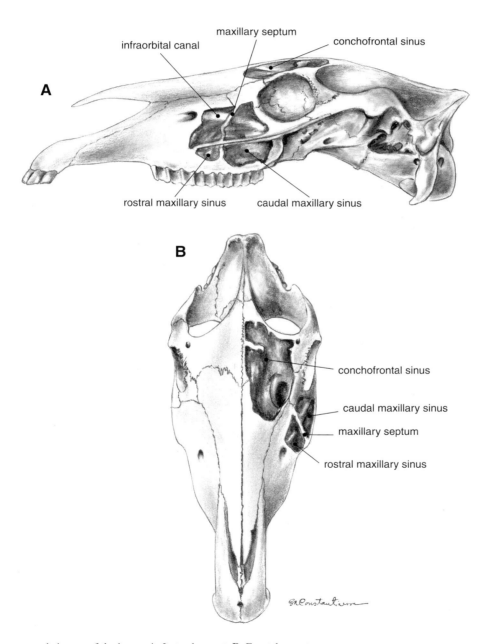

Fig. H7.28. The paranasal sinuses of the horse. **A.** Lateral aspect. **B.** Frontal aspect.

The **rostral** and **caudal maxillary sinuses** are separated by the **maxillary septum** only in the horse. They extend dorsal and ventral to the **facial crest**, but the approach is always dorsal to this landmark. The rostral sinus opens freely into the ventral conchal sinus. The caudal sinus communicates with the frontal and sphenopalatine sinuses and opens into the middle nasal meatus.

The **conchofrontal sinus**, specific to the horse, is the result of communication between the **frontal sinus** and the **dorsal conchal sinus**.

The **sphenopalatine sinus**, also specific to the horse, is a combination of the **sphenoid** and the **palatine sinuses**.

The **ventral conchal sinus** is the cavity enclosed by the caudal part of the ventral concha. It opens into the middle nasal meatus.

The **middle conchal sinus** is the cavity enclosed by the largest of the ethmoturbinates, part of the middle concha.

The clinical correlation of the paranasal sinuses will be detailed in the Modlab H7, at the end of this chapter.

Start the study of the central nervous system. Turn the head so that the sectioned side is up and examine first the median/sagittal aspect of the **brain** and **spinal cord**.

Examine the **leptomeninges** (the **pia mater** and the **arachnoid**) and the **pachymeninx** (the **dura mater**). The spinal cord, intimately surrounded by the pia mater, is anchored to the dura mater by symmetrical **denticulate ligg.** The dura mater that separates the two **cerebral hemispheres** is called the **falx cerebri**. It fills most of the **cerebral longitudinal fissure**. The **cerebrum** is separated from the **cerebellum** by the **tentorium cerebelli membranaceum** (attached to the **tentorium cerebelli osseum**, the osseous shelf formed by the **tentoric process** of the **occipital**, **interparietal**, and **parietal bones**). The **hypophysis** is protected and anchored within the **hypophyseal fossa** by the **diaphragma sellae**, the horizontal extension of the dura mater, partially separating the hypophysis from the brain (Fig. H7.29A).

On the same aspect of the brain, systematically identify the structures belonging to the telencephalon, diencephalon, mesencephalon, metencephalon, and myelencephalon in a rostrocaudal sequence (Fig. H7.29B).

Identify the following structures of the *telencephalon*:

- The four lobes of each hemisphere: frontal, parietal, temporal, and occipital
  - gyri
  - sulci
  - fissures
- The **olfactory bulb**, which sends the **filla olfactoria** (the first cranial nerve) through the **cribriform plate** of the ethmoid bone

- The **corpus callosum** with
  - The **body**—in the middle, between the genu and the splenium
  - The **genu**—rostrally
  - The **splenium**—caudally
  - The **rostrum**, connecting the genu to the **lamina terminalis grisea**, which closes the third ventricle rostrally, dorsal to the **optic chiasm**
- The **rostral commissure**
  *Note*. The corpus callosum and the rostral commissure are two of the white substance connections between the two halves of the **cerebrum** (the other connection is the caudal commissure).
- The **fornix**; this is a unique X-shaped structure with arcuate fibers that connects the hippocampus to the mamillary body and consists of
  - The **body**, nonsymmetrical, acting as part of the floor of the lateral ventricles, and the roof of the third ventricle of the brain
  - The symmetrical **crura** (sing. **crus**), caudally, starting from the hippocampus
  - The symmetrical **columns**, rostrally, extending up to the mamillary body
- The **septum pellucidum**, the median, vertical wall of white matter between the corpus callosum (dorsally) and the fornix (ventrally). It separates the two lateral ventricles from each other.

Remove the septum pellucidum and enter the lateral ventricle; on the floor of the **lateral ventricles (first and second),** identify rostrally the **nucleus caudatus,** and caudally the **hippocampus**. They are separated by the **tela choroidea** (a layer of pia mater), supporting the **choroid plexus**, which produces the **cerebrospinal fluid**.

Continue by exploring the structures of the *diencephalon*, which consists of five major components: thalamus, epithalamus, hypothalamus, metathalamus, and subthalamus (which is located between the thalamus and the substantia nigra). Only some structures belonging to these components can be identified on the median section of the brain, as follows:

- The **interthalamic adhesion**, part of the *thalamus* and appearing circular on the section; it is surrounded by the **third ventricle**. The **interventricular foramen** allows communication between the lateral ventricles and the third ventricle. Explore the third ventricle and identify the following recesses: **optic, neurohypophyseal, pineal,** and **suprapineal**. On the roof of the third ventricle the tela choroidea and choroid plexus can be seen.

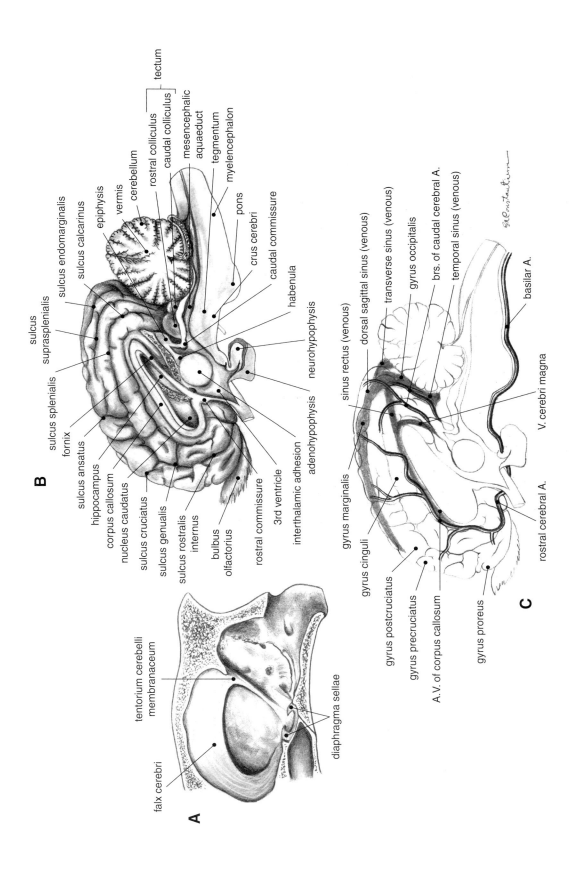

Fig. H7.29. The brain cavity and the encephalon, horse. **A.** Encephalic dura mater. **B.** Encephalon, sagittal aspect. **C.** Arterial supply to the encephalon, sagittal aspect.

- The **epiphysis (pineal body)**, part of the *epithalamus* and anchored to the thalamus by the **habenula**
- The **hypophysis (the pituitary gland)**, the **infundibulum**, **tuber cinereum** (the gray tubercle) (see Fig. H7.30), the **mamillary body** (see Fig. H7.30), the **optic chiasm** (see Fig. H7.30), and the **optic tract** (see Fig. H7.30), all structures belonging to the *hypothalamus*. The hypophysis consists of two main parts: the **adenohypophysis** (the glandular part) and the **neurohypophysis** (the nervous part). The latter is attached to the hypothalamus by the **infundibulum**. The **intermediate part** of the hypophysis is sometimes visible.

The *mesencephalon* (see Fig. H7.29B) consists of the cerebral peduncle and tectum. The cerebral peduncle consists of the crus cerebri and tegmentum. Identify them on your specimen:

- The **tectum** is the most dorsal part of the mesencephalon and consists of **colliculus rostralis** (opticus) and **colliculus caudalis** (acusticus); together they are called the **lamina quadrigemina** and represent the roof of the mesencephalon. They are separated from the rest of the structures by the **mesencephalic aquaeduct**; this narrow duct is the communication between the third and the fourth ventricles.
- The **tegmentum**, just below the aquaeduct, is the dorsal part of the **cerebral peduncle**. The ventral part of the peduncle is the **crus cerebri**; they are separated from each other by the **substantia nigra**.

The transitional area between the tectum and the epiphysis is the **caudal commissure**.

*Remember!* The corpus callosum, the rostral commissure, and the caudal commissure are the only structures (white matter) that connect the two halves of the cerebrum.

The *metencephalon* consists of two main structures: the pons (ventrally), and the cerebellum (dorsally). The cerebellum also covers the medulla oblongata, which is continuous rostrally with the pons. The pons, the medulla oblongata, and the cerebellum enclose the fourth ventricle.

- The **pons** contributes to the floor of the fourth ventricle (the rostral part).
- The **cerebellum** shows the nine **lobules** of the **vermis**: **lingula, lobulus centralis, culmen, declive, folium vermis, tuber vermis, pyramid, uvula**, and **nodulus** (starting from over the fourth ventricle and moving in a rostrodorsal, then clockwise, direction).
- Part of the roof of the fourth ventricle is the **rostral medullary velum**, an ependymal lamella between the

rostral cerebellar peduncle and the lingula (there is also a caudal medullary velum, part of the myelencephalon).

The *myelencephalon* is represented by the medulla oblongata and the caudal medullary velum:

- The **medulla oblongata** is the caudal part of the floor of the fourth ventricle.
- The **caudal medullary velum** closes the fourth ventricle caudally.
- The **fourth ventricle** contains a tela choroidea and a choroid plexus. It continues caudally with the **central canal** of the **spinal cord.**

On the midsection, identify the veins (including the sinuses) and the arteries of the brain. Veins include the **dorsal sagittal sinus**, within the falx cerebri; the **sinus rectus**; the **V. of corpus callosum**; the **V. cerebri magna**; the **transverse sinus**; the **temporal sinus** and so on. Arteries include the **basilar** and **caudal cerebral Aa.**, the **A. of the corpus callosum,** and so on (Fig. H7.29C).

Examine the **gyri** (sing. **gyrus**) and **sulci** (sing. **sulcus**, or groove) of the medial aspect of the cerebral hemisphere and the distribution of the white and gray matter in the cerebellum (see Fig. H7.29B).

Carefully remove the brain and the spinal cord from the cranial cavity and the vertebral canal, respectively. With a fine scissors, free the hypophysis from the diaphragma sellae. Place the brain and the spinal cord on a tray with the ventral side up and identify the structures in the same order that they were examined on the midsection (Fig. H7.30A).

However, before proceeding, observe that the cranial cavity is divided into two compartments (**cerebral** and **cerebellar**) by the tentorium cerebelli osseum and membraneceum.

On the ventral aspect of the *telencephalon,* identify the olfactory bulb, the **olfactory peduncle**, the **lateral** and **medial olfactory tracts** bordering the **olfactory tubercle,** the **piriform lobe**, and the **lateral** and **medial olfactory grooves**. All these structures belong to the **rhinencephalon** (the olfactory brain). The lateral olfactory groove separates the olfactory brain from the hemisphere. The olfactory bulb is the origin of the **olfactory Nn. (CN I)**.

The *diencephalon* consists of the optic chiasm, the optic tract, the tuber cinereum with the infundibulum and the hypophysis, and the mamillary body. The optic chiasm is the crossing point of the **optic Nn. (CN II)**.

The *mesencephalon* shows the two symmetrical cerebral crura (sing. crus), separated from each other by the

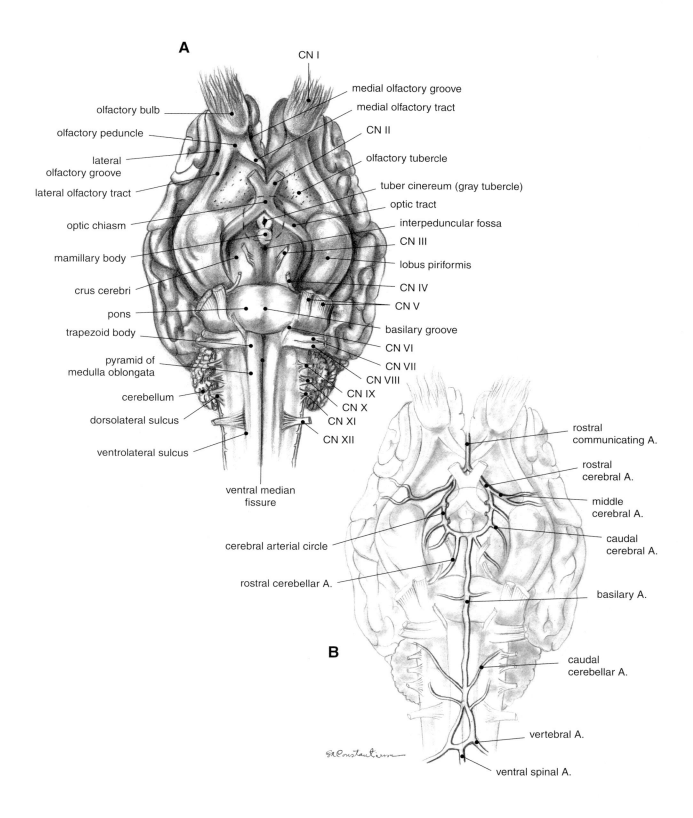

**A**

CN I

medial olfactory groove

medial olfactory tract

CN II

olfactory tubercle

tuber cinereum (gray tubercle)

optic tract

interpeduncular fossa

CN III

lobus piriformis

CN IV

CN V

basilary groove

CN VI

CN VII

CN VIII

CN IX

CN X

CN XI

CN XII

olfactory bulb

olfactory peduncle

lateral olfactory groove

lateral olfactory tract

optic chiasm

mamillary body

crus cerebri

pons

trapezoid body

pyramid of medulla oblongata

cerebellum

dorsolateral sulcus

ventrolateral sulcus

ventral median fissure

rostral communicating A.

rostral cerebral A.

middle cerebral A.

caudal cerebral A.

basilary A.

caudal cerebellar A.

vertebral A.

ventral spinal A.

cerebral arterial circle

rostral cerebellar A.

**B**

Fig. H7.30. The brain of the horse. **A.** Ventral structures of the brain. **B.** Arterial and venous supply of the brain, ventral aspect.

interpeduncular fossa (each cerebral crus is part of the cerebral peduncle). The **oculomotor N. (CN III)** originates from the ventral aspect of the crus cerebri, whereas the **trochlear N. (CN IV)** originates from the tectum (the most dorsal component of the mesencephalon) and surrounds the mesencephalon in a ventral direction; it arises between the crus cerebri and the pons.

The ventral *metencephalon* exposes the pons with the **basilary groove** in the middle, and the **trigeminal N. (CN V)** on the lateral sides. The lateral lobes of the cerebellum exceed the limits of the medulla oblongata laterally.

The ventral aspect of the *medulla oblongata* shows the following structures: the symmetrical **pyramids**, separated by the **ventral median fissure**, the **trapezoid body** (parallel with the caudal border of the pons), and the **ventrolateral** and **dorsolateral sulci**.

The **intermediofacial N. (CN VII)** and the **vestibulocochlear N. (CN VIII)** originate from the lateral extent of the trapezoid body. The **abducent N. (CN VI)** and the **hypoglossal N. (CN XII)** leave the medulla oblongata from the ventrolateral sulcus, whereas the **glossopharyngeal N. (CN IX)**, the **vagus N. (CN X)**, and the **accessory N. (CN XI)** leave from the dorsolateral sulcus.

*Note*. The accessory N. has two roots: cranial and spinal.

On the ventral aspect, the choroid plexus of the fourth ventricle is also visible between the lateral borders of the medulla oblongata and the cerebellum.

Identify the following vessels: the **ventral spinal A.** (lying within the **ventral median fissure** of the spinal cord) and the anastomosis with the **vertebral Aa.**, the basilary A., the **caudal cerebellar A.**, the **rostral cerebellar A.**, the caudal cerebral A., the **middle cerebral A.**, the **rostral cerebral A.**, the **caudal communicating A.** (between the internal carotid and the basilar Aa.), and the **cerebral arterial circle** (the circle of Willis, around the hypophysis and the optic chiasm) (Fig. H7.30B).

Turn the brain lateral side up. Identify the olfactory brain and the hemisphere, which are the only components of the *telencephalon* from this perspective. The olfactory brain consists of the olfactory bulb, olfactory peduncle, lateral olfactory tract, olfactory trigone, and the piriform lobe. *Notice* the CN I at the rostral end of the olfactory bulb. On the lateral aspect of the hemisphere examine the gyri, sulci, and fissures, as they are illustrated in Figure H7.31A.

The *diencephalon* consists of the optic chiasm, the hypophysis with the infundibulum and tuber cinereum, and the mamillary body. The **lateral and medial geniculate bodies (the metathalamus) and the epiphysis** can be seen either by reflecting the caudal pole of the hemisphere rostrally or by removing the hemisphere. *Notice* the CN II (Fig. H7.32).

The *mesencephalon* shows the cerebral peduncle, rostral and caudal colliculi (sing. colliculus), CN III and CN IV, and the **rostral cerebellar peduncle** (see Fig. H7.32).

The *metencephalon* consists of the pons, the **middle cerebellar peduncle**, the lateral lobe of the cerebellum, CN V, and the trapezoid body with CN VII and CN VIII (see Fig. H7.32).

The *myelencephalon* contains the pyramid, the **caudal cerebellar peduncle**, the ventrolateral sulcus with the CN VI and CN XII, and the dorsolateral sulcus with the CN IX, CN X, and CN XI (see Fig. H7.32).

Before removing the cerebellum, examine the dorsal aspect of the hemisphere and identify the sulci and the gyri. Some of them are continuous on the lateral or medial side of the hemisphere (Fig. H7.31B).

Remove the cerebellum by transecting the three cerebellar peduncles: rostral (from the dorsal aspect of the mesencephalon), middle (from the pons), and caudal (from the dorsal aspect of medulla oblongata). The dorsal aspect of the medulla oblongata and the floor of the fourth ventricle are now exposed. The medulla oblongata exposes the **fasciculus gracilis**, on both sides of the **(dorsal) median sulcus**, and the **fasciculus cuneatus**, lateral to the previous fascicle (Fig. H7.33A).

Remove the **striate body**, with the **hippocampus (Amon's horn)**, to fully expose the structures shown in Fig. H7.33A.

Before taking the next step, review the structures of the **corpus striatum** (striate body), an important extrapyramidal center represented by **basal nuclei**, connected by cords of gray matter and separated from each other and the surroundings by fibers (white matter).

The basal nuclei consist of the following structures:

- The nucleus caudatus
- The **nucleus lentiformis**, divided by the **lateral medullary lamina** into
  – **Putamen** (laterally) and
  – **Pallidum** (medially)
- The **capsula interna** (white matter), which separates the caudate nucleus from the lentiform nucleus
- The **capsula externa** (also a white matter), which separates the lentiform nucleus from the **claustrum**
- The **claustrum**, which separates the putamen from the **insula**
- The **capsula extrema**, white matter between the claustrum and the cortex

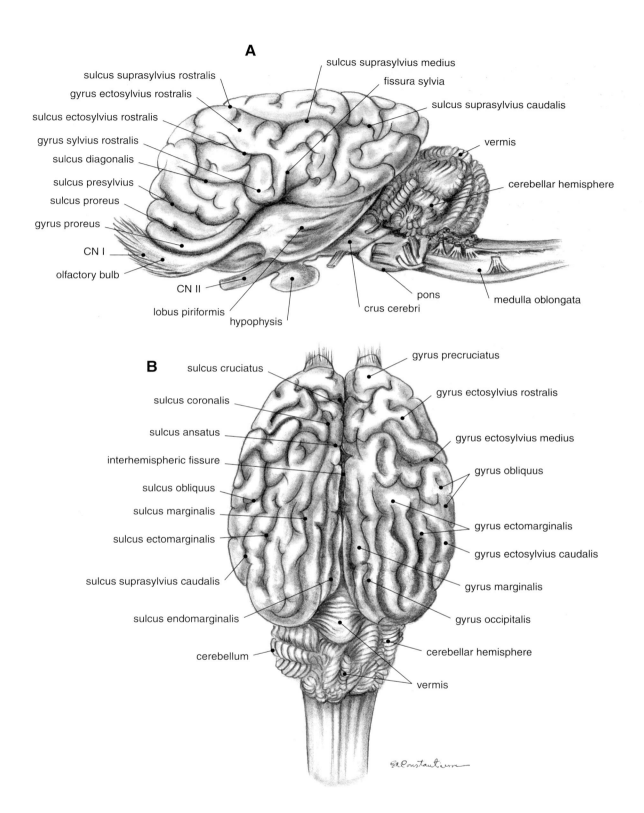

**A**

sulcus suprasylvius rostralis
gyrus ectosylvius rostralis
sulcus ectosylvius rostralis
gyrus sylvius rostralis
sulcus diagonalis
sulcus presylvius
sulcus proreus
gyrus proreus
CN I
olfactory bulb
CN II
lobus piriformis
hypophysis

sulcus suprasylvius medius
fissura sylvia
sulcus suprasylvius caudalis
vermis
cerebellar hemisphere
pons
crus cerebri
medulla oblongata

**B**

sulcus cruciatus
sulcus coronalis
sulcus ansatus
interhemispheric fissure
sulcus obliquus
sulcus marginalis
sulcus ectomarginalis
sulcus suprasylvius caudalis
sulcus endomarginalis
cerebellum

gyrus precruciatus
gyrus ectosylvius rostralis
gyrus ectosylvius medius
gyrus obliquus
gyrus ectomarginalis
gyrus ectosylvius caudalis
gyrus marginalis
gyrus occipitalis
cerebellar hemisphere
vermis

Fig. H7.31. Brain of the horse. **A.** Lateral aspect. **B.** Dorsal aspect.

With a brain knife make a transverse section in the hemisphere at the level of, and in the middle of, the caudate nucleus (Fig. H7.33B).

Using the other half of the brain make a horizontal section through the hemisphere at the level of the floor of the lateral ventricle and identify the structures illustrated in Figure H7.33C.

Make a second horizontal section (parallel with and ventral to the previous section) at the level of the rostral commissure and identify the structures illustrated in Figure H7.33D.

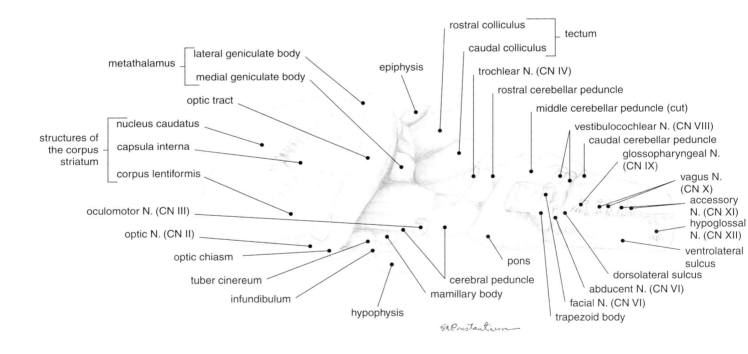

Fig. H7.32. The brain stem of the horse, left lateral view.

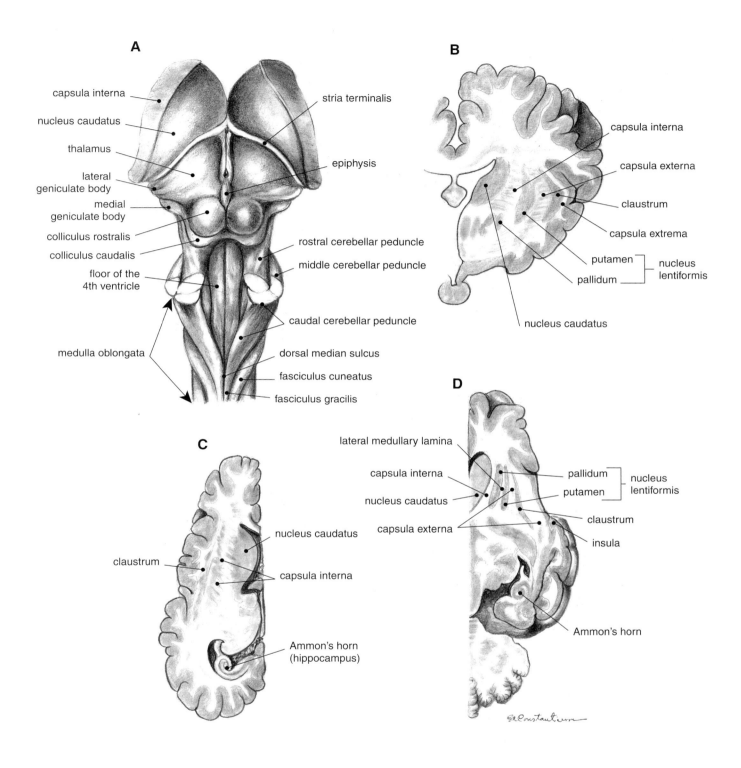

Fig. H7.33. Brain of the horse. **A.** Brain stem, dorsal aspect. **B.** Striate body, transverse section. **C.** Striate body, longitudinal section through the floor of the lateral ventricle. **D.** Striate body, longitudinal section through the rostral commisure.

## MODLAB H7

Approaching a live horse with care, attempt to palpate the structures listed at the beginning of this chapter.

Check the following *landmarks* and *approaches* of the most clinically relevant anatomical structures for physical examination and/or clinical interventions.

1. **Facial A. V.** and **parotid duct** (Fig. H7.34A)
   A. *Landmarks*: rostral border of the masseter M.; the notch of the mandible for the facial vessels, and the facial tubercle
   B. *Approach*: through the skin, superficial fascia of the head, and cutaneous faciei M., along the rostral border of the masseter M., and from the notch for the facial vessels halfway to the facial tubercle

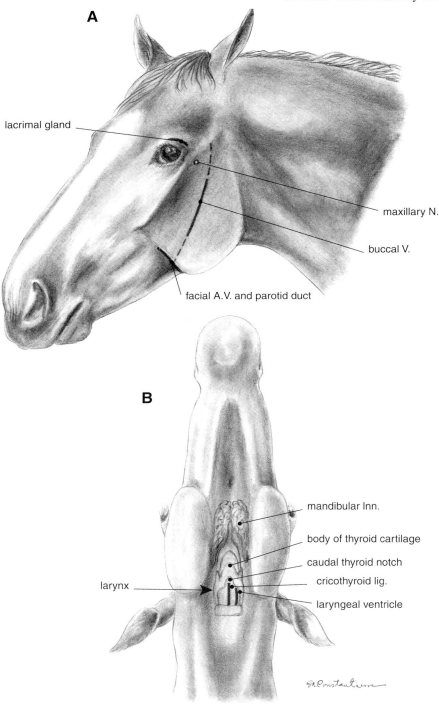

Fig. H7.34. Landmarks for physical examination and/or clinical approach to the head, horse. **A.** Structures in the ocular and masseteric areas. **B.** Laryngeal structures, ventral view.

*Caution*. In a rostrocaudal direction, the relationship between the vessels and the duct is: **A**rtery, **V**ein, and **P**arotid duct.

**The facial artery is commonly used for palpation of a pulse or arterial blood gas measurements at the notch mentioned above, on the medial aspect of the body of the mandible.**

2. **Lacrimal gland** (Fig. H7.34A)

   A. *Landmarks*: zygomatic process of the frontal bone, the orbital rim, the superior eyelid

   B. *Approach*: through the superior eyelid, along the orbital rim of the zygomatic process of the frontal bone, deep on the medial aspect of the process, lying in the **fossa for the lacrimal gland**

3. **Mandibular lnn.** (Fig. H7.34B)

   A. *Landmarks*: the intermandibular space, the notch for the facial vessels, the basihyoid bone and the lingual process

   B. *Approach*: through the skin and superficial fascia of the head, in the intermandibular space, 5 cm caudal to the notch for the facial vessels

   **These lymph nodes are commonly enlarged in infectious upper respiratory disease caused by *Streptococcus equi* ("strangles").**

4. **Larynx** (Figs. H1.17 and H7.34B)

   A. *Landmarks*: ramus of the mandible, tendon of the sternocephalicus M., linguofacial V.

   B. *Approach*: Keep the head of the horse in extension and approach the larynx through the skin and omohyoideus M. It is palpable at the level of the ramus of the mandible, where the sternocephalicus M. is attached.

5. **Cricothyroid lig.** (Fig. H7.34B)

   A. *Landmarks*: **body of the thyroid cartilage** (the laryngeal prominence), **caudal thyroid notch**, cricoid arch

   B. *Approach*: between the three landmarks, on the ventral midline of the larynx

6. **Laryngeal ventricle** (Fig. H7.34B)

   A. *Landmarks*: caudal thyroid notch, thyroid laminae, cricoid arch with the cricothyroid lig.

   B. *Approach*: between the three landmarks, on the medial aspect of the thyroid lamina, and within the larynx (**for surgical approach in roaring**). The laryngeal ventricle cannot be palpated externally, but can be readily viewed endoscopically.

7. **Maxillary N.** (Fig. H7.34A)

   A. *Landmarks*: facial crest and lateral canthus of the eye

   B. *Approach*: A needle can be inserted perpendicular to and through the skin, superficial fascia of the head, and masseter M., ventral to the facial crest, at the level of the lateral canthus of the eye.

   *Caution*. The nerve travels between the foramen rotundum and pterygopalatine fossa, on the deep side of the maxillary A. The needle should reach the narrow space between the **maxillary tubercle** (on the caudal extent of maxilla) and the coronoid process of the mandible. The nerve block of the maxillary N. will anesthetize the following structures: (1) all superior teeth; (2) the skin of the head between the eye, facial crest, commissure of the lips, upper lip, and the dorsal midline of the head; and (3) the mucosa of the hard palate.

8. **Infraorbital N.** (Fig. H7.35)

   A. *Landmarks*: infraorbital foramen, facial crest and tubercle, medial canthus of the eye

   B. *Approach*: Reflect the **levator labii superioris M.** dorsally and insert a needle through the skin and **levator nasolabialis M.** in a rostrocaudal direction; the needle should be held close to the surface of the head to enter the infraorbital foramen.

   *Notice* that the infraorbital foramen is located at the rostral intersection of two lines: a line traced from the medial canthus rostrally and parallel to the facial crest, and a line extending dorsally from the facial tubercle. The infraorbital foramen can also be palpated approximately 2.5 cm dorsal to the midpoint of a line connecting the facial tubercle and the nasoincisive notch. A practical method to palpate the infraorbital foramen (on the left side of the head) is to feel the nasoincisive notch with the middle finger of the left hand, and the facial tubercle with the thumb. The second finger will touch the foramen midway between the other two landmarks. The nerve block of the infraorbital N. will anesthetize different structures according to the length of the needle. With a short needle, only the skin of the head, mentioned above, and the upper incisors and canine tooth will be desensitized. A needle penetrating deep into the infraorbital canal will block the first two to four upper cheek teeth.

   **The infraorbital N. is sometimes anesthetized in the clinical work-up of headshaking syndrome (trigeminal neuralgia). Sometimes, an attempt is made to destroy the affected nerve by injecting a sclerosing agent.**

9. **Inferior alveolar N.** (Fig. H7.35)

   A. *Landmarks*: Viborg's triangle, lateral canthus of the eye, occlusal surface of the cheek teeth, notch for facial vessels, temporomandibular joint

B. *Approach*:

*Note*. The **mandibular foramen** is located at the intersection of the caudal extent of the occlusal surface of the cheek teeth, with the perpendicular line drawn from the lateral canthus.

α. A needle should be introduced through Viborg's triangle toward the mandibular foramen along the medial aspect of the mandible and between the pterygoid fossa and the medial pterygoideus M.

β. A needle should be inserted in a ventrodorsal position on a line between the notch for facial vessels and the rostral limit of the temporomandibular joint, and between the pterygoid fossa and the medial pterygoideus M.

γ. A needle should be inserted medial to the ventral border of the mandible in the direction of the perpendicular line that is drawn from the lateral canthus and between the pterygoid fossa and the medial pterygoideus M.

10. **Mental N.** (Fig. H7.35)
    A. *Landmarks*: mental foramen, commissure of the lips, tendon of **depressor labii inferioris M.**, orbicularis oris M.
    B. *Approach*: Reflect the tendon of depressor labii inferioris M. ventrally, at the level of the commissure of the lips (ventral to orbicularis oris M.), and insert a needle through the skin in a rostrocaudal direction toward the mental foramen; hold the needle close to the surface of the head. With a short needle, only the chin, the lower lip, the lower incisors, and the lower canine tooth will be desensitized. A long needle, penetrating deep into the **mandibular canal** will block the first two to four lower cheek teeth.

11. **Facial** and **auriculotemporal Nn.** (Fig. H7.36A)
    A. *Landmarks*: facial crest, temporomandibular joint, caudal border of ramus mandibulae
    B. *Approach*: through the skin, 2–4 cm ventral to the temporomandibular joint. The nerves emerge from

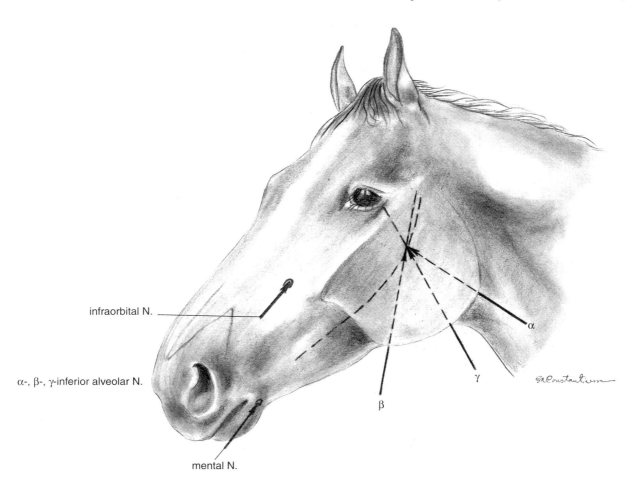

infraorbital N.

α-, β-, γ-inferior alveolar N.

mental N.

Fig. H7.35. Landmarks for physical examination and/or clinical approach to the head, horse.

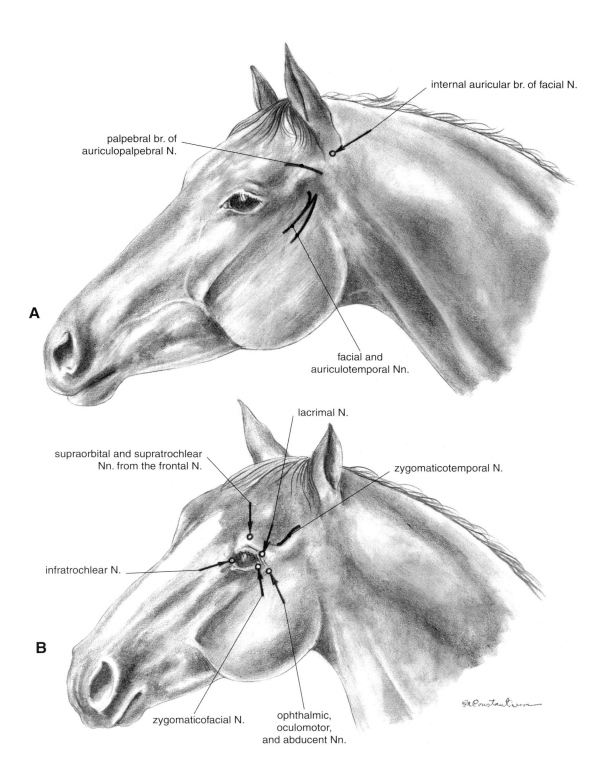

Fig. H7.36. Landmarks for physical examination and/or clinical approach to the head, horse. **A.** Structures around the temporomandibular joint.
**B.** Structures around the eye.

under the parotid gland in a rostral direction, parallel to the facial crest.

*Notice* that the auriculotemporal N. is situated dorsal to the facial N. on the surface of the masseter M., separated by the transverse facial A. and V.

12. **Palpebral branch of the auriculopalpebral N.** (Fig. H7.36A)
   A. *Landmarks*: temporomandibular joint, zygomatic arch, base of external ear
   B. *Approach*: A needle should be inserted in a dorsorostral direction between the skin and the zygomatic arch, dorsocaudal to the temporomandibular joint, and midway between the joint and the base of external ear.

13. **Internal auricular branch of facial N.** (Fig. H7.36A)
   A. *Landmarks*: external acoustic meatus, base of auricle
   B. *Approach*: A needle should be inserted perpendicularly through the skin and caudal to the external acoustic meatus (palpable), at the base of the ear.

14. **Supraorbital and supratrochlear Nn.** (Fig. H7.36B)
   A. *Landmarks*: zygomatic process of the frontal bone, supraorbital foramen
   B. *Approach*: A needle should be inserted in a vertical position through the skin, **levator anguli oculi medialis M.**, and **supraorbital foramen** (palpable). The frontal N. passes through the foramen and branches into the supraorbital N. (caudally) and the supratrochlear N. (rostrally).

15. **Zygomaticotemporal N.** (Fig. H7.36B)
   A. *Landmarks*: dorsal border of zygomatic arch, zygomatic processes of the frontal and temporal bones
   B. *Approach*: through the skin and parallel to the dorsal border of the zygomatic arch, in a rostrocaudal direction from the angle between the zygomatic processes of the frontal and temporal bones

16. **Lacrimal N.** (Fig. H7.36B)
   A. *Landmarks*: lateral canthus of the eye, upper eyelid
   B. *Approach*: through the skin of the upper eyelid at the level of the lateral canthus of the eye

17. **Zygomaticofacial N.** (Fig. H7.36B)
   A. *Landmarks*: temporal process of zygomatic bone, ventral rim of the orbita, lower eyelid
   B. *Approach*: through the skin of the lower eyelid, at the dorsal border of the temporal process of the zygomatic bone (which corresponds to the ventral rim of the orbita)

18. **Infratrochlear N.** (Fig. H7.36B)
   A. *Landmarks*: medial canthus of the eye, the **caudal lacrimal process**
   B. *Approach*: through the skin at the medial canthus of the eye, close to the caudal lacrimal process (palpable)

19. **Ophthalmic, oculomotor,** and **abducent Nn.** (sometimes also the **trochlear N.**) (Fig. H7.36B)
   A. *Landmarks*: facial crest, lateral canthus of the eye
   B. *Approach* (two techniques):
      a. A needle should be inserted through the skin and masseter M., ventral to the facial crest at the level of the lateral canthus of the eye and toward the opposite temporomandibular joint.
      b. A needle should be introduced in a manner similar to that for the maxillary N. (see no. 7, above); however, the position of the needle is oblique ventrodorsally at a 10-degree angle.
   *Note.* The nerves emerge from the **orbital fissure**, which is located 1 cm dorsal to foramen rotundum (the exit point for the maxillary N.).

20. **Ventral nasal meatus** (Fig. H7.37A)
   A. *Landmarks*: **ventral commissure of the nostril**, nasal septum, ventral nasal concha, floor of the nasal cavity
   B. *Approach*: A flexible gastric tube or an endoscope may be introduced into the ventral nasal meatus just above the ventral commissure of the nostril and firmly pressed against the nasal septum (medially) and the floor of the nasal cavity (ventrally). With this procedure, the ventral nasal concha will not be touched.
   *Caution.* The gastric tube must be introduced slowly and carefully to avoid entering the larynx and trachea. A flexible bronchoalveolar lavage tube similar to the nasogastric tube may also pass, but for the tube to enter the trachea/bronchi, the head must be extended. Passage of the tube into the esophagus is facilitated by flexing of the head and neck. Proper esophageal placement must be confirmed by palpating the tube within the esophagus.

21. **Paranasal sinuses** (Fig. H7.37B)
   The only sinuses readily accessible to a clinical intervention are the conchofrontal and maxillary sinuses.

*The conchofrontal sinus*
   A. *Landmarks*: middorsal line of the head, base of zygomatic process of frontal bone, dorsal rim of orbita, medial canthus of the eye, facial tubercle
   B. *Approach*: Through the skin within the area that extends from the middorsal line of the head to the base of the zygomatic process of frontal bone, along the dorsal rim of orbita; from the medial canthus of the eye, trace a convex line in a rostrodorsal direction to the middorsal line, midway between the orbita and the facial tubercle.

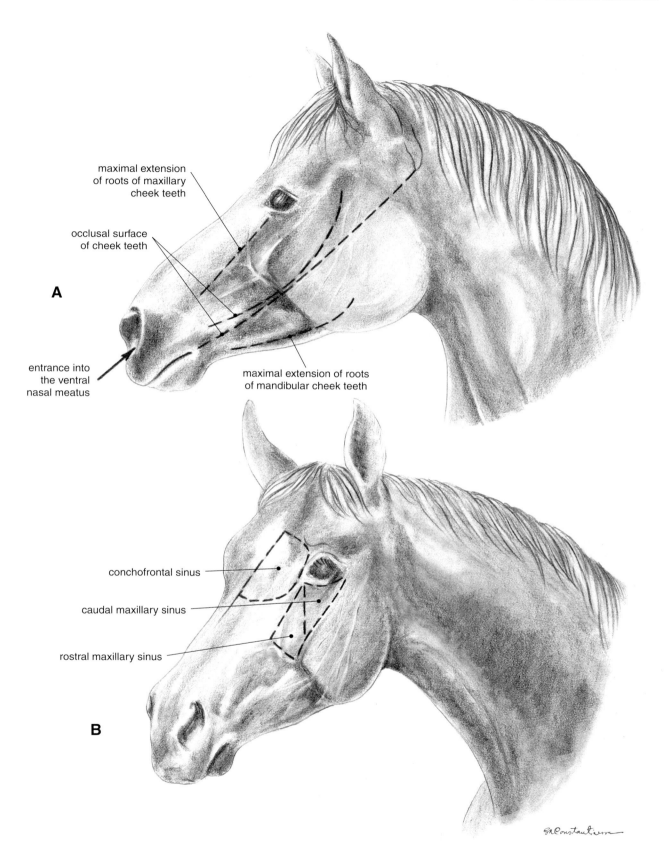

maximal extension
of roots of maxillary
cheek teeth

occlusal surface
of cheek teeth

**A**

entrance into
the ventral
nasal meatus

maximal extension of roots
of mandibular cheek teeth

conchofrontal sinus

caudal maxillary sinus

rostral maxillary sinus

**B**

Fig. H7.37. Landmarks for physical examination and/or clinical approach to the head, horse. **A.** Approach to the teeth and nasal cavity. **B.** Paranasal sinuses.

*Caution*. In older specimens, the caudal extent of the sinus exceeds the orbita caudally.

### The *caudal maxillary sinus*

A. *Landmarks*: rostral rim of orbita, medial canthus of the eye, facial crest and tubercle
B. *Approach*: through the skin and the **malaris** and levator labii superioris Mm., within the area outlined between the medial canthus of the eye, along the rostral rim of the orbita and the facial crest, a few centimeters caudal to the facial tubercle

### The *rostral maxillary sinus*

A. *Landmarks*: medial canthus of the eye, facial crest and tubercle, and infraorbital foramen
B. *Approach*: reflect the levator labii superioris M. dorsally and approach the sinus within the area rostral to the previous sinus and between the medial canthus of the eye, the infraorbital foramen, and the facial tubercle

22. **Linguofacial V.** (Fig. H7.38)
    A. *Landmarks*: jugular groove, angle of the mandible
    B. *Approach*: through the skin and cutaneous faciei M., between the cranial extent of the jugular groove and the angle of mandible

    **Ventral to the linguofacial V. is a triangular area outlined by the vein and the sternomandibularis M., the so-called Whitehouse approach to the guttural pouch. Ventral to it, on the midventral line of the same area, the modified Whitehouse approach is shown.**

    **The modified Whitehouse approach is commonly used to approach the dorsolateral aspect of the larynx during laryngoplasty ("tie back") procedures, and the ventrolateral aspect of the**

**guttural pouch when surgical drainage of the guttural pouch is required.**

23. **Viborg's triangle** (Fig. H7.38)
    A. *Landmarks and approach*: linguofacial V., caudal border of ramus of the mandible, tendon of sternomandibularis M.

    *Caution*. When the head of the horse is held in extension, this area is practically free of major vessels and nerves and corresponds to the most ventral extent of the guttural pouch in abnormal conditions, such as empyema.

    *The triangle is also a landmark for the surgical intervention on the guttural pouch called the Viborg's approach (see above). Distal to the linguofacial V., two other approaches to the guttural pouch are outlined: the Whitehouse approach and the modified Whitehouse approach.*

24. **Occipitohyoideus M.** (Fig. H7.38)
    A. *Landmarks*: jugular process of occipital bone, stylohyoid angle of the stylohyoid bone
    B. *Approach*: through the skin and aponeurosis of the **cleidomastoideus M.**, between the jugular process and the stylohyoid angle of the stylohyoid bone

    *This muscle is a landmark for performing either the hyovertebrotomy approach or the approach of Chabert-Fromage in a surgical intervention on the guttural pouch.*

    *Note* The Viborg's approach and the approach of Chabert-Fromage are known together as the Dietrich's approach in the surgical procedure of hyovertebrotomy.

25. **Great auricular N.** (Fig. H7.38)
    A. *Landmark*: **wing of atlas** (palpable caudoventral to the base of the ear)
    B. *Approach*: through the skin and aponeurosis of the **splenius M.**, along the border of the wing of atlas

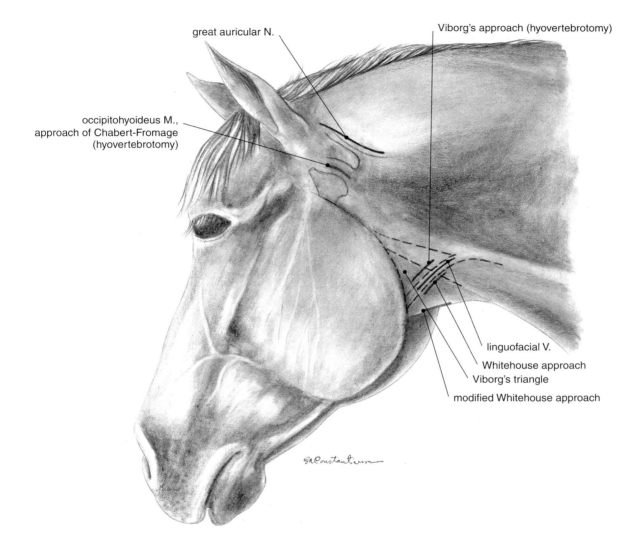

great auricular N.

Viborg's approach (hyovertebrotomy)

occipitohyoideus M.,
approach of Chabert-Fromage
(hyovertebrotomy)

linguofacial V.
Whitehouse approach
Viborg's triangle
modified Whitehouse approach

Fig. H7.38. Landmarks for physical examination and/or clinical approach to the head, horse (parotid region). *Note:* The landmarks and approaches to the guttural pouch are outlined.

Table H7.3 shows the average age of fusion of the epiphyses of all bones. This table is helpful for radiological, clinical, and necropsy purposes.

Table H7.3. The Revised Table with the Average Age of Fusion of the Epiphyses

| The Bone | The Ossification Center, which Is Fused | Horse | Ox | Small Ruminants | Pig | Dog |
|---|---|---|---|---|---|---|
| Occipital | Exoccipital-basioccipital | 3–6 mo. | 10–12 mo. | 6 mo. | 8–10 mo. | 2½–3 mo. |
| | Exoccipital-squama | 12–15 mo. | | | | 3–4 mo. |
| | Interparietal-squama | 1–2 yr. | b.b. | a.b. | absent | b.b. |
| Presphenoid | Body + wings | b.b. | | | | |
| Basisphenoid | Body + wings | 6 mo. | 6 mo. | 3–4 yr. | 12 mo. | 3–4 yr. |
| | Pre- and Basisphenoid | 2–4 yr. | 2½–4 yr. | 4–5 yr. | 6–12 mo. | 1–2 yr. |
| | Spheno-occipital | 3–5 yr. | 2 yr. | 1–2 yr. | 1–2 yr. | 8–10 mo. |
| Parietal | Interparietal suture | 15–36 mo. | 6 mo. | 1 mo. | 6–15 mo. | 2–3 yr. |
| Frontal | Interfrontal suture | 5–7 yr. | Incomplete | 5–7 yr. | 1–2 yr. | 3–4 yr. |
| Temporal | Petrotympanic | 2–4 mo. | At birth | Never or very late | 6 mo. | |
| | Petrosquamous | Never or very late | 2–4 mo. | 4–6 mo. | At birth | 2–3 yr. |
| Mandible | Centers of each bone | b.b. | | | | |
| | Fusion of the two bones | 6 mo. | Never complete | | After birth | Never or very late |
| Vertebrae | Body epiphyses | 4½–5 yr. | 4½–5 yr. | 4–5 yr. | 4–7 yr. | 1½–2 yr. |
| Scapula | Coracoid center | 10–12 mo. | 7–10 mo | 10–11 mo | 1 yr | 5–8 mo |
| Humerus | Proximal extremity | 42 mo. | 42–48 mo. | 30–40 mo. | 42 mo. | 12–15 mo. |
| | Distal extremity | 15–18 mo. | 15–20 mo. | 9–11 mo. | 12 mo. | 7–8 mo. |
| Radius | Proximal extremity | 15–18 mo. | 12–15 mo. | 8–10 mo. | 12 mo. | 9–10 mo. |
| | Distal extremity | 42 mo. | 40–48 mo. | 40–60 mo. | 42 mo. | 10–12 mo. |
| Ulna | Proximal extremity | 42 mo. | 42 mo. | 20–40 mo. | 42 mo. | 7–8 mo. |
| | Distal extremity | 2–3 mo. to radius | 3 yr. | 35–40 mo. | 3 yr. | 9–12 mo. |
| Metacarpals | Distal extremity | 15 mo. | 24–30 mo. | 30–36 mo. | 2 yr. | 6–7 mo. |
| Prox. phalanx | Proximal extremity | 12–15 mo. | 20–24 mo. | 10–16 mo. | 13 mo. | 6–7 mo. |
| Middle phalanx | Proximal extremity | 10–12 mo. | 15–18 mo. | 12–18 mo. | 1 yr. | 6–7 mo. |
| Coxal | Main centers + acetabular | 10–12 mo. | 7–10 mo. | 10 mo. | 1 yr. | 6 mo. |
| | Ischiatic tuberosity | 4–5 yr. | 5 yr. | 4–5 yr. | 6–7 yr. | 10–12 mo. |
| | Iliac crest | 4½–5 yr. | 5 yr. | 4½–5 yr. | 6–7 yr. | 2–3 yr. |
| Femur | Proximal extremity | 3 yr. | 3 yr. | 36–40 mo. | 3 yr. | 9–12 mo. |
| | Distal extremity | 42 mo. | 42 mo. | 40–42 mo. | 42 mo. | 9–12 mo. |
| Tibia | Proximal extremity | 42 mo. | 4 yr. | 50–55 mo. | 42 mo. | 10–12 mo. |
| | Distal extremity | 2 yr. | 24–30 mo. | 25–35 mo. | 2 yr. | 9–10 mo. |
| Fibula | Proximal extremity | | 42 mo. to tibia | | 42 mo. | 10–12 mo. |
| Calcaneus | Tuberosity | 3 yr. | | | 24–30 mo. | 6–7 mo. |

*Source:* After Barone 1999.
*Note:* mo. = month(s); yr. = year(s); b.b. = before birth; a.b. = after birth.

# Large
# Ruminants

# R 1

## The Neck

Before starting the dissection of the muscles of the neck, review the systematization of the cervical muscles, presented in Table R1.1.

The cervical vertebrae are illustrated in Figure R1.1.

*Identify and palpate the following structures as landmarks for physical examination and/or clinical approach: the intercornual protuberance, the cranial angle of the scapula, the manubrium sterni, the wing of atlas, the jugular groove, and the superficial cervical ln.*

Table R1.1. Muscles of the Neck, Horse and Large Ruminants

**Dorsal Muscles of the Neck** (dorsal to the cervical vertebrae)

*1st layer*
 – trapezius p. cervicalis
 – omotransversarius
    (cleidotransversus in Eq.)
*2nd layer*
 – rhomboideus cervicis
 – splenius
 – serratus ventralis cervicis
*3rd layer*
 – iliocostalis cervicis (from
    iliocostalis thoracis)                    (erector spinae)
 – longissimus cervicis
 – longissimus atlantis (from
    longissimus thoracis)
 – longissimus capitis
 – semispinalis capitis (from
    semispinalis thoracis)                    (transversospinalis)
*4th layer*
 – multifidi cervicis
 – spinalis cervicis (from spinalis
    thoracis)                                 (erector spinae)
 – intertransversarii cervicis
 – rectus capitis dorsalis major
    (superficial and deep fascicles)
 – rectus capitis dorsalis minor
 – obliquus capitis cranialis
 – obliquus capitis caudalis

**Ventral Muscles of the Neck** (ventral to the cervical vertebrae)

*Superficial muscles*
 – cleidobrachialis
 – cleidocephalicus
    • mastoid part (cleidomastoideus)
    • occipital part (cleidooccipitalis—only in Ru.)
 – clavicular intersection
 – sternocephalicus
    • mandibular part (sternomandibularis)
    • mastoid part (sternomastoideus—only in Ru.)
 – sternohyoideus and sternothyroideus
 – omohyoideus
*Deep muscles*
 – longus capitis
 – longus colli
 – rectus capitis ventralis
 – rectus capitis lateralis
 – scalenus dorsalis (only in Ru.)
 – scalenus medius
 – scalenus ventralis

**To palpate the superficial cervical ln., identify the supraspinatus M. and place the fingertips along the cranial border of this muscle, one hand proximal to the shoulder joint. Press firmly and slip your hand in a cranial direction. The superficial cervical ln., a large structure up to 10–12 cm long and 3–4 cm wide, will be felt. This lymph node is prone to inflammation (lymphadenitis) in case of a positive reaction to the tuberculine (*the tuberculine is a revelatory substance that is injected i.d.—intradermally—to detect a possible TBC, or tuberculosis infection*).**

Make a skin incision on the middorsal line of the neck, from the intercornual protuberance to the cranial angle of the scapula. From the cranial end of the incision make a second incision caudal to the base of the ear and perpendicular to the ventral midline. From the caudal end of the first incision make a third incision to the manubrium sterni around the shoulder joint.

When skinning the cervical region in the large ruminants, the very thin and adherent cutaneous colli M. may remain attached to the skin.

Remove the **superficial lamina of the cervical fascia** and expose the superficial muscles as they are shown in Figure R1.2. Identify and save the **accessory N.**, the **great** auricular N., the **transverse nerve of the neck (transverse cervical N.)**, and the **external jugular V.**

*Notice* that in the large ruminants the **cleidocephalicus M.** consists of two parts: the **mastoid part** and the **occipital part**. They usually are called the cleidomastoideus and the cleidooccipitalis Mm. Also, the **sternocephalicus**

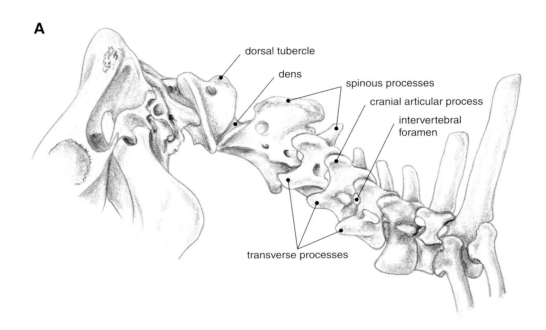

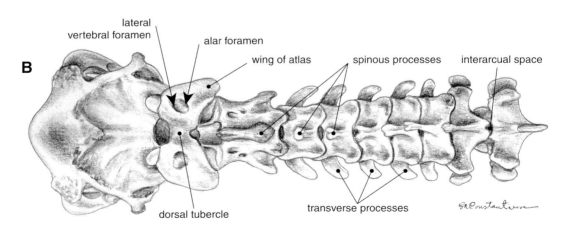

Fig. R1.1. Cervical vertebrae, large ruminants. **A.** Lateral view. **B.** Dorsal view.

**M.** has two parts: the **mandibular part** and the **mastoid part**. They are known as the sternomandibularis and the sternomastoideus Mm. The **jugular groove** is bordered by the cleidomastoideus M. (dorsally), the sternomandibularis M. (ventrally), and the sternomastoideus M. (on the deep side).

The **omohyoideus M.** is very short and thin in comparison to that of the horse, and it does not separate the external jugular V. from the structures included in the **carotid sheath**.

Transect the cleidooccipitalis and cleidomastoideus Mm. and separate them from the adjacent structures. Transect the sternomastoideus M. and carefully separate it from the external jugular V. and the carotid sheath. Dissect the carotid sheath and identify the **common carotid A.**, the **vagosympathetic trunk**, the **recurrent laryngeal N.** (see Fig. R1.3), and **the internal jugular V.** Reflect the external jugular V. and the sternocephalicus M. to expose the **trachea**, the **lobe of the thyroid gland**, the **esophagus,** and the **deep cervical lnn.**

Transect the **trapezius M. pars cervicalis** 2 cm ventral and parallel to the dorsal midline. Transect the **omotransversarius M.** and reflect the stumps. Carefully dissect the caudal stump of the latter and separate it from the **super-**

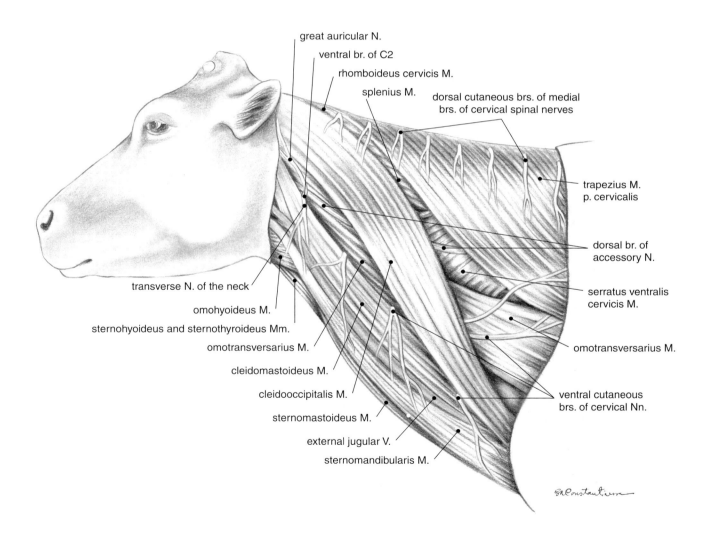

Fig. R1.2. Superficial structures of the neck, large ruminants, lateral aspect.

ficial cervical ln. and the **prescapular branches of the superficial cervical A. and V.** All structures exposed after transecting these muscles are shown in Figure R1.4.

*Notice* that the **longus atlantis M.** is part of the **intertransversarii cervicis Mm.** It is not listed in the *N.A.V.* but is mentioned in many anatomy books.

Transect the **splenius** and **semispinalis Mm.** separately, parallel to the ventral border of the **rhomboideus cervicis M.** Transect the cranial aponeuroses of these muscles and reflect them ventrally. Transect the cranial attachment of the **longissimus capitis M.** and reflect it caudally. These

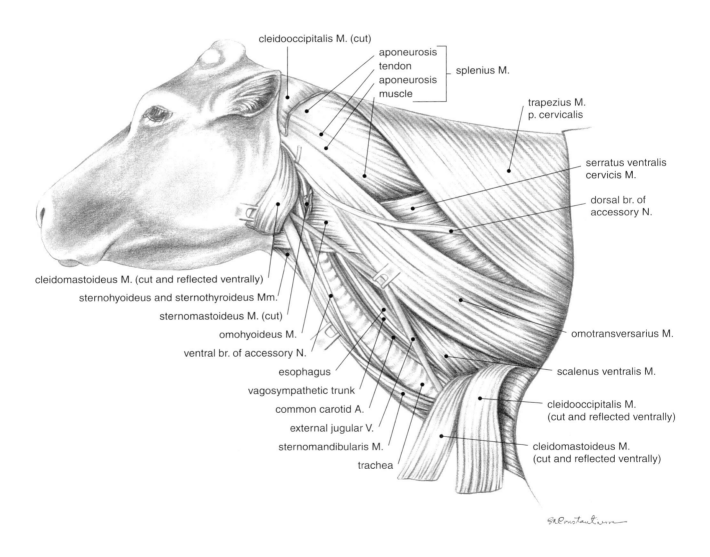

Fig. R1.3. Structures of the neck, large ruminants, lateral aspect, second plane.

deep structures (as they are shown in Fig. R1.5) will be clearly exposed following removal of the thoracic limb.

*Remember!* Among the large domestic animals only the large ruminants and the pig constantly show **scalenus dorsalis**, **scalenus medius**, and **scalenus ventralis Mm.**

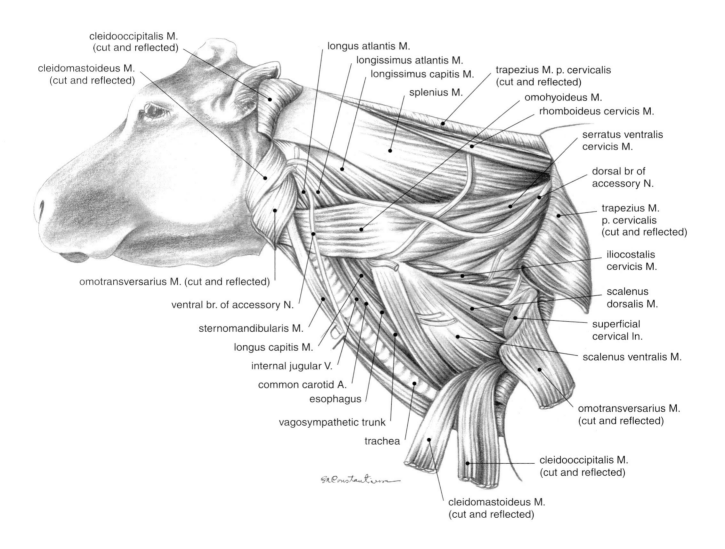

cleidooccipitalis M.
(cut and reflected)

cleidomastoideus M.
(cut and reflected)

longus atlantis M.

longissimus atlantis M.

longissimus capitis M.

splenius M.

trapezius M. p. cervicalis
(cut and reflected)

omohyoideus M.

rhomboideus cervicis M.

serratus ventralis
cervicis M.

dorsal br of
accessory N.

trapezius M.
p. cervicalis
(cut and reflected)

iliocostalis
cervicis M.

scalenus
dorsalis M.

superficial
cervical ln.

scalenus ventralis M.

omotransversarius M.
(cut and reflected)

cleidooccipitalis M.
(cut and reflected)

cleidomastoideus M.
(cut and reflected)

omotransversarius M. (cut and reflected)

ventral br. of accessory N.

sternomandibularis M.

longus capitis M.

internal jugular V.

common carotid A.

esophagus

vagosympathetic trunk

trachea

Fig. R1.4. Structures of the neck, large ruminants, lateral aspect, third plane.

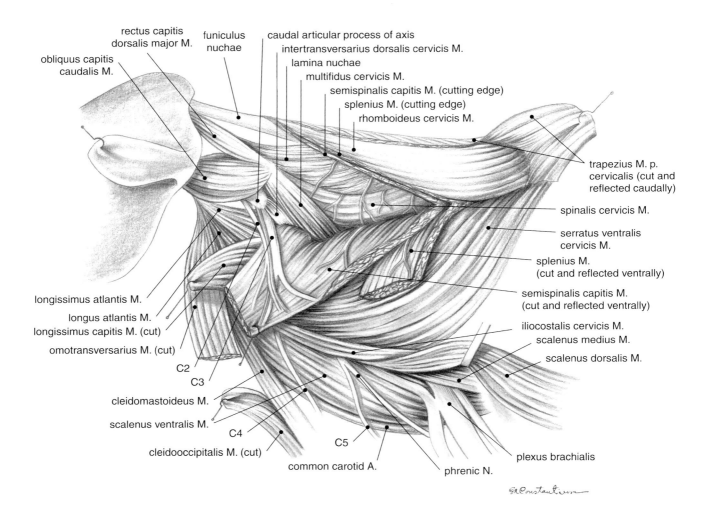

rectus capitis
dorsalis major M.

funiculus
nuchae

caudal articular process of axis

intertransversarius dorsalis cervicis M.

obliquus capitis
caudalis M.

lamina nuchae

multifidus cervicis M.

semispinalis capitis M. (cutting edge)

splenius M. (cutting edge)

rhomboideus cervicis M.

trapezius M. p.
cervicalis (cut and
reflected caudally)

spinalis cervicis M.

serratus ventralis
cervicis M.

splenius M.
(cut and reflected ventrally)

semispinalis capitis M.
(cut and reflected ventrally)

iliocostalis cervicis M.

scalenus medius M.

scalenus dorsalis M.

longissimus atlantis M.

longus atlantis M.

longissimus capitis M. (cut)

omotransversarius M. (cut)

C2

C3

cleidomastoideus M.

scalenus ventralis M.

C4

cleidooccipitalis M. (cut)

C5

common carotid A.

phrenic N.

plexus brachialis

Fig. R1.5. Structures of the neck, large ruminants, lateral aspect, fourth plane.

# R 2

# The Thorax and Thoracic Viscera

Before beginning the dissection, review the systematization of the muscles of the dorsal aspect of the body and the thorax shown in Table R2.1.

The **thoracic vertebrae** are illustrated from the lateral perspective in Figure R2.1A. The proximal part of a **rib** is illustrated from the cranial perspective in Figure R2.1B, and from the medial perspective in Figure R2.1C. The sternum is illustrated from the lateral and dorsal perspectives in Figures R2.1D and R2.1E, respectively.

The **costovertebral** and **sternocostal joints** are similar to those of the horse (see Fig. H2.2C,D).

Outline and/or palpate the following structures: the ribs, the **costal arch**, the tips of the **spinous processes of the thoracic vertebrae**, the **triceps brachii M.**, the **olecra-**

non, the **caudal angle of scapula**, and the **shoulder joint**. They are all landmarks for similar approaches as those mentioned in the horse.

Continue the skin incision from the dorsal extent of the cranial border of the scapula to the **spinous process of the last thoracic vertebra** on the dorsal midline. Continue the incision alongside the last rib to the corresponding **costochondral junction** and perpendicular to the midventral line. From the **manubrium sterni** make an incision on the midventral line to meet the previous incision. Reflect the skin ventrally. Similar to the horse, skin the area carefully to separate the skin from the cutaneous muscles and the superficial fasciae. Dissect and reflect them ventrally after examining the cutaneous nerves.

Table R2.1. Muscles of the Dorsal Aspect of the Body and Thorax, Horse and Large Ruminants

**Dorsal Muscles**

*(Extrinsic muscles of thoracic limb and epaxial muscles)*

- trapezius p. thoracica (+ cervical part)
- latissimus dorsi
- rhomboideus thoracis (+ cervicis)
- serratus dorsalis cranialis
- serratus dorsalis caudalis

  ***Erector spinae M.***

- iliocostalis
  • iliocostalis thoracis and lumborum (+ cervicis)
- longissimus
  • longissimus thoracis and lumborum (+ atlantis + capitis)
- spinalis
  • spinalis thoracis (+ cervicis)

  ***Transversospinalis M.***

- semispinalis
  • semispinalis thoracis (+ capitis – biventer and complexus)
- multifidi
- rotatores

  ***Interspinales Mm.***

  ***Intertransversarii Mm.***

- intertransversarii thoracis and lumborum (+ cervicis)

**Muscles of the Thorax**

- superficial pectoral
  • descending pectoral
  • transverse pectoral
- deep pectoral (ascending pectoral)
- subclavius
- serratus ventralis thoracis (+ serratus ventralis cervicis)
- levatores costarum
- external intercostal Mm.
- internal intercostal Mm.
- retractor costae
- transversus thoracis
- rectus thoracis

  ***Diaphragm***

- pars lumbalis
  • crus dextrum
  • crus sinistrum
- pars costalis
- pars sternalis
  • aortic hiatus
  • esophageal hiatus
  • diaphragmatic cupula
  • tendinous center (centrum tendineum)
  • foramen of caudal vena cava

Dissect the **thoracic part of the trapezius M.**, carefully protecting the aponeurosis of the **latissimus dorsi M.** Dissect the latter and separate it from the **triceps** **brachii** and **tensor fasciae antebrachii Mm.** The aponeurosis of the latissimus dorsi M. overlaps the caudal extent of the scapular cartilage (Fig. R2.2A).

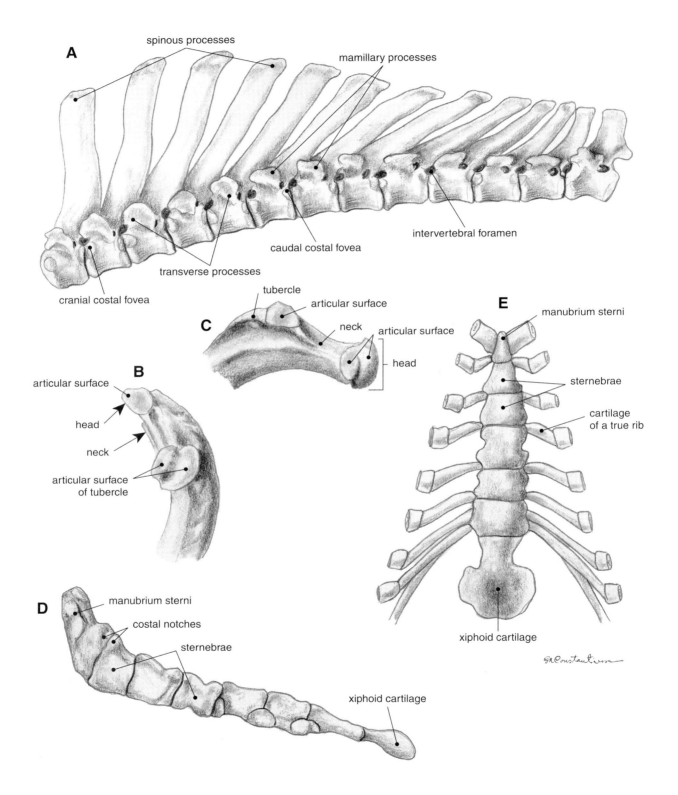

Fig. R2.1. Thoracic, vertebrae, ribs, and sternum, large ruminants. **A.** Thoracic vertebrae, left lateral aspect. **B.** Proximal part of a rib, cranial aspect. **C.** Proximal part of a rib, medial aspect. **D.** Sternum, left lateral aspect. **E.** Sternum, dorsal aspect.

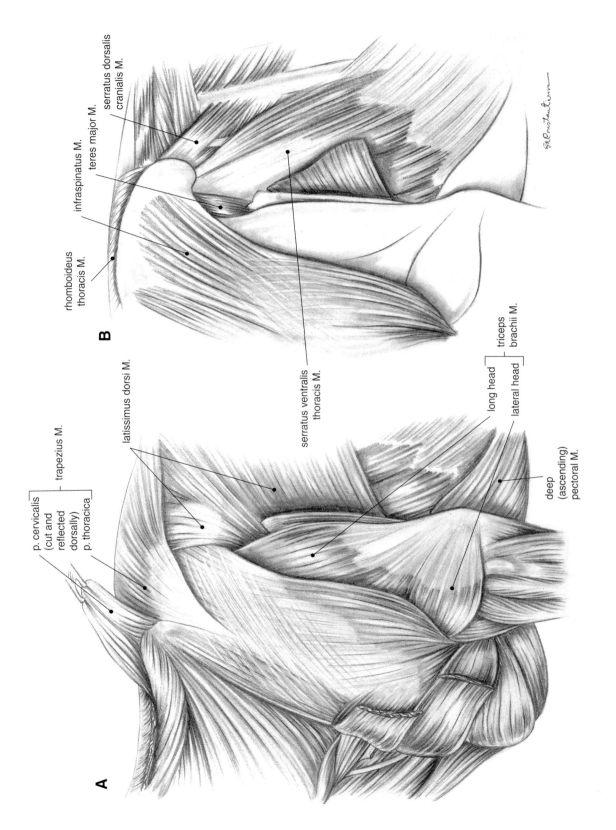

Fig. R2.2. Muscles of the shoulder and thorax, large ruminants, left side. **A.** Superficial structures. **B.** Deep structures.

*Notice* the sudden transition between the muscular fibers and the aponeurosis of the latissimus dorsi muscle.

Dissect the **deep (ascending) pectoral**, **serratus ventralis thoracis** and the **external abdominal oblique Mm.** The serratus ventralis is protected by a strong fascia, whereas the external abdominal oblique is protected by the **tunica flava abdominis (abdominal tunic)**, which is thicker than in the horse.

Transect the scapular attachment of the thoracic part of the trapezius M. and reflect the muscle dorsally. Transect the muscular part of the latissimus dorsi M., leaving 10–15 cm of it attached to the forelimb; either reflect the remnant of the muscle dorsally, or transect it from its attachment on the **supraspinous lig.** The muscles exposed are shown in Figure R2.2B.

Remove the forelimb following similar procedures to those of the horse. The entire serratus ventralis M., the three **scaleni Mm.**, the **rectus thoracis** and **iliocostalis cervicis Mm.** are still attached to the thorax (Fig. R2.3).

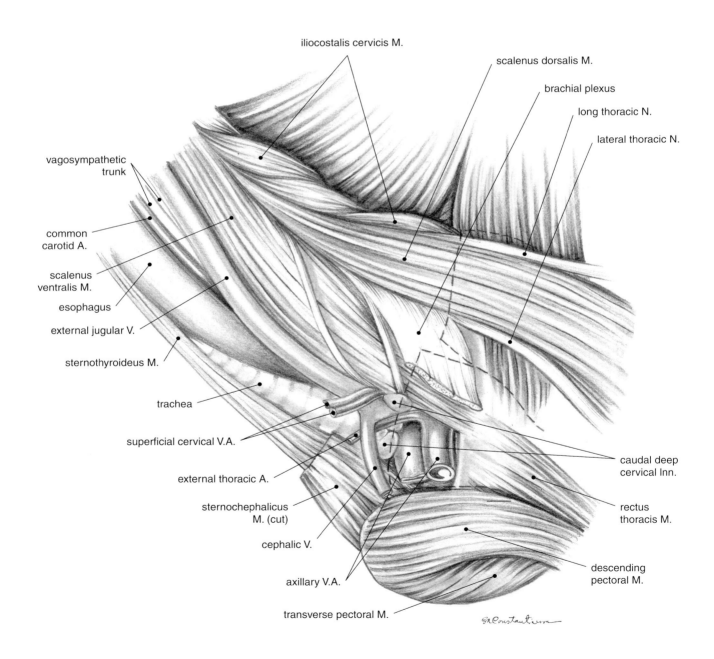

Fig. R2.3. Superficial structures of the thoracic inlet, large ruminants, left aspect, after removing the thoracic limb. Interrupted line outlines the omotransversarius M. (dorsal) and the braciocepalic M. (ventral) both cut.

*Notice* that in the large ruminants there are three scaleni: the **scalenus ventralis**, the **scalenus medius** and the **scalenus dorsalis Mm.** The first two are similar to those of the horse. The scalenus medius is overlapped by the scalenus dorsalis. In order to expose the scalenus medius, the scalenus dorsalis should be reflected dorsally. The latter is a long muscle, attached to the first three to four ribs.

On both sides transect the scalenus ventralis and scalenus medius Mm. and with a rib cutter remove most of the first rib; with your finger protect the soft structures located on the medial side of the rib as you transect and remove it.

Continue the dissection of the structures included within the **carotid sheath**.

*Caution.* The **vagosympathetic trunk** is located dorsal and close to the **common carotid A.** Isolate it from the artery. Near the thoracic inlet the **cervical sympathetic trunk** separates from the **vagus N.** and ends at the **middle cervical ggl.** The relationship between the first rib and the middle cervical ggl. is very similar on both sides.

The **cervicothoracic ggl.**, on the left side is located in the first intercostal space (Fig. R2.4), whereas on the right side it appears close to the first rib; most of the

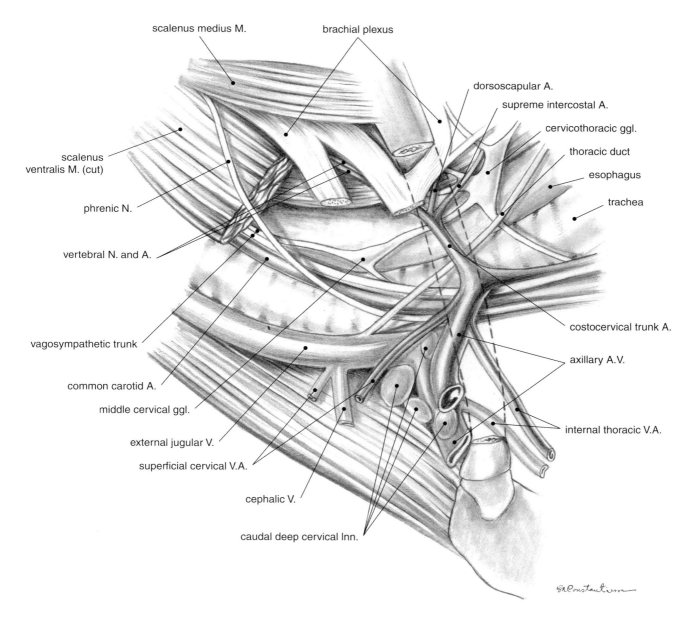

Fig. R.2.4. Deep structures of the thoracic inlet, large ruminants, left side. Broken line outlines the first rib.

ganglion is located on the medial aspect of the rib (Fig. R2.5).

If the base of the scapula is attached to the body transect the serratus ventralis M. as close to the remnant of the scapula as possible, and reflect the base of the scapula dorsally to dissect the deep structures. *Notice* that the **rhomboideus cervicis and thoracis Mm.** are still attached to scapula. The **dorsoscapular lig.**, the entire **serratus dorsalis cranialis M.** and the transition of the **epaxial mus-** cles from the thoracic to the cervical area are now exposed.

Remove the **serratus dorsalis cranialis** and the serratus ventralis Mm., and carefully dissect the **dorsal branches of the thoracic Nn.**, with their medial and lateral branches.

Transect the epaxial muscles (which are similar to those of the horse) to expose the deep structures of the area (see Fig. H2.6). Remove an **external intercostal**

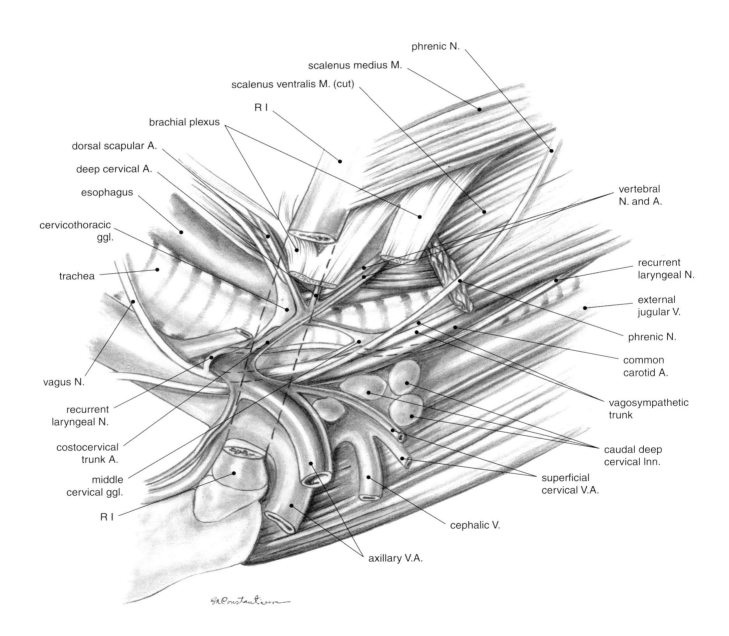

Fig. R2.5. Deep structures of the thoracic inlet, large ruminants, right side. Broken line outlines the first rib.

M. to expose the **internal intercostal M.** and the **intercostal A.V.N.**

The relationship of internal organs of the thorax and abdomen to the chest wall are important in the evaluation of illness or reduced production in ruminants. The auscultation borders of the lungs of ruminants differ from horses due to the size and location of the abdominal viscera and the location of the lungs. In the standing ruminant, a line drawn from the point of the tuber coxae to the 11th rib space is the caudodorsal most aspect of the lung (tip of diaphragmatic lobe). A line drawn from the point of the shoulder (scapulohumeral joint) to the ninth rib space is the ventral border of the middle portion of the lung field. A line from the elbow to the fifth rib space is the cranioventral most portion of the lung field. Combined auscultation and percussion of both lung fields is important in recognizing common pulmonary disorders such as bronchopneumonia (reduced lung field size ventrally) or pneumothorax (reduced lung field size dorsally). Overinflation of the lung periodically occurs and can be recognized as lung fields that exceed the aforementioned borders.

Liver biopsy is an often-used procedure to diagnose disorders of liver function or deficiencies of micronutrients. Liver biopsy is performed in the standing ruminant with adequate restraint by locating the liver using a line drawn from the point of the right hip (tuber coxae) to the point of the right shoulder (scapulohumeral joint) and clipping/prepping the skin over the line where it intersects with the 9–11th rib spaces. After sterile preparation of this area, and local anesthetic infusion [note: it is important to use a 1.5 inch (3.8 cm) 18–20 gauge needle to infuse local anesthetic into the skin, subcutaneous tissues, intercostal muscles and parietal pleura to reduce anxiety and discomfort to the patient]; a no. 15 scalpel blade is used to make a skin incision (stab) to reduce drag of biopsy instrument through skin. The biopsy instrument (Tru-cut®; Biopty®) is introduced into the skin and is directed toward the opposite shoulder. The needle passes through the skin, intercostal muscles, parietal pleura, diaphragm, parietal peritoneum, visceral peritoneum and into the right lobe of the liver. Multiple biopsies that range in size from 5–40 mg of tissue may be acquired with few adverse effects.

The large ruminants are prone to development of traumatic reticulo-peritonitis and pericarditis due to the nature of the proximal digestive tract (nasal planum), how they prehend feed and the presence of foreign objects in the feed. If the animal develops pericarditis (foreign body penetration of the reticulum, diaphragm, lungs and/or pericardium), accumulation of purulent fluid can be associated with cardiac failure due to elevated pericardial pressure, and restriction due to accumulation of massive fibrin deposits on the pericardial sac and epicardium. The classic approach to this problem is to anesthetize the skin and subcutaneous tissues over the left fifth rib from the mid-thorax to the costo-chondral junction. After skin incision, the latissimus dorsi and serratus muscles are incised or spread to allow access to the rib. The periosteum over the rib is incised in an H-pattern to allow for passage of obstetrical wire around the rib. The rib is removed by cutting either at top and bottom of the periosteal incision or by cutting at the top and breaking the lower portion of the rib by hand. The deeper layer of periosteum is often adherant to the endothoracic fascia, parietal pleura and pericardium in this location; however, some recommend suturing these layers (periosteum, endothoracic fascia, pleura) together with surgical gut prior to incising the pericardium. Once incised, the purulent fluid can be drained and manual exploration of the pericardial sac for foreign bodies can be performed. Drainage may be facilitated by introduction of large volumes of sterile polyionic fluids to reduce viscosity of the exudate. This is generally a salvage procedure in animals of high genetic value or for late pregnancy cows with valuable calves close to parturition.

Leaving the fourth, sixth, ninth, and last two ribs in place (R IV, R VI, R IX, R XII, and R XIII), remove the other ribs and the intercostal muscles in a similar manner to the horse.

Examine the lungs and identify the lobes, notches, and fissures; examine the **pericardium** and the **diaphragm** on the left side (see Fig. R2.6A) and on the right side (see Fig. R2.6B). Remove the lungs transecting the bronchi and the vessels as you did in the horse.

*Caution.* While removing the lungs identify the **tracheal bronchus** of the right lung, located within the **cranial mediastinum**. Pay special attention to the **accessory lobe** (of the right lung), the **plica venae cavae** and the **caudal vena cava**, all structures of the right side. Also pay special attention to the **cranial part of the right cranial lobe of the lung**, which passes underneath the trachea from the right into the left half of the thoracic cavity.

The caudal vena cava is often a site of abscessation and pulmonary embolic disease associated with metastasis of hepatic abscesses into the thorax. Although sometimes present, hemoptysis, anemia, and melena are generally considered to be poor prognostic indicators in pulmonary embolic disease. Radiographic evaluation of the caudal thorax in the cow is sometimes beneficial in diagnosis of metastatic pulmonary abscessation in animals with compatible clinical signs (anemia, hemoptysis and melena).

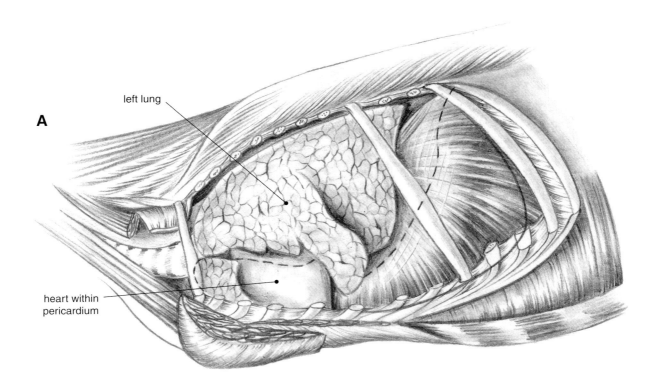

left lung

**A**

heart within
pericardium

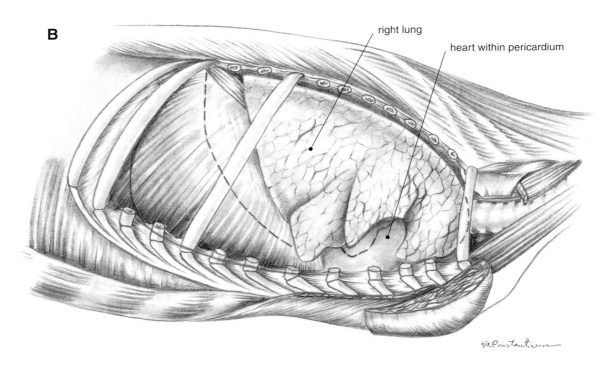

**B**

right lung

heart within pericardium

Fig. R2.6. The thoracic cavity with the lungs and the heart in situ, large ruminants: Broken line, normal extension of the lung in living specimen; heavy line, line of pleural reflection. **A.** Left aspect. **B.** Right aspect.

Dissect the vessels and the nerves on both sides and *notice* the differences from the horse:

- On both sides, all the dorsally oriented branches of the **subclavian Aa.** (the **supreme intercostal**, **dorsoscapular**, **deep cervical** and **vertebral Aa.**—in a caudocranial order) originate from the **costocervical trunk A.** (Even though a **costocervical trunk V.** is not listed in the *N.A.V.*, it is mentioned in some anatomy books.)
- An **internal jugular V.** is present.
- There are **two azygous Vv.** in the large ruminants: a **left** (R2.7) and a **right azygos V.** (see Fig. R2.8).

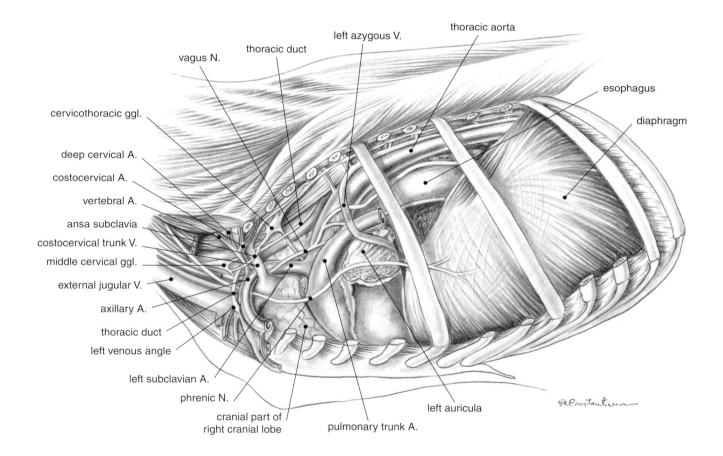

Fig. R2.7. Heart, vessels, and nerves within the thoracic cavity, large ruminants, left side.

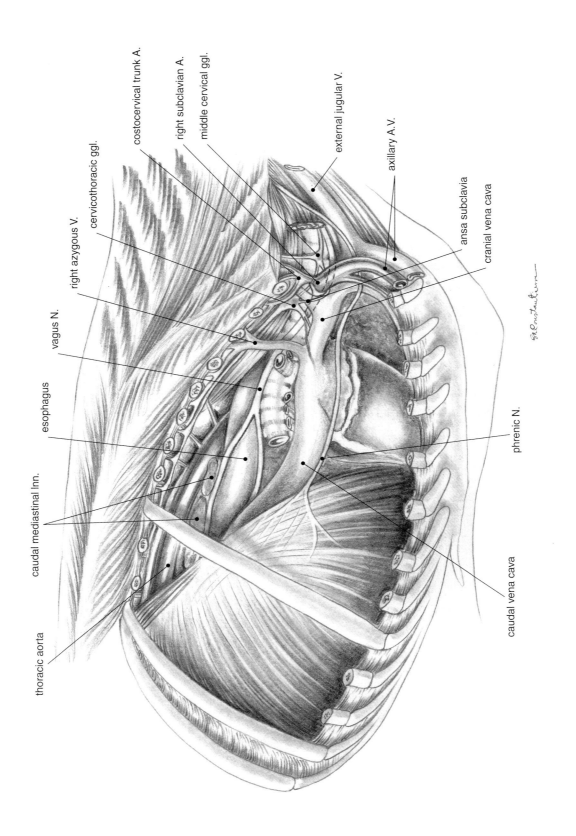

costocervical trunk A.

right subclavian A.

middle cervical ggl.

external jugular V.

axillary A.V.

ansa subclavia

cranial vena cava

cervicothoracic ggl.

right azygous V.

vagus N.

esophagus

caudal mediastinal lnn.

thoracic aorta

phrenic N.

caudal vena cava

Fig. R2.8. Heart, vessels, and nerves within the thoracic cavity, large ruminants, right side.

Remove the heart from the thoracic cavity in a manner similar to that described for the horse. Examine the two lungs and *notice* the different number of lobes and their fissures: the **cranial and caudal parts of both left and right lobes**, and the **middle (cardiac) lobe of the right lung**. Examine the tracheal bronchus.

*Notice* the most distinct feature that differentiates the lungs of the large ruminants from those of the small ruminants, namely the **polyhedral design** on the surface of *all* the lobes (similar to the pig). Identify the so-called impressions of other structures on both the costal and medial sides of the lungs (Figs. R2.9 and R2.10).

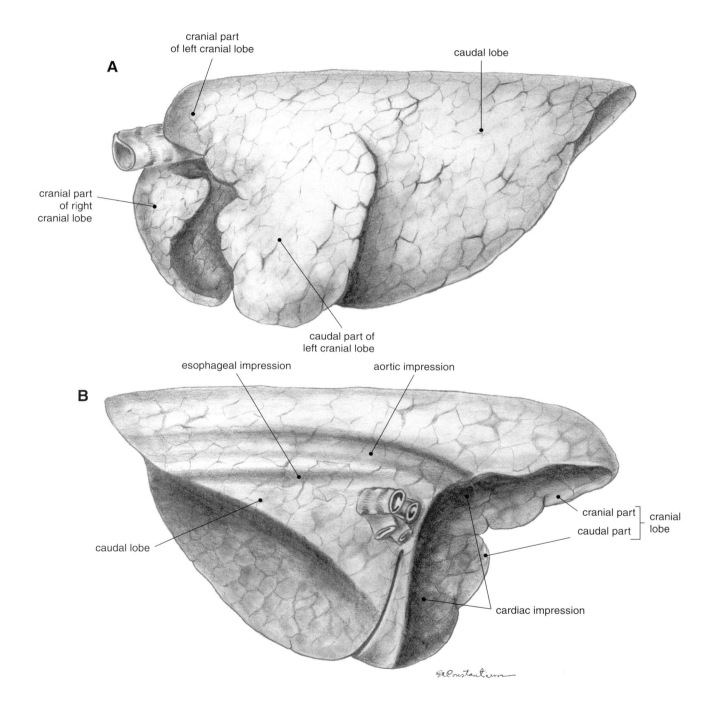

Fig. R2.9. Lungs of the large ruminants. **A.** Left lung, lateral aspect. **B.** Left lung, medial aspect.

Examine and identify the external and internal structures of the heart using the horse as a model (see Figs. R2.11–R2.14).

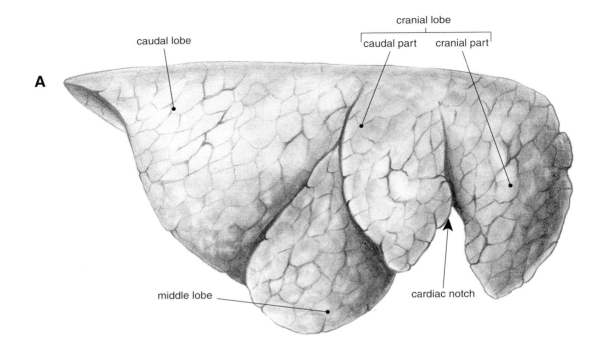

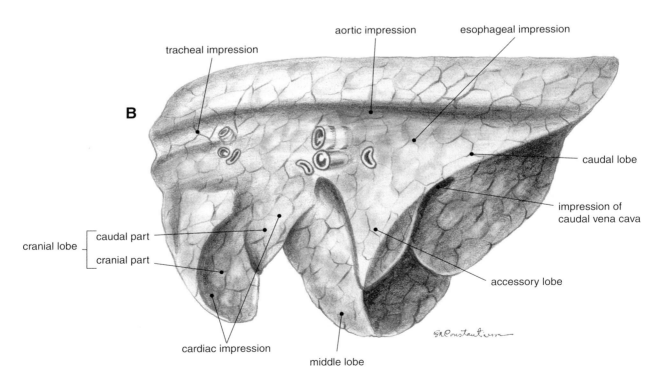

Fig. R2.10. Lungs of the large ruminants. **A.** Right lung, lateral aspect. **B.** Right lung, medial aspect.

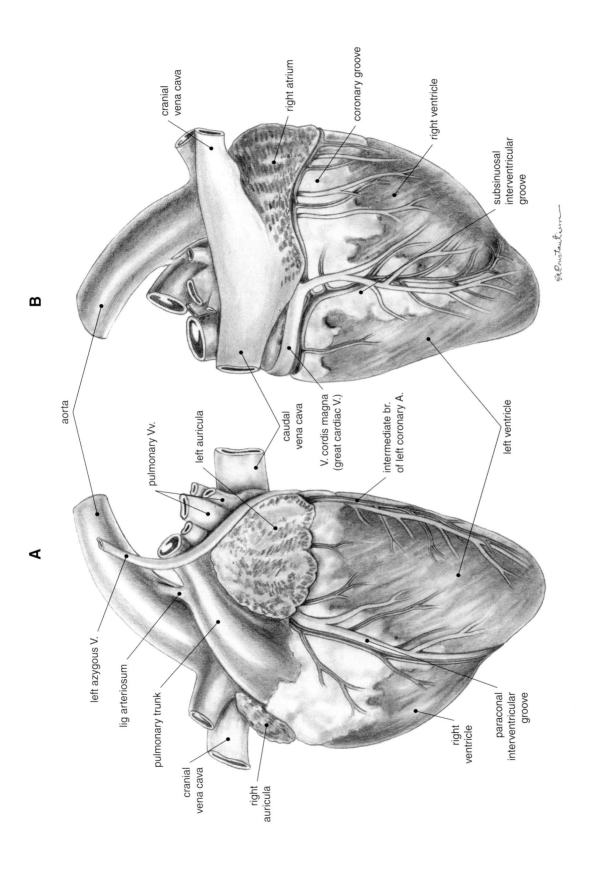

**B**

cranial vena cava

right atrium

coronary groove

right ventricle

subsinuosal interventricular groove

caudal vena cava

V. cordis magna (great cardiac V.)

intermediate br. of left coronary A.

left ventricle

**A**

aorta

left azygous V.

lig arteriosum

pulmonary trunk

cranial vena cava

right auricula

pulmonary Vv.

left auricula

right ventricle

paraconal interventricular groove

Fig. R2.11. Heart of the large ruminants. **A.** Left (auricular) aspect. **B.** Right (atrial) aspect.

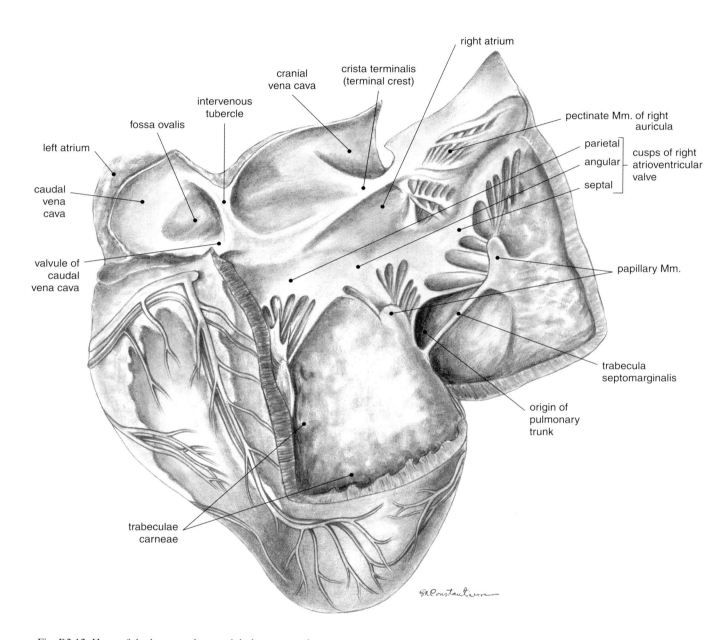

Fig. R2.12. Heart of the large ruminants, right heart opened.

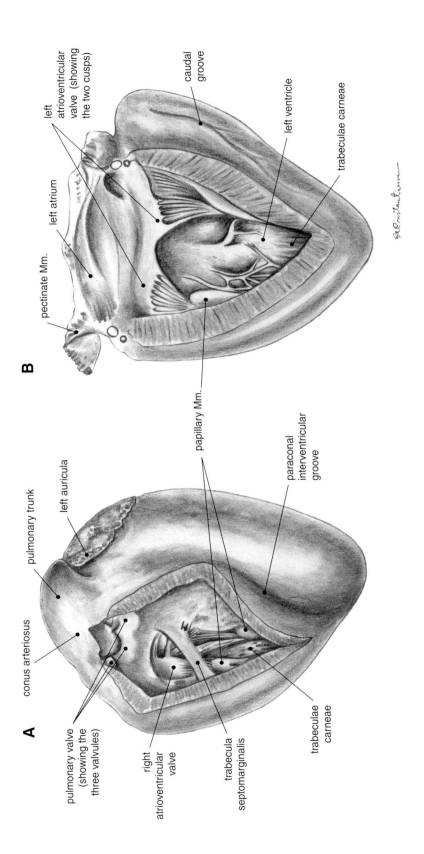

**B**

left
atrioventricular
valve (showing
the two cusps)

caudal
groove

left atrium

left ventricle

pectinate Mm.

trabeculae carneae

papillary Mm.

**A**

pulmonary trunk

conus arteriosus

left auricula

paraconal
interventricular
groove

pulmonary valve
(showing the
three valvules)

right
atrioventricular
valve

trabecula
septomarginalis

trabeculae
carneae

Fig. R2.13. Heart of the large ruminants. **A.** Right ventricle opened. **B.** Left heart opened.

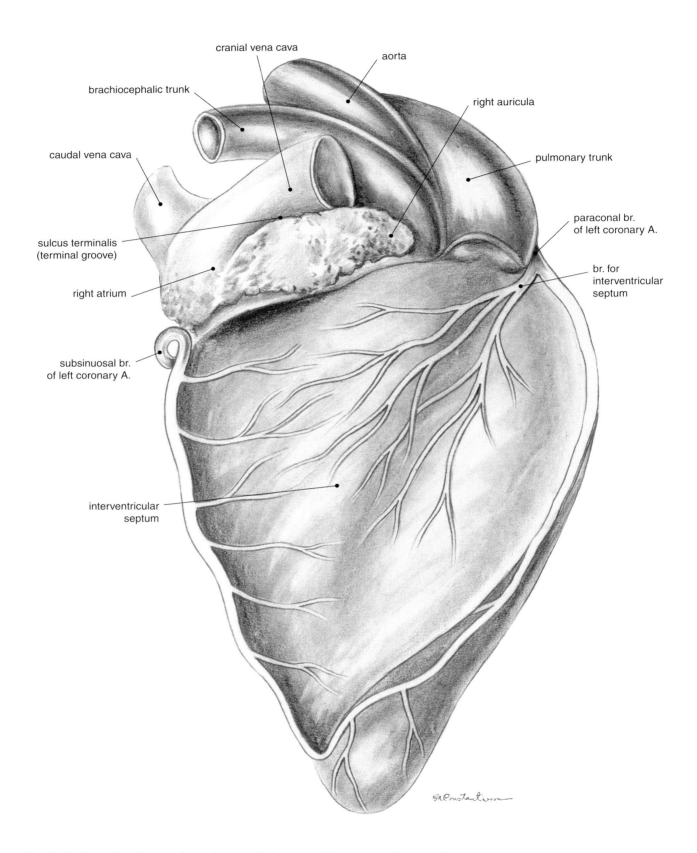

cranial vena cava

aorta

brachiocephalic trunk

right auricula

caudal vena cava

pulmonary trunk

paraconal br.
of left coronary A.

sulcus terminalis
(terminal groove)

br. for
interventricular
septum

right atrium

subsinuosal br.
of left coronary A.

interventricular
septum

Fig. R2.14. Heart of the large ruminants, interventricular septum (right ventricle is removed).

# R 3

# The Abdomen and Abdominal Viscera

The systematization of the abdominal muscles is shown in the Table R3.1.

The **lumbar vertebrae** are illustrated in Figure R3.1.

Reflect the skin from the abdomen ventrally as was performed in the horse.

Carefully dissect the **dorsolateral cutaneous branches** and **ventral branches** of the **costoabdominal** and the **first two lumbar spinal Nn.,** listed together as **thoracolumbar Nn.** (see Fig. R3.2).

**The standing approach to the ruminant abdomen is usually by a right or left paralumbar approach. Anesthesia of the flank—including the paralumbar fossa—for standing surgical exploration is commonly performed using an inverted L (line block), or**

Table R3.1. Abdominal Muscles, Horse and Large Ruminants

**Ventral Abdominal Muscles**
– rectus abdominis
  • rectus sheath
    ◦ external lamina
    ◦ internal lamina
– external abdominal oblique
  • superficial inguinal ring
  • arcus inguinalis
  • deep inguinal ring
  • femoral lamina
– internal abdominal oblique
  • deep inguinal ring
  • cremaster M.
– transversus abdominis
– tunica flava abdominis (abdominal tunic)
– linea alba
  • umbilical ring

**Dorsal Abdominal Muscles**
– quadratus lumborum
– intertransversarii lumborum
– iliopsoas
  • iliacus
  • psoas major
– psoas minor

**paravertebral/paralumbar anesthesia. The proximal paravertebral block (Farquharson method) anesthetizes the segmental sensory and muscular branches innervating the paralumbar fossa on either side soon after the nerves exit the intervertebral foramina. The distal paravertebral nerve blocks (Magda's method) anesthetize the dorsal and ventral nerve branches as they course near the lumbar transverse processes. The procedure involves anesthesia of the 13th thoracic and first and second lumbar Nn. In the proximal paravertebral method, after the animal is clipped and prepped for surgery, the transverse process of $L_1$ is located, and a needle (16 gauge, 1 inch) is inserted approximately 1–1.5 inches (2.5–3.5 cm) off of the dorsal midline into the skin and used as a guide to allow passage of a 6–8 inch (18–20 gauge) needle. The longer needle is advanced until the transverse process is located, and then the needle is advanced forward or backward until the space between $T_{13}$ and $L_1$ is located. At this time, approximately 10 ml of anesthetic are infiltrated into the region to anesthetize the 13th thoracic nerve. The procedure is repeated for L1 and L2, using the transverse processes of $L_1$ and $L_2$ as a guide. The distal approach requires local anesthetic (skin bleb) placement over the transverse process of $L_1$, $L_2$, and $L_4$. After local anesthesia of the skin, a 3.5 inch (9–10 cm), 18 gauge, spinal needle is introduced perpendicular to the tips of the transverse processes until the needle reaches the bone; the needle is advanced dorsally over the process, and approximately 5–15 ml of local anesthetic is deposited as the needle is passed toward midline. The needle is then backed off to the skin and passed under the transverse process, and the infusion of 5–15 ml of local anesthetic is repeated. The process is repeated dorsally and ventrally over the transverse processes of $L_2$ and $L_4$ to ensure adequate anesthesia of the 13th thoracic and first and second lumbar Nn. (see Fig. R3.3A,B).**

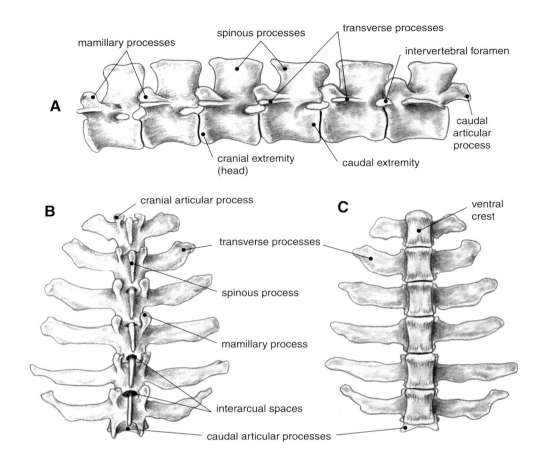

mamillary processes

spinous processes

transverse processes

intervertebral foramen

caudal articular process

A

cranial extremity (head)

caudal extremity

B

cranial articular process

transverse processes

spinous process

mamillary process

interarcual spaces

caudal articular processes

C

ventral crest

Fig. R3.1. Lumbar vertebrae, large ruminants. **A.** Left lateral view. **B.** Dorsal view. **C.** Ventral view.

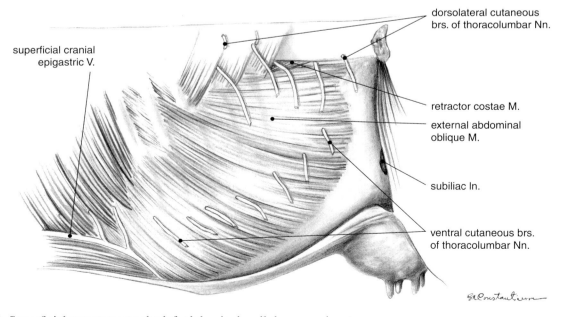

superficial cranial epigastric V.

dorsolateral cutaneous brs. of thoracolumbar Nn.

retractor costae M.

external abdominal oblique M.

subiliac ln.

ventral cutaneous brs. of thoracolumbar Nn.

Fig. R3.2. Superficial structures on the left abdominal wall, large ruminants.

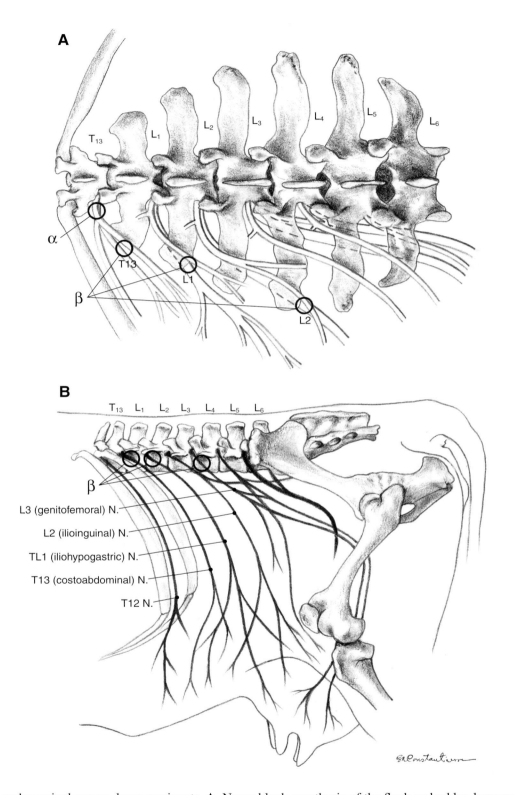

Fig. R3.3. Lumbar spinal nerves, large ruminants. **A.** Nerve block anesthesia of the flank and udder, large ruminants, dorsal aspect. **B.** The nerves supplying the flank and udder, large ruminants, left lateral aspect. α = Farquharson method; β = Magda's method.

Dissect the caudal extent of the **cutaneous trunci M.** and reflect it ventrally. Palpate and dissect the **subiliac ln.**, which is in a similar location and position to that in the horse. Then identify the **lateral cutaneous femoral N.** and the caudal branches of the **deep circumflex iliac A.V.**

Similarly to the dissection of the horse, dissect a small area of the **abdominal tunic (tunica flava abdominis)** and sever the muscular attachments and the aponeurosis of the **external abdominal oblique M.**, reflecting the muscle ventrally. The **retractor costae** and the **internal abdominal oblique Mm.** are now exposed. Identify the nerves lying on the external abdominal oblique M. (Fig. R3.4A).

**Flank approaches are best made approximately 3 inches caudal to the 13th rib and approximately 3 inches ventral to the lumbar transverse processes. Additionally, care to prevent incising the caudal-most aspect of the paralumbar fossa is recommended to prevent incision of the external and internal abdominal oblique and the transversus abdominis Mm. The approach to the left or right side of the abdomen requires knowledge of the layers that must be incised in order to gain access to the peritoneal cavity. The skin and subcutaneous structures are incised, allowing visualization of the fascial layer covering the external abdominal oblique. This muscle layer can be either sharply incised with a scalpel or bluntly dissected (grid technique) to expose the deeper internal abdominal oblique Mm. Incising the internal abdominal oblique M. provides access to the transversus abdominus M. and, finally, the transverse fascia and parietal peritoneum. When the approach is made to incise the transverse fascia and peritoneum on either side of the animal, care should be used in animals with abdominal distension to prevent incising the duodenum (right side; in greater omentum) or rumen (left side).**

Transect the origin and insertions on the ribs of the internal abdominal oblique M. and reflect it ventrally. Identify the nerves running vertically over the **transversus abdominis M.** (Fig. R3.4B). Transect the transversus abdominis M. and reflect it ventrally, saving the **transverse fascia** and the **parietal peritoneum**. Examine and transect the transverse fascia and the parietal peritoneum to enter the peritoneal cavity and start exploring the viscera.

Gently reflect the **psoas major and minor Mm.** ventral to the **transverse processes of the lumbar vertebrae** and expose part of the proximal segments of the ventral branches of the **nerves L1** and **L2** lying between them, and the **quadratus lumborum** and **intertransversarii lumborum Mm.** Transect the intertransversarii lumborum Mm., the **intertransverse ligg.**, and the quadratus lumborum M. up to the **intervertebral foramina** to expose the ventral branch joining the dorsal branch of each lumbar nerve.

As for the horse, here is a brief description of the post-diaphragmatic viscera of the digestive system.

The *esophagus* opens on the roof of the stomach, at the border between the rumen and the reticulum.

The *stomach* is multicompartmented, consisting of the rumen, reticulum, omasum, and abomasum.

The *rumen,* almost entirely filling the left side of the peritoneal cavity, has a capacity of 110–235 liters (in adult animals and depending on the individual size and breed). The parietal aspect is against the left abdominal wall and the floor of the abdominal cavity, whereas the visceral aspect comes in contact with the reticulum, omasum, abomasum, liver, and intestines. A dorsal curvature and a ventral curvature, cranial and caudal extremities, and several grooves are also seen on the surface. The left and right longitudinal grooves are continuous with the cranial and caudal grooves (transversely oriented) and surround the rumen completely. There are left and right accessory grooves, shorter than and dorsal to the longitudinal grooves. The four main grooves separate the dorsal sac from the ventral sac of the rumen and correspond inside to four pillars: left and right, cranial and caudal. The cranial extremity of the dorsal sac is called ruminal atrium (cranial sac of the rumen), and it communicates with the reticulum over the ruminoreticular fold (of the mucosa), which corresponds outside to the ruminoreticular groove. The cranial extremity of the ventral sac, called the ruminal recess, is the cranial end of this sac. The caudal extremities of both dorsal and ventral sacs are called the dorsal and ventral blind sacs. They are separated from the dorsal and ventral sacs by the coronary grooves (outside) and the coronary pillars (inside). Therefore, the cranial groove, corresponding to the cranial pillar, separates the ruminal atrium from the ruminal recess, whereas the caudal groove, corresponding to the caudal pillar, separates the blind sacs from one another. The four pillars outline the communication between the dorsal and the ventral sacs, called intraruminal ostium. The cranial pillar sends two branches each, to the right and to the left. One branch will meet the middle branch of the caudal pillar, building the right and left longitudinal pillars, horizontally oriented. The other branch, much shorter and dorsal to the previous branch is the accessory pillar (right and left). The longitudinal and accessory pillars correspond outside to the longitudinal and accessory grooves. The longitudinal and accessory pillars on each side outline a triangular area called insula. The caudal pillar sends three pairs of branches: right and left dorsal, middle, and ventral branches. The dorsal and the ventral branches are the coronary pillars, whereas the middle branches contribute to the formation of the longitudinal pillars. The mucosa of the rumen is provided with conical and foliate papillae.

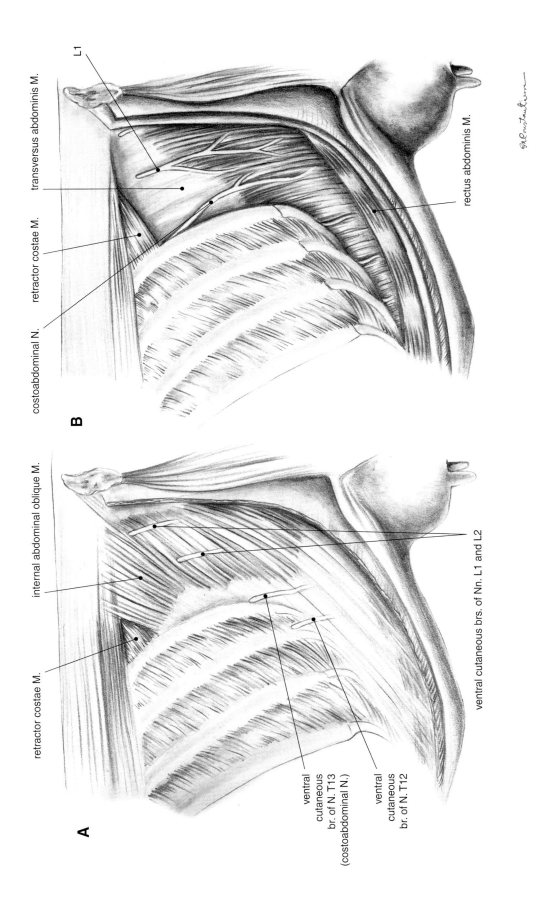

Fig. R3.4. Structures of the left abdominal wall, large ruminants. **A.** Second level. **B.** Third level.

The *reticulum*, in continuation with the ruminal atrium, is in intimate contact with the diaphragm and the floor of the abdominal cavity. One has access to it on both sides of the specimen. The reticulum is separated from the rumen by the ruminoreticular groove and fold, respectively. The esophageal ostium is continuous with the gastric groove. In ruminants, the gastric groove is divided into three segments: reticular, omasal, and abomasal. The reticular groove has two lips, right and left, which cross each other in an X-shaped manner. The reticular mucosa is honeycomb-shaped, with cells separated by walls called crests. There are conical papillae in the cells and on the free borders of the crests. The reticulum communicates with the omasum through the reticuloomasal ostium.

The *omasum* is located on the right side of the abdominal cavity, between the reticulum and the abomasum. It has a spherical shape, a body, a curvature, and a base, a parietal aspect, and a visceral aspect. The curvature is dorsally oriented, caudally and to the right. The base faces cranially and to the left. The body is between the curvature and the base. The parietal aspect is facing the liver, whereas the visceral aspect comes in contact with the rumen. Inside the base, the short omasal groove connects the reticular groove to the abomasal groove (the three segments of the gastric groove). The omasal groove opens into the abomasum through the omasoabomasal ostium. A transversely oriented omasal pillar can be identified at the level of this ostium. The mucosal folds of the omasum are characteristic. There are many different parallel folds of four various sizes, from the highest to the lowest, separated by interlaminar recesses. On the surface, the laminae are provided with thickened papillae.

The *abomasum* is the glandular compartment of the stomach, while the rumen, reticulum, and omasum, collectively called proventriculus, act as a mechanical stomach. The abomasum has a parietal aspect against the abdominal wall; a visceral aspect against the rumen; a greater curvature ventrally; a lesser curvature dorsally; a fundus as the initial part; the body in the middle; and the pyloric part caudally, at the end of the abomasum. Large spiral folds of the mucosa are found in the longitudinal axis of the abomasum. The abomasal groove follows the lesser curvature. The pyloric sphincter is not well developed, but a prominence called the torus pyloricus is present on the lesser curvature of the pylorus.

The *duodenum* has the same parts as in the horse, with species-specific differences. The cranial part is vertically oriented, starts with the ampulla, and ends at the cranial flexure. The sigmoid loop is present. Outside, the cranial duodenum makes the connection between the lesser omentum, cranially, and the superficial wall of the greater omentum, caudally. Inside, the major duodenal papilla at around 50 cm from the pylorus bears only the choledochus (the common bile duct), because there is no pancreatic duct in the large ruminants. Outside, the major duodenal papilla corresponds to the sigmoid loop. From the cranial flexure, the descending part of the duodenum, horizontally oriented, marks the connection between the superficial and the deep walls of the greater omentum. The minor duodenal papilla, where the accessory pancreatic duct opens, is located 30–40 cm distal to the major duodenal papilla. From the caudal flexure, the ascending part of duodenum starts. It is not quite clear whether a transverse part exists. From the duodenojejunal flexure, the jejunum starts.

The *jejunum* is as long as up to 40 m, with a reduced diameter, and is suspended by a long mesojejunum. It lies on the deep wall of the greater omentum, within the supraomental recess, on the right side of the rumen.

The *ileum* is short and is attached to the cecum by the ileocecal fold. The ileal ostium is provided with the ileal papilla and a sphincter.

The *cecum,* like the other segments of the large intestines, has no haustrae or bands. It is horizontally located, slightly curved ventrally. The body ends with the apex oriented caudally. The cecocolic ostium is very wide and makes the transition to the ascending colon.

The *ascending colon* is divided into the following segments:

- The proximal loop
- The spiral loop
  - centripetal coils
  - central flexure
  - centrifugal coils
- The distal loop

The *proximal loop* is S-shaped and is located dorsal to the cecum.

The *spiral loop* is vertically oriented, in direct continuation of the proximal loop. It starts with two to three *centripetal coils,* changes direction at the level of the *central flexure* and ends with two to three *centrifugal coils.* The coils are very close to each other, and the entire spiral loop is located on the left side of the mesentery.

The *distal loop* is the last segment of the ascending colon. It is the direct continuation of the spiral loop, is S-shaped, and is located dorsal to the proximal loop.

The *transverse colon* is that part of the large intestines that surrounds the cranial mesenteric A. cranially and is positioned transversely from right to left.

The *descending colon* is craniocaudally oriented, usually on the left side and dorsal to the distal loop.

The *sigmoid colon*, specific to the large ruminants is an S-shaped curve just before the rectum starts.

The *liver* is vertically oriented, with the right lobe dorsally and the left lobe ventrally. It has the fewest number of lobes possible: left, quadrate, and right. In addition, there is the caudate lobe, with a small papillary process and a large caudate process. The gall bladder is present and is very large, far exceeding the ventral border of the liver (oriented to the right side).

The *pancreas* has a body, a right lobe, and a left lobe. In addition, the uncinate lobe, specific to the ruminants, is a hooked process that extends medially from the right lobe around the caudodorsal surface of the portal V. The pancreatic notch surrounds the portal V. In the large ruminants only the accessory pancreatic duct is present.

On the *left side,* cut off ribs IX and XII and remove the **intercostal Mm.** from the last intercostal space. Incise the **diaphragm** at the costal attachments, and leave the left

portion of a median strip extending over the cranial border of the **spleen**. To avoid damaging the **phrenicosplenic lig.,** palpate it between the diaphragm and the dorsocaudal extremity of the spleen.

Identify the **dorsal sac of the rumen**, the **ruminal atrium (cranial sac of the rumen)**, the **caudodorsal blind sac of the rumen**, the **left longitudinal groove** and the **superficial wall of the greater omentum** attached to it, the **left accessory groove**, the **cranial** groove, the **caudal groove**, the **reticulum**, the **ruminoreticular groove**, and the **fundus of the abomasum** (the dilation of the abomasum that touches the ruminal atrium) (Fig. R3.5). Introduce your right hand between the caudal extent of the superficial wall of the greater omentum and the pelvic inlet, and palpate the continuity of the greater omentum toward the right side.

The abdominal topography (the projection of viscera on the left lateral wall of the abdomen) is as follows (Fig. R3.5):

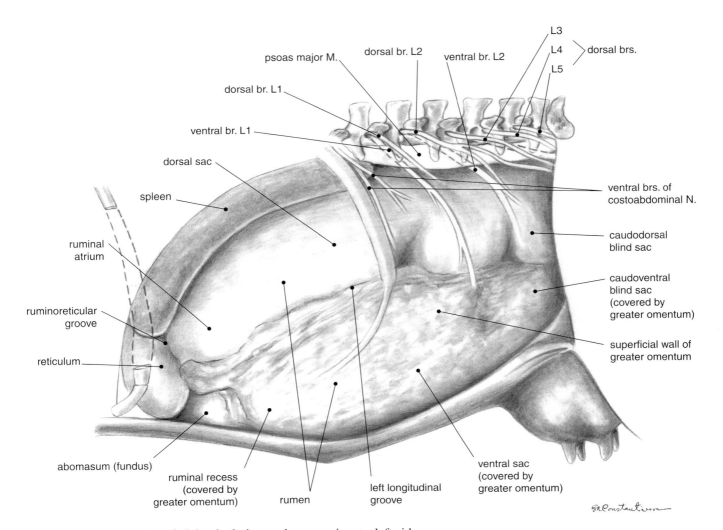

Fig. R3.5. Topography of abdominal viscera, large ruminants, left side.

## Rumen

- Almost the entire wall of the abdominal cavity

*Notice* that the ventral sac of the rumen is covered by the superficial wall of the greater omentum.

**Exploration of the left side of the abdomen of the ruminant is often required for correction of left displacement of the abomasum. There is nothing aside from the spleen between the left body wall and the rumen in the normal animal. If a gas/fluid-distended viscus is palpable, it is the abomasum, and your exploratory was successful. From the standing right flank approach, the surgeon locates the caudal-most extent of the superficial wall of the greater omentum and passes the left hand axial (toward midline) to it, locating the right kidney. Below and axial to the kidney sits the axial (medial) surface of the rumen. Once the rumen is located, the left hand is passed caudally and ventral to the kidney and ureters until the left body wall is palpable. The abomasum is palpable between the rumen and left body wall on this side. From the left flank approach, the abomasum is obvious once the incision is made through the parietal peritoneum.**

**Left or right flank approaches to the uterus are commonly used for standing cesarian section in cattle. The choice is often based upon the surgeon's experience and potentially on presurgical evaluation, such as pregnant horn and/or torsion of the uterus. The left approach has the advantage of the large rumen preventing the small intestine or other viscera from slipping outside the abdomen. The right approach is often preferred by some surgeons due to the ability to perform a more complete abdominal exploratory.**

## Spleen

- Between the diaphragm and the ruminal atrium, 10 cm wide and exceeding the last rib by 5–10 cm

## Reticulum

- Between the diaphragm, ruminal atrium, abomasum, and spleen, between ribs VI and VII or VIII

**The reticulum is important to evaluate during the exploratory of the ruminant and can be evaluated from either the left or right approach. It is most easily palpated from the right side by passing the left arm forward and ventral to the omental sling until a loose structure with internal honeycombs is palpated cranial and medial to the abomasum. It should be freely movable.**

## Abomasum

- Between the reticulum, ruminal atrium, and ruminal recess, on the floor of the abdominal cavity

**This structure is often filled with dirt, sand, rocks and other material; however, if empty, it is easily located by gently lifting the organ by tension on the omental sling until the pyloric portion of the abomasum is evident. Tension on the omentum with the right hand allows passage of the left hand along the greater curvature until the omasal-abomasal orifice is located. Assessment of the reticulum, omasum, and abomasum is also possible using ultrasound guidance, by placing the ultrasound probe head on the ventral abdomen caudal and to the right of the xiphoid cartilage. Careful examination of the area (several minutes) provides the observer with information regarding movement of the reticulum and abomasum in cases where inflammation may be reducing movement of these gastric compartments.**

On the *right side,* remove the same ribs and intercostal Mm. as you did on the left side. Most of the viscera are covered by the **greater omentum**. The two major components of the greater omentum in ruminants are the superficial wall and the **deep wall**. The superficial wall originates from the left longitudinal groove of the rumen (Fig. R3.6). The deep wall originates from the right longitudinal groove of the rumen. Both of them surround several abdominal viscera and continue on the right side inside of the body wall. Their relationship is shown in a cross section in Figure R3.7. Before reaching the duodenum, the superficial and the deep walls fuse with each other. After removal of the ribs and the intercostal Mm., only the superficial wall is exposed. It lies between the pelvic inlet, the **descending part of the duodenum**, the gall bladder, the **cranial part of the duodenum**, the **pylorus**, and the

**greater curvature of the abomasum**. The **mesoduodenum** suspends the descending part of the duodenum and covers the **right lobe of the pancreas** (see Fig. R3.8A).

Carefully reflect the right lobe of the liver as much as possible. Identify the **cranial flexure of the duodenum**, the cranial part of the duodenum with the **sigmoid loop** and the **pylorus** (Fig. R3.8B). The ligament attaching the cranial part of the duodenum to the liver is the **hepatoduodenal lig.**, which continues on the **omasum** and **abomasum** as the **hepatogastric lig.**

*Remember!* The **lesser omentum** consists of the hepatoduodenal and hepatogastric ligaments.

The lesser omentum, passing over the cranial part of the duodenum, the pylorus, and the abomasum, continues caudally with the superficial wall of the greater omentum. Slip your left hand over the superficial wall of the greater omentum in a caudal direction and continue to feel the omentum toward the left side to check the continuity of this structure.

Both the superficial and deep walls of the greater omentum consist of two apposing laminae (see Fig. R3.7). Introduce your hand between the superficial and the deep walls, into the **omental bursa**. Explore the **supraomental recess** in a caudal direction and your hand will feel a cul de sac called **caudal recess.** Pass your hand in the opposite (cranial) direction up to the cranial part of the duodenum. This is still the omental bursa. Cranial to the duodenum your hand will slip between the lesser omentum (on the right side of the body) and the rumen (on the left side), into the **vestibule** of the omental bursa. Within the most cranial extent of the vestibule, the omasum can be palpated. *Notice* that the **omental (epiploic) foramen** opens into the vestibule.

With your hand still within the omental bursa, palpate the attachment of the deep wall to the superficial wall before reaching the descending part of the duodenum (see Fig. R3.8A). Transect the superficial wall and expose the omental bursa. Either the **proximal** or the **distal loop of**

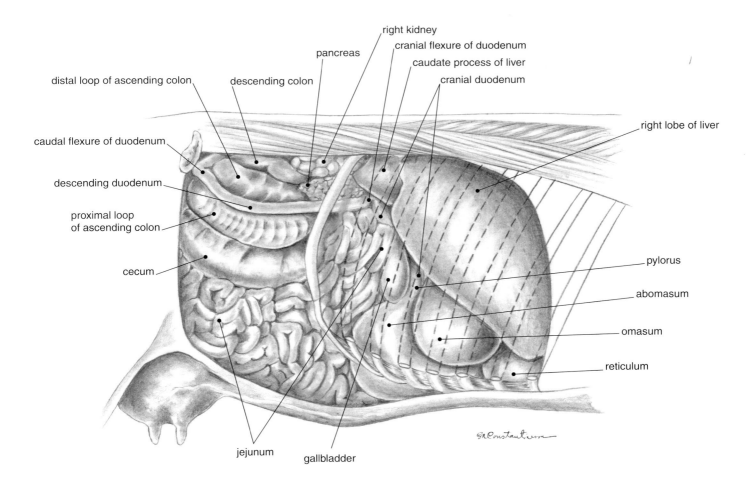

Fig. R3.6. Topography of abdominal viscera, large ruminants, right side.

the ascending colon, the **cecum** (see Fig. R3.9A), and the **jejunum** are now exposed. Sometimes, in embalmed specimens, the caudal extent of the proximal loop of the ascending colon, of the cecum, and/or of the jejunum exceeds the supraomental recess caudally and is visible between the greater omentum and the **pelvic inlet**.

Reflect the **caudate process of the liver** and continue to reflect the **right lobe of the liver**, identifying the **portal V.** between the **body of the pancreas** and the **hilus of the liver**. Introduce a finger over the mesoduodenum and the portal V. through the omental (epiploic) foramen into the omental bursa (see Fig. R3.9B). *Notice* the transition between the mesoduodenum and the hepatoduodenal lig.

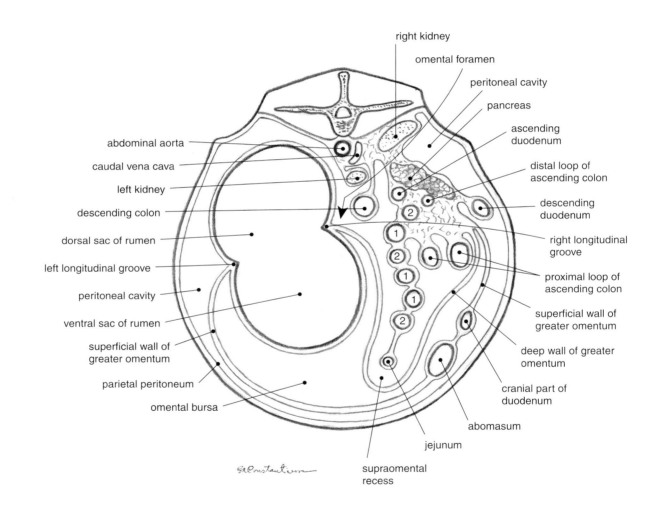

Fig. R3.7. Cross section through the flank, large ruminants. *Key:* 1-Centripetal coils of the spiral loop. 2-Centrifugal coils of the spiral loop.

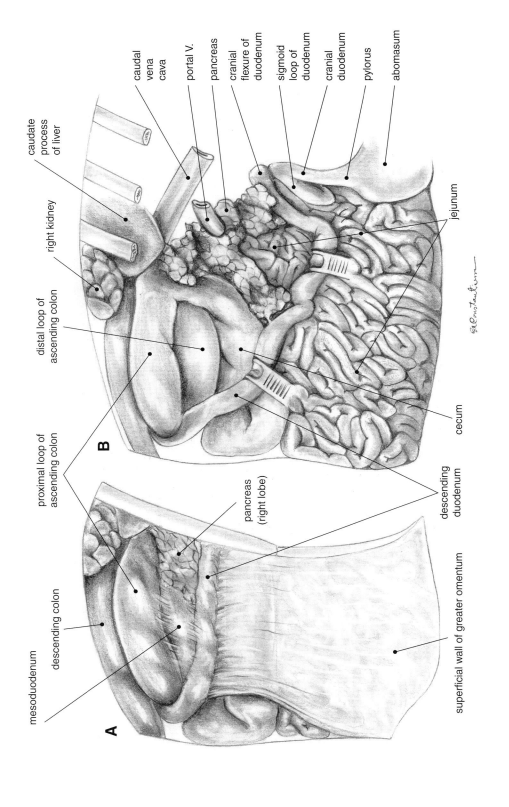

Fig. R3.8. Abdominal viscera in situ, large ruminants, right side. **A.** Viscera in situ in the flank. **B.** After removing the superficial wall of the greater omentum and the liver.

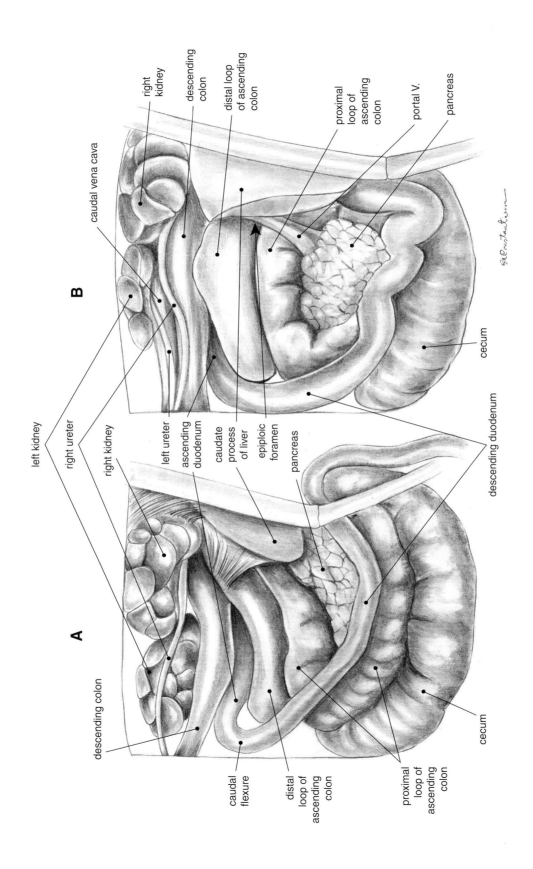

Fig. R3.9. Abdominal viscera in situ, large ruminants, right side. **A.** The descending duodenum was reflected to expose the pancreas. **B.** The portal vein and epiploic foramen are exposed.

*Note.* The omental foramen is a narrow passage between the peritoneal cavity and the omental bursa, outlined dorsally by the **caudal vena cava**, ventrally by the portal V., cranially by the **caudate process of the caudate lobe of the liver**, and caudally by the **pancreas**.

The abdominal topography on the right side of the abdominal cavity follows:

## Liver

- Between the diaphragm and a convex line joining the last rib dorsally (where the caudate process of the caudate lobe is found) to rib VI ventrally

## Gall Bladder

- Between ribs X and XI, ventral to the liver

## Reticulum

- At the cranioventral end of the liver, between ribs VI and VII, and the floor of the abdominal cavity

## Omasum

- Caudal to the reticulum, between ribs VII and X in their ventral half

## Abomasum

- Following the omasum in the next two intercostal spaces, limited by the costal arch, the gall bladder, and the ventral wall of the abdominal cavity

## Duodenum

- Cranial part in the 10th intercostal space
- Descending part lying horizontally in the flank, from the caudate process of the liver to the tuber coxae (see Figs. R3.6, R3.8, R3.9)
- Caudal flexure close to tuber coxae

## Pylorus

- Between the abomasum and cranial part of the duodenum, ventral to the gall bladder

## Ascending Colon

- Proximal loop lying in the flank, ventral to the duodenum
- Distal loop lying in the flank, dorsal to the duodenum

## Pancreas (the right lobe) (see Figs. R3.8, R3.9)

- Between the distal loop of the ascending colon, the descending colon, the descending part of duodenum, the kidney, and the caudate process of the liver

## Descending Colon (see Figs. R3.8, R3.9)

- Dorsal to the pancreas and the distal loop of the ascending colon

## Cecum (see Figs. R3.8, R3.9)

- In the flank in an almost horizontal position, ventral to the proximal (sometimes to the distal) loop of the ascending colon and dorsal to the level of the last costochondral joint

## Jejunum

- Lying in the remainder of the flank and up to the duodenum, gall bladder, and abomasum

## Right Kidney (see Figs. R3.8, R3.9)

- On the dorsal wall of the abdominal cavity, between the last rib and the transverse process of second lumbar vertebra

Before incising the diaphragm, locate the **right triangular lig. of the liver** (it extends from the caudodorsal border of the **right lobe of the liver** to the dorsolateral abdominal wall). Preserve the ligament and continue the incision of the diaphragm, leaving a right portion of a 2–3 cm wide median strip to the right of the **caudal vena cava**. The vein courses between the liver and the diaphragm toward the **foramen of caudal vena cava**. Palpate the right fold of the **coronary lig.** on the diaphragmatic aspect of the liver up to the foramen of caudal vena cava; then palpate the **falciform lig.** to the right, running toward the **umbilicus**.

Palpate, isolate, and transect the **hepatorenal lig.** Bluntly isolate the **kidneys** and the **adrenal glands** (with the corresponding vessels), the **ureters**, and the **renal lnn.** by removing the **perirenal fat (adipose capsule)**. Examine the **renal lobes**, which are characteristic for the large ruminants.

There are several different techniques for exenteration.

*In one technique*, the liver is removed first, followed by the intestinal mass, and finally the stomach with the pancreas, the duodenum, and the spleen.

*In another technique*, the intestinal mass is first removed, followed by the stomach, duodenum, pancreas, spleen, and liver as a unit. There are *two choices:* to remove first the stomach with the duodenum, pancreas, and spleen as a unit, and then the liver, or vice versa.

The authors suggest removing the intestinal mass first and leaving the liver until the end.

The stomach can be removed together with the duodenum, pancreas, spleen, *and* liver as a unit, especially when a study of the three main branches of the celiac A. is needed.

***Do not attempt to remove the entire stomach until it is emptied by removing the ruminal and reticular ingesta. Explore the internal configuration of the rumen and reticulum either now or later.***

Transect the mesoduodenum. Double ligate the duodenum at the caudal flexure and transect it between the ligatures. Identify the **sigmoid colon**, double ligate it, and transect it between the ligatures. Transect the **descending mesocolon**. Identify and transect the root of the **mesentery** and the **cranial mesenteric A.** Cranial to the artery and surrounding it is the **transverse colon**. Transect the **transverse mesocolon** and the attachment of the deep wall of the greater omentum on the transverse colon. Transect the cranial extent of the superficial wall of the greater omentum on the cranial part of the duodenum and the greater curvature of the abomasum. Transect the portal V. as close as possible to the **pancreatic notch** and remove the intestinal mass.

*Note.* The pancreatic notch allows the passage of the portal V. on its way to the liver.

The **spiral loop of the ascending colon** is now exposed. Attempt to reconstitute the natural position of the intestines lying on the table. Then spread out the jejunum with the mesojejunum and identify the **centripetal** and **centrifugal coils (gyri)** and the **central flexure** of the spiral

loop; they are close to one another. The jejunum surrounds the spiral loop and continues on the ileum, whose **ileocecal fold** connects its greater curvature to the **cecum**. Identify the **jejunal lnn.,** which are close to the lesser curvature of the jejunum. Examine the **distal loop of the ascending colon**, the transverse colon, and the descending colon.

The spiral loop and its relationships to the jejunum, mesojejunum, and left kidney can be examined in situ much better from the left side, after removing the rumen. The disadvantage of this technique, however, is the difficulty in exposing the arteries.

Return to the previous position (with the right side of the intestines exposed) and identify each segment of the small and large intestine, the major branches of the cranial mesenteric A., and their divisions and anastomoses. There are some correlations between the names of the arteries and the structures supplied. The *branches* that are called **"colic"** supply the first half of the ascending colon (the proximal loop and the centripetal coils of the spiral loop), whereas the *arteries* that are called **"right colic"** supply the second half of the ascending colon (the centrifugal coils and the distal loop). The **middle colic A.** supplies the middle segment of the colon, or the transverse colon. The **mesenteric ileal branch** supplies the ileum at the lesser curvature (corresponding to the attachment of the mesentery), while the **antimesenteric ileal branch** supplies the ileum at the greater curvature (the opposite side of the mesentery, where the ileocolic fold is attached).

Also clinically important are the anastomoses between the **caudal pancreaticoduodenal A.** and the **cranial pancreaticoduodenal A.** (from the gastroduodenal A. of the hepatic A.), and between the middle colic A. and the **left colic A.** (from the **caudal mesenteric A.**). The anastomoses are highlighted in Figure R3.10 by circles.

After the intestines are removed, the attachment of the deep wall of the greater omentum on the right longitudinal groove of the rumen becomes visible.

With the stomach still in place, make a longitudinal incision in the dorsal sac of the rumen on the left side, from the **dorsal coronary groove** to the ruminal atrium. Take out the ruminal ingesta and wash and examine the interior of the rumen and reticulum, starting with the **cardia** and the **reticular groove** (sulcus). Examine the reticular groove (see Fig. R3.11), which is the first segment of the **ventricular groove**.

*Notice* that the ventricular groove consists of three segments corresponding to three different compartments of the stomach: the reticular, the omasal, and the abomasal grooves (sulci).

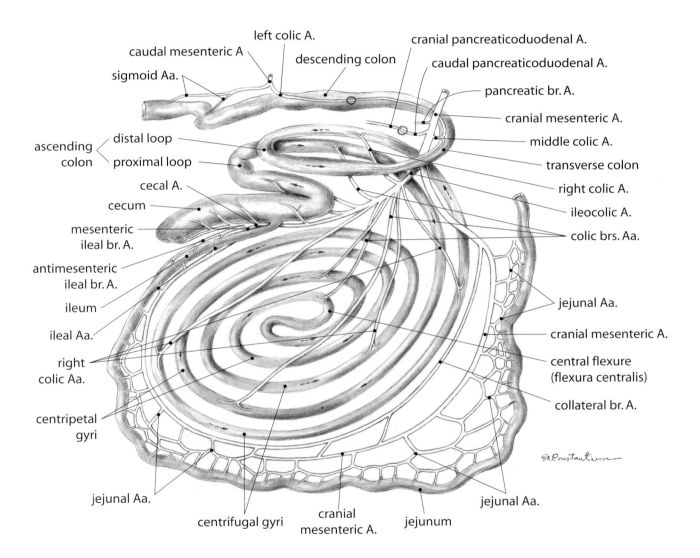

Fig. R3.10. Cranial and caudal mesenteric arteries in the large ruminants. The arterial anastomoses are indicated by circles.

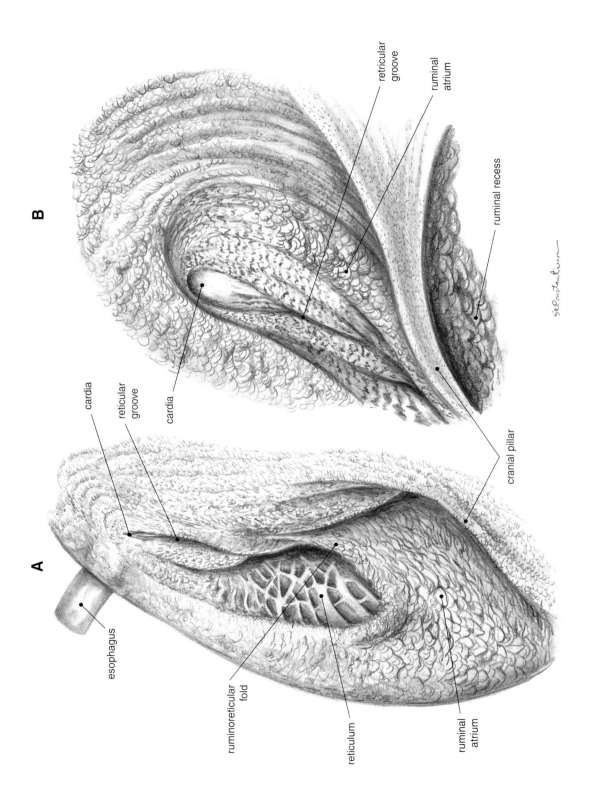

Fig. R3.11. Reticular groove (sulcus), large ruminants. **A.** General view. **B.** Details of the origin of reticular groove.

The two lips of the reticular groove are muscular. In suckling calves, the two lips transform the groove into a canal, allowing the milk to pass through it directly into the abomasum, with one condition: the calves must swallow the milk either from the udder or from a baby bottle, and not from a bucket. In bucket feeding, the amount of milk swallowed and the greediness of the calves make impossible the maintenance of the canal, and the milk drops into the rumen. This compartment of the stomach is underdeveloped and unable to perform any type of digestion, especially the enzymatic digestion of milk; consequently, a certain degree of indigestion occurs. At this age the only compartment of the stomach capable of enzymatic digestion is the abomasum. At about two months of age the rumen has a capacity comparable to that of the abomasum. In adults the reticular groove can be transformed into a canal following treatment with certain chemical substances that stimulate this process. The procedure is used in the treatment of some diseases of the omasum, abomasum, and small or large intestine, for bypassing the rumen.

Next, inspect the compartments of the rumen (dorsal and **ventral sacs**, dorsocaudal and **ventrocaudal blind sacs**, ruminal atrium or **cranial sac of rumen** and **ruminal recess**) and the structures separating them (**folds and pillars**) (Fig. R3.12).

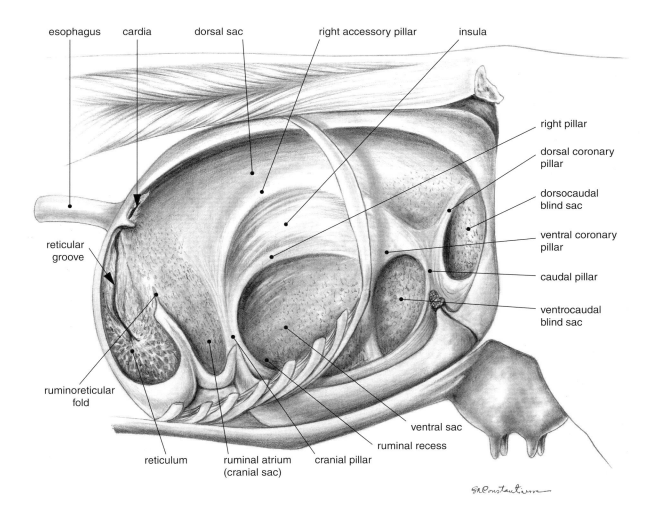

Fig. R3.12. Internal configuration of the rumen and reticulum, large ruminants.

Examine the **ruminoreticular fold** and look at the corresponding ruminoreticular groove (on the surface of rumen). The **cranial pillar** (horizontally oriented) corresponds outside to the **cranial groove**. The **right longitudinal pillar** and the **right accessory pillar** correspond to the **right longitudinal groove** and to the **right accessory groove** that, together, outline the **insula**. The **left longitudinal pillar** and the **left accessory pillar** correspond to the **left longitudinal groove** and the **left accessory groove**, respectively. The **caudal pillar** (horizontally oriented) corresponds to the **caudal groove**, whereas the **coronary pillars** (dorsal and ventral) correspond to the **coronary grooves** (dorsal and ventral) (Fig. R3.13).

*Notice* that the coronary pillars originate from the caudal pillar, and the coronary grooves from the caudal extents of the right and left longitudinal grooves. The caudal groove and the coronary grooves separate the ruminal sacs from the blind sacs.

In the next step, remove the emptied stomach (only the omasum and abomasum are still filled with ingesta) together with the spleen, the cranial and descending parts of the duodenum, the pancreas, the liver, and the corresponding segments of the abdominal aorta and caudal vena cava. Transect the ventral and dorsal attachments of the diaphragm (the sternal part and the crura). Transect the aorta and the caudal vena cava cranial to the right kidney, but before the point where they exit from the **aortic hiatus** and reach the liver, respectively. Transect the **esophagus** caudal to the **esophageal hiatus**, the place where it enters into the abdominal cavity. Free the liver, the spleen, and the rumen from any attachment to the dorsal wall of the abdominal cavity and remove all viscera mentioned above. The liver, spleen, and the diaphragm in situ are illustrated in Figure R3.14A, and the diaphragmatic aspect of the liver in Figure R3.14B.

Place the viscera on a table and try to arrange them in their natural position. Identify the **celiac A.**, the two **dorsal and ventral vagal trunks**, and the **greater splanchnic N.**

**In cattle, the vagal indigestion syndrome is a functional disturbance of the normal motility of the first three compartments of the stomach (rumen, reticulum, and omasum), of the abomasum, or of all compartments. On physical examination from behind the cow, marked ruminal distension in the left sublumbar fossa and the right ventral abdomen causes the so-called "papple shape," on the left side looking like a pear,**

**and on the right side like an apple** (*pear + apple = papple*).

Identify and dissect the branches of the main arteries (**splenic**, **left gastric**, and **hepatic**). *Notice* the absence of the **splenic hilus**.

*Notice* the anastomoses between the **left gastric A.** and the **right gastric A.**, between the **left gastroepiploic A.**, and the **right gastroepiploic A.**, and between the **caudal** and **cranial pancreaticoduodenal Aa.**, shown by circles in Figure R3.15. Dissect the vagal trunks and the **celiac ganglia** and **plexuses**. Identify the **ruminal, reticular, omasal, abomasal,** and **portal lnn.**

Make a continuous incision on the greater curvature of the reticulum, omasum, and abomasum including the **pylorus**. Take out the ingesta and wash the interior of these viscera. Examine the **reticular, omasal,** and **abomasal grooves**, as parts of the gastric groove (see Fig. R3.11). Examine the inside characteristics of all compartments of the stomach, and *notice* the ruminal pillars and sacs (see Fig. R3.12), the cellular (honeycomb) aspect of the reticulum, the four categories of the **omasal folds (laminae)** provided with marginal thickenings, the **omasal pillar**, the **spiral folds of the abomasum** (see Fig. R3.16), the **pyloric sphincter**, and the **torus pyloricus**. (The torus pyloricus is a protuberance in the pylorus formed by the circular muscle fibers at the end of the lesser curvature of the pylorus.)

Pull the descending part of the duodenum ventrally together with the right lobe of the pancreas and identify and isolate the **accessory pancreatic duct** (see Fig. R3.17A). Make a longitudinal incision on the greater curvature of the duodenum, and expose the **minor duodenal papilla** (see Fig. R3.17B).

Examine the kidneys and the **adrenal glands**, and **notice** the twisted shape of the left kidney (as a consequence of the pressure of the rumen from the left to the right). Examine the relationship between the **hilus** and the three structures entering and exiting the kidneys (the **renal A.**, **renal V.**, and **ureter**, respectively), as well as the direction of the renal vessels. Make a longitudinal section through each kidney at the level of the hilus and examine the **minor** and **major calices** (sing. calix), the **cortex** and **medulla** of each **renal lobe**, and the **renal papilla** of each **renal pyramid** (see Fig. R3.18). *Notice* that the renal pyramid and papilla are parts of the medulla. *There is no renal pelvis in the large ruminants!*

*Notice* that the large ruminants have a lobated, multipyramidal type of kidney.

**A**

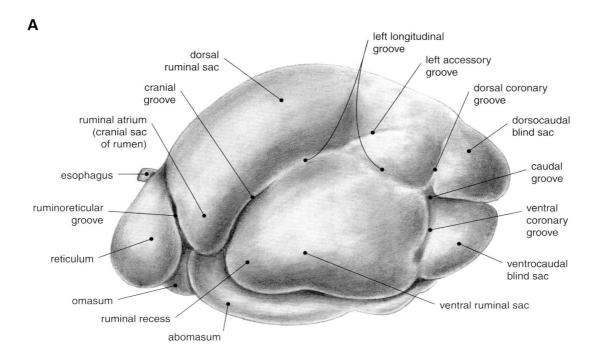

left longitudinal groove

left accessory groove

dorsal coronary groove

dorsal ruminal sac

cranial groove

dorsocaudal blind sac

ruminal atrium (cranial sac of rumen)

esophagus

caudal groove

ruminoreticular groove

ventral coronary groove

reticulum

ventrocaudal blind sac

omasum

ruminal recess

ventral ruminal sac

abomasum

**B**

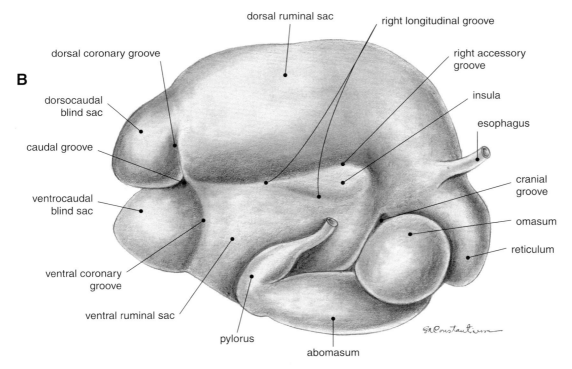

dorsal ruminal sac

right longitudinal groove

dorsal coronary groove

right accessory groove

dorsocaudal blind sac

insula

caudal groove

esophagus

ventrocaudal blind sac

cranial groove

ventral coronary groove

omasum

reticulum

ventral ruminal sac

pylorus

abomasum

Fig. R3.13. The compartments of the stomach, large ruminants. **A.** Left aspect. **B.** Right aspect.

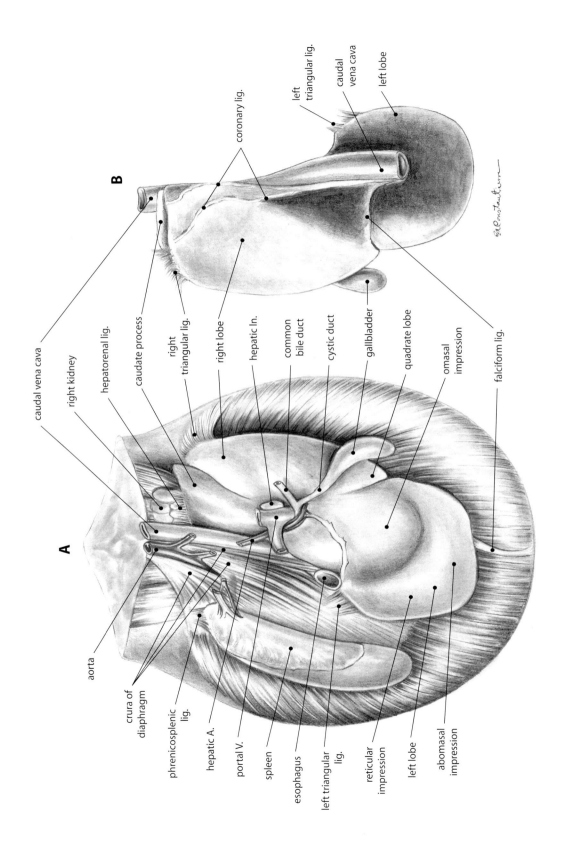

**B**

coronary lig.

left
triangular lig.

caudal
vena cava

left lobe

caudal vena cava

right kidney

hepatorenal lig.

caudate process

right
triangular lig.

right lobe

hepatic ln.

common
bile duct

cystic duct

gallbladder

quadrate lobe

omasal
impression

falciform lig.

**A**

aorta

crura of
diaphragm

phrenicosplenic
lig.

hepatic A.

portal V.

spleen

esophagus

left triangular
lig.

reticular
impression

left lobe

abomasal
impression

Fig. R3.14. The liver and spleen, large ruminants. **A.** Visceral aspect of liver and spleen in situ. **B.** Diaphragmatic aspect of liver.

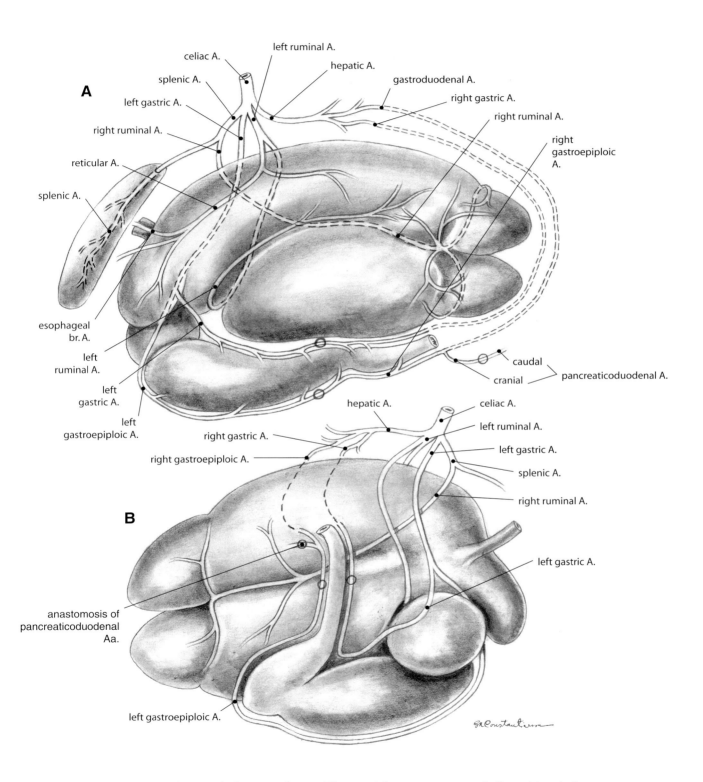

Fig. R3.15. Arterial supply of stomach, large ruminants. The arterial anastomoses are indicated by circles.
**A.** Left aspect. **B.** Right aspect.

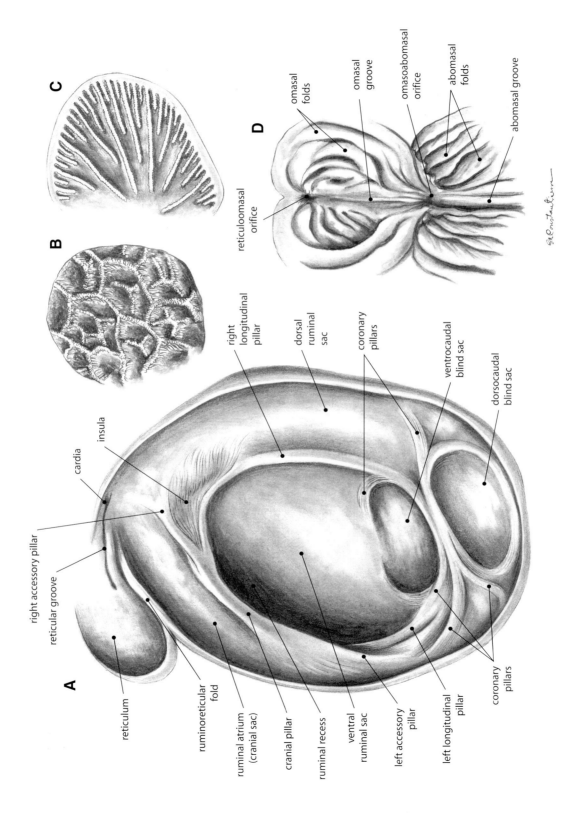

Fig. R3.16. Internal configuration of all four compartments of the stomach, large ruminants. **A.** Opened stomach (the roof of the dorsal sac is removed). **B.** Reticulum. **C.** Omasum. **D.** Omasum and abomasum.

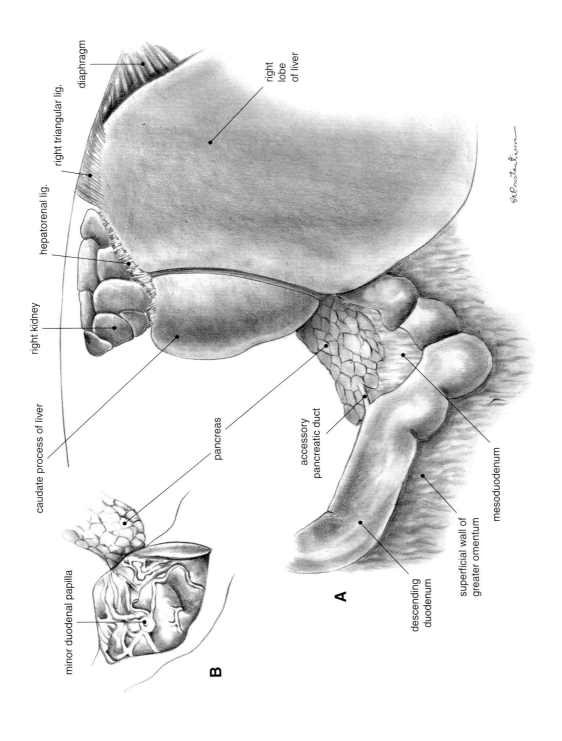

Fig. R3.17. Pancreas, large ruminants. **A**. Accessory pancreatic duct. **B**. Minor duodenal papilla.

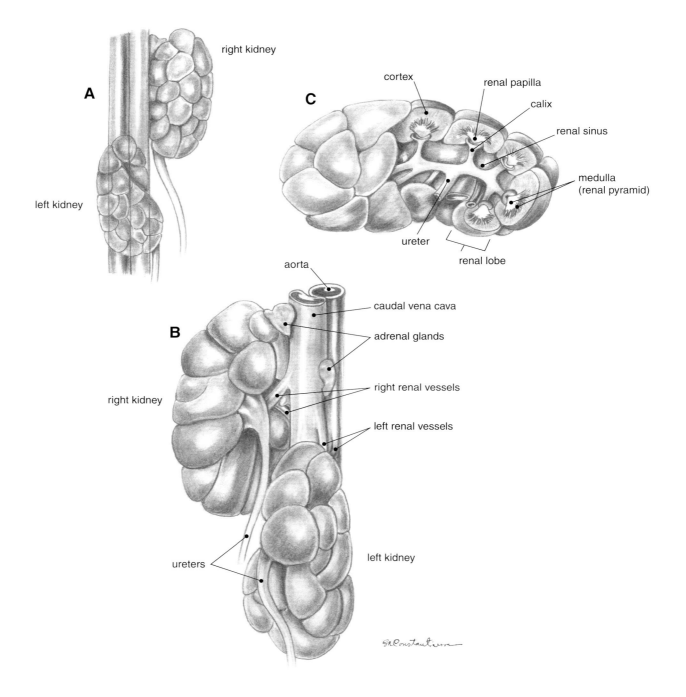

Fig. R3.18. Kidneys, large ruminants. **A.** Dorsal view. **B.** Ventral view. **C.** Internal aspect of right kidney.

# R 4

# The Pelvis, Pelvic Viscera, Tail, and External Genitalia

For systematization of the muscles of the pelvis and tail, see Table R4.1.

The bones of the pelvis and tail, the **coxal bones**, and the **sacrum**, respectively, are illustrated in Figures R4.1 and R4.2. The **caudal vertebrae** are illustrated in Figure R4.3.

**The ventral sacral foramina are important landmarks for performing the "subsacral anesthesia" (Fig. R4.4), blocking the viscera supplied by the pudendal and caudal rectal Nn. The procedure is necessary during dystocia (in the cow and the mare) and physical examination of the glans penis (in the bull and the stallion) and for different diagnostic procedures and treatment applications on the urogenital apparatus. Landmarks and approach were detailed in Modlab H4, item 7, for the horse; the technique is demonstrated at the end of Modlab R1, in this chapter.**

Table R4.1. Muscles of the Pelvis and Tail, Large Ruminants

**Muscles of the Pelvis**

*Lateral/external aspect*
– superficial gluteus (superficial gluteal M.) incorporated with gluteobiceps M.
– middle gluteus (middle gluteal M.)
– piriformis
– accessory gluteus (accessory gluteal M.)
– deep gluteus (deep gluteal M.)

*Internal aspect*
– external obturator
  • intrapelvic part
– gemelli
– quadratus femoris

**Muscles of the Tail**
– coccygeus
– sacrocaudalis dorsalis medialis
– sacrocaudalis dorsalis lateralis
– intertransversarii dorsales
– intertransversarii ventrales
– sacrocaudalis ventralis lateralis
– sacrocaudalis ventralis medialis

The **obturator membrane** and **canal**, the **sacrosciatic lig.** with the **greater** and **lesser ischiatic foramina**, the **sacroiliac joint** (including the **ventral**, **dorsal**, and **interosseous sacroiliac ligg.**), and the **pelvic symphysis** are similar to those in the horse (see Fig. H4.6). The hip joint will be exposed in the Chapter R5, The Pelvic Limb. The pelvimetry is illustrated in Figure R4.5.

**Fetal–pelvic size incompatibility has been identified as the leading cause of dystocia. Internal pelvic area measurements are taken prior to the breeding season or at the time of pregnancy examination to estimate the pelvic area of calving. The internal pelvic height (the vertical diameter) and the internal pelvic width (the transverse diameter) are taken in consideration to estimate the pelvic area of calving. The pelvic axis, the conjugate diameter, and the pelvic inclination are also measured to assess the normal size of the pelvic canal during parturition (birth).**

For the dissection of the pelvis, pelvic viscera, tail, and external genitalia in the large ruminants, a procedure similar to that performed in the horse is suggested. However, many characteristics are unique to the large ruminants.

The pattern of relationships of the **pelvic inlet** and the ventral abdominal muscles (with their tendons and aponeuroses) is easily adaptable from the horse to the large ruminants. In addition, the techniques of dissection and separation of the pelvis from the abdominal cavity (including the viscera, vessels, and nerves) are very similar to those of the horse.

However, starting with the terminal branching of the abdominal aorta, some differences are encountered. For instance, the **internal iliac Aa.** originate from a common trunk; the **uterine A.** is a branch of the **umbilical A.** (and not of the external iliac, as in the horse); the **caudal mesenteric A.** originates far caudally, at the same level as the paired **external iliac Aa.**; the **cremasteric A.** is a branch of the **pudendoepigastric trunk** (and not of the external iliac, as in the horse); and *no* **obturator A.** is present in ruminants. (The systematization of the major

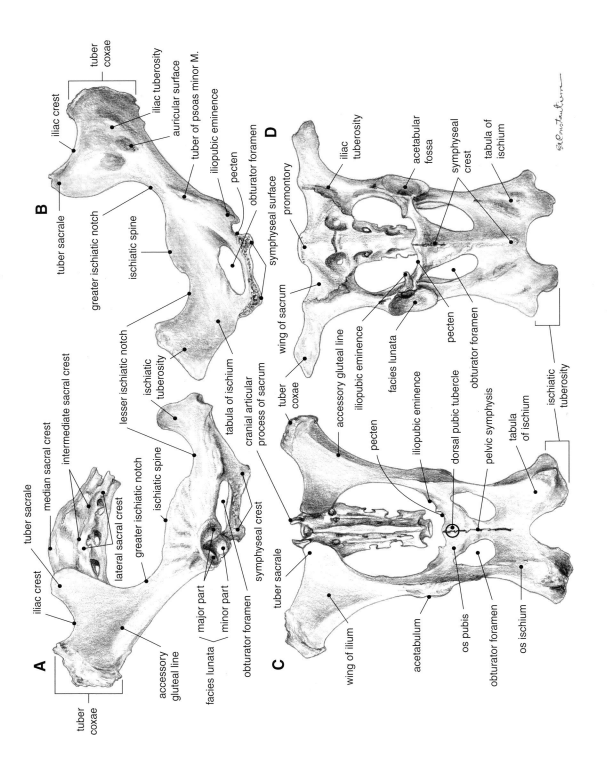

Fig. R4.1. Coxal bones with sacrum, large ruminants. **A.** Left lateral aspect. **B.** Left medial aspect. **C.** Dorsal aspect. **D.** Ventral aspect.

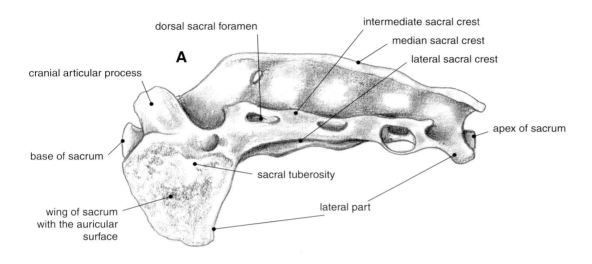

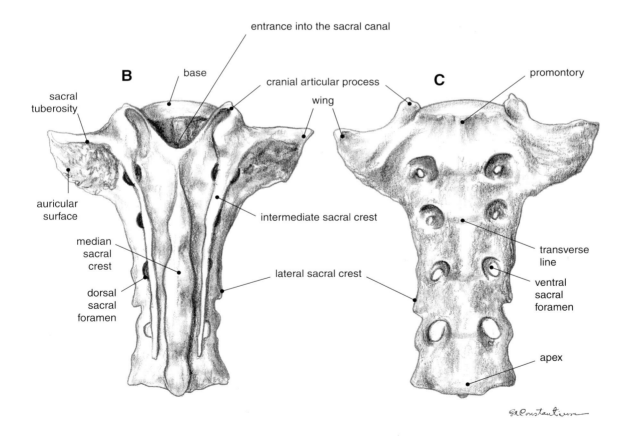

Fig. R4.2. Sacrum, large ruminants. **A.** Left lateral aspect. **B.** Dorsal aspect. **C.** Ventral aspect.

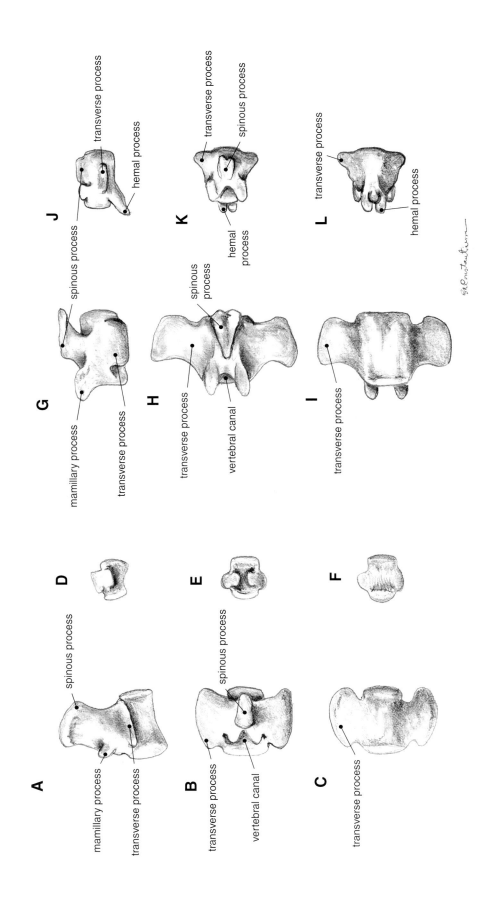

Fig. R4.3. Caudal vertebrae, horse (A–F) and large ruminants (G–L). *First vertebra, horse:* **A.** Left lateral view. **B.** Dorsal view. **C.** Ventral view. *Fourth vertebra, horse:* **D.** Left lateral view. **E.** Dorsal view. **F.** Ventral view. *First vertebra, large ruminants:* **G.** Left lateral view. **H.** Dorsal view. **I.** Ventral view. *Fourth vertebra, large ruminants:* **J.** Left lateral view. **K.** Dorsal view. **L.** Ventral view.

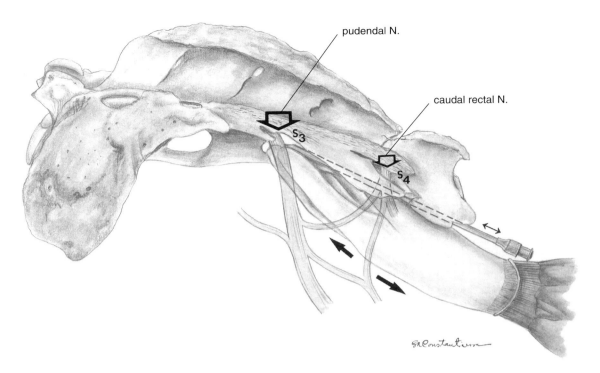

Fig. R4.4. Landmarks for performing the subsacral anesthesia (introduced by P. Popescu et al. 1958) in the large ruminants.

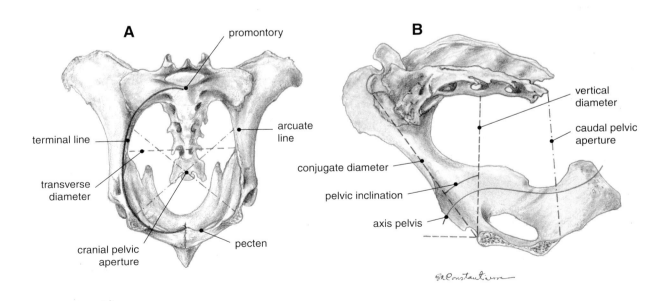

Fig. R4.5. Pelvimetry in the cow. **A.** Cranial view. **B.** Right coxal bone, medial view.

branches of the internal iliac A. in the male and in the female ruminant, according to the *N.A.V.,* is shown in Table R4.2.)

*In the cow* there are many differences from the mare, including location, position, blood supply, and each segment of the genital apparatus, including the **udder**. All internal genitalia of the cow lie within the pelvic cavity; in multiparous specimens, the **ovaries**, **uterine tubes**, and the cranial extent of the **uterine horns** exceed the pelvic inlet, extending onto the floor of the abdominal cavity.

Examine the shape of the uterine horns, which are similar to the ram's horns. They are connected to each other by the **dorsal** and **ventral intercornual ligg.** (Fig. R4.6).

**The intercornual ligg. are important structures during the transrectal examination of the ovaries and the uterine tubes of multiparous specimens, in which these viscera slip into the abdominal cavity. Pulling the intercornual ligg. with a finger will bring the whole internal genitalia to rest in the pelvic cavity and make them approachable for examination.**

Examine the uterine tubes and the ovaries. The **broad lig.** is well developed, especially the **proximal mesovarium**, which is 25–30 cm long. The **ovarian bursa** is located lateral and cranial to the ovary.

Perform the dissection of *the bull.*

Table R4.2. Major Branches of Internal Iliac A., Male and Female Large Ruminants

| Male | Female |
|---|---|
| – umbilical A. | – umbilical A. |
| • cranial vesical Aa. | • uterine A. |
| | • cranial vesical Aa. |
| – iliolumbar A. | – iliolumbar A. |
| – cranial gluteal A | – cranial gluteal A. |
| – prostatic A. | – vaginal A. |
| • A. of ductus deferens | • uterine br. |
| – caudal vesical A. | – caudal vesical A. |
| • ureteric br. | • ureteric br. |
| • urethral A. | • urethral br. |
| | • middle rectal A. |
| | • dorsal perineal A. |
| | – caudal rectal A. |
| | – dorsal labial br. |
| – caudal gluteal A. | – caudal gluteal A. |
| – internal pudendal A. | – internal pudendal A. |
| • urethral A. | • urethral A. |
| | • vestibular A. |
| | • ventral perineal A. |
| | – caudal rectal A. |
| | – dorsal labial and mammary br. |
| • A. of penis | • A. of clitoris |
| – A. of bulbus penis | – deep A. of clitoris |
| – deep A. of penis | – dorsal A. of clitoris |
| – dorsal A. of penis | |

*Notice* that the ruminants do *not* have a **cranial A. of the penis**.

The **prepuce** of the ox is also different. Examine the **preputial orifice**, and dissect the area from the **xiphoid process** to the **scrotum** to expose the **cranial** and **caudal preputial Mm**. Identify the **preputial laminae**. Pull the penis out of the prepuce and examine the **glans** and the **free part of the penis**, twisted to the left side. The **raphe of the penis** is obliquely oriented from the left ventral to the right aspect of the glans, paralleling the most distal extent of the **urethra (the urethral process)** and the **urethral orifice** (see Fig. R4.7A–C).

**The glans penis and the free part of the penis are examined for penile fibropapillomatosis, or warts, caused by the *bovine papillomavirus*; for the persistent penile frenulum; and for different types of inflammation (including that of the prepuce).**

**The persistent penile frenulum is a band of tissue that extends from the prepuce to the ventral aspect of the penis near the glans, and results from the failure of the fused penis and prepuce to separate at puberty.**

Make a longitudinal incision on the dorsal aspect of the penis between the glans and the attachment of the prepuce to the free part of the penis. Dissect the **apical lig.** (see Fig. R4.7D), which is responsible for the twisted (spiral) free part of the penis. This ligament has thicker fibers on the left side.

**Premature spiraling prevents intromission. To prevent this anomaly, the apical lig. is shortened and sutured to the tunica albuginea of the penis.**

Examine the entire length of penis and *notice* the **sigmoid flexure**, an S-shaped double flexure of the penis caudal to the testicles. The **retractor penis M.** is attached to the ventral bend of the sigmoid flexure (see Fig. R4.8).

Make a unilateral longitudinal **scrotodartoic** incision and bluntly free the **internal spermatic fascia** together with the **vaginal tunic** and the **spermatic cord** from the **external spermatic fascia** (for details look at the similar procedure in the horse—pages 82, 84 and 85). Transect the **lig. of the tail of the epididymis**, examine the **cremaster M.** protected by the **cremasteric fascia**, and look at the position of the **testicle** within the **testicular tunics** (see Fig. R4.9).

**The technique used here to expose all of the above-mentioned structures is also used as the "closed castration," the surgical technique of castration suggested by the authors. The "open castration" exposes the vaginal canal (see below) and, implicitly, creates the possibility of an infection spreading into the peritoneal cavity.**

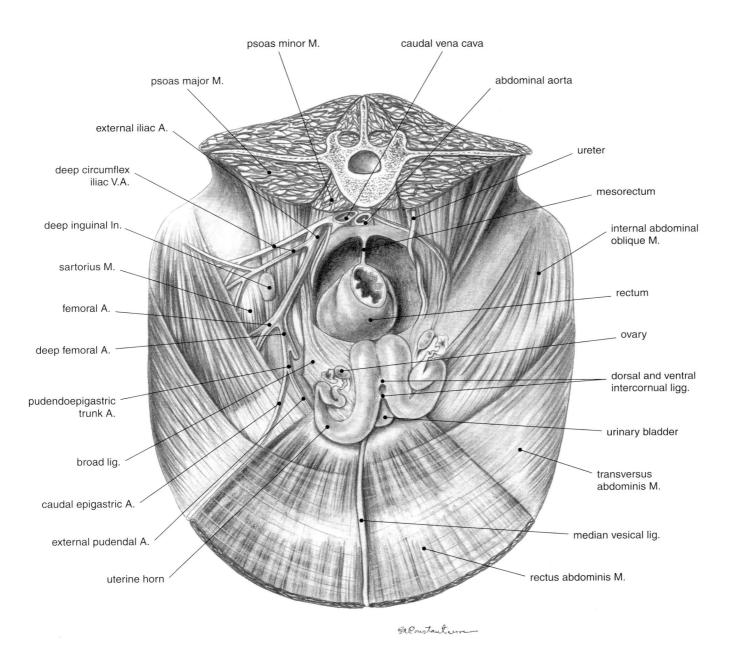

psoas minor M.

caudal vena cava

psoas major M.

abdominal aorta

external iliac A.

ureter

deep circumflex
iliac V.A.

mesorectum

deep inguinal ln.

internal abdominal
oblique M.

sartorius M.

rectum

femoral A.

ovary

deep femoral A.

dorsal and ventral
intercornual ligg.

pudendoepigastric
trunk A.

urinary bladder

broad lig.

transversus
abdominis M.

caudal epigastric A.

median vesical lig.

external pudendal A.

rectus abdominis M.

uterine horn

Fig. R4.6. Pelvic inlet in the cow, cranial view.

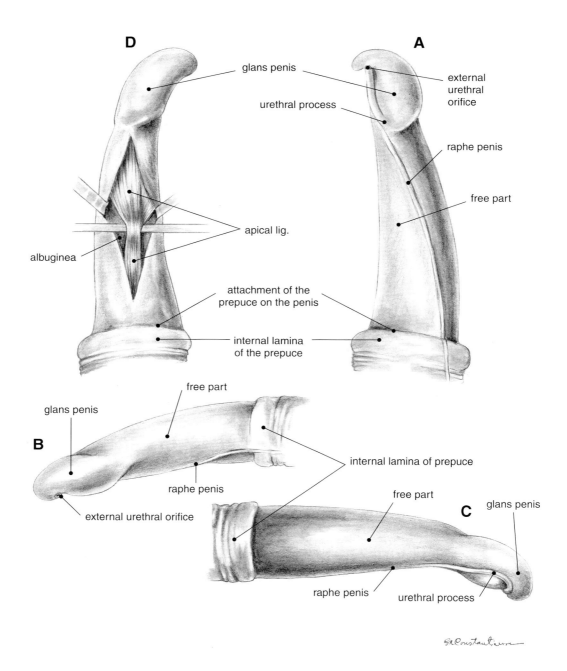

Fig. R4.7. Penis of the bull. **A.** Ventral aspect. **B.** Left lateral aspect. **C.** Right lateral aspect. **D.** Dorsal aspect with the apical ligament.

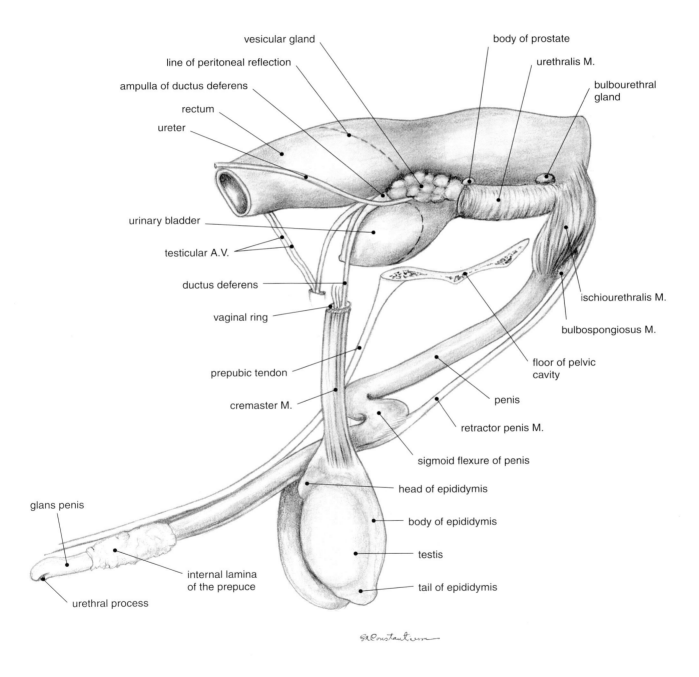

Fig. R4.8. Genital apparatus, bull, left lateral aspect (redrawn in pencil from Barone 1978).

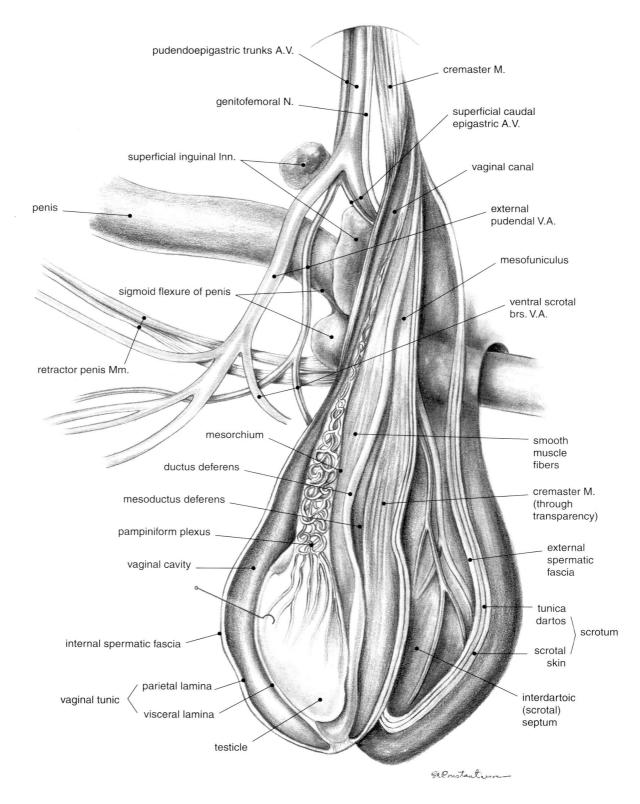

Fig. R4.9. Right spermatic cord and adjacent structures in the bull.

Palpate the **ductus deferens** and make a longitudinal incision in the internal spermatic fascia and the **parietal lamina** of the vaginal tunic, on the opposite side of the ductus deferens (cranially). The **vaginal canal** and the **vaginal cavity** are now opened, showing the **spermatic cord,** composed of the ductus deferens held by the **mesoductus deferens,** the **testicular A. and V. (the pampiniform plexus),** and smooth muscle fibers, all surrounded by the **mesorchium**. The mesoductus deferens and the

mesorchium are parts of the **visceral lamina** of the vaginal tunic. The transition between the parietal and the visceral laminae of the vaginal tunic is the **mesofuniculus** (Fig. R4.9).

Examine the testicle, the **epididymis** with the **head, body,** and **tail,** the **testicular bursa**, the ductus deferens, and the **proximal** and the **distal mesorchium** with the vessels and smooth muscle fibers (Fig. R4.10), and compare them with those of the horse.

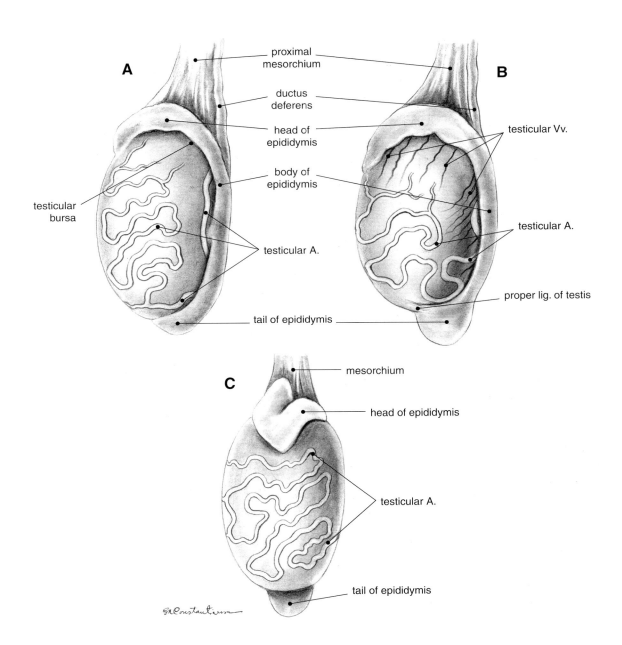

Fig. R4.10. Left testicle with vascular supply, bull. **A.** Caudolateral aspect with arteries. **B.** Caudolateral aspect with arteries and veins. **C.** Cranial view.

In the female specimens, examine the external aspect of the **udder**, the **intermammary sulcus**, and the **mammary papillae (the teats)**.

*Remember!* The udder is the collective term for all the **mammary glands** in the ruminants and the horse. There are four mammary glands or "quarters" in the large ruminants.

In the dissection of the udder, first identify the two structures of the **mammary suspensory apparatus**: the **lateral laminae** and the **medial laminae** (Fig. R4.11A,B).

Identify and look at the **external inguinal ring**. The cranial part of the lateral laminae of the suspensory apparatus originates from the **lateral crus** of this ring. Examine the medial aspect of the **gracilis** and **adductor Mm.**, and the **symphyseal tendon** (the median tendon of origin of these two muscles). The caudal part of the lateral laminae of the suspensory apparatus originates from the symphyseal tendon.

Dissect and check the elasticity of the **abdominal tunic** that intimately covers the external abdominal oblique M., with which it exchanges some fibers. The medial laminae of the suspensory apparatus originate mostly from the abdominal tunic, while the caudal part originates from the symphyseal tendon.

Carefully remove one-half of the udder from its base and from the symmetrical half, exposing the superficial inguinal ring. There are several structures passing through the ring, such as the **external pudendal A.** and **V.** and the **genitofemoral N.**, as well as the **superficial inguinal lnn. (the mammary lnn.)**, subcutaneously located and draining the udder and the vulva.

Dissect the blood supply to the udder: the **superficial caudal epigastric A.**, as a branch of the external pudendal A. that anastomoses with the **superficial cranial epigastric A.**, and the **dorsal labial and mammary branch**, as a branch of the **ventral perineal A.** The veins discharging the blood from the udder pass through the external pudendal V., the **superficial caudal epigastric V. (the cranial mammary V.)**, and the **ventral labial V. (the caudal mammary V.)**. The superficial caudal epigastric V. (see Fig. R4.12) joins the superficial cranial epigastric V. The cranial and caudal superficial epigastric Vv. are also collectively known as the **subcutaneous abdominal V. (the milk V.)**. There is a palpable ring called the **milk well**, where the superficial cranial epigastric V. perforates the abdominal wall to empty into the **internal thoracic V.**

Reexamine the ventral cutaneous branches of the **iliohypogastric**, **ilioinguinal**, and **pudendal Nn.**, which supply the skin of the udder, and the **genitofemoral N.**, which supplies the glandular system of the udder.

Make an incision in a mammary papilla in its longitudinal axis and examine the wall, which is composed of three layers: the skin, a musculovascular layer, and a mucosal layer. At the base of the teat, examine the venous ring. Inspect the **papillary duct (the teat canal)** surrounded by the **papillary sphincter** and the **papillary part of the lactiferous sinus (the teat sinus)**. Continue the incision within the mammary gland and expose the **glandular part of the lactiferous sinus** and the **glandular tissue** (see Fig. R4.11B,C). Also inspect the **lactiferous ducts**.

For the dissection of the pelvic walls, the identification of the same landmarks as in the horse is suggested.

*Notice* that in the ruminants the **greater trochanter** is not divided into cranial and caudal parts, the **ischiatic tuberosity** has three processes (dorsal, lateral, and ventral), and the **third trochanter** is *absent*.

After skinning, branches of the lumbar nerves similar to those in the horse are exposed. As in the horse, the **lateral cutaneous femoral N.**, cutaneous branches of the **tibial N.**, and the **caudal cutaneous sural N.** are visible on the caudoventral extent of the **gluteobiceps M.** and over the intermuscular space between the gluteobiceps M. and the **semitendinosus M.** The most important nerves within the area are the **proximal** and **distal cutaneous branches of the pudendal N.**, which become superficial in different areas: the proximal branch cranial to the dorsal process of the ischiatic tuberosity, and the distal branch surrounding the ventral process of the ischiatic tuberosity (see Fig. R4.13).

The blood and nerve supply to the perineal region in the cow is shown in Figure R4.14.

Follow the same instructions suggested for the horse and dissect the pelvic walls.

Before starting the dissection, try to identify the muscles through the transparency of the gluteal fascia.

*Notice* that in ruminants there are the following differences from the horse:

- The **superficial gluteal M.** shows only the caudal part, which is fused with the biceps femoris M. in the so-called **gluteobiceps M.** (see Fig. R4.15).
- The gluteobiceps M. has two distinct portions: a cranial part attached to the sacrum and the **sacrosciatic lig.**, and a caudal part attached to the ischiatic tuberosity.
- The **tensor fasciae latae M.** is more developed than in the horse because the cranial part of the superficial gluteal M. is included.
- The semitendinosus M. has *no* vertebral attachment.

After dissecting the muscles of the rump and the laterocaudal muscles of the thigh, continue the dissection of the deep structures, as they are shown in Figures R4.15–R4.18.

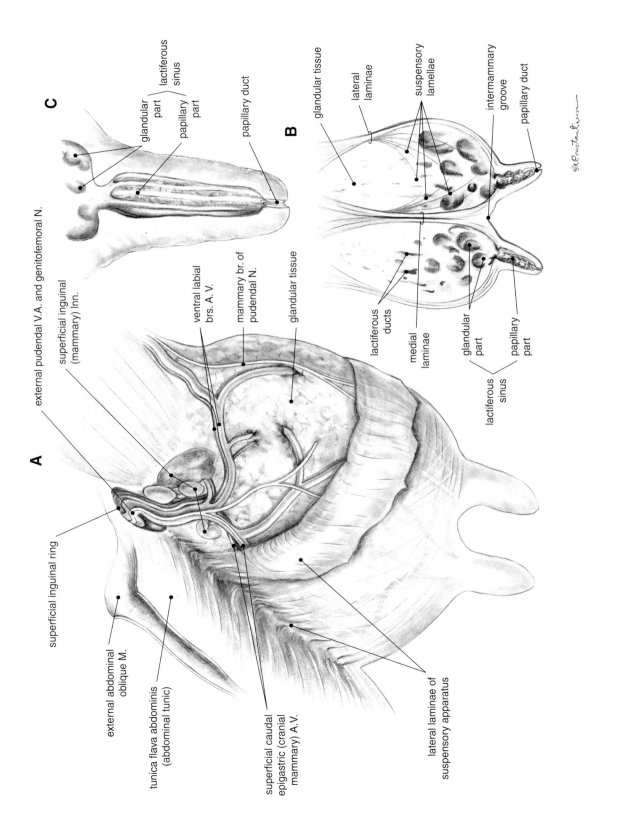

Fig. R4.11. Mammary gland (udder), cow. **A.** Left lateral aspect with vessels and lymph nodes. **B.** Suspensory apparatus. **C.** Papilla (teat).

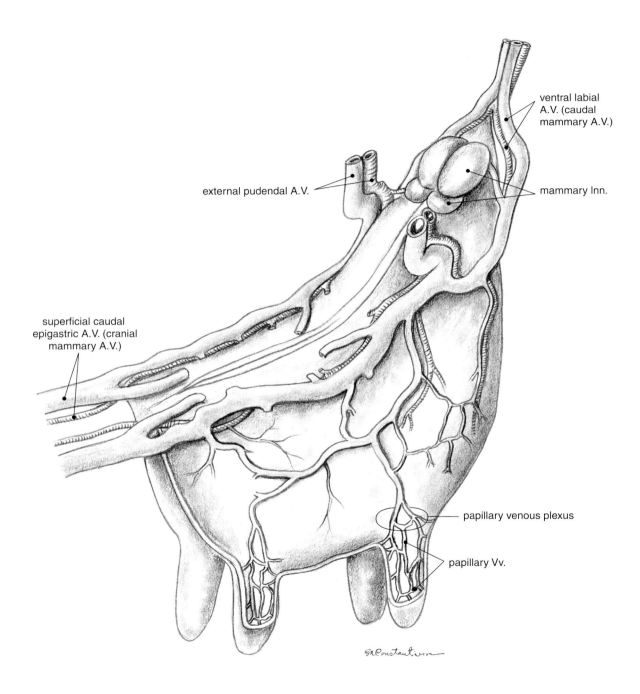

ventral labial
A.V. (caudal
mammary A.V.)

external pudendal A.V.

mammary lnn.

superficial caudal
epigastric A.V. (cranial
mammary A.V.)

papillary venous plexus

papillary Vv.

Fig. R4.12. Blood supply to the udder, cow (redrawn in pencil from Barone 1978).

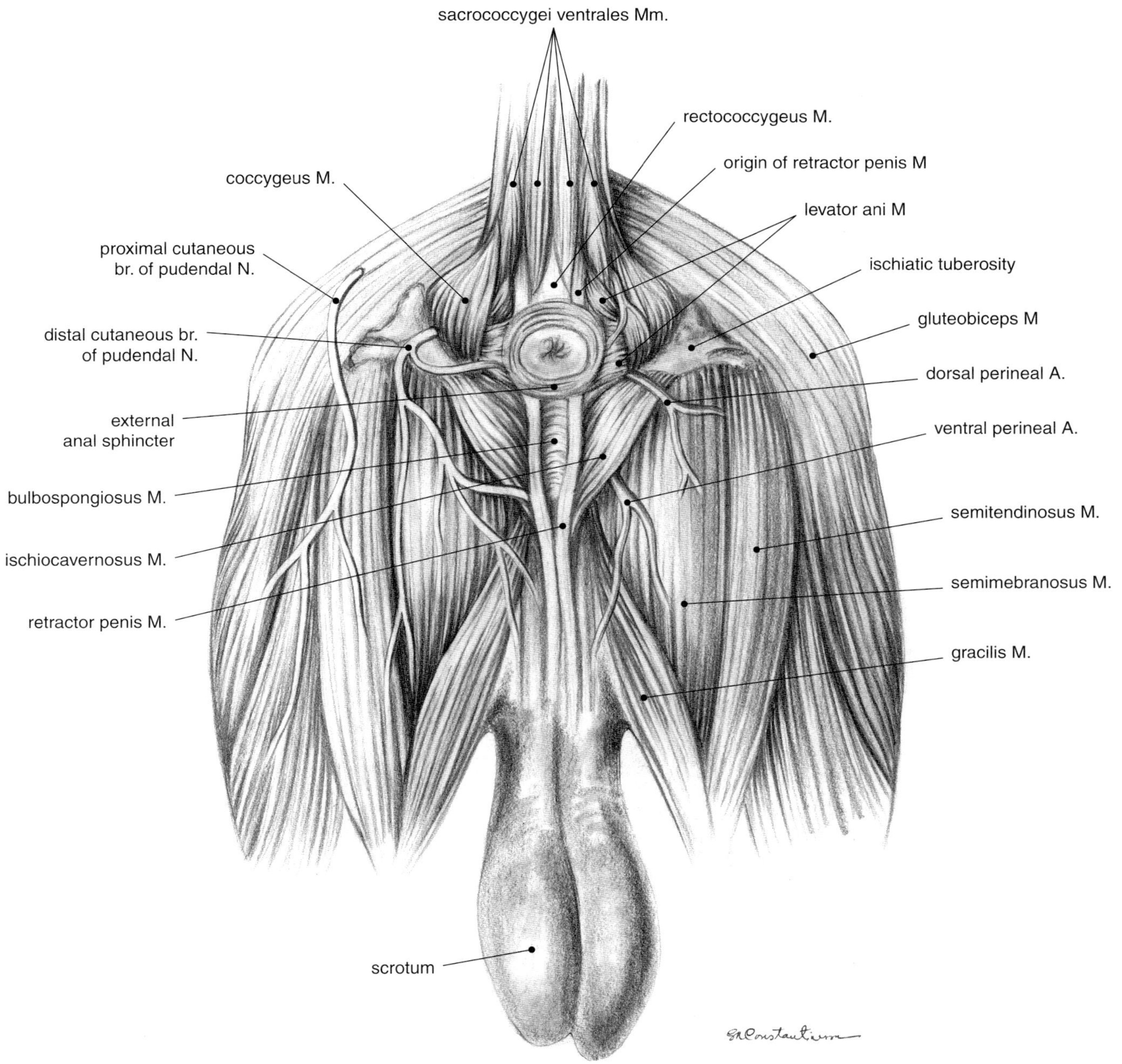

Fig. R4.13. Perineal region, bull.

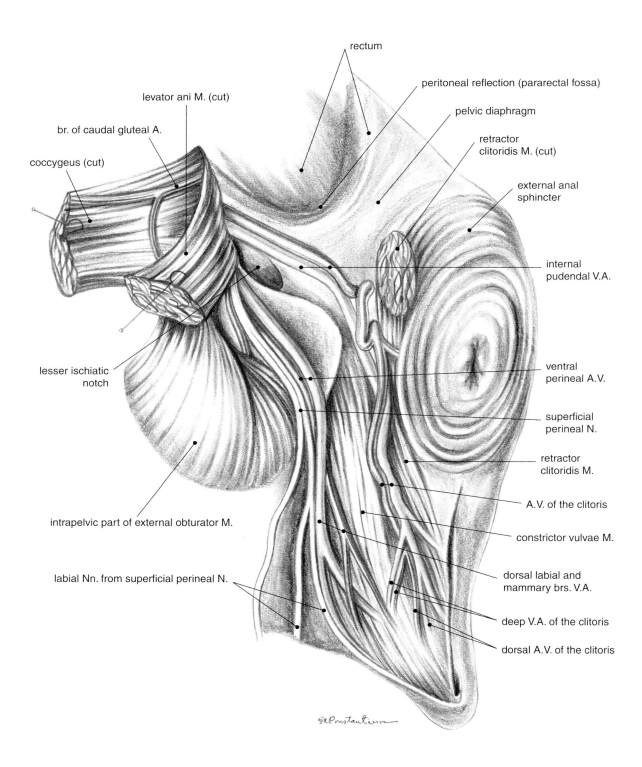

rectum

peritoneal reflection (pararectal fossa)

pelvic diaphragm

retractor clitoridis M. (cut)

external anal sphincter

internal pudendal V.A.

levator ani M. (cut)

br. of caudal gluteal A.

coccygeus (cut)

lesser ischiatic notch

ventral perineal A.V.

superficial perineal N.

retractor clitoridis M.

A.V. of the clitoris

constrictor vulvae M.

intrapelvic part of external obturator M.

dorsal labial and mammary brs. V.A.

labial Nn. from superficial perineal N.

deep V.A. of the clitoris

dorsal A.V. of the clitoris

Fig. R4.14. Blood and nerve supply to the perineal region, cow, left lateral aspect.

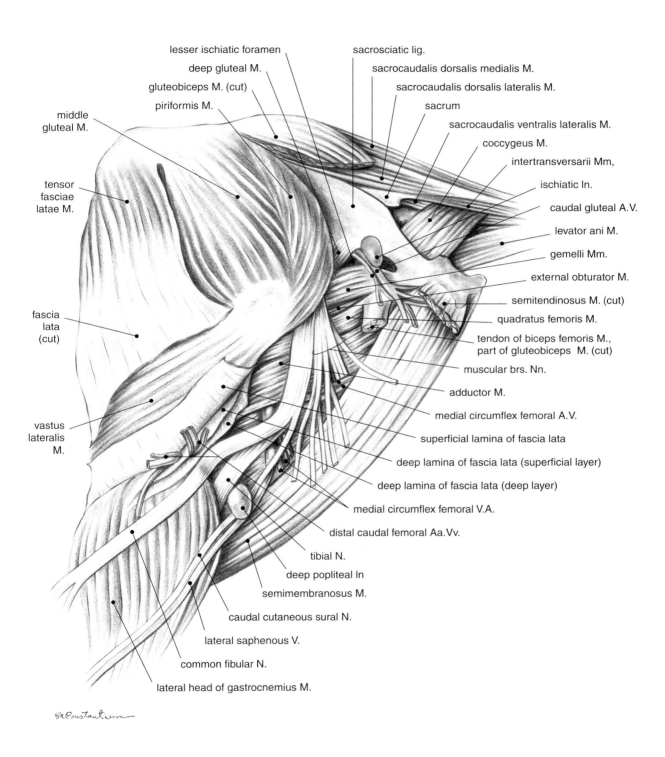

Fig. R4.15. Deep left lateral structures of croup and thigh, large ruminants.

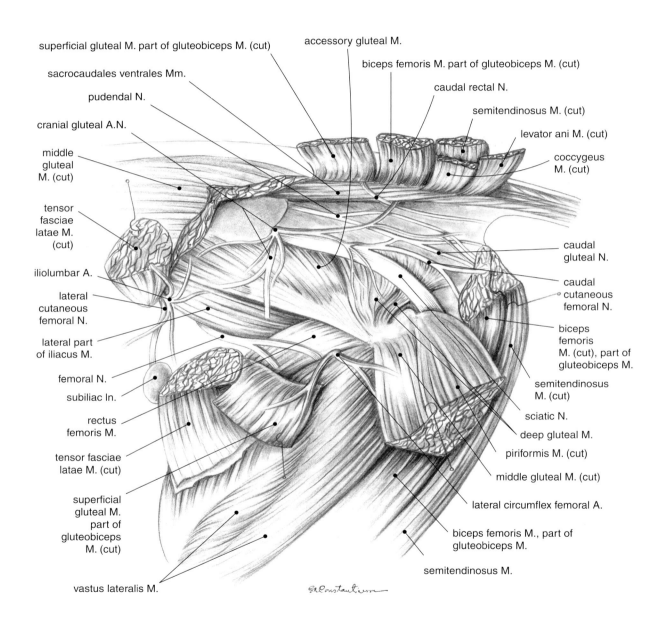

superficial gluteal M. part of gluteobiceps M. (cut)

sacrocaudales ventrales Mm.

pudendal N.

cranial gluteal A.N.

middle gluteal M. (cut)

tensor fasciae latae M. (cut)

iliolumbar A.

lateral cutaneous femoral N.

lateral part of iliacus M.

femoral N.

subiliac ln.

rectus femoris M.

tensor fasciae latae M. (cut)

superficial gluteal M. part of gluteobiceps M. (cut)

vastus lateralis M.

accessory gluteal M.

biceps femoris M. part of gluteobiceps M. (cut)

caudal rectal N.

semitendinosus M. (cut)

levator ani M. (cut)

coccygeus M. (cut)

caudal gluteal N.

caudal cutaneous femoral N.

biceps femoris M. (cut), part of gluteobiceps M.

semitendinosus M. (cut)

sciatic N.

deep gluteal M.

piriformis M. (cut)

middle gluteal M. (cut)

lateral circumflex femoral A.

biceps femoris M., part of gluteobiceps M.

semitendinosus M.

Fig. R4.16. Deep structures of left pelvis, large ruminants, lateral aspect.

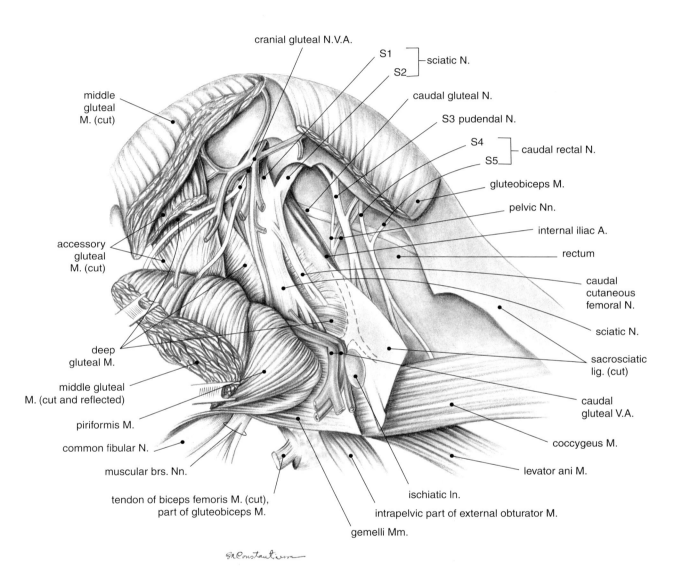

cranial gluteal N.V.A.

S1

sciatic N.

S2

caudal gluteal N.

middle
gluteal
M. (cut)

S3 pudendal N.

S4

caudal rectal N.

S5

gluteobiceps M.

pelvic Nn.

internal iliac A.

accessory
gluteal
M. (cut)

rectum

caudal
cutaneous
femoral N.

sciatic N.

sacrosciatic
lig. (cut)

deep
gluteal M.

caudal
gluteal V.A.

middle gluteal
M. (cut and reflected)

coccygeus M.

piriformis M.

levator ani M.

common fibular N.

muscular brs. Nn.

tendon of biceps femoris M. (cut),
part of gluteobiceps M.

ischiatic ln.

intrapelvic part of external obturator M.

gemelli Mm.

Fig. R4.17. The deepest structures of left pelvis, large ruminants, lateral aspect.

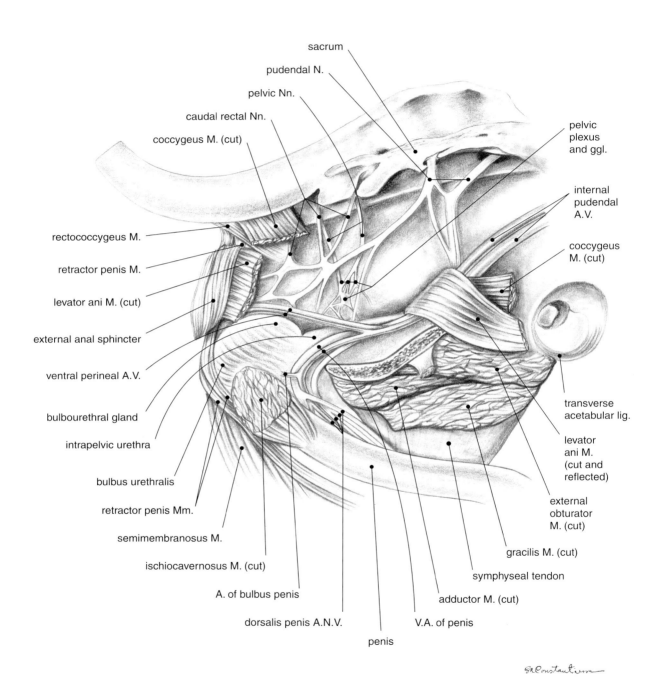

sacrum

pudendal N.

pelvic Nn.

caudal rectal Nn.

coccygeus M. (cut)

pelvic plexus and ggl.

internal pudendal A.V.

coccygeus M. (cut)

rectococcygeus M.

retractor penis M.

levator ani M. (cut)

external anal sphincter

ventral perineal A.V.

bulbourethral gland

intrapelvic urethra

bulbus urethralis

retractor penis Mm.

semimembranosus M.

ischiocavernosus M. (cut)

A. of bulbus penis

dorsalis penis A.N.V.

penis

V.A. of penis

adductor M. (cut)

symphyseal tendon

gracilis M. (cut)

external obturator M. (cut)

levator ani M. (cut and reflected)

transverse acetabular lig.

Fig. R4.18. The deepest structures of the pelvis in large ruminants, medial aspect.

Pay attention to the nerves of the sacral part of the lumbosacral plexus (**cranial gluteal, sciatic, caudal cutaneous femoral, caudal gluteal, pudendal, and caudal rectal Nn.:** Fig. R4.16 and, after sacrosciatic lig. has been cut, Fig. R4.17). The pelvic Nn.—parasympathetic—build up the **pelvic plexus**. The **pelvic ggl.** is always present (Fig. R4.18).

*Remember!* The **hypogastric Nn.** from the **caudal mesenteric ggl.** (sympathetic) join the pelvic plexus but do not synapse within the pelvic ggl. because the hypogastric Nn. and the pelvic Nn. belong to separate and specific components of the autonomic nervous system.

Be prepared to remove the male or female genital apparatus after reading the instructions given for the same procedures in the horse.

The entire male genital apparatus is illustrated in Figures R4.8 (profile) and R4.19 (dorsal view). Compare the **vesicular glands,** the **prostate**, and the **bulbourethral**

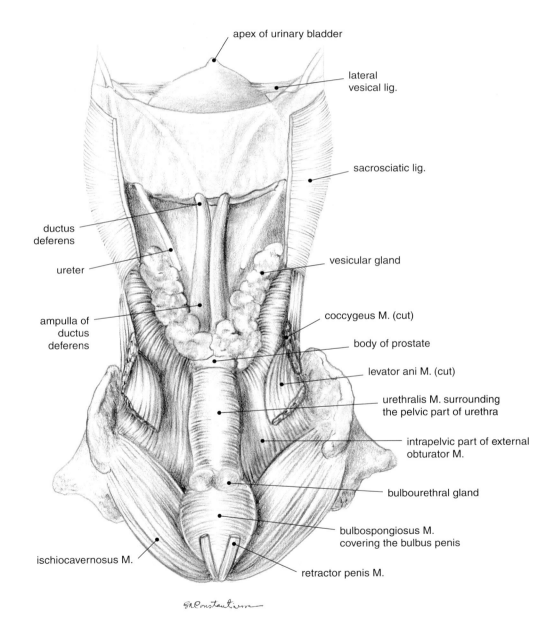

apex of urinary bladder

lateral vesical lig.

sacrosciatic lig.

ductus deferens

ureter

vesicular gland

ampulla of ductus deferens

coccygeus M. (cut)

body of prostate

levator ani M. (cut)

urethralis M. surrounding the pelvic part of urethra

intrapelvic part of external obturator M.

bulbourethral gland

bulbospongiosus M. covering the bulbus penis

ischiocavernosus M.

retractor penis M.

Fig. R4.19. Genital apparatus, bull, dorsal view (modified and redrawn in pencil from Barone 1978 and Nickel, Schummer, Seiferle, and Sack 1979).

glands with those of the horse. *Remember!* The vesicular glands of the horse are called seminal vesicles. Make a longitudinal section within the **pelvic urethra**, the **urethral isthmus**, and the **penile urethra**, and explore the **urethral diverticulum** (Fig. R4.20).

During the catheterization of the urinary bladder or a search for urethral calculi, the catheter may progress into the urethral diverticulum during retrograde passage. Pulling back the catheter and trying again is advisable.

Alternatively, a urinary catheter with a semiflexible wire may be used to stiffen the catheter enough to allow passage into the bladder. If the urethral diverticulum is encountered, passing a second catheter into the urethra while the first catheter remains in the diverticulum may allow passage of the second catheter proximally and into the bladder. Retrograde passage of urinary catheters into the bladder is extremely difficult in large and small ruminants alike. Often perineal surgery (urethrotomy, urethrostomy, penile amputation) or exploratory laparotomy for bladder repair or to place a catheter or tube into the bladder is advisable.

Make several transverse sections of the penis and identify the **corpus cavernosum penis** and the **albuginea**, the **corpus spongiosum penis**, the penile urethra, and the **bulbospongiosus M.** Compare them with those of the horse.

The female genital apparatus is shown in Figure R4.21. *Notice* the following important features that are *not* found in the mare:

- The **caruncles**, eminences of the **endometrium**; they enlarge in pregnancy and receive the **chorionic villi** of the **cotyledons** (of the **placenta**) to form the so-called **placentomes**.
- The **circular folds** of the **cervix** and the sinuosal **cervical canal**
- The **vaginal ridges** around the cervix in the **vaginal fornix**
- The openings of the **Gärtner's ducts** (remnants of the embryonic **mesonephric ducts**)
- The **major vestibular glands**
- The **suburethral diverticulum** (see Fig. R4.22)

During the catheterization of the urinary bladder, or during the endoscopic explorations of the urinary bladder, it is advisable to introduce the index finger of one hand within the suburethral diverticulum and with the other hand to pass the catheter or the endoscope over the index finger. By doing so, the catheter or the endoscope does not enter the suburethral diverticulum.

## MODLAB R1

In cattle, the reproductive tract, including the cervix, uterus, and ovaries in cows and the base of the penis, prostate, vesicular glands, and ampullae of the deferent ducts in bulls, is readily palpable by rectal exploration. The urinary bladder is palpable ventral to the reproductive tract; when distended, it is an obvious structure, but it is flaccid when empty and may be overlooked. By sweeping the hand along the craniodorsal aspect of the ilium, at 2 o'clock and 10 o'clock, just cranial and lateral to the arcuate line, the deep inguinal (iliofemoral) lnn. can be palpated. These lymph nodes normally have the size and shape of a walnut.

At 4 o'clock and 8 o'clock, cranial and ventral to the arcuate line, the deep inguinal rings are palpable in the bulls. Inguinal hernias are uncommon but may occur and cause intestinal strangulation. From midline to the left and cranially, the rumen is palpable. To the right of the rumen, usually on the midline, is the lobated left kidney, which hangs in a position at about the level of the anus. Pyelonephritis may be palpable as enlargement of the kidney; a painful response to palpation supports this diagnosis. Ventral and to the right of the kidney is the region where the small intestine and the cecum may be palpated. Often, the right side of the abdomen feels fairly empty in healthy animals.

There are several methods for nerve block anesthesia of the pudendal and caudal rectal Nn. in cattle. Among them, the method of Larson (1953) seems to be the most recommended. This method indicates three or even four points of approach to the nerves. No precise landmarks are suggested, and the method, as described in Westhues and Fritsch (1964, 177–179), is complicated and takes a long time. In 1958, a new method, the so-called "subsacral anesthesia," was described by P. Popescu et al. (a Romanian team; this is not the P. Popesko, author of the *Atlas of the Topographical Anatomy of the Domestic Animals*). This technique is simple and is based on the transrectal digital palpation of the $S_3$ and $S_4$ ventral sacral foramina: "The infiltration of the pudendal and hemorrhoidal (N.A. caudal rectal) nerves as they leave the sacrum in the third and fourth ventral sacral foramina appears technically easier than Larsen's method" (Westhues and Fritsch 1964, 179) (see Fig. R4.3).

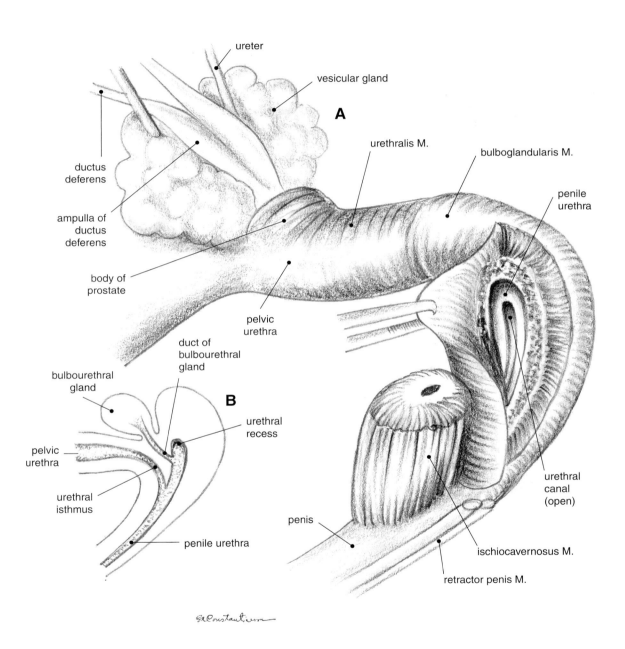

Fig. R4.20. The urethral diverticulum, bull (redrawn from Garrett 1987). **A.** Topography of urethral diverticulum. **B.** Schematic representation of a median section.

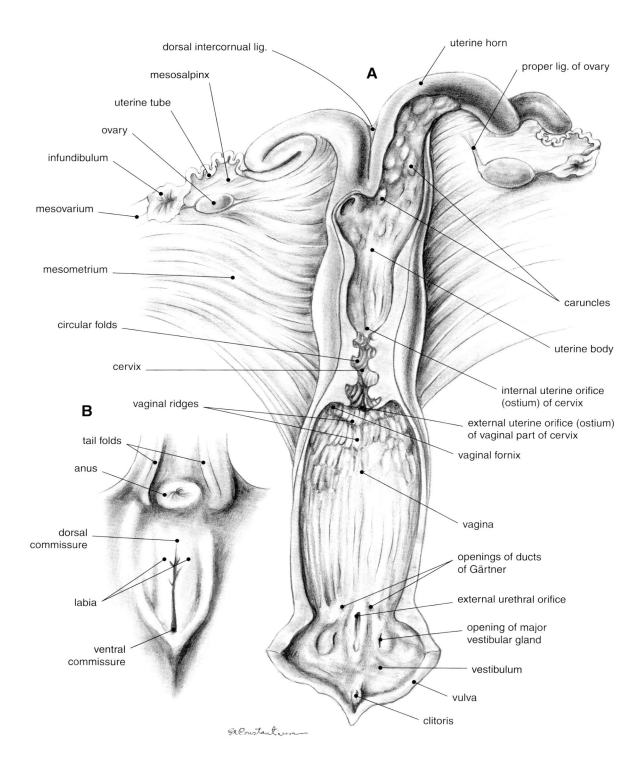

dorsal intercornual lig.

mesosalpinx

uterine tube

ovary

infundibulum

mesovarium

mesometrium

circular folds

cervix

**A**

uterine horn

proper lig. of ovary

caruncles

uterine body

internal uterine orifice (ostium) of cervix

external uterine orifice (ostium) of vaginal part of cervix

vaginal fornix

**B**

vaginal ridges

tail folds

anus

dorsal commissure

labia

ventral commissure

vagina

openings of ducts of Gärtner

external urethral orifice

opening of major vestibular gland

vestibulum

vulva

clitoris

Fig. R4.21. Genital apparatus, cow. **A.** Genital tract (dorsal aspect). **B.** Vulva.

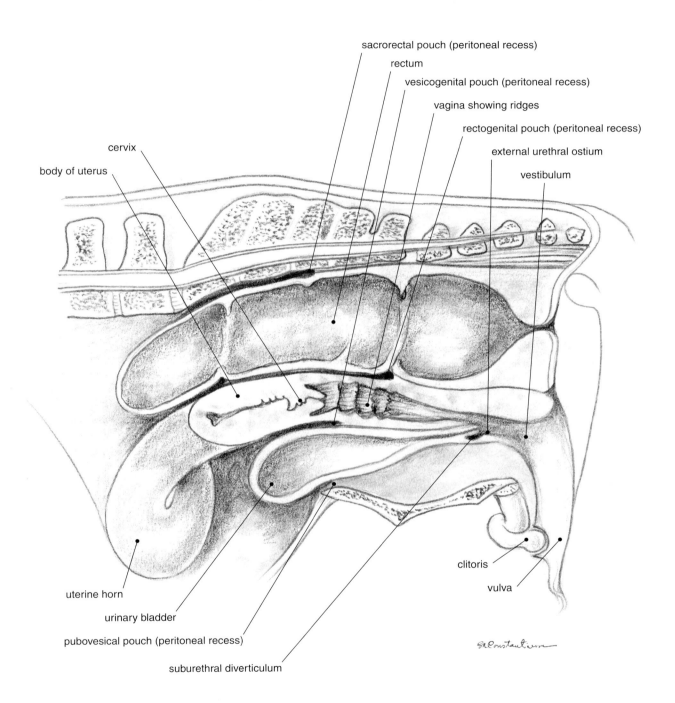

Fig. R4.22. Sagittal section within the pelvic cavity, cow (modified and redrawn in pencil from Barone 1978).

# R 5

## The Pelvic Limb

The bones of the pelvic limb, the **femur** and the **patella**, the **tibia** and **fibula**, the **tarsal** and **metatarsal bones** are illustrated in Figures R5.1–R5.6. A comparison between the hip joints of the horse and the ox is shown in Figure H5.6B,C. The phalanges will be illustrated in Chapter R6, The Thoracic Limb.

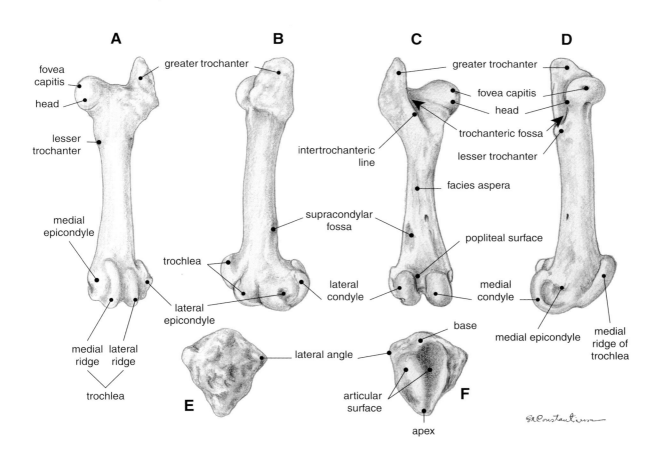

Fig. R5.1. Left femur and patella, large ruminants. Femur: **A.** Cranial aspect. **B.** Lateral aspect. **C.** Caudal aspect. **D.** Medial aspect. **E.** Patella, cranial aspect. **F.** Patella, caudal aspect.

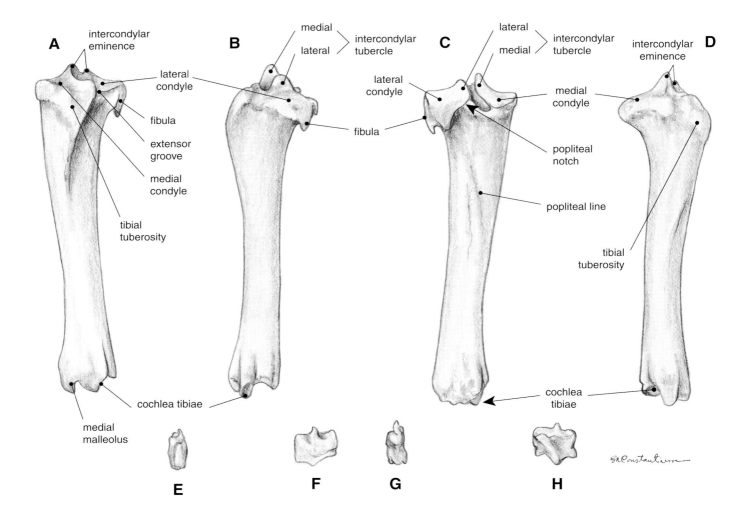

Fig. R5.2. Left tibia and malleolar bone, large ruminants. Left Tibia: **A.** Cranial aspect. **B.** Lateral aspect. **C.** Caudal aspect. **D.** Medial aspect. **E.** Malleolar bone, cranial aspect. **F.** Malleolar bone, lateral aspect. **G.** Malleolar bone, caudal aspect. **H.** Malleolar bone, medial aspect.

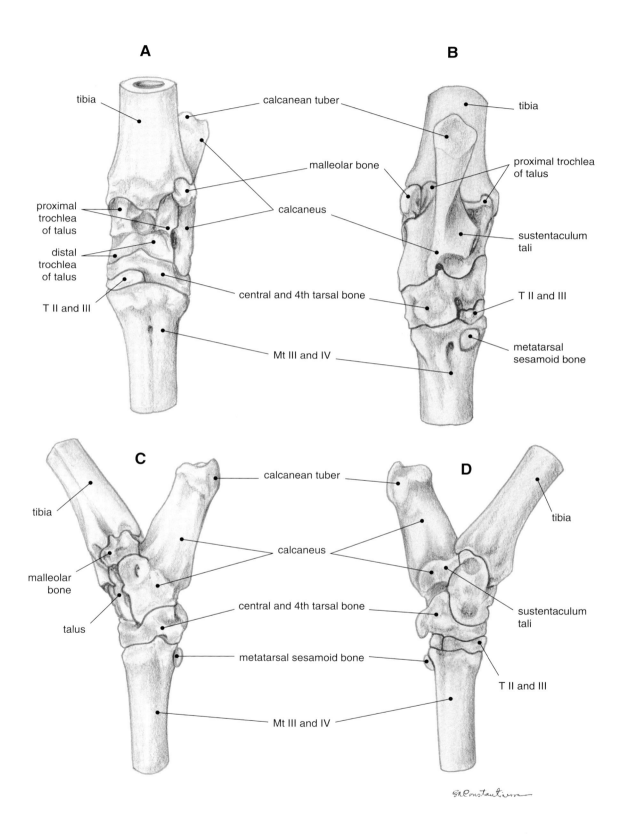

Fig. R5.3. Tarsal bones, large ruminants, left limb. **A.** Dorsal aspect. **B.** Plantar aspect. **C.** Lateral aspect. **D.** Medial aspect.

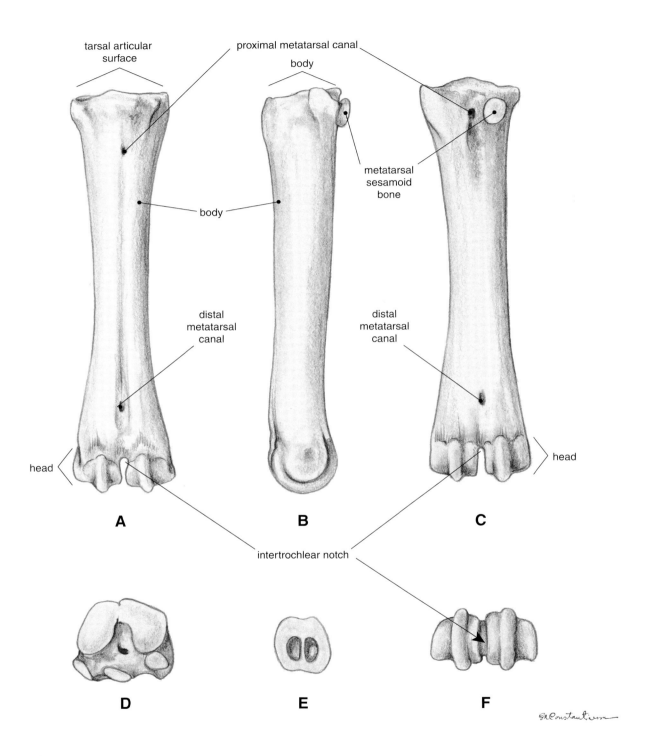

Fig. R5.4. Left metatarsal bones, large ruminants. **A.** Dorsal aspect. **B.** Lateral aspect. **C.** Plantar aspect. **D.** Tarsal articular surface. **E.** Transverse section, body. **F.** Head.

*As in the procedure for the horse, first identify the following structures used as landmarks: the greater trochanter, the lateral and medial epicondyles of the femur, the trochlea of the femur, the patella, the three patellar ligaments, the lateral and medial condyles of the tibia, the tibial tuberosity, the craniomedial surface of tibia, the common calcanean tendon, the calcaneus and the calcanean tuber, the distal end of the lateral ridge of the trochlea of the talus, the malleolar bone, the third and fourth metatarsal bones (fused), the tendons of the interosseous, deep digital flexor, and superficial digital flexor Mm., the paired dewclaws, the metatarsophalangeal joints (fetlock joint), the first phalanx (pastern), the coronet (the narrow area along the dorsal border of each hoof), and the hooves.*

Separate the two pelvic limbs using the same technique as in the horse (see page 127), and examine the **vertebral canal** and the **spinal cord** (Fig. R5.5). The most noticeable difference between the horse and the large ruminants is that the medullary cone ends at the lumbosacral junction in the horse.

The systematization of the muscles of the pelvic limb is shown in Table R 5.1 and the nerve supply to the muscles of the pelvic limb is shown in Table R5.2.

Here are the differences between the ruminants and the horse as far as the muscles of the pelvic limb are concerned:

- There is *no* articularis coxae M.
- The biceps femoris M. is fused with the caudal part of the superficial gluteal M. in the gluteobiceps M.; the corresponding cranial part of the superficial gluteal M. of the horse is fused with the tensor fasciae latae M.
- There is *no* fibrous ring in the proximal part of the gracilis M. for any vein.
- There is *no* accessory lig. of the head of femur, and consequently no split attachment of the pectineus M.
- There is only one adductor M. (the adductor major and minor are fused).
- There is *no* internal obturator M. (the corresponding muscle of the horse is the intrapelvic part of the external obturator M. in the ox).
- There is an additional fibularis longus M.
- There are two tendons of the long digital extensor M.
- There are several muscle bundles between the superficial and the deep digital flexor Mm., known as the interflexor Mm.
- There are *no* lumbricales Mm.
- Interosseous Mm. III and IV are fused in a single structure.

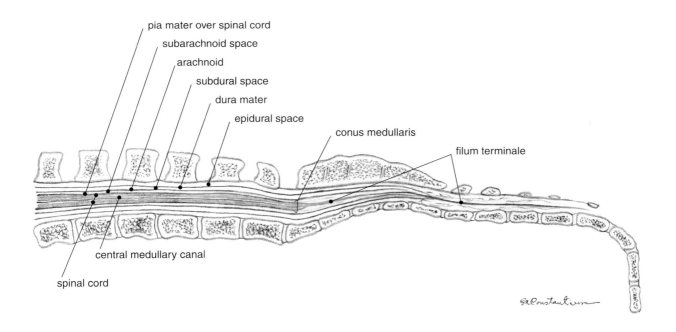

Fig. R5.5. Conus medullaris and associated structures in large ruminants, median section (schematic) (modified after Nickel, Schummer, and Seiferle, 1984, vol. 4).

Table R5.1. Muscles of the Pelvic Limb, Large Ruminants

**Thigh**

*Cranial aspect*
  – tensor fasciae latae, fused with cranial part of superficial gluteal M.
  – quadriceps femoris M.
    • rectus femoris
    • vastus lateralis
    • vastus intermedius
    • vastus medialis

*Caudolateral aspect*
  – biceps femoris, fused with caudal part of superficial gluteal M. in gluteobiceps M.
  – semitendinosus
  – semimembranosus

*Medial aspect*
  – superficial muscles
    • sartorius
    • gracilis
  – deep muscles
    • pectineus
    • adductors
      ○ long adductor, fused with pectineus
      ○ major adductor and minor adductor, fused

**Crus**

*Cranial aspect*
  – cranial tibial
  – fibularis tertius ⎫ with proximal action (on the hock)
  – fibularis longus ⎬
  – long digital extensor ⎫ with distal action (on the digits)
  – lateral digital extensor ⎭

*Caudal aspect*
  – superficial muscles
    • triceps surae (gastrocnemius—lateral and medial heads, and soleus), with proximal action (on the hock)
    • superficial digital flexor, with distal action (on the digits)
      ○ sleeve at the level of metatarsophalangeal joint, by fusion with the accessory lig. of interossei Mm.
  – deep muscles
    • popliteus [with proximal action (on the crus)]
    • deep digital flexor [with distal action (on the digits)]
      ○ lateral digital flexor
      ○ medial digital flexor
      ○ caudal tibial

*Autopodium*
  – extensor digitorum brevis
  – interossei lateralis and medialis Mm. (III and IV fused)
    • accessory lig. fused with the superficial digital flexor tendon

Follow the same technique as in the horse (see pages 128, 133, and following) and identify each structure on the medial aspect of the pelvis, including the **intrapelvic portion of the external obturator M.** Transect the **femoral lamina** over the **femoral triangle** in the long axis of the thigh and expose the **vastus medialis, sartorius,** **pectineus,** and **gracilis Mm.** Dissect the **femoral A.V., and N.** and their branches (see Fig. R5.6).

*Note.* Do not expect to find the **deep inguinal (iliofemoral) lnn.** in the femoral triangle, as in the horse. They are located on the **external iliac A.,** just before the origin of the **deep femoral A.,** within the abdominal cavity. Dissect the **medial circumflex femoral A.,** which is a continuation of the deep femoral A.

Transect the gracilis M., reflect it, and expose the **adductor** and **semimembranosus Mm.** *Notice* that there is only one adductor M. in ruminants (the major and minor adductors are fused; the long adductor is still fused with the pectineus M.).

Dissect the **rectus femoris M.,** the attachments of the **semitendinosus** and semimembranosus Mm. on the **stifle joint,** and the **calcanean tendon of the semitendinosus M.**

Turn the limb lateral side up. Reflect the **biceps femoris** and the semitendinosus Mm. ventrally and identify the **gemelli, quadratus femoris,** and **external obturator Mm.** The vessels and nerves are similar to those of the horse.

*Notice* that in ruminants the gemelli Mm. look like a single muscle because there is no tendon of the internal obturator M. to pass between them. The corresponding internal obturator M. of the horse is called in ruminants the intrapelvic portion of the external obturator M., whose tendon passes through the **obturator foramen** and joins the external obturator M.

If your instructor asks you to examine the **hip joint,** transect the **deep gluteal** and gemelli Mm. from the femur attachments and reflect them carefully off the joint capsule. Transect the quadratus femoris and the external obturator Mm. from their femoral attachments and reflect them. Transect the origin of the rectus femoris M. and reflect the muscle ventrally. Make an incision in the joint capsule and explore the **acetabular cavity.** Identify the **lig. of the head of the femur** and the **transverse acetabular lig.** (see Fig. H5.6A,C).

Continue the dissection on the lateral aspect of the crus. Outline the two (not three, as in the horse) **extensor retinaculae** and remove the **crural fasciae,** saving the vessels and nerves (see Fig. R5.7). In comparison to the horse, one additional structure found in the large ruminants is the **fibularis (peroneous) longus M.** You will also find the branching of the **lateral saphenous V.** in **cranial** and **caudal branches.** The lateral saphenous V. and the caudal branch are accompanied by the **caudal cutaneous sural N.** (see Fig. R5.8).

Transect the fibularis longus and the long digital extensor Mm. to fully expose the route of both the **superficial** and **deep fibular (peroneal) Nn.** (see Fig. R5.9).

Table 5.2. Muscles and Nerve Supply, Pelvic Limb, Horse and Large Ruminants.

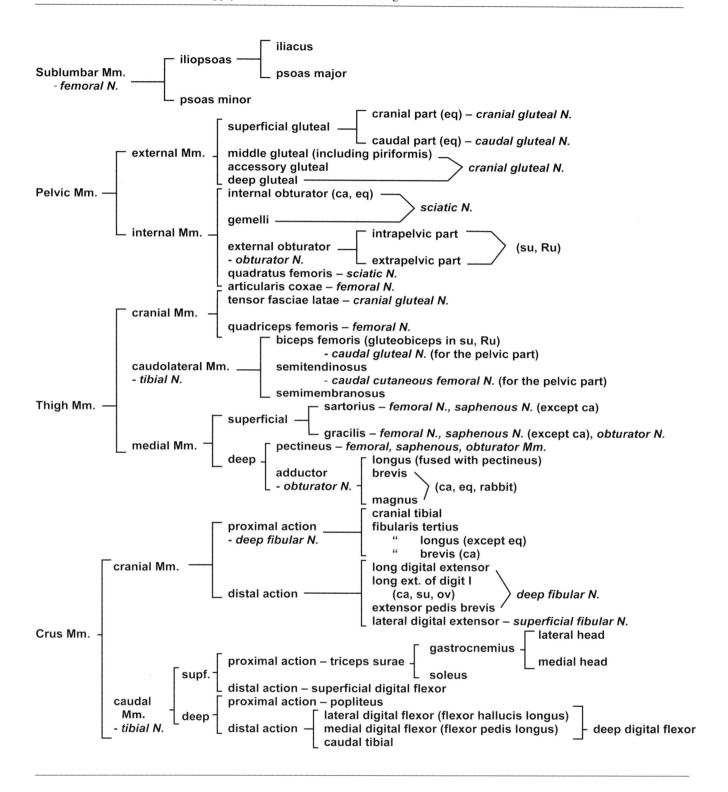

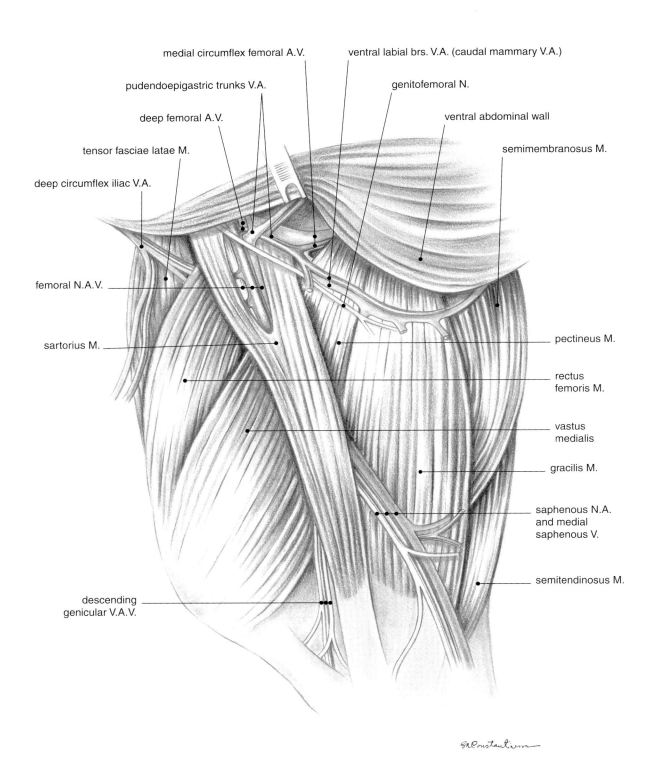

medial circumflex femoral A.V.

pudendoepigastric trunks V.A.

deep femoral A.V.

tensor fasciae latae M.

deep circumflex iliac V.A.

ventral labial brs. V.A. (caudal mammary V.A.)

genitofemoral N.

ventral abdominal wall

semimembranosus M.

femoral N.A.V.

sartorius M.

pectineus M.

rectus femoris M.

vastus medialis

gracilis M.

saphenous N.A. and medial saphenous V.

semitendinosus M.

descending genicular V.A.V.

Fig. R5.6. Superficial structures of the right thigh, large ruminants, medial aspect.

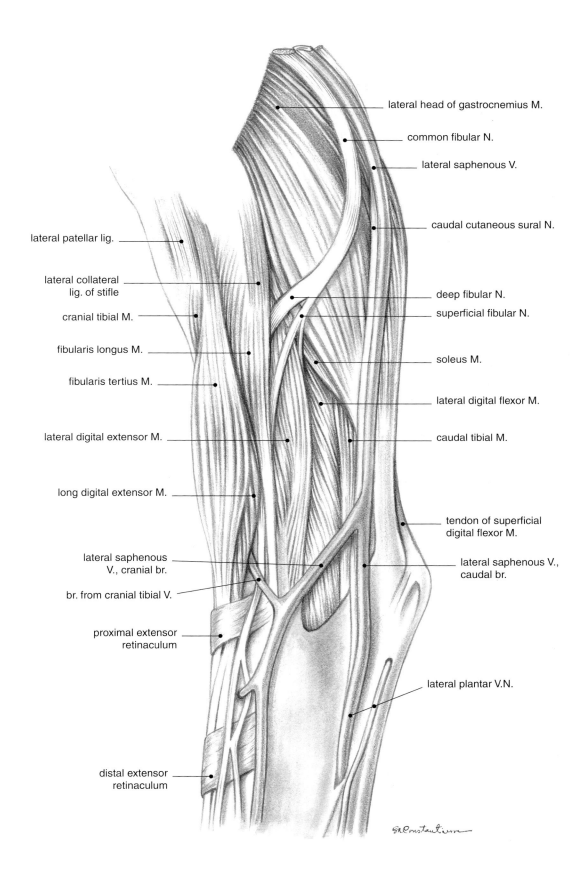

lateral head of gastrocnemius M.

common fibular N.

lateral saphenous V.

caudal cutaneous sural N.

lateral patellar lig.

lateral collateral lig. of stifle

deep fibular N.

cranial tibial M.

superficial fibular N.

fibularis longus M.

soleus M.

fibularis tertius M.

lateral digital flexor M.

lateral digital extensor M.

caudal tibial M.

long digital extensor M.

tendon of superficial digital flexor M.

lateral saphenous V., cranial br.

lateral saphenous V., caudal br.

br. from cranial tibial V.

proximal extensor retinaculum

lateral plantar V.N.

distal extensor retinaculum

Fig. R5.7. Craniolateral aspect of crus and hock, large ruminants.

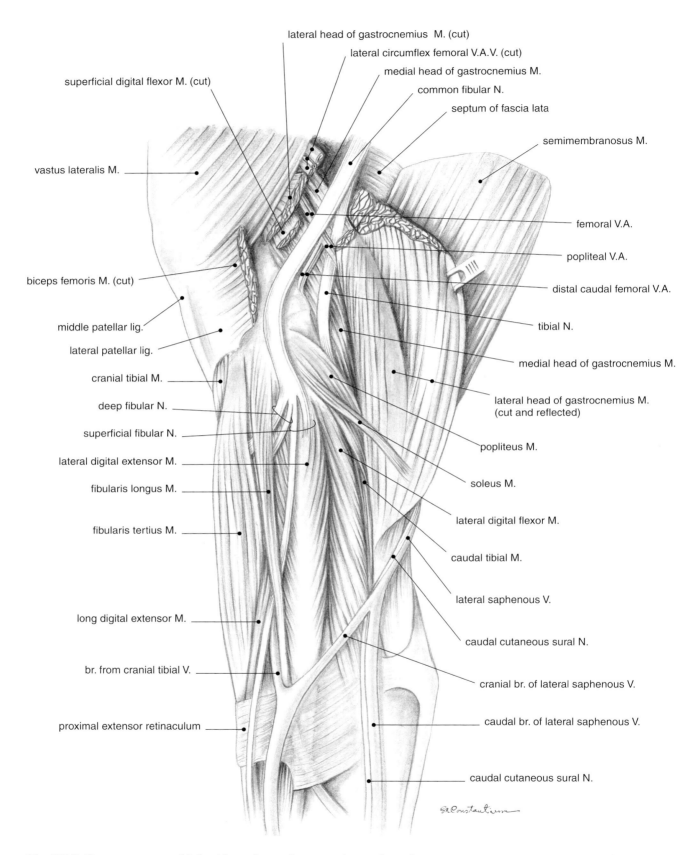

lateral head of gastrocnemius M. (cut)

lateral circumflex femoral V.A.V. (cut)

medial head of gastrocnemius M.

common fibular N.

septum of fascia lata

semimembranosus M.

superficial digital flexor M. (cut)

vastus lateralis M.

femoral V.A.

popliteal V.A.

biceps femoris M. (cut)

distal caudal femoral V.A.

middle patellar lig.

tibial N.

lateral patellar lig.

medial head of gastrocnemius M.

cranial tibial M.

lateral head of gastrocnemius M. (cut and reflected)

deep fibular N.

superficial fibular N.

popliteus M.

lateral digital extensor M.

soleus M.

fibularis longus M.

lateral digital flexor M.

fibularis tertius M.

caudal tibial M.

lateral saphenous V.

long digital extensor M.

caudal cutaneous sural N.

br. from cranial tibial V.

cranial br. of lateral saphenous V.

proximal extensor retinaculum

caudal br. of lateral saphenous V.

caudal cutaneous sural N.

Fig. R5.8. Deep structures of left stifle and crus, large ruminants, lateral aspect.

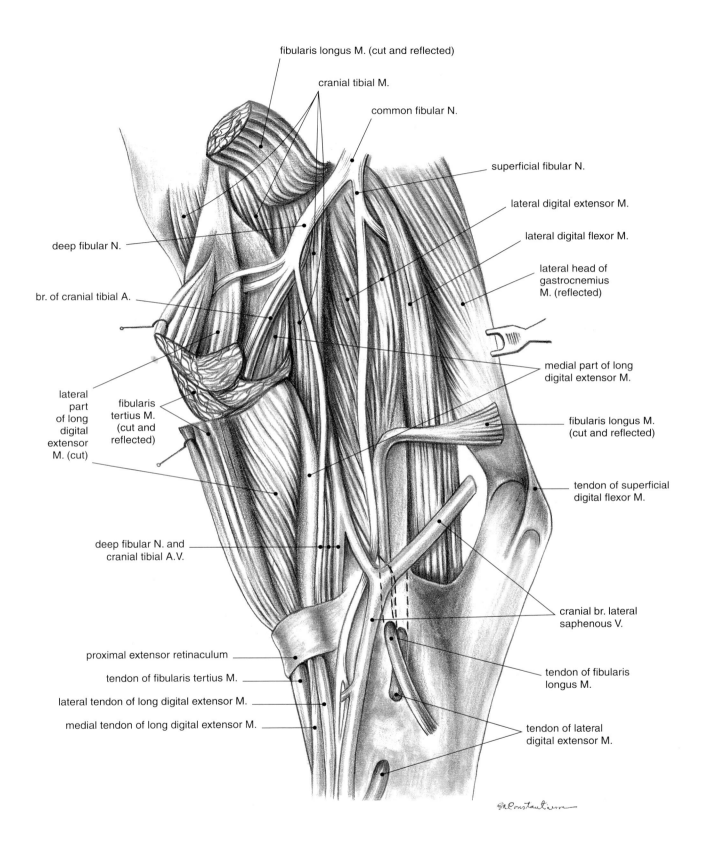

fibularis longus M. (cut and reflected)

cranial tibial M.

common fibular N.

superficial fibular N.

lateral digital extensor M.

lateral digital flexor M.

lateral head of gastrocnemius M. (reflected)

deep fibular N.

br. of cranial tibial A.

medial part of long digital extensor M.

lateral part of long digital extensor M. (cut)

fibularis tertius M. (cut and reflected)

fibularis longus M. (cut and reflected)

tendon of superficial digital flexor M.

deep fibular N. and cranial tibial A.V.

cranial br. lateral saphenous V.

proximal extensor retinaculum

tendon of fibularis tertius M.

lateral tendon of long digital extensor M.

medial tendon of long digital extensor M.

tendon of fibularis longus M.

tendon of lateral digital extensor M.

Fig. R 5.9. Left lateral aspect of crus, large ruminants.

*Notice* that the long digital extensor M. has two portions that continue as two distinct tendons, one medial, and one lateral. In some books there is a wrong classification of this muscle as the long digital extensor (the portion that continues with the lateral tendon) and the medial digital extensor (the portion that continues with the medial tendon).

On the caudal aspect of the stifle trace the **femoral A.** and its branches, then the **popliteal A.** which ends in the **cranial** and **caudal tibial Aa.** To better expose the cranial tibial A., transect the popliteus M. and continue the dissection of the popliteal A. *Notice* that the cranial tibial A. in the ox is at least twice as large as the caudal tibial A.

On the medial aspect of the crus, remove the crural fasciae and expose the superficial muscles, vessels, and nerves (Fig. R5.10A). The **medial saphenous V.** normally has only one branch, the **caudal branch**, which anastomoses with the lateral saphenous V.

To expose the **tibial N.** reflect the **saphenous A.** and **N.** and the medial saphenous V. and transect the distal attachments of the semitendinosus and semimembranosus Mm. (Fig. R5.10A).

In the tarsometatarsal area, dissect the tendons, vessels, and nerves on the lateral aspect (see Fig. R5.11A) and on the medial aspect (see Fig. R5.11B).

Dissect one by one the **stifle** and the **hock joints** in a similar manner to that used in the horse (see pages 140, 142–144). Disarticulate the joints and examine the bones.

Look at the location and the relationships of the **dewclaws** to the other structures.

## Modlab R2

*Anatomoclinical landmarks for physical examination and clinical approach to the pelvic limb in the large ruminants.*

Lame cows have been more susceptible to other diseases. Local and/or intraarticular analgesia is essential in the diagnosis or treatment of many causes of lameness. Pelvic limb analgesia, extending from immediately distal to the hock and including the digits, can be induced by desensitizing the common fibular and the tibial nerves.

The common fibular N. is approached immediately caudal to the lateral condyle of tibia as it courses in a cranioventral direction. This large nerve can be readily palpated in cattle with thin skin, making the injection site easy to identify.

The tibial N. can be palpated just between the deep and the superficial muscles of the caudal aspect of the crus, namely between the deep digital flexor and the common calcanean tendon. The site for desensitizing the tibial N. is about 10 cm proximal to the calcanean tuber. The tibial N. is highly myelinated, and although it lies closer to the medial aspect of the crus, where it is easier to block, it requires injections from both medial and lateral sides.

Knuckling is observed when the analgesic drug is injected around the common fibular N. and on the medial and lateral sides of the tibial N.

The sites for blocking these two nerves are shown in Figure R5.12.

The nerves supplying sensory innervation to the digit may be blocked with four separate injections, but this is technically more difficult than the common fibular and tibial nerve blocks already described. The four separate injections block specific nerves, all branches of the common fibular and tibial Nn. They are shown in Figure R5.13.

Under field conditions, it is often easier and simpler to perform a ring block in the upper third of the metatarsal region.

Intravenous regional analgesia, using either dorsal common digital V. III or the cranial and/or caudal branches of the lateral saphenous V., is the method of choice for performing most surgical digital procedures (see Fig. R5.14).

The injection into the lateral saphenous V. or any of its branches (cranial or caudal) is effective as long as the placement of the tourniquet is proximal to the site of injection (*a tourniquet is an instrument, usually a piece of flat or tubular rubber used for the compression of a blood vessel by application around a limb to prevent the flow of blood—in our case from the distal area*) (Fig. R5.14).

Arthroscopy, arthrocentesis, and intraarticular analgesia can be performed in all joints of the pelvic limb. The sites for those procedures are shown in Figures R5.15–R5.17.

The deep popliteal ln. is subject to meat inspection in the slaughterhouse and/or farmers' market.

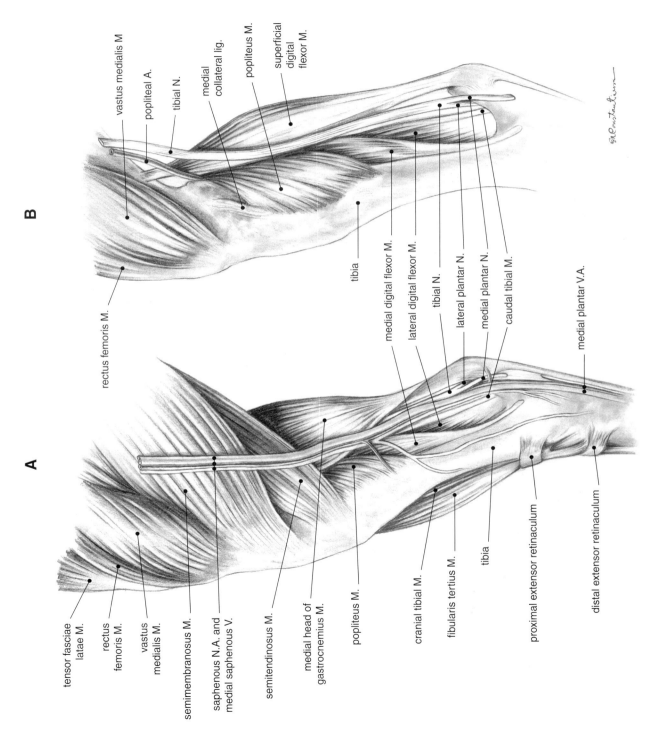

Fig. R5.10. Structures of the right crus, large ruminants. **A.** Medial aspect, superficial structures. **B.** Medial aspect, deep structures.

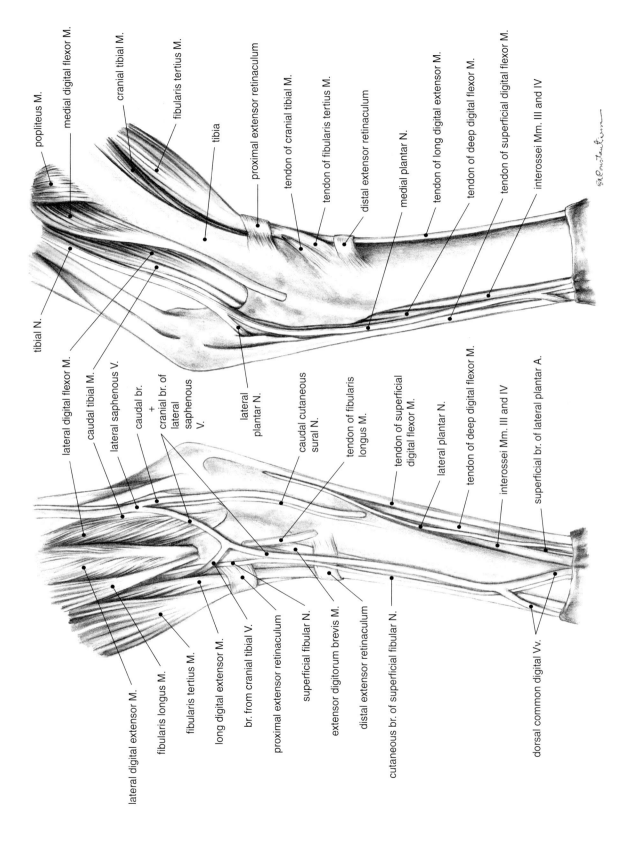

Fig. R5.11. Structures of left tarsometatarsal area, large ruminants. **A.** Lateral aspect. **B.** Medial aspect.

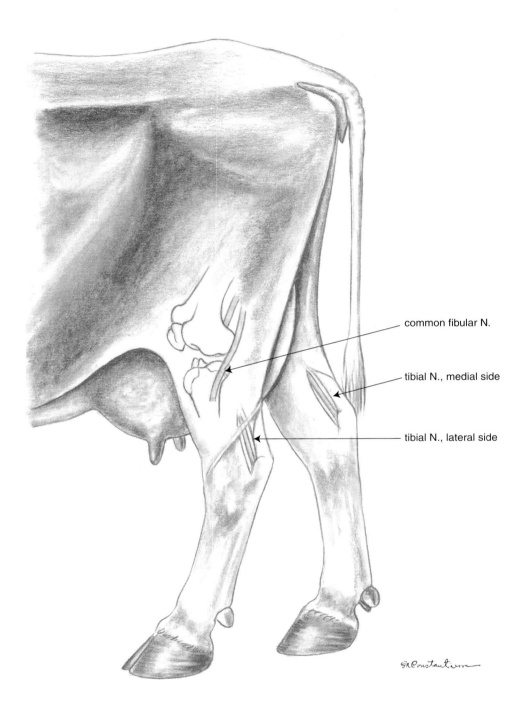

common fibular N.

tibial N., medial side

tibial N., lateral side

Fig. R5.12. Sites for blocking the common fibular and tibial nerves, large ruminants.

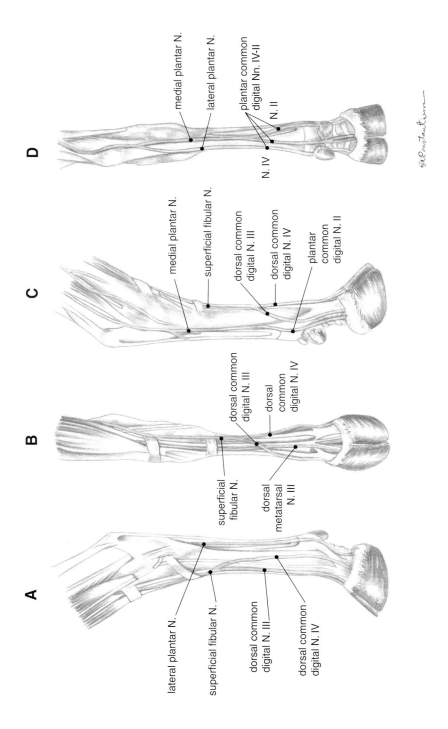

Fig. R5.13. Nerve block sites for digital analgesia, left pelvic limb, large ruminants. **A.** Lateral aspect. **B.** Dorsal aspect. **C.** Medial aspect. **D.** Plantar aspect.

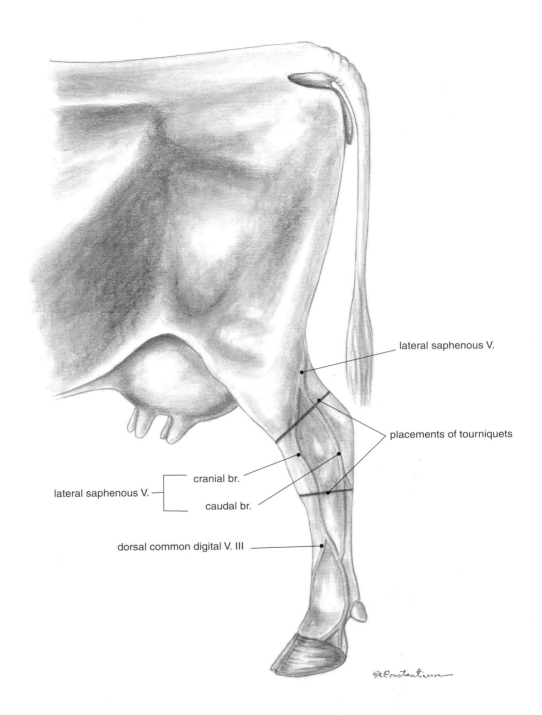

lateral saphenous V.

placements of tourniquets

lateral saphenous V. — cranial br.

caudal br.

dorsal common digital V. III

Fig. R5.14. Intravenous regional analgesia in the large ruminants, using the lateral saphenous vein.

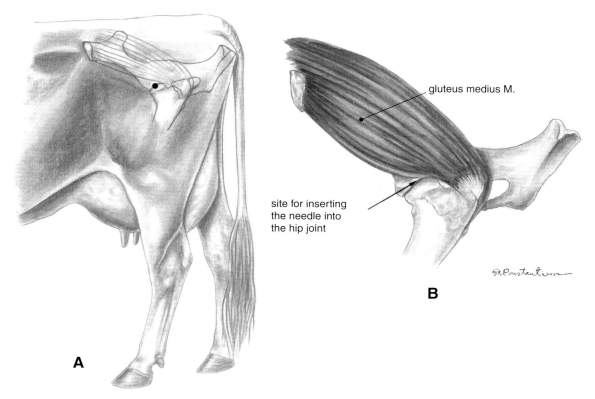

Fig. R5.15. Site for performing arthroscopy, arthrocentesis, and intraarticular analgesia in the hip joint of the ox. **A.** Hip joint. **B.** Anatomical structures involved.

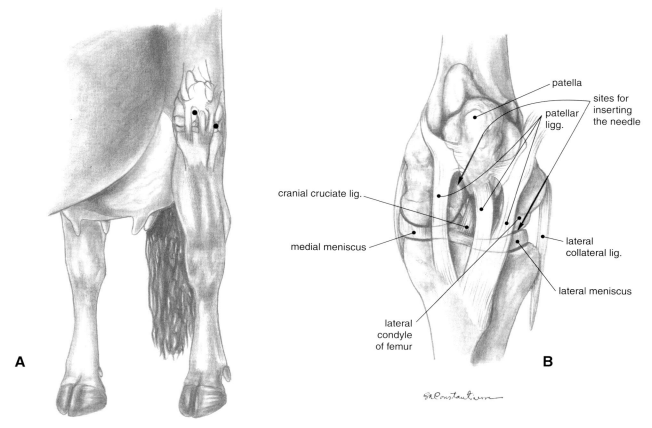

Fig. R5.16. Sites for performing arthroscopy, arthrocentesis, and intraarticular analgesia in the stifle joint of the ox. **A.** Stifle joint. **B.** Anatomy of the stifle joint (cranial aspect).

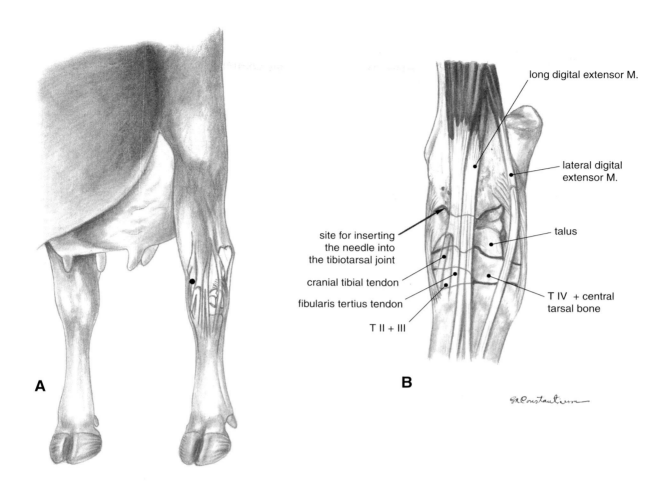

long digital extensor M.

lateral digital
extensor M.

site for inserting
the needle into
the tibiotarsal joint

talus

cranial tibial tendon

fibularis tertius tendon

T IV  + central
tarsal bone

T II + III

**A**

**B**

Fig. R5.17. Site for performing arthroscopy, arthrocentesis, and intraarticular analgesia in the hock joint of the ox. **A.** Hock joint. **B.** Anatomy of the hock (dorsal aspect).

# R 6

## The Thoracic Limb

Before starting the dissection look at the bones of a skeleton. The **scapula**, **humerus**, **radius and ulna**, **carpal bones, metacarpal bones**, and **phalanges and sesamoid bones** are illustrated in Figures R6.1–R6.6. The **scapulohumeral**, **elbow**, **carpal**, **fetlock**, and **digital joints** are illustrated in Figures R6.7–R6.10.

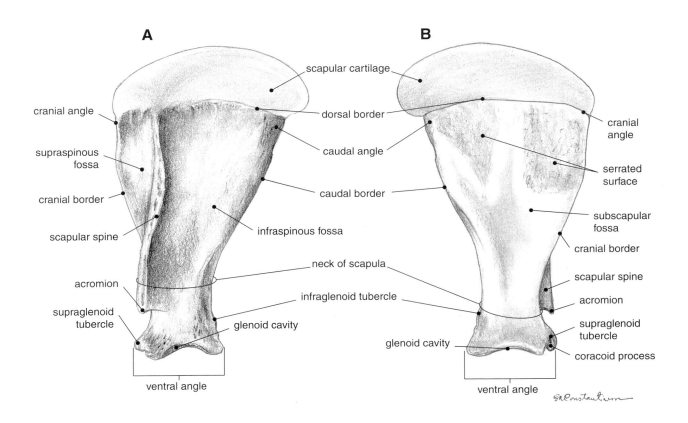

**A**

- scapular cartilage
- cranial angle
- supraspinous fossa
- dorsal border
- caudal angle
- cranial border
- caudal border
- scapular spine
- infraspinous fossa
- neck of scapula
- acromion
- infraglenoid tubercle
- supraglenoid tubercle
- glenoid cavity
- ventral angle

**B**

- scapular cartilage
- cranial angle
- serrated surface
- subscapular fossa
- caudal border
- cranial border
- scapular spine
- acromion
- glenoid cavity
- supraglenoid tubercle
- coracoid process
- ventral angle

Fig. R6.1. Left scapula, large ruminants. **A.** Lateral aspect. **B.** Medial aspect (costal surface).

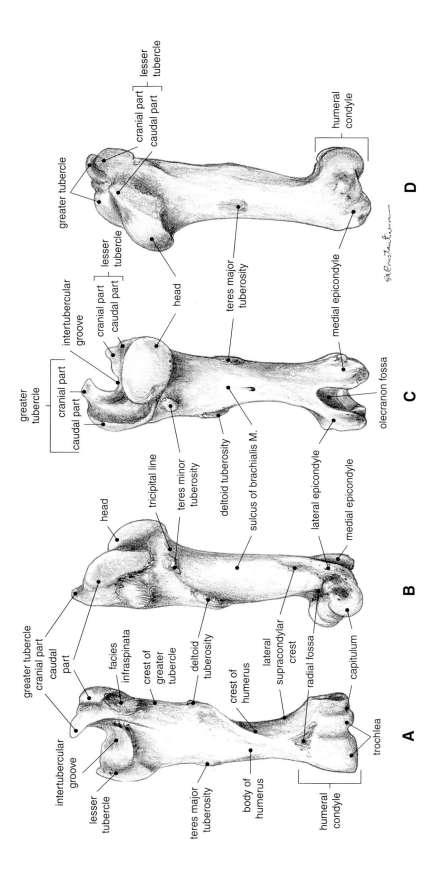

Fig. R6.2. Left humerus, large ruminants. **A**. Cranial aspect. **B**. Lateral aspect. **C**. Caudal aspect. **D**. Medial aspect.

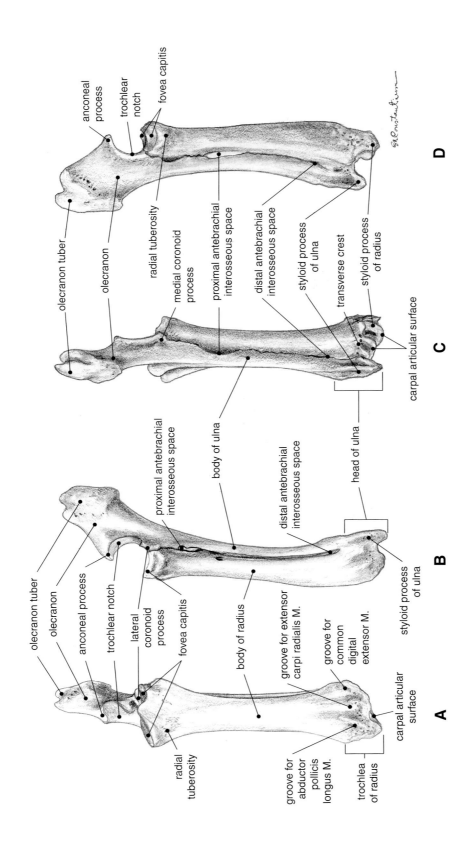

Fig. R6.3. Left radius and ulna, large ruminants. **A.** Cranial aspect. **B.** Lateral aspect. **C.** Caudal aspect. **D.** Medial aspect.

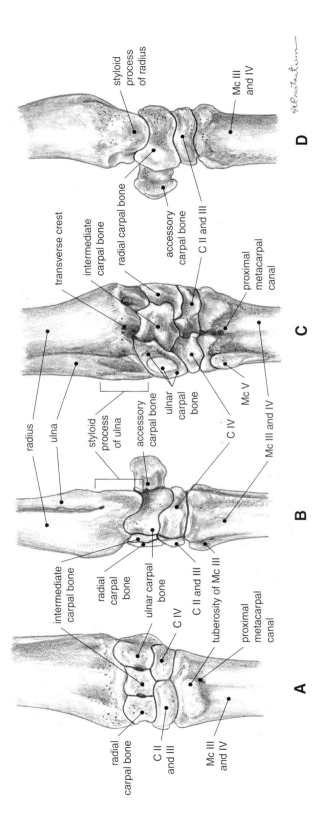

Fig. R6.4. Left carpal bones, large ruminants. **A.** Dorsal aspect. **B.** Lateral aspect. **C.** Palmar aspect (the accessory carpal bone has been removed). **D.** Medial aspect.

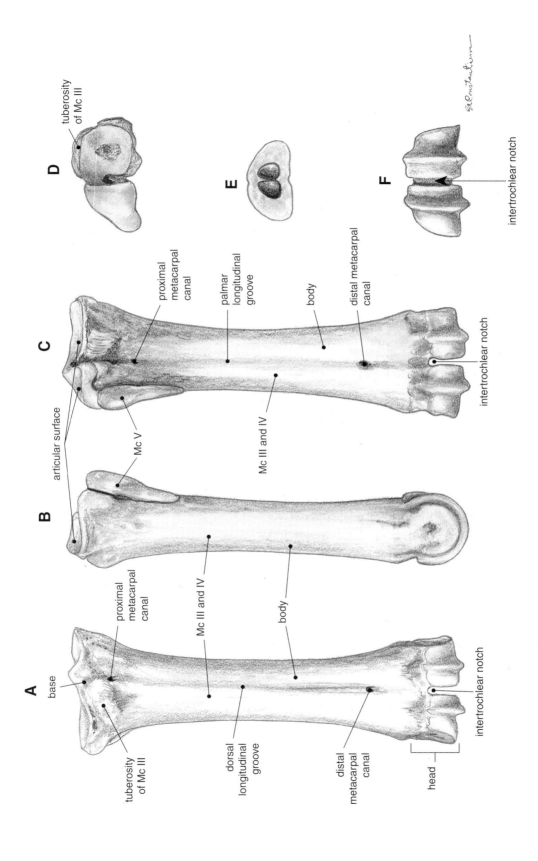

Fig. R6.5. Left metacarpal bones, large ruminants. **A.** Dorsal aspect. **B.** Lateral aspect. **C.** Palmar aspect. **D.** Articular surface of Mc III and IV (dorsal view). **E.** Transverse section through the body of Mc III and IV. **F.** Head of Mc III and IV (ventral view).

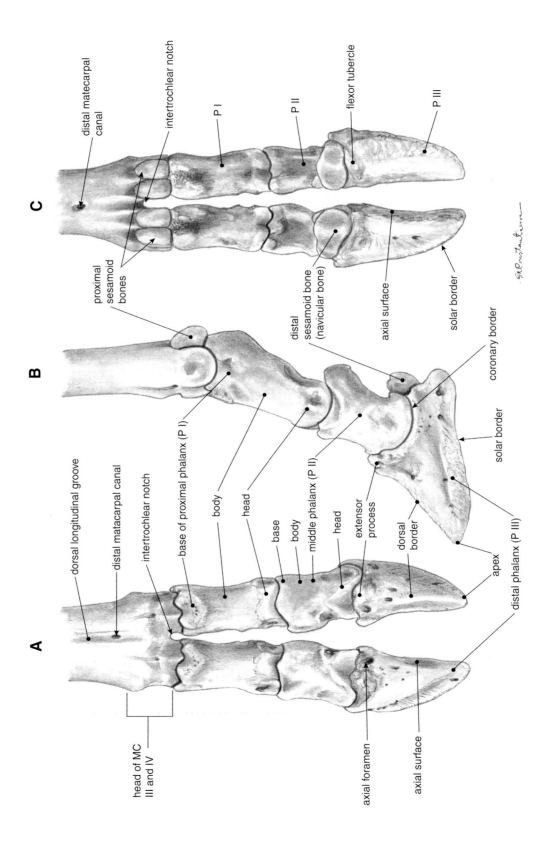

Fig. R6.6. Bones of the digits of the thoracic limb in the large ruminants. **A.** Dorsal aspect. **B.** Lateral aspect. **C.** Palmar aspect.

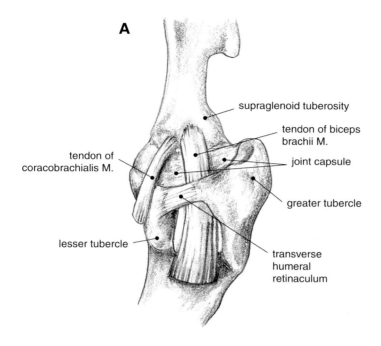

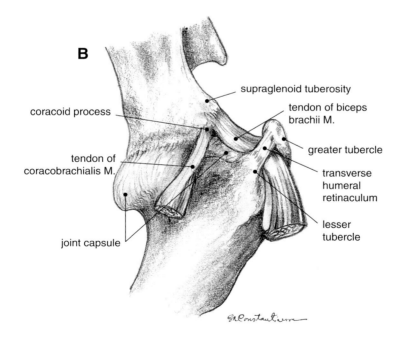

Fig. R6.7. Left scapulohumeral (shoulder) joint in the large ruminants. **A.** Cranial aspect. **B.** Medial aspect.

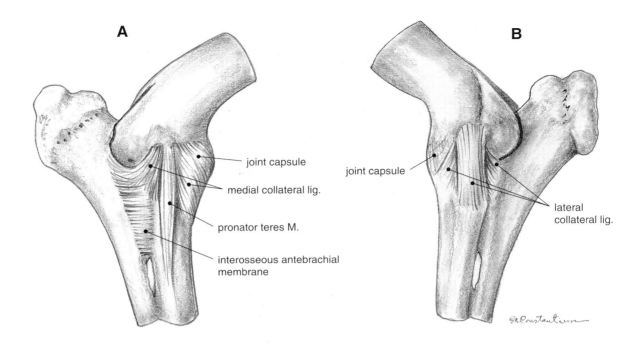

Fig. R6.8. Left humeroradioulnar (elbow) joint in the large ruminants. **A.** Medial aspect. **B.** Lateral aspect.

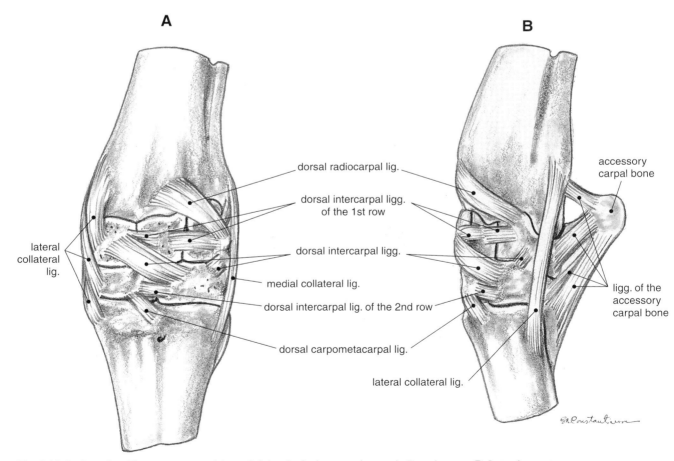

Fig. R6.9. Left antebrachiocarpometacarpal (carpal) joints in the large ruminants. **A.** Dorsal aspect. **B.** Lateral aspect.

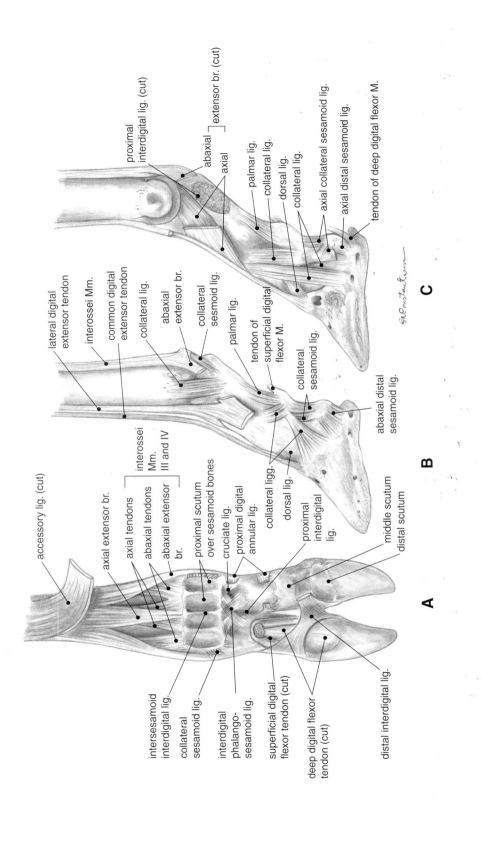

intersesamoid interdigital lig.

collateral sesamoid lig.

interdigital phalango-sesamoid lig.

superficial digital flexor tendon (cut)

deep digital flexor tendon (cut)

distal interdigital lig.

accessory lig. (cut)

axial extensor br.

axial tendons

abaxial tendons

abaxial extensor br.

interossei Mm. III and IV

proximal scutum over sesamoid bones

cruciate lig.

proximal digital annular lig.

collateral ligg.

dorsal lig.

proximal interdigital lig.

middle scutum

distal scutum

lateral digital extensor tendon

interossei Mm.

common digital extensor tendon

collateral lig.

abaxial extensor br.

collateral sesamoid lig.

palmar lig.

tendon of superficial digital flexor M.

collateral sesamoid lig.

abaxial distal sesamoid lig.

proximal interdigital lig. (cut)

abaxial ⎤ extensor br. (cut)
axial ⎦

palmar lig.

collateral lig.

dorsal lig.

collateral lig.

axial collateral sesamoid lig.

axial distal sesamoid lig.

tendon of deep digital flexor M.

**A**

**B**

**C**

Fig. R6.10. The interosseous muscles, digital ligaments, and tendons in the large ruminants. **A.** Palmar aspect. **B.** Abaxial aspect. **C.** Axial aspect.

*As in the horse, first identify the following clinically important structures used as landmarks, first on the lateral aspect, then on the medial aspect.*

*On the lateral aspect: the cranial and caudal angles of scapula, the scapular spine and the acromion, the supraglenoid tubercle, the greater tubercle of the humerus, the tendons of the biceps brachii and infraspinatus Mm., the deltoid tuberosity, the olecranon, the elbow, the lateral epicondyle of humerus, the accessory carpal bone, the carpal joint, the styloid process of ulna, the accessoriometacarpal lig., the metacarpal bones, the tendons of interossei Mm. III and IV, the deep digital flexor (DDF) and superficial digital flexor (SDF) Mm., the dewclaw, the fetlock joint, the pastern, the coronet, and the hoof. There are also in the forearm three external vertical grooves separating muscles from each other: the groove separating the extensor carpi radialis from the common digital extensor, the groove separating the common digital extensor from the lateral digital extensor, and the goove separating the lateral digital extensor from the extensor carpi ulnaris Mm. (in craniocaudal order).*

*On the medial aspect identify the elbow, the medial epicondyle of the humerus, the radial tuberosity, the body of the radius, the styloid process of the radius, the carpal joint, and the bones, joints, and tendons that were already identified on the lateral side of the forelimb. The vertical grooves separating the muscles, in craniocaudal order, are between the extensor carpi radialis M. and the radius, between the radius and the flexor carpi radialis M., and between the flexor carpi radialis and flexor carpi ulnaris Mm.*

Before beginning the dissection of the limb, review the systematization of the muscles and nerves listed in Tables R6.1 and R6.2.

In a manner similar to that used for the horse, skin the limb to the fetlock and remove the hoof, either with a saw and pliers or by boiling (see the procedure described in the section on the horse, page 165). Skin the digital area.

Turn the limb medial side up and identify the pectoral muscles, which were previously dissected and transected. *Notice* that in the large ruminants the **subclavius M.** is very small in comparison to that in the horse. It extends from the first costal cartilage to the medial aspect of the **brachiocephalicus M.**, just cranial to the shoulder joint (see Fig. R6.11).

Pull up the brachial plexus and attempt to identify the nerves in conjunction with the muscles. The same muscles, vessels, and nerves dissected in the horse are present in the cow. Identify the **axillary ln. of the first rib** on the medial aspect of the supraspinatus M. close to the shoulder joint (if it did not remain attached to the lateral wall of the thorax in the first intercostal space); it is sometimes

### Table R6.1. Muscles of the Thoracic Limb, Large Ruminants

**Shoulder**

*Lateral aspect*
– deltoideus
– supraspinatus
– infraspinatus
– teres minor

*Medial aspect*
– teres major
– subscapularis
– coracobrachialis

**Arm**

*Cranial aspect*
- biceps brachii
  • lacertus fibrosus
- brachialis

*Caudal aspect*
– triceps brachii
  • long head
  • lateral head
  • medial head
  • accessory head
– anconeus
– tensor fasciae antebrachii

**Forearm**

*Craniolateral aspect*
– extensor carpi radialis ⎫
– abductor pollicis longus ⎬ muscles with proximal action (to the carpus)
– extensor carpi ulnaris ⎭
  (ulnaris lateralis)
– common digital extensor ⎫
– lateral digital extensor ⎬ muscles with distal action (to the digit)
– accessory muscles of the ⎭
  common and lateral digital
  extensors

*Caudomedial aspect*
– flexor carpi ulnaris [with proximal action
  (to the carpus)]
  • humeral head
  • ulnar head
– flexor carpi radialis [with proximal action
  (to the carpus)]
– pronator teres (atrophied) [with proximal action
  (to the carpus)]
– superficial digital flexor [with distal action
  (to the digit)]
  • superficial part
  • deep part
  • sleeve at the level of metacarpophalangeal joint, by fusion
    with the accessory lig. of interossei Mm.
– deep digital flexor [with distal action (to the digit)]
  • humeral head
  • ulnar head
  • radial head
– interflexorii Mm.

**Autopodium**
– interossei lateralis and medialis Mm. (III and IV fused)
  • accessory lig. fused with the superficial digital flexor tendon

Table R6.2. Muscles and Nerve Supply, Thoracic Limb, Horse and Large Ruminants

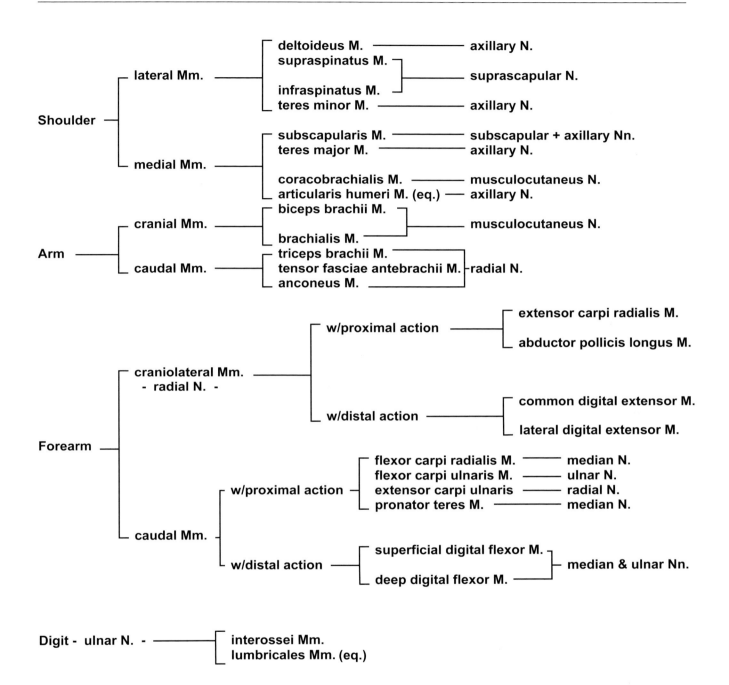

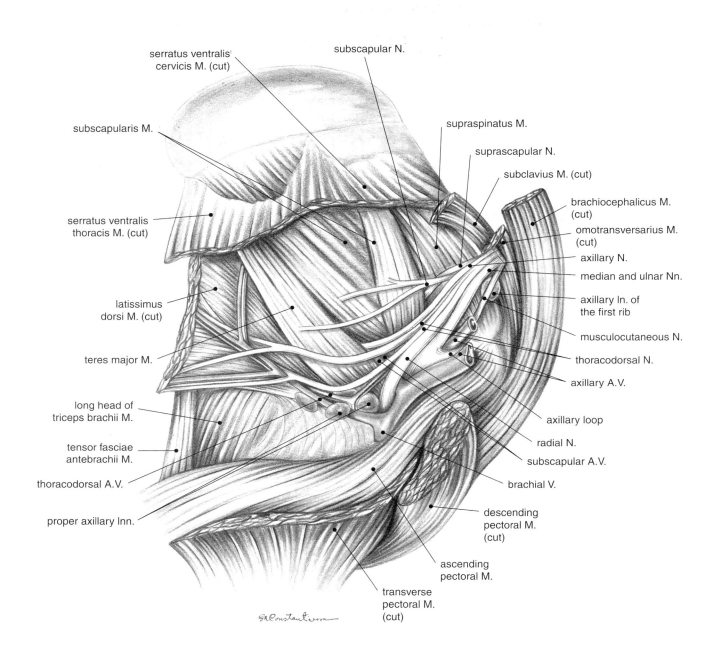

serratus ventralis
cervicis M. (cut)

subscapular N.

subscapularis M.

supraspinatus M.

suprascapular N.

subclavius M. (cut)

serratus ventralis
thoracis M. (cut)

brachiocephalicus M.
(cut)

omotransversarius M.
(cut)

axillary N.

median and ulnar Nn.

latissimus
dorsi M. (cut)

axillary ln. of
the first rib

musculocutaneous N.

teres major M.

thoracodorsal N.

axillary A.V.

long head of
triceps brachii M.

axillary loop

radial N.

tensor fasciae
antebrachii M.

subscapular A.V.

brachial V.

thoracodorsal A.V.

descending
pectoral M.
(cut)

proper axillary lnn.

ascending
pectoral M.

transverse
pectoral M.
(cut)

Fig. R6.11. Brachial plexus and adjacent structures of left thoracic limb, large ruminants, medial aspect.

absent. The **proper axillary lnn.** are located caudal to the shoulder joint. The **accessory axillary ln.,** often absent, is located on the dorsal border of the **ascending pectoral M.** Dissect all structures shown in Figure R6.11.

*Notice* that *no* **cubital ln.** is present in the large ruminants, as it is in the horse.

Separate and remove the pectoral muscles to expose the medial aspect of the arm. Identify and dissect the following structures of the shoulder in a craniocaudal order: the **supraspinatus, subscapularis, teres major,** and **latissimus dorsi Mm.** The **suprascapular A., V.,** and **N.** penetrate between the supraspinatus and subscapularis Mm. The **subscapular N.** supplies the muscle with the same name. The **axillary N.** and **subscapular A.** and **V.** penetrate between the subscapularis and teres major Mm. (see Fig. R6.12).

In the brachial area, identify, in the same craniocaudal order, the **biceps brachii, coracobrachialis,** and **tensor fasciae antebrachii Mm.** (in the superficial layer) (see Fig. R6.12), the **brachialis M.,** and the **long, medial and accessory heads of the triceps brachii M.** (in the deep layer). To expose the origin of the biceps brachii M., transect the supraspinatus M. at the level of the suprascapular N. Dissect the deep aspect of the distal part of the muscle and reflect it. Transect its medial attachment on the **lesser tubercle of the humerus** and expose the **intertubercular bursa** under the tendon of the biceps brachii M. *Notice* that the tendon is bound down by the **transverse humeral retinaculum,** in a manner similar to that seen in the dog (see Fig. R6.7).

The **brachial A.** and **V.** run parallel to the caudal border of the coracobrachialis M., accompanied by the **musculocutaneous, median, ulnar,** and **radial Nn.** *Notice* that there is a loop between the musculocutaneous and median Nn., called **axillary loop,** around the **axillary A.** The **proximal muscular branch of the musculocutaneous N.** penetrates between the two portions of the coracobrachialis M., accompanied by the **cranial circumflex humeral A.** and **V.,** and ends in the biceps brachii M. The **distal muscular branch of the musculocutaneous N.** supplies the **brachialis M.** It is accompanied by the **bicipital A.** and **V.** and the **transverse cubital A.** (Fig. R6.13).

Identify the **deep brachial A.** and **V.,** accompanied by the radial N., on their way between the humerus, **triceps brachii, teres major,** and **latissimus dorsi Mm.** (see Fig. R6.12). Proximal to the elbow, identify the **collateral ulnar A.** and **V.** (see Fig. R6.17).

Turn the limb lateral side up. Identify the **cleidobrachialis M.** (the caudal component of the **brachiocephalicus M.),** separated from the **descending pectoral M.** by the **cephalic V.** Reflect both muscles to expose the attachment of the ascending pectoral M. on the greater tubercle of the humerus, and the tendon of the biceps brachii M. Identify the **deltoideus M.** with both the **acromial** and **scapular parts.** Do not attempt to separate the aponeurotic fusion of the scapular part with the **axillary fascia.** *Notice* that the axillary fascia intermingles with the **infraspinatus M.** First, carefully outline the caudal border of the scapular part of the deltoideus M. and save the **axillary N.** on its way to supply the brachiocephalicus M. and then become the **cranial cutaneous antebrachial N.** The axillary N. is accompanied by the **caudal circumflex humeral A.** Carefully separate the long head from the **lateral head** of the triceps brachii M. to save the **lateral cutaneous antebrachial N.** (branch of the radial N.), several centimeters caudal to the cranial cutaneous antebrachial N. (see Fig. R6.14).

Transect the deltoideus M. from the **deltoid tuberosity** and reflect it to fully expose the axillary N. Transect the lateral head of the triceps brachii M. in the middle, reflect the stumps, and expose the radial N. and the **collateral radial A.** (and **V.**) (see Fig. R6.15).

Transect the (superficial) tendon of the infraspinatus M., leaving a short portion attached to the **facies infraspinata.** Reflect the muscle and explore the **subtendinous bursa of the infraspinatus M.,** between the reflected tendon and the caudal part of the **greater tubercle of the humerus.** There is, in addition, a deep part of the tendon, attached to the border of the greater tubercle. Caudal and deep to the infraspinatus M., identify the **teres minor M.** The joint capsule of the shoulder is overlapped by these two muscles (see Fig. R6.16).

Turn the limb again so the medial side is up. Continue the dissection of the cephalic V. caudoventrally in an oblique direction, accompanied by the cranial cutaneous antebrachial N. and the **medial cutaneous antebrachial N.** The latter joins the vein after exiting between the biceps brachii M. and the **lacertus fibrosus** (see Fig. R6.17).

*Remember!* The lacertus fibrosus is the connection between the tendons of the biceps brachii and extensor carpi radialis Mm. and is a landmark for blocking the medial cutaneous antebrachial N.

The cephalic V. is the result of the confluence between the **accessory cephalic V.** and the **radial V.** (see Fig. R6.17).

On the medial aspect of the elbow identify the median N. and the brachial A. and V. crossing the site and entering under the **pronator teres** and **flexor carpi radialis Mm.,** accompanied by the **median cubital V.** (see Fig. R6.17). Identify and dissect all structures shown in Figure R6.17.

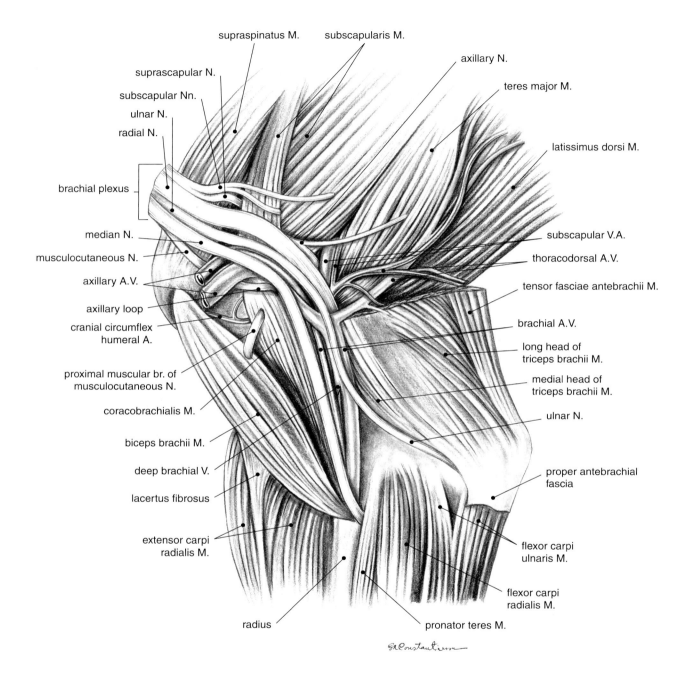

supraspinatus M.

subscapularis M.

axillary N.

suprascapular N.

teres major M.

subscapular Nn.

latissimus dorsi M.

ulnar N.

radial N.

brachial plexus

median N.

subscapular V.A.

musculocutaneous N.

thoracodorsal A.V.

axillary A.V.

tensor fasciae antebrachii M.

axillary loop

brachial A.V.

cranial circumflex
humeral A.

long head of
triceps brachii M.

medial head of
triceps brachii M.

proximal muscular br. of
musculocutaneous N.

ulnar N.

coracobrachialis M.

biceps brachii M.

proper antebrachial
fascia

deep brachial V.

lacertus fibrosus

flexor carpi
ulnaris M.

extensor carpi
radialis M.

flexor carpi
radialis M.

radius

pronator teres M.

Fig. R6.12. Vessels and nerves of medial shoulder and arm, and adjacent structures of right thoracic limb, large ruminants.

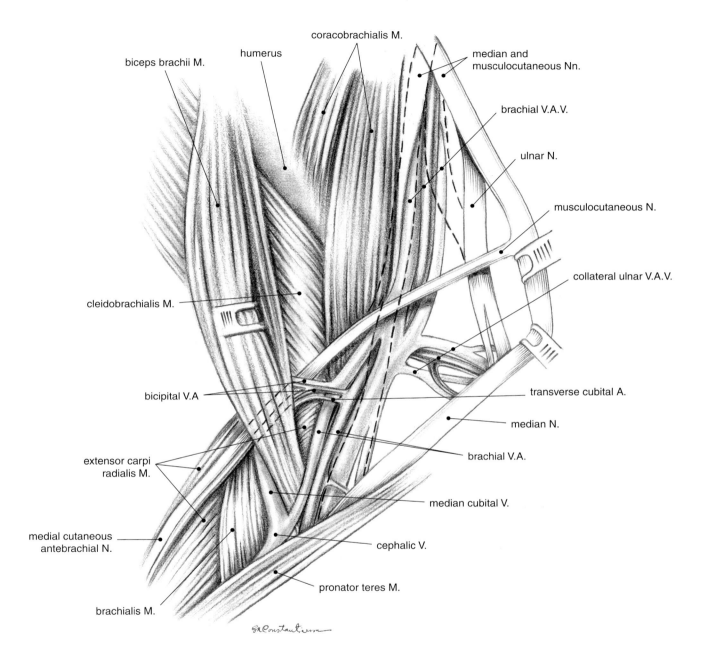

Fig. R6.13. Vessels, nerves, and muscles of elbow of right thoracic limb, large ruminants, medial aspect.

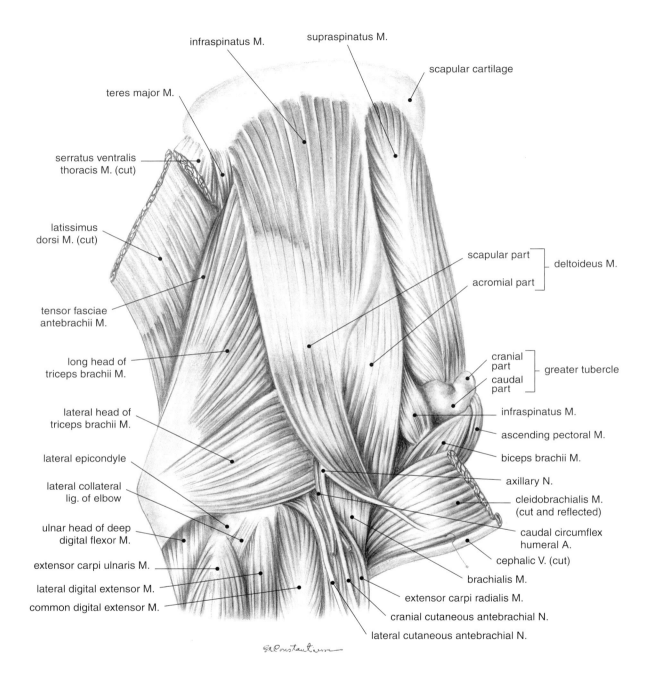

infraspinatus M.

supraspinatus M.

scapular cartilage

teres major M.

serratus ventralis
thoracis M. (cut)

latissimus
dorsi M. (cut)

tensor fasciae
antebrachii M.

long head of
triceps brachii M.

lateral head of
triceps brachii M.

lateral epicondyle

lateral collateral
lig. of elbow

ulnar head of deep
digital flexor M.

extensor carpi ulnaris M.

lateral digital extensor M.

common digital extensor M.

scapular part ⎤
acromial part ⎦ deltoideus M.

cranial
part ⎤
caudal
part ⎦ greater tubercle

infraspinatus M.

ascending pectoral M.

biceps brachii M.

axillary N.

cleidobrachialis M.
(cut and reflected)

caudal circumflex
humeral A.

cephalic V. (cut)

brachialis M.

extensor carpi radialis M.

cranial cutaneous antebrachial N.

lateral cutaneous antebrachial N.

Fig. R6.14. Superficial structures of lateral shoulder of right thoracic limb, large ruminants.

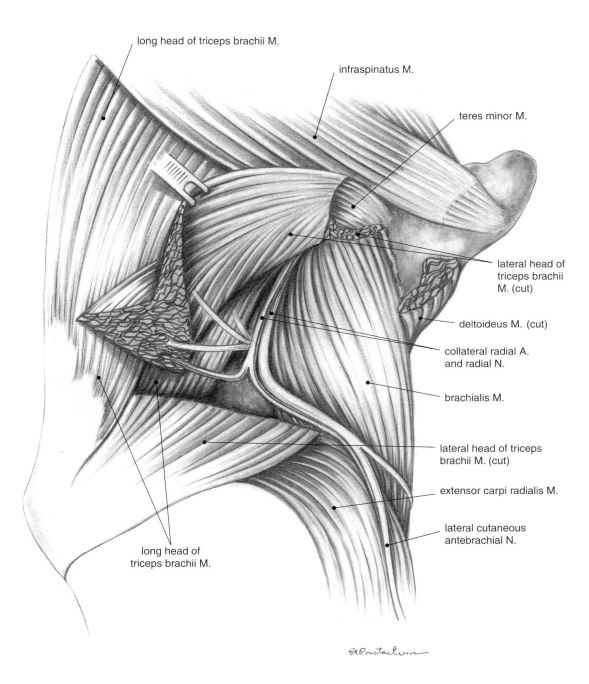

long head of triceps brachii M.

infraspinatus M.

teres minor M.

lateral head of triceps brachii M. (cut)

deltoideus M. (cut)

collateral radial A. and radial N.

brachialis M.

lateral head of triceps brachii M. (cut)

extensor carpi radialis M.

lateral cutaneous antebrachial N.

long head of triceps brachii M.

Fig. R6.15. Deep structures of right lateral shoulder, large ruminants.

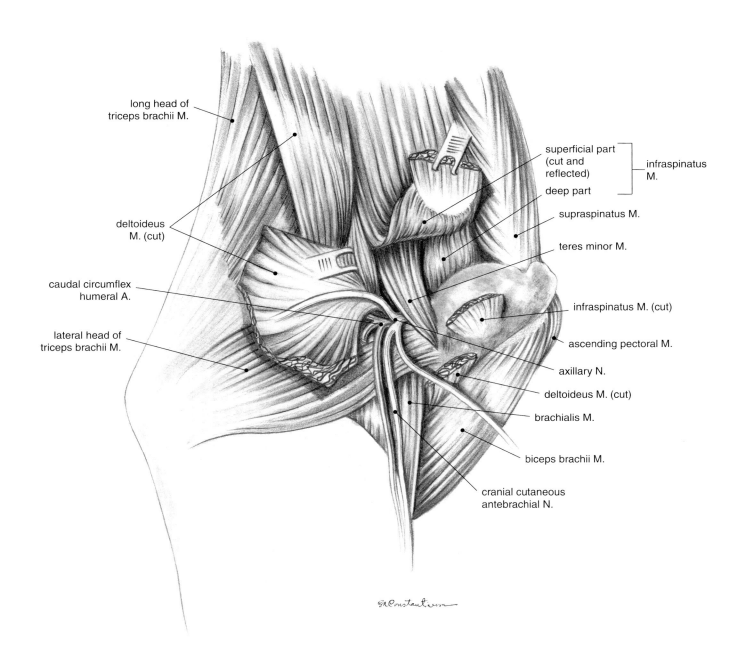

long head of
triceps brachii M.

superficial part
(cut and
reflected)
deep part

infraspinatus
M.

supraspinatus M.

deltoideus
M. (cut)

teres minor M.

caudal circumflex
humeral A.

infraspinatus M. (cut)

ascending pectoral M.

lateral head of
triceps brachii M.

axillary N.

deltoideus M. (cut)

brachialis M.

biceps brachii M.

cranial cutaneous
antebrachial N.

Fig. R6.16. Deeper structures of right lateral shoulder, large ruminants.

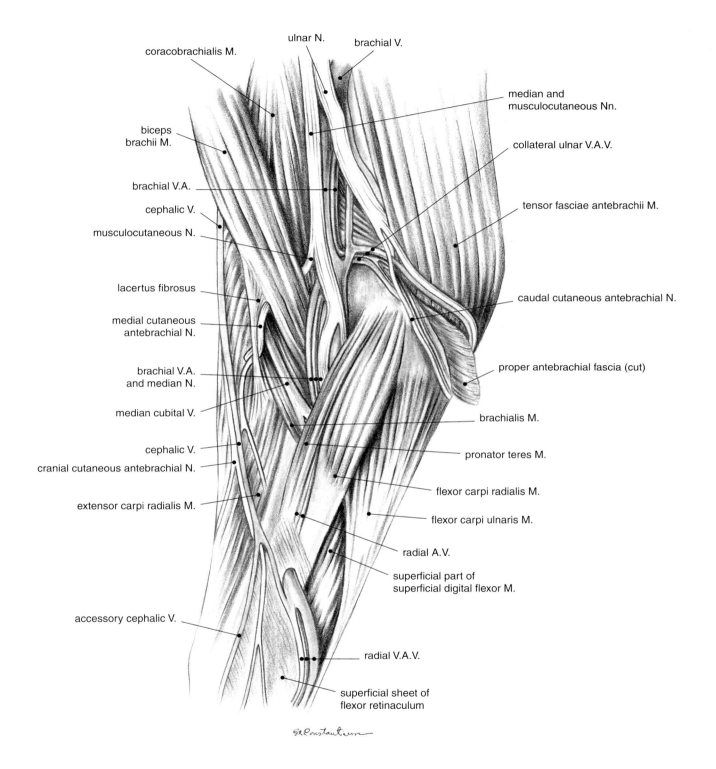

coracobrachialis M.

ulnar N.

brachial V.

median and
musculocutaneous Nn.

collateral ulnar V.A.V.

biceps
brachii M.

brachial V.A.

cephalic V.

tensor fasciae antebrachii M.

musculocutaneous N.

lacertus fibrosus

medial cutaneous
antebrachial N.

caudal cutaneous antebrachial N.

brachial V.A.
and median N.

proper antebrachial fascia (cut)

median cubital V.

brachialis M.

cephalic V.

pronator teres M.

cranial cutaneous antebrachial N.

flexor carpi radialis M.

extensor carpi radialis M.

flexor carpi ulnaris M.

radial A.V.

superficial part of
superficial digital flexor M.

accessory cephalic V.

radial V.A.V.

superficial sheet of
flexor retinaculum

Fig. R6.17. Superficial structures of the arm and forearm of the right thoracic limb, large ruminants, medial aspect.

Transect the **flexor carpi radialis M.** in the middle and reflect the stumps. The last branches of the **brachial A.**, the distribution of the **median N.**, and the **median** and **radial Aa.** are shown in Figure R6.18. The **superficial** and **deep parts of the superficial digital flexor (SDF) M.** are also exposed (Fig. R6.19). Identify and dissect all structures shown in Figures R6.18 and R6.19.

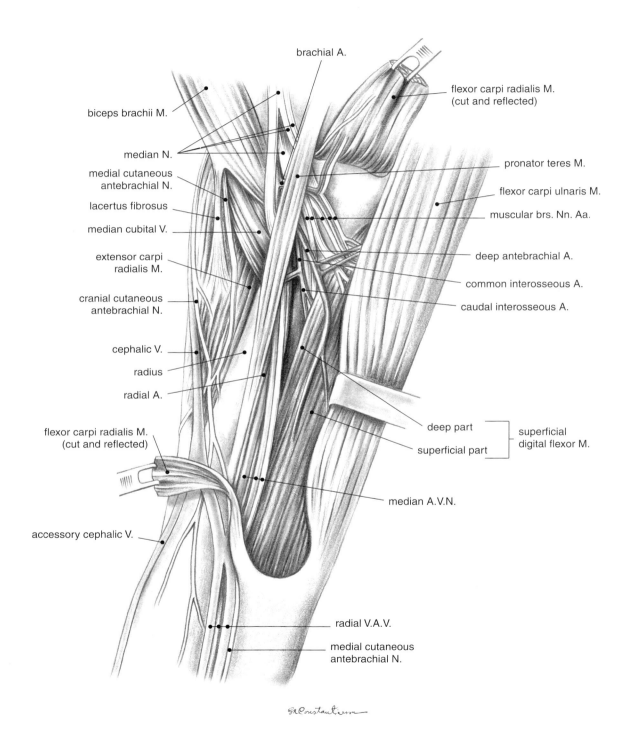

Fig. R6.18. Deep structures of the elbow and forearm of the right thoracic limb, large ruminants, medial aspect.

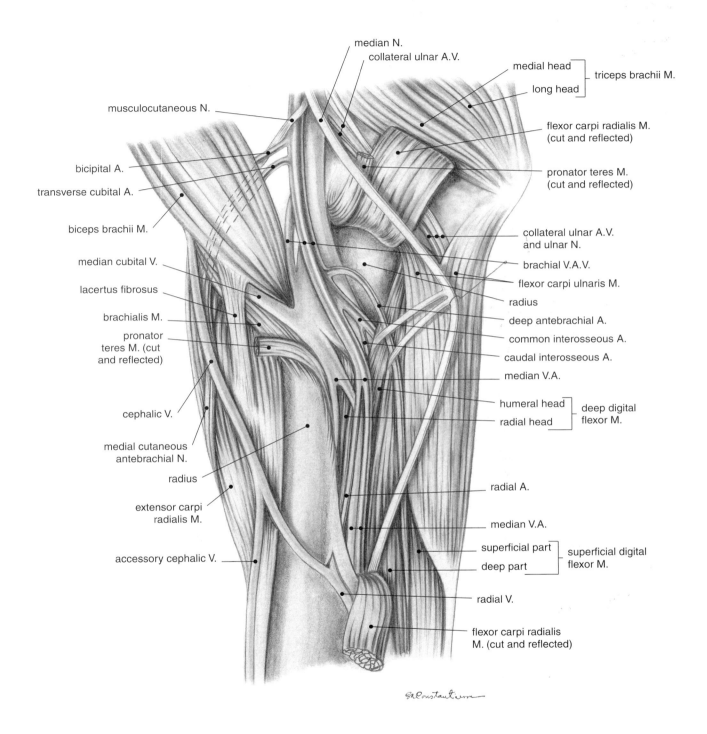

median N.
collateral ulnar A.V.
medial head
long head
triceps brachii M.
musculocutaneous N.
flexor carpi radialis M.
(cut and reflected)
bicipital A.
pronator teres M.
(cut and reflected)
transverse cubital A.
biceps brachii M.
collateral ulnar A.V.
and ulnar N.
median cubital V.
brachial V.A.V.
lacertus fibrosus
flexor carpi ulnaris M.
radius
brachialis M.
deep antebrachial A.
pronator
teres M. (cut
and reflected)
common interosseous A.
caudal interosseous A.
median V.A.
cephalic V.
humeral head
deep digital
flexor M.
radial head
medial cutaneous
antebrachial N.
radius
radial A.
extensor carpi
radialis M.
median V.A.
superficial part
superficial digital
flexor M.
deep part
accessory cephalic V.
radial V.
flexor carpi radialis
M. (cut and reflected)

Fig. R6.19. Deeper structures of right elbow and forearm, large ruminants, medial aspect.

Transect the **flexor carpi ulnaris M.** and reflect the stumps. Separate the two parts of the SDF and expose the **humeral head**, the **ulnar head**, and the **radial head of the deep digital flexor (DDF) M.** Identify the **interflexorii Mm.,** which connect the humeral head of the DDF and the deep part of SDF (Fig. R6.20).

Trace the ulnar N. from the elbow to the carpus on the caudal border of the forearm. It runs between the flexor carpi ulnaris and the **extensor carpi ulnaris Mm.** Before leaving the elbow, the ulnar N. delivers the **caudal cutaneous antebrachial N.** (see Fig. R6.17). Proximal to the carpus, the ulnar N. splits into the **dorsal branch** and the **palmar branch**.

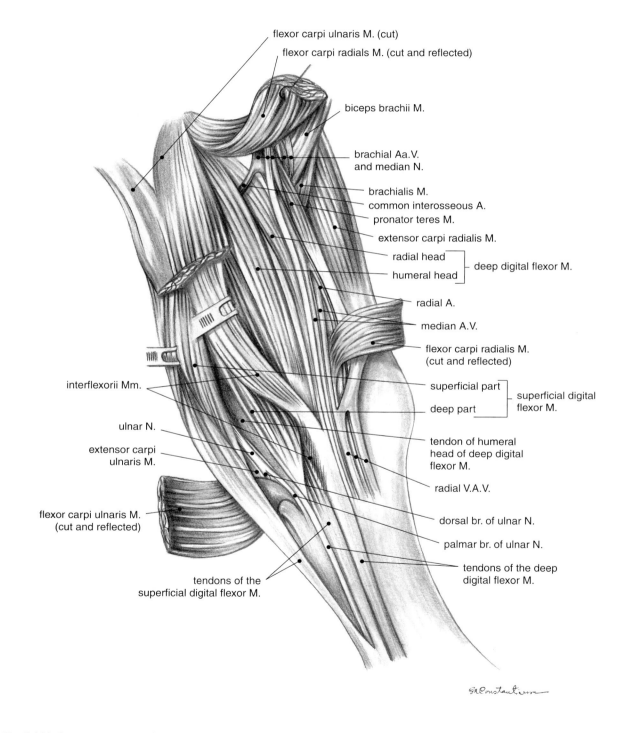

Fig. R6.20. Deepest structures of right forearm, large ruminants, medial aspect.

Turn the limb lateral side up. Remove the antebrachial fascia and expose the muscles shown in Figure R6.21. Pay attention to the **common digital extensor M.,** consisting of two parts that continue with two separate tendons, one lateral and one medial. These two tendons and the tendon of the **lateral digital extensor M.** will be shown on the dorsal aspect of the digits.

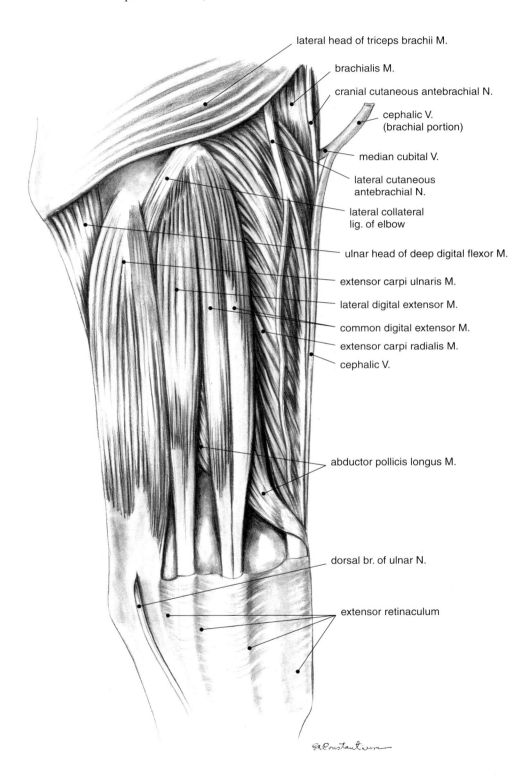

lateral head of triceps brachii M.

brachialis M.

cranial cutaneous antebrachial N.

cephalic V.
(brachial portion)

median cubital V.

lateral cutaneous
antebrachial N.

lateral collateral
lig. of elbow

ulnar head of deep digital flexor M.

extensor carpi ulnaris M.

lateral digital extensor M.

common digital extensor M.

extensor carpi radialis M.

cephalic V.

abductor pollicis longus M.

dorsal br. of ulnar N.

extensor retinaculum

Fig. R6.21. Superficial structures of right forearm, large ruminants, lateral aspect.

Transect the common digital extensor M. and reflect the stumps to expose the **accessory M. of the common digital extensor M.** (not listed in the *N.A.V.*) and all the other structures illustrated in Figure R6.22.

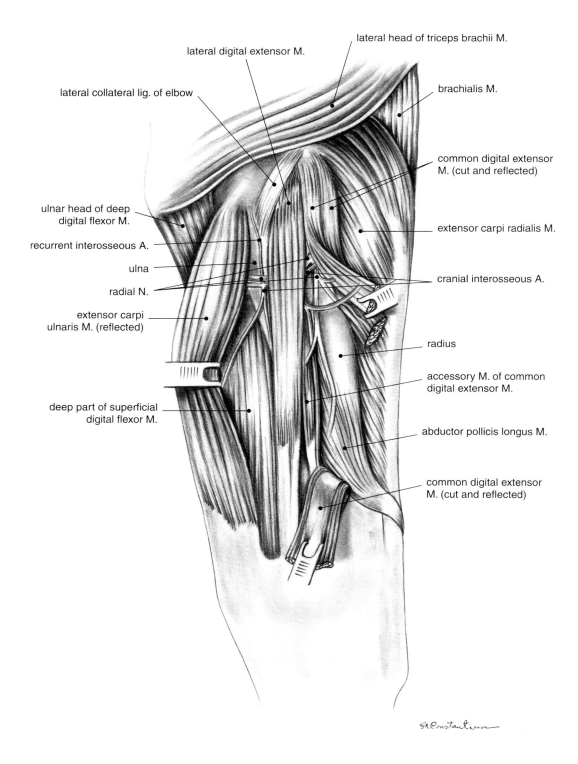

Fig. R6.22. Deep structures of right forearm, large ruminants, lateral aspect.

Turn the limb so the dorsal side of the autopodium is up. *Remember!* The cranial aspect of the autopodium is called "dorsal," while the caudal aspect is called "palmar."

The continuation of the antebrachial fascia on the dorsal carpal area is called the **extensor retinaculum**. It binds down all tendons gliding over the carpus, between the retinaculum and the dorsal carpal joint capsule. As in the horse, separating walls are built up between the retinaculum and the joint capsule. They allow each tendon to glide within one space surrounded by its tendon sheath, with the exception of both tendons of the common digital extensor, which pass together within one space.

Trace the three extensor tendons in the metacarpal and the digital areas and notice that the lateral tendon of the common digital extensor M. splits in the digital area into two symmetrical thin and cylindrical tendons. They end on the **extensor processes** of the third phalanges of digits III and IV. The medial tendon of the common digital extensor M. and the tendon of the lateral digital extensor M. are wide, thin, and symmetrical, and they attach on the dorsal aspect of all phalanges.

The attachments of all tendons on the proximal sesamoid bones and phalanges are shown in Figure R6.23. Around the fetlock, the lateral tendon of the common digital extensor M. and the tendon of the lateral digital extensor M. fuse with the corresponding **axial** and **abaxial extensor branches of the interossei Mm.** Dissect them with the accompanying vessels and nerves (see Fig. R6.24A).

*Note.* The **autopodium** includes the **basipodium** (the carpal or tarsal region), the **metapodium** (the metacarpal or metatarsal region), and the **acropodium** (the digital regions).

According to the *Nomina Anatomica Veterinaria,* the generic names of the arteries, veins, and nerves of the autopodium are as follows.

The superficial Aa., Vv., and Nn. of the metapodium are designated *common digital.* The deep structures are termed *metacarpal/metatarsal.* Digital structures that originate from the bifurcation of common digital Aa., Vv., and Nn. are called *proper digital.* They are called *axial/abaxial* in species with more than one digit. The abaxial digital vessels of the most lateral and/or medial digits originate from other sources and are called *abaxial digital.* Digital Nn. originating from some other source than the bifurcation of the common digital Nn. are called simply *digital.*

In the large ruminants, on the dorsal aspect of the metapodium, identify the **superficial branch of the radial N.,** branching into **dorsal common digital Nn. II** and **III,** and the **dorsal branch of the ulnar N.,** becoming **dorsal common digital N. IV.** The axial and abaxial digital nerves are named as shown in Figure 6.24A. The superficial branch of the radial N. and the dorsal common digital N. III are paralleled by **dorsal common digital V. III,** similar to the **dorsal common digital V. IV** that accompanies its corresponding nerve. **Dorsal metacarpal A. III** is protected within the **dorsal longitudinal groove of metacarpal bone III–IV.** It will anastomose with the **interdigital A.**

Turn the limb so that the palmar aspect of the autopodium is up. The **proper (deep) antebrachial fascia** continues in the carpal area as the **flexor retinaculum.** The flexor retinaculum has two sheets: superficial and deep. Between the two sheets passes the superficial part of the SDF tendon, accompanied by a bursa. Make a vertical incision through the superficial sheet of the flexor retinaculum and expose this tendon and its tendon sheath. Trace the cephalic V. proximal to the carpus and make an incision through the same sheet of the flexor retinaculum to expose the **radial V.,** which is the origin of the cephalic V. Also expose the **radial A.**

Make a vertical incision through the deep sheet of the flexor retinaculum and open the **carpal canal.** Identify the deep part of the SDF tendon and the tendon of the DDF. They are protected by individual bursae. The median A., V., and N. accompany the tendons (see Fig. R6.25).

The **palmar fascia** is thick and is firmly attached to the borders of **metacarpal bones III** and **IV** and the borders of the **interossei Mm.** Make a midlongitudinal incision through the fascia and expose the two tendons of the SDF that fuse in a unique tendon in the middle of metacarpus. After fusion, the SDF bifurcates and sends one tendon for each digit. Each tendon of the SDF is fused with the corresponding accessory lig. of interossei Mm. III and IV. By fusing with each other, they provide a symmetrical sleeve proximal to the fetlock joint for the DDF tendons to pass through.

In the distal third of the metacarpal area, the median N. splits into a **medial** and a **lateral branch.** The medial branch bifurcates into **palmar common digital N. II** and **axial palmar digital N. III.** The lateral branch gives off the **axial palmar digital N. IV** and a **communicating branch** to **palmar common digital N. IV.** A **communicating branch** between the two branches of the median N. may also be present, obliquely crossing the median A. and V. (see Fig. R6.25). The axial and abaxial digital (proper) Nn. are named according to the previously shown rules (see Fig. R6.24B).

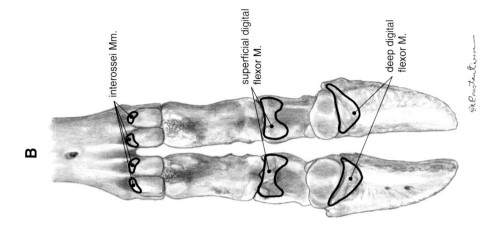

interossei Mm.

superficial digital
flexor M.

deep digital
flexor M.

**B**

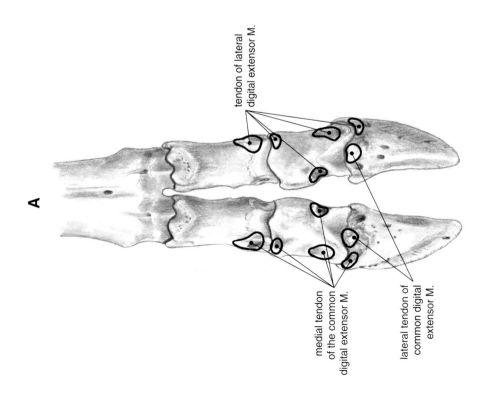

tendon of lateral
digital extensor M.

**A**

medial tendon
of the common
digital extensor M.

lateral tendon of
common digital
extensor M.

Fig. R6.23. Areas of tendinous attachments on phalanges and sesamoid bones, left thoracic limb, large ruminants. **A.** Dorsal aspect. **B.** Palmar aspect.

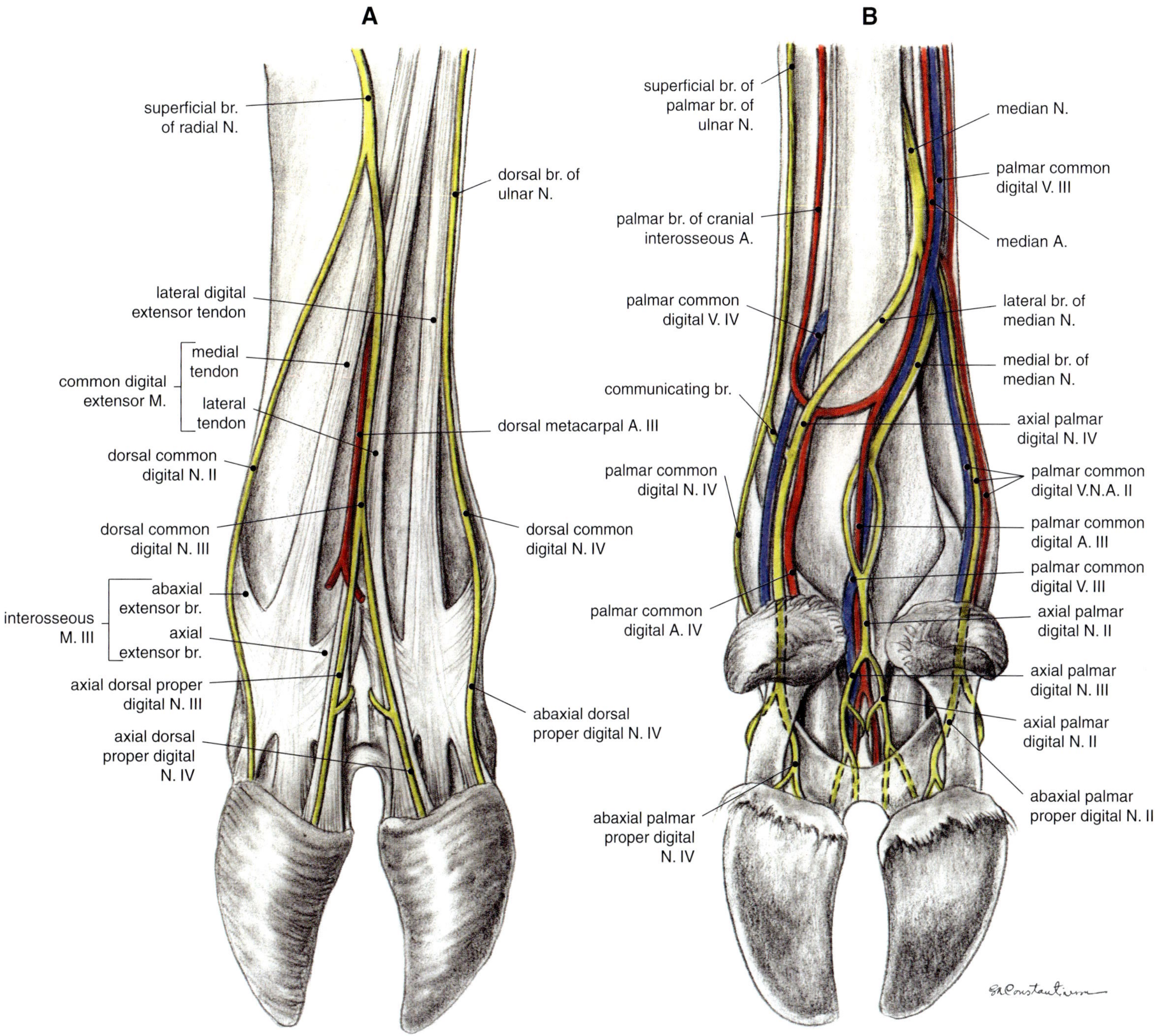

**B**

median N.

palmar common
digital V. III

median A.

lateral br. of
median N.

medial br. of
median N.

axial palmar
digital N. IV

palmar common
digital V.N.A. II

palmar common
digital A. III

palmar common
digital V. III

axial palmar
digital N. II

axial palmar
digital N. III

axial palmar
digital N. II

abaxial palmar
proper digital N. II

superficial br. of
palmar br. of
ulnar N.

palmar br. of cranial
interosseous A.

palmar common
digital V. IV

communicating br.

dorsal metacarpal A. III

palmar common
digital N. IV

dorsal common
digital N. IV

palmar common
digital A. IV

abaxial dorsal
proper digital N. IV

abaxial palmar
proper digital
N. IV

**A**

dorsal br. of
ulnar N.

superficial br.
of radial N.

lateral digital
extensor tendon

medial
tendon

lateral
tendon

common digital
extensor M.

dorsal common
digital N. II

dorsal common
digital N. III

interosseous
M. III

abaxial
extensor br.

axial
extensor br.

axial dorsal proper
digital N. III

axial dorsal
proper digital
N. IV

Fig. R6.24. Tendons, vessels, and nerves of the left metacarpophalangeal region in the large ruminants. **A.** dorsal aspect. **B.** Palmar aspect.

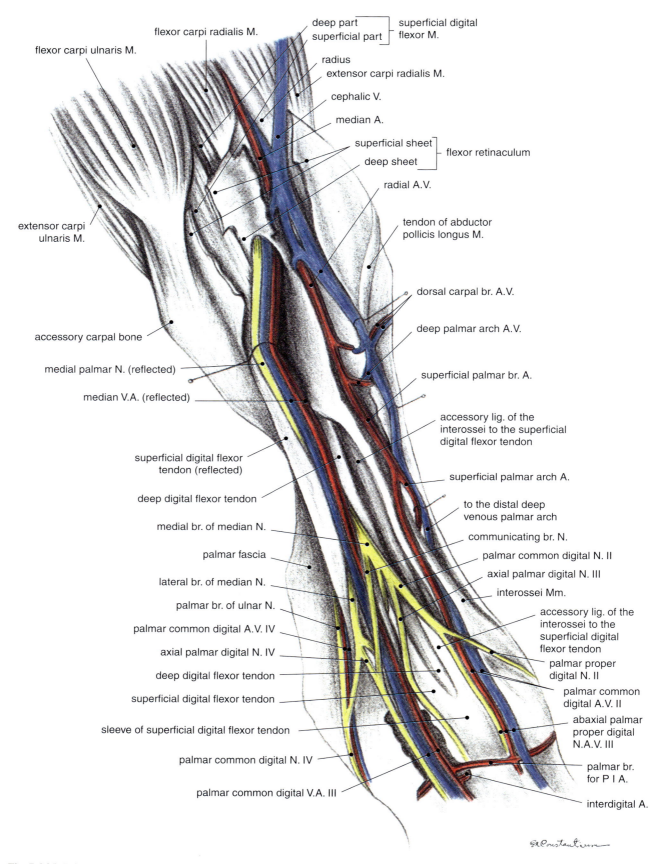

flexor carpi ulnaris M.

flexor carpi radialis M.

deep part
superficial part ⎤ superficial digital flexor M.

radius

extensor carpi radialis M.

cephalic V.

median A.

superficial sheet
deep sheet ⎤ flexor retinaculum

radial A.V.

tendon of abductor pollicis longus M.

extensor carpi ulnaris M.

dorsal carpal br. A.V.

deep palmar arch A.V.

accessory carpal bone

medial palmar N. (reflected)

superficial palmar br. A.

median V.A. (reflected)

accessory lig. of the interossei to the superficial digital flexor tendon

superficial digital flexor tendon (reflected)

superficial palmar arch A.

deep digital flexor tendon

to the distal deep venous palmar arch

medial br. of median N.

communicating br. N.

palmar common digital N. II

palmar fascia

axial palmar digital N. III

lateral br. of median N.

interossei Mm.

palmar br. of ulnar N.

accessory lig. of the interossei to the superficial digital flexor tendon

palmar common digital A.V. IV

palmar proper digital N. II

axial palmar digital N. IV

palmar common digital A.V. II

deep digital flexor tendon

superficial digital flexor tendon

abaxial palmar proper digital N.A.V. III

sleeve of superficial digital flexor tendon

palmar br. for P I A.

palmar common digital N. IV

palmar common digital V.A. III

interdigital A.

Fig. R6.25. Palmar structures of left carpus and metacarpus, large ruminants, medial aspect.

The median A. is paralleled on both sides of the metacarpal area by two **superficial branches** that end together in the **superficial palmar arch**. **Palmar metacarpal Aa. II**, **III**, and **IV** also empty into this arch.

From the superficial palmar arch arise the **palmar common digital Aa. II**, **III**, and **IV**. The branches of these arteries on the palmar, axial, and abaxial aspects are shown in Figure R6.26.

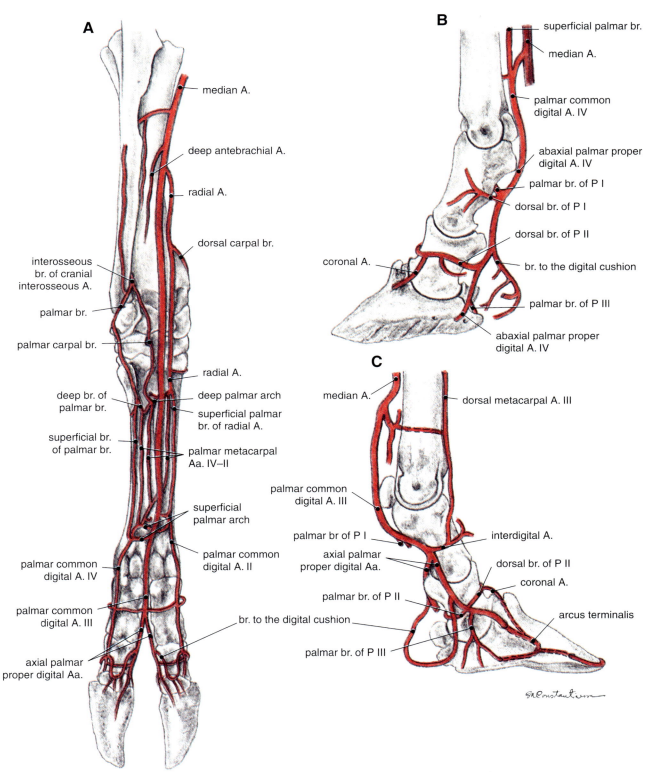

Fig. R6.26. Arteries of the distal left forelimb in the large ruminants. **A.** Palmar aspect. **B.** Abaxial aspect. **C.** Axial aspect.

Return to the carpal area where interossei Mm. III and IV originate, and send an accessory lig. to the SDF. Identify all the tendon branches of these muscles as they are shown in Figure R6.27.

Dissect the **fascia of the digital cushion** and the **lig. of the ergot** of one digit. Dissect the **palmar annular lig.**, the **proximal and distal digital annular ligg.**, and the **proximal and distal interdigital ligg.** (Figs. R6.10A and R6.28A).

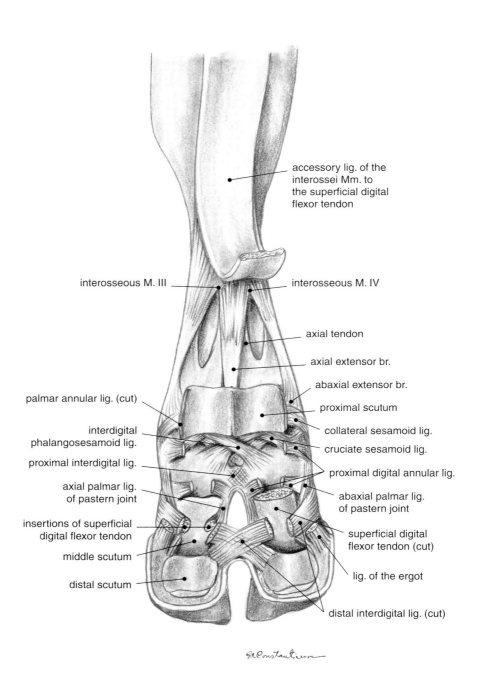

Fig. R6.27. The interossei muscles, right thoracic limb, in the large ruminants.

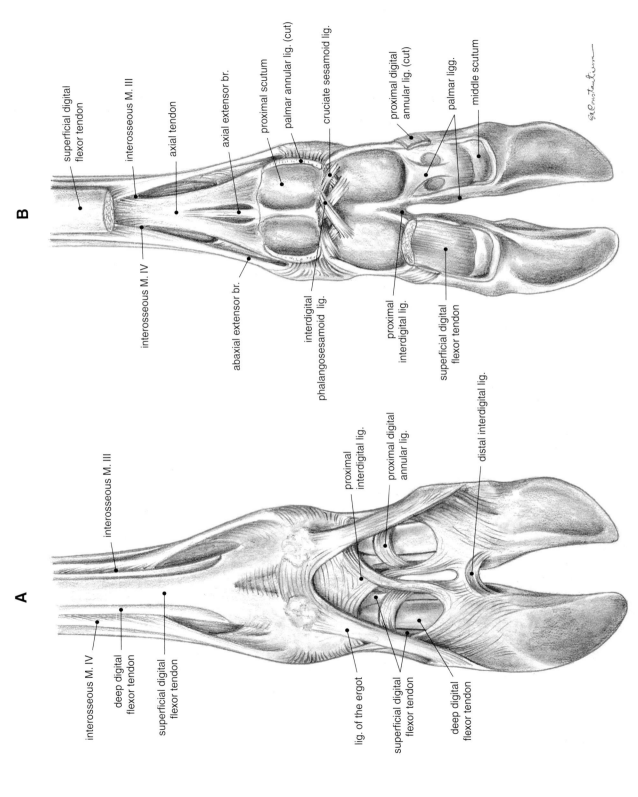

**B**

superficial digital flexor tendon

interosseous M. III

axial tendon

axial extensor br.

proximal scutum

palmar annular lig. (cut)

cruciate sesamoid lig.

proximal digital annular lig. (cut)

palmar ligg.

middle scutum

interosseous M. IV

abaxial extensor br.

interdigital phalangosesamoid lig.

proximal interdigital lig.

superficial digital flexor tendon

**A**

interosseous M. III

proximal interdigital lig.

proximal digital annular lig.

distal interdigital lig.

interosseous M. IV

deep digital flexor tendon

superficial digital flexor tendon

lig. of the ergot

superficial digital flexor tendon

deep digital flexor tendon

Fig. R6.28. Palmar aspect of digital area, left thoracic limb, in the large ruminants. **A.** Superficial structures. **B.** Deep structures.

Remove the tendons of the SDF and DDF and identify first the **proximal scutum** (on the palmar aspect of the paired **proximal sesamoid bones**). Carefully transect the attachments of SDF on the **middle scutum**, the **transverse lamina** of the DDF on P II, and the distal attachment of DDF on the **flexor tubercle**. Also examine the **distal scutum** covering the flexor aspect of the **navicular bone (the distal sesamoid bone)** (see Fig. R6.27B).

Examine the structures of the digital organ. Only the differences between the large ruminants and the horse are discussed.

The two symmetrical **hooves (claws)** correspond to the digits and, when in close apposition, look similar to a horse hoof. Each hoof has an axial and an abaxial surface (including a **dorsal part**, the **heel,** and the **bulb of the heel**) (Fig. R6.29A,B). The ruminants' hooves bear *no bars or frogs.* There are *no cartilages of the hooves.* Only the **wall** and **sole** are present. The sole is reduced to the area within the angle of inflection of the wall and continues without a distinct limit with the bulb of the heel. A very reduced **white zone** is observed (Fig. R6.29D).

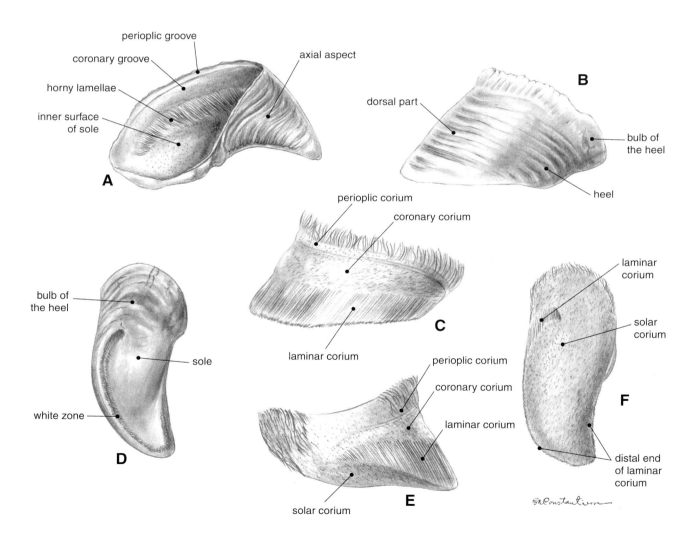

Fig. R6.29. The hoof and corium of digit, large ruminants. **A.** Internal aspect of hoof. **B.** Abaxial aspect of wall of hoof. **C.** Corium of digit, abaxial aspect. **D.** Solar aspect of hoof. **E.** Corium of digit, axial and ventral aspects. **F.** Solar corium of digit.

Inside the hooves, the **perioplic and coronary grooves** are wider, but not as deep as in the horse. The **horny lamellae** are as numerous as the lamellae of the laminar corium (Fig. R6.29A).

The live tissue (the corium), namely the **perioplic corium** and the **coronary corium** are thicker than in the horse. The lamellae of the **laminar corium** are much shorter but much more numerous (1,000–1,300). No secondary lamellae are observed (Fig. R6.29C,E).

Only the digital cushion is covered by the corium (the **solar corium**) (Fig. R6.29F). It is much reduced compared to the digital cushion in the horse and is *not* protected by a frog.

**Dewclaws** are present in the large ruminants. They resemble the main claws and cover one to two vestigial phalanges.

## MODLAB R3

*Anatomoclinical landmarks for physical examination and clinical approach of the thoracic limb in the large ruminant are discussed below.*

**Bovine lameness is a classical multifactorial problem. Local and/or intraarticular analgesia are essential in the diagnostic or the surgical treatment of many causes of lameness. Although practitioners often prefer to perform a ring block just distal to the carpus, thoracic limb analgesia can be induced by blocking the median and ulnar Nn. and the nerves supplying sensory innervation to the forearm, carpus, metacarpus (and phalanges): the cranial, lateral, caudal, and medial cutaneous antebrachial Nn.**

**The proximal site for the median N. block is on the medial aspect of the forearm, 5–8 cm distal to the elbow, between the radius and the cranial border of the flexor carpi radialis (Fig. R6.30A).**

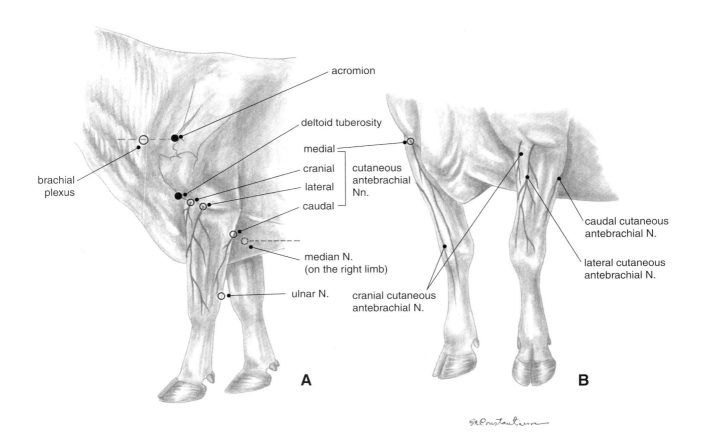

Fig. R6.30. Sites and landmarks for blocking the brachial plexus, the median and ulnar nerves, and the cutaneous antebrachial nerves.

The proximal site for the ulnar N. block is just under the skin and proper antebrachial fascia, 10–12 cm proximal to the accessory carpal bone, in the groove between the extensor and the flexor carpi ularis (see Fig. R6.30A).

The following are the sites for blocking the cutaneous antebrachial Nn. in the forearm (there is a distal site for blocking the lateral cutaneous antebrachial N., which is not shown here) (see Fig. R6.30).

The cranial cutaneous antebrachial N. (branch of the axillary) is blocked ventrocaudal to the deltoid tuberosity. The lateral cutaneous antebrachial N. (from the superficial branch of the radial N.) is blocked at the ventral border of the lateral head of the triceps brachii, 5 cm from the deltoid tuberosity. The caudal cutaneous antebrachial N. (branch of the ulnar) is blocked 15 cm distal to the olecranon on the caudal border of the forearm, on the line between the elbow and the accessory carpal bone. The medial cutaneous antebrachial N. (branch of the musculocutaneous) is blocked on the lacertus fibrosus as a landmark, immediately cranial to the cephalic V. over the cranial aspect of the radius.

The sites for the nerve block of the dorsal branch of the ulnar N., of the superficial branch of the radial N. on the dorsal aspect of metacarpus, and of the lateral and medial palmar nerves are shown in Figure R6.31.

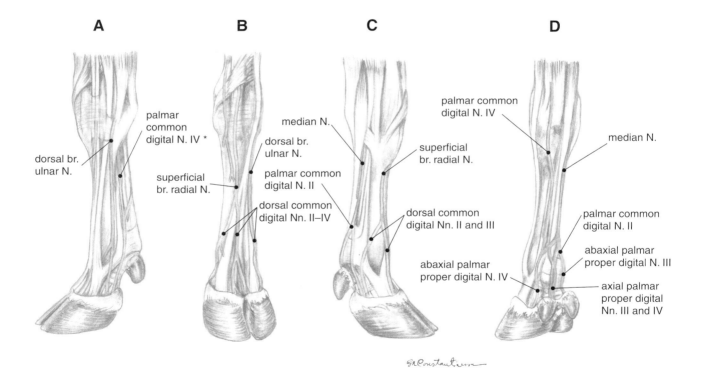

Fig. R6.31. Nerve block sites for digital analgesia, left thoracic limb, large ruminants. **A.** Lateral aspect. **B.** Dorsal aspect. **C.** Medial aspect. **D.** Palmar aspect. * = continuation of the superficial branch of the palmar branch of the ulnar nerve.

The brachial plexus block is another alternative for the whole limb. This block can be approached by locating the tips of the transverse processes of the last three cervical vertebrae. At this site the needle is inserted horizontally through the skin in the direction of the acromion (of the scapula) and directed caudally until the tip contacts the cranial edge of the first rib (see Fig. R6.30A).

Under field conditions, intravenous regional analgesia using the radial V. is the method of choice to perform most surgical digital procedures.

Arthroscopy, arthrocentesis, and intraarticular analgesia can be performed in all joints of the thoracic limb. The sites for those procedures are shown in Figures R6.32–R6.35.

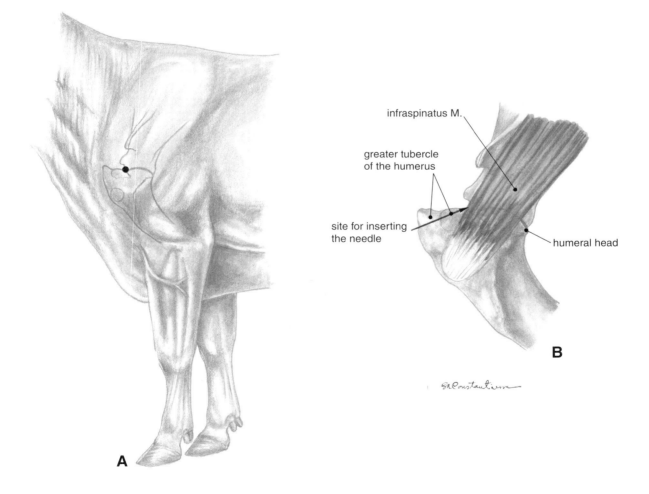

Fig. R6.32. Site for performing arthroscopy, arthrocentesis, and intraarticular analgesia in the shoulder joint of the ox. **A.** Shoulder joint. **B.** Anatomy of the shoulder joint, lateral aspect.

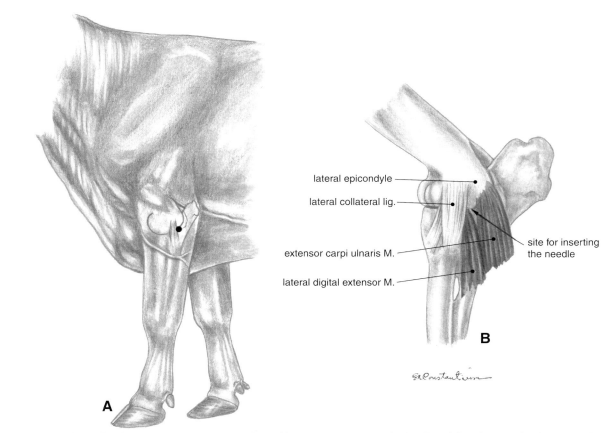

Fig. R6.33. Site for performing arthroscopy, arthrocentesis, and intraarticular analgesia in the elbow joint of the ox. **A.** Elbow joint. **B.** Anatomy of the elbow joint, lateral aspect.

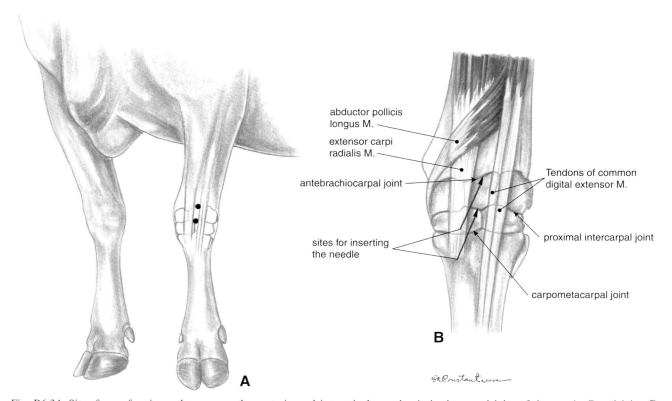

Fig. R6.34. Sites for performing arthroscopy, arthrocentesis, and intraarticular analgesia in the carpal joint of the ox. **A.** Carpal joint. **B.** Anatomy of the carpal joint, dorsal view.

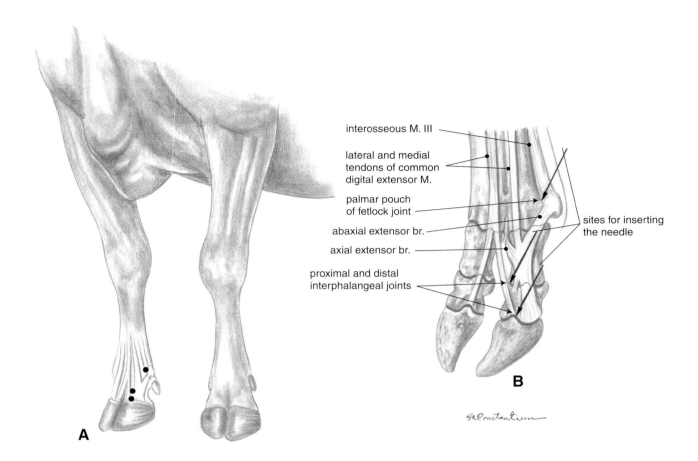

interosseous M. III

lateral and medial tendons of common digital extensor M.

palmar pouch of fetlock joint

abaxial extensor br.

axial extensor br.

proximal and distal interphalangeal joints

sites for inserting the needle

A

B

Fig. R6.35. Sites for performing arthroscopy, arthrocentesis, and intraarticular analgesia in the digital joints of the ox. **A.** Digital joints. **B.** Anatomy of the digital joints, dorsomedial aspect.

# R 7

# The Head

Compare the skull of a large ruminant with the skull of a horse and attempt to identify similar structures as they were described in Chapter H7 (see page 207).

On the skull in a lateral view (Fig. R7.1) *notice* that no **superior incisors** are present (the same in the small ruminants); the **infraorbital foramen** is located in a rostral position (dorsal to the first upper premolar); the **facial crest** is irregular, and therefore the **facial tubercle** looks like an isolated structure; the **temporal fossa** is deep and narrow and is bordered dorsally by the **temporal line**; the **parietal bone** is reduced and lies on the bottom of the temporal fossa; a **cornual process** is present, even in dehorned individuals; the **tympanic bulla** is well developed and extends to the level of the distal end of the **paracondylar (jugular) process of the occipital bone**; the **muscular process of the temporal bone** is well developed.

Within the **orbita,** identify the three foramina of the **pterygopalatine fossa** (in dorsoventral order), the **sphenopalatine, maxillary,** and **caudal palatine foramina** (sing. foramen); the well-developed and irregular **pterygoid crest** and the foramina located rostral to the pterygoid crest, which are, in dorsoventral order, the orbital opening of the **supraorbital canal**, the **ethmoidal foramen**, the **optic canal**, and the **foramen orbitorotundum** (only the last three structures are located within the **pterygoid fossa**).

Compare the **mandible** of the ox (Fig. R7.2) with that of the horse.

*Note*. In the ruminants, large and small alike, the **lower canine teeth** migrated rostrally and joined the incisors; therefore, there are four symmetrical incisive teeth and no upper canine teeth.

In a frontal view (Fig. R7.3), the **frontal bones** exceed the rostral limits of the orbitae and fill the rest of the skull, up to and including the **intercornual protuberance**; the frontal opening of the supraorbital canal continues rostrally and caudally with the **supraorbital groove (sulcus)**.

In a ventral view—the base of the skull (Fig. R7.4)—several characteristics should be noted. Again, there are no superior incisive or canine teeth; the **major palatine foramen** on the **hard palate** (the rostral openings of the **major palatine canal**) belongs only to the **palatine bone** and is located very close to the symmetrical foramen; the **choanae** (sing. choana) are narrow; a well-developed **lacrimal bulla** is located within the orbita; there is no **foramen lacerum** in ruminants, but the **oval foramen** is present; a very narrow **petrooccipital fissure** (between the **temporal bone** and the **basioccipital**) communicates caudally with the **jugular foramen**. Identify the tympanic bulla and the muscular process of the temporal bone. Identify the **mastoid process**, the **styloid process**, the **stylomastoid foramen,** and the prominent **muscular turbercle.**

Compare the brain cavity of the ox with that of the horse.

On the head examine the **planum nasolabiale**, a rostral structure common to the upper lip and nostrils and specific to the large ruminants. It contains glands, but not hair. The nasal cartilages are not palpable. Examine the relationship between the **horns** (or cornual processes) and the **ears.**

Split the head of your specimen into two halves and skin and dissect them, following the same procedure as described in the dissection of the horse (see pages 216–220).

Turn the skinned head lateral side up and dissect the muscles, arteries, veins, nerves, salivary glands, and lymph nodes as they are illustrated in Fig. R7.5. For a systematic presentation of the muscles of the head see Table R7.1.

There are some obvious characteristics in the large ruminants, as follows.

There is a **frontalis M.,** wide and thick. The **sternomandibularis M.** is attached to the mandible rostral to the **masseter M.,** passing over some vessels and nerves. The **facial N.** delivers a **buccal branch,** similar to that of the horse, and the **mandibular marginal branch (ramus**

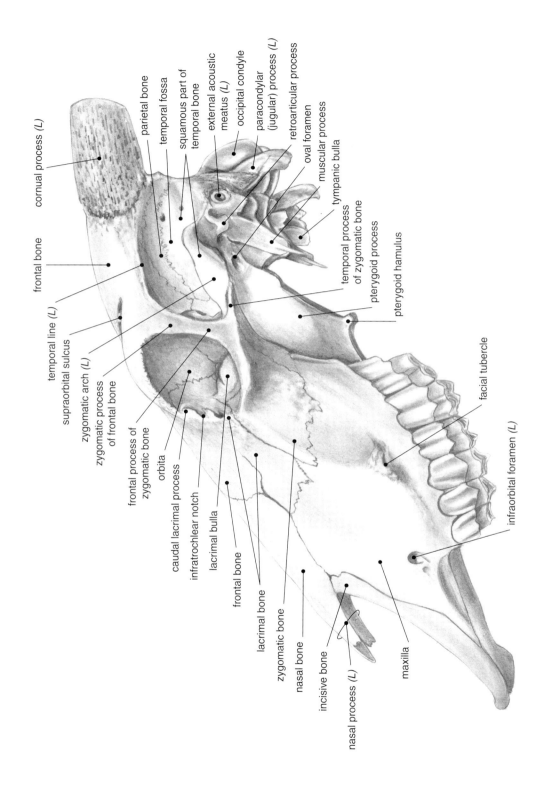

Fig. R7.1. Ox skull, lateral aspect, without mandible. (L) = landmark for physical examination and/or clinical approach.

cornual process (L)

frontal bone

temporal line (L)

supraorbital sulcus

zygomatic arch (L)

zygomatic process
of frontal bone

frontal process of
zygomatic bone

orbita

caudal lacrimal process

infratrochlear notch

lacrimal bulla

frontal bone

lacrimal bone

zygomatic bone

nasal bone

incisive bone

nasal process (L)

maxilla

parietal bone

temporal fossa

squamous part of
temporal bone

external acoustic
meatus (L)

occipital condyle

paracondylar
(jugular) process (L)

retroarticular process

oval foramen

muscular process

tympanic bulla

temporal process
of zygomatic bone

pterygoid process

pterygoid hamulus

facial tubercle

infraorbital foramen (L)

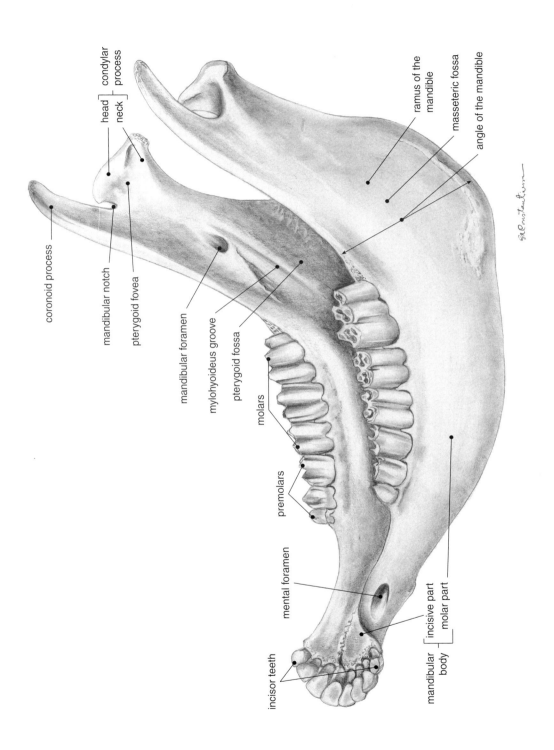

coronoid process

head ⎤
neck ⎦ condylar process

mandibular notch

pterygoid fovea

mandibular foramen

mylohyoideus groove

pterygoid fossa

molars

premolars

mental foramen

incisor teeth

ramus of the mandible

masseteric fossa

angle of the mandible

mandibular body ⎡ incisive part
⎣ molar part

Fig. R7.2. The mandible, large ruminants, dorsolateral view.

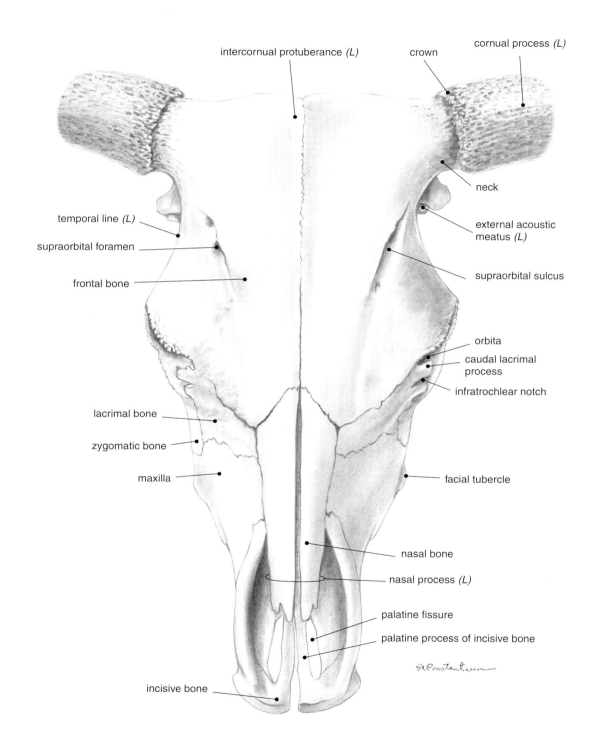

intercornual protuberance *(L)*

crown

cornual process *(L)*

neck

temporal line *(L)*

external acoustic meatus *(L)*

supraorbital foramen

frontal bone

supraorbital sulcus

orbita

caudal lacrimal process

infratrochlear notch

lacrimal bone

zygomatic bone

maxilla

facial tubercle

nasal bone

nasal process *(L)*

palatine fissure

palatine process of incisive bone

incisive bone

Fig. R7.3. Ox skull, frontal aspect. *(L)* = landmarks for physical examination and/or clinical approach.

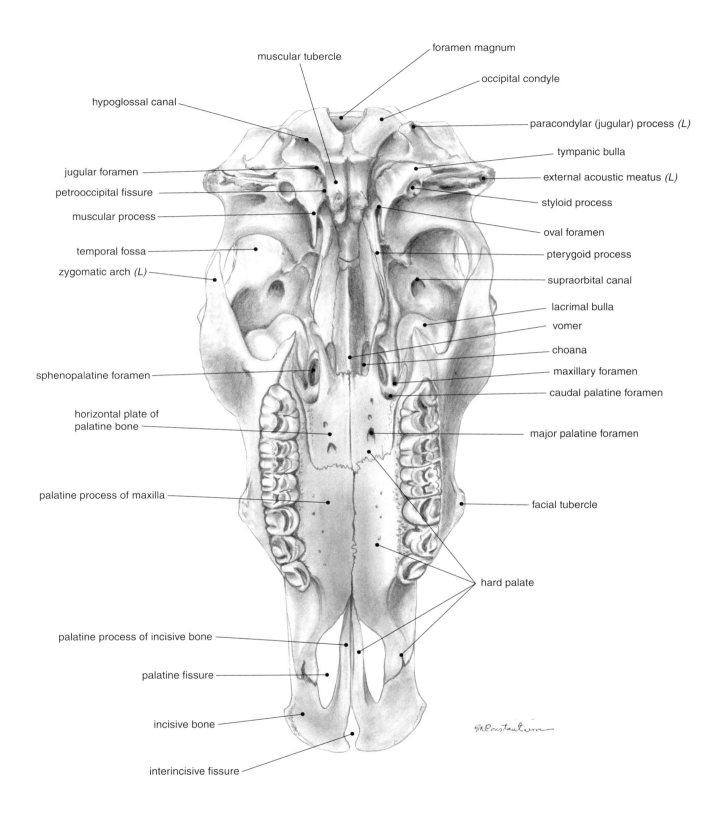

muscular tubercle

foramen magnum

occipital condyle

hypoglossal canal

paracondylar (jugular) process *(L)*

tympanic bulla

jugular foramen

external acoustic meatus *(L)*

petrooccipital fissure

styloid process

muscular process

oval foramen

temporal fossa

pterygoid process

zygomatic arch *(L)*

supraorbital canal

lacrimal bulla

vomer

choana

sphenopalatine foramen

maxillary foramen

caudal palatine foramen

horizontal plate of
palatine bone

major palatine foramen

palatine process of maxilla

facial tubercle

hard palate

palatine process of incisive bone

palatine fissure

incisive bone

interincisive fissure

Fig. R7.4. Ox skull, ventral aspect, without mandible. *(L)* = landmark for physical examination and/or clinical approach.

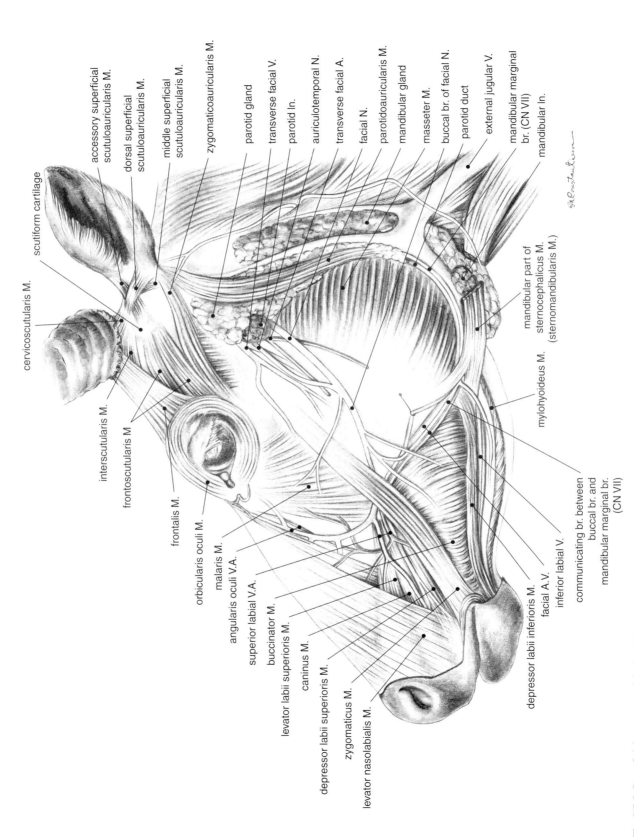

accessory superficial scutuloauricularis M.

dorsal superficial scutuloauricularis M.

middle superficial scutuloauricularis M.

zygomaticoauricularis M.

parotid gland

transverse facial V.

parotid ln.

auriculotemporal N.

transverse facial A.

facial N.

parotidoauricularis M.

mandibular gland

masseter M.

buccal br. of facial N.

parotid duct

external jugular V.

mandibular marginal br. (CN VII)

mandibular ln.

scutiform cartilage

cervicoscutularis M.

interscutularis M.

frontoscutularis M

frontalis M.

orbicularis oculi M.

malaris M.

angularis oculi V.A.

superior labial V.A.

buccinator M.

caninus M.

levator labii superioris M.

depressor labii superioris M.

zygomaticus M.

levator nasolabialis M.

depressor labii inferioris M.

facial A.V.

inferior labial V.

communicating br. between buccal br. and mandibular marginal br. (CN VII)

mylohyoideus M.

mandibular part of sternocephalicus M. (sternomandibularis M.)

Fig. R7.5. Superficial structures of the head, lateral aspect, large ruminants.

Table R7.1. Muscles of the Head, Horse, and Large
Ruminants

**Facial Muscles**
– frontalis *(except eq)*
– lateralis nasi
– dilatator naris apicalis
– orbicularis oculi
– levator anguli oculi medialis
– retractor anguli oculi lateralis *(except eq)*
– malaris
– incisivus superior
– incisivus inferior
– mentalis
– orbicularis oris
– depressor anguli oris
– zygomaticus
– levator nasolabialis
– levator labii superioris
– caninus
– depressor labii superioris *(except eq)*
– depressor labii inferioris
– buccinator

**Muscles of Mastication**
– masseter
– temporalis
– pterygoideus medialis
– pterygoideus lateralis
– digastricus
  • pars occipitomandibularis *(only in eq)*

**Muscles of the Ear**
– auriculares rostrales
  • scutuloauriculares superficiales
  • scutuloauriculares profundi
  • frontoscutularis
  • zygomaticoscutularis
  • zygomaticoauricularis
– auriculares dorsales
  • interscutularis
  • parietoscutularis
  • parietoauricularis
– auriculares caudales
  • cervicoscutularis
  • cervicoauricularis superficialis
  • cervicoauricularis medius
  • cervicoauricularis profundus
– auriculares ventrales
  • parotidoauricularis
  • styloauricularis

**marginalis mandibulae)**, which surrounds the ventral border of the masseter M. It communicates with the buccal branch at the rostral border of the masseter M., under the **zygomaticus M.** The two parts of the **levator nasolabialis M.** are separated by three muscles: the **levator labii superioris** and **caninus Mm.** (found also in the horse) and the **depressor labii superioris M.** These three

muscles send rostrally a multitude of tendons. The **parotid ln.** is very large, but its location is similar to that in the horse (see Figs. R7.5 and R7.6).

Carefully dissect all the superficial structures illustrated in Figure R7.6, then reflect and remove the parotid gland. Dissect the structures in a manner similar to that used in the horse; they are illustrated in Figure R7.7. *Notice* the common origin of the buccal branch and the mandibular marginal branch (from CN VII); the fibrous band separating the **external carotid A.** from the deepest structures (the **stylohyoid bone**); the **stylohyoideus M.,** whose origin is tendinous and is *not* split, as it is in the horse. The other structures are similar to those of the horse.

*Notice* that there is no **occipitomandibular part of the digastricus M.** in ruminants.

Reflect the veins and the **lateral retropharyngeal ln.,** transect the **digastricus M.,** and reflect the stumps to expose the deepest structures of the parotid area, as they are illustrated in Figure R7.8.

Dissect the **cornual A. and V.** (branches of the superficial temporal A. and V.) and the **cornual N.,** branch of either the **zygomatic N.** or **lacrimal N.** (see Fig. R7.9A). They run together parallel to the temporal line (see Fig. 7.9B).

Focus your attention on the ear. Skin it carefully and dissect the muscles, identifying the four groups that were dissected in the horse (Fig. H7.5).

Prepare the head for removal of the mandible, in a procedure similar to that used for the horse (pages 220 and 224, Fig. H7.15).

For better understanding of the cranial nerves, Table R7.2 shows the foramina through which these nerves pass in and out of the cranial cavity, the quality of the fibers that they carry, and some observations.

The deep structures of the head are illustrated in Figures R7.10 and R7.11. They are very similar to those of the horse. The following are the major differences between the large ruminants and the horse.

The biggest difference is the presence of both **monostomatic** and **polystomatic sublingual salivary glands**. The monostomatic gland is located rostral to the polystomatic gland. The **styloglossus M.** has intimate contact with the polystomatic gland, whereas the **geniohyoideus** and the **mylohyoideus Mm.** come in contact with the monostomatic gland.

*Remember!* In the horse there is only the polystomatic sublingual salivary gland.

The monostomatic gland empties the saliva through the **major sublingual duct**, which accompanies the **mandibular duct** and opens on, or near, the **sublingual caruncle**. The mandibular duct runs parallel to the ventral border of the styloglossus M.

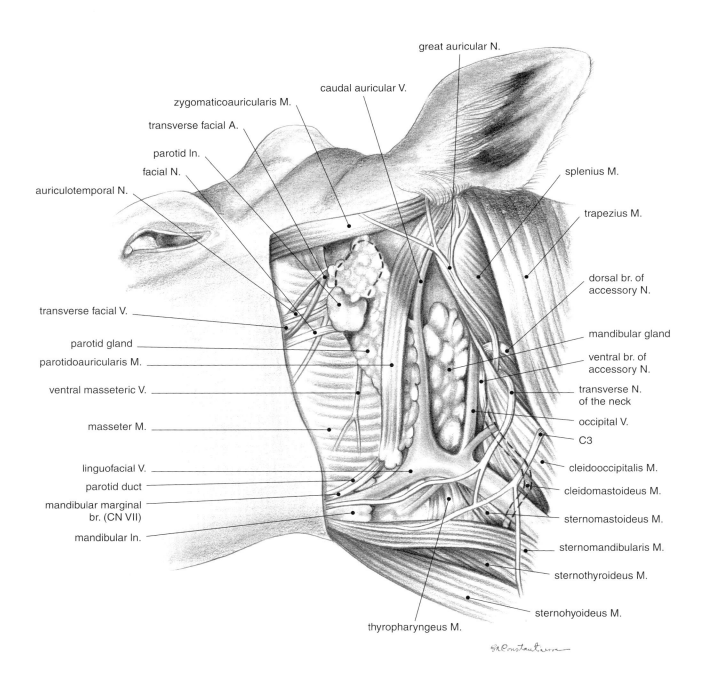

Fig. R7.6. Superficial structures in the parotid region, large ruminants.

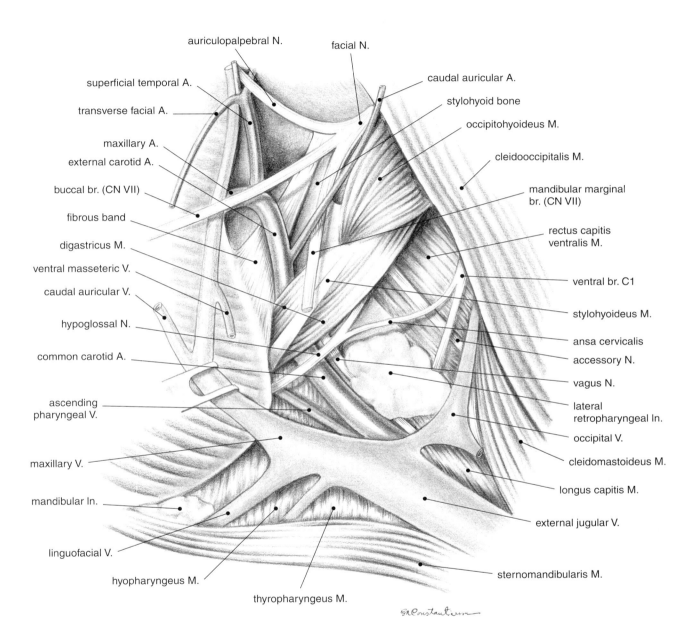

auriculopalpebral N.

facial N.

superficial temporal A.

caudal auricular A.

transverse facial A.

stylohyoid bone

occipitohyoideus M.

maxillary A.

cleidooccipitalis M.

external carotid A.

buccal br. (CN VII)

mandibular marginal
br. (CN VII)

fibrous band

digastricus M.

rectus capitis
ventralis M.

ventral masseteric V.

ventral br. C1

caudal auricular V.

stylohyoideus M.

hypoglossal N.

ansa cervicalis

accessory N.

common carotid A.

vagus N.

ascending
pharyngeal V.

lateral
retropharyngeal ln.

occipital V.

maxillary V.

cleidomastoideus M.

longus capitis M.

mandibular ln.

external jugular V.

linguofacial V.

hyopharyngeus M.

sternomandibularis M.

thyropharyngeus M.

Fig. R7.7. Deep structures adjacent to the facial nerve and external carotid artery, left side, large ruminants.

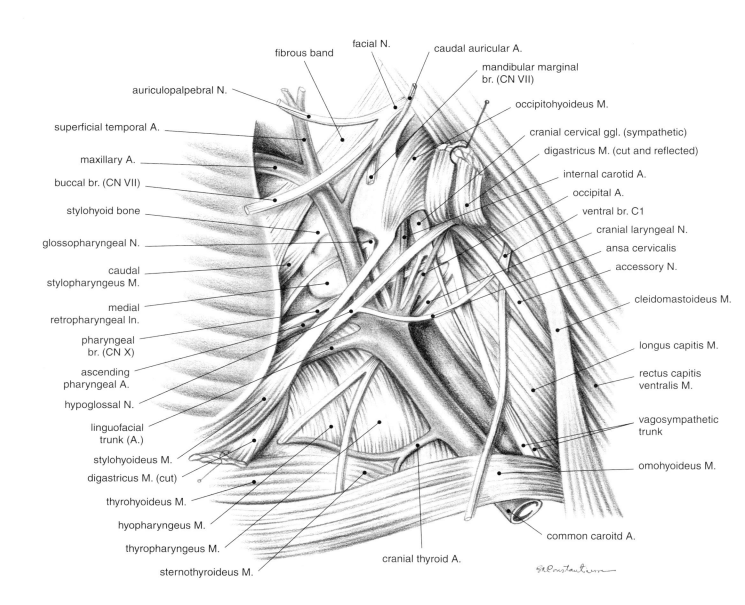

fibrous band

facial N.

caudal auricular A.

mandibular marginal br. (CN VII)

auriculopalpebral N.

occipitohyoideus M.

superficial temporal A.

cranial cervical ggl. (sympathetic)

maxillary A.

digastricus M. (cut and reflected)

buccal br. (CN VII)

internal carotid A.

stylohyoid bone

occipital A.

glossopharyngeal N.

ventral br. C1

caudal stylopharyngeus M.

cranial laryngeal N.

ansa cervicalis

medial retropharyngeal ln.

accessory N.

pharyngeal br. (CN X)

cleidomastoideus M.

ascending pharyngeal A.

longus capitis M.

hypoglossal N.

rectus capitis ventralis M.

linguofacial trunk (A.)

vagosympathetic trunk

stylohyoideus M.

digastricus M. (cut)

omohyoideus M.

thyrohyoideus M.

hyopharyngeus M.

thyropharyngeus M.

common caroitd A.

sternothyroideus M.

cranial thyroid A.

Fig. R7.8. Deepest structures of the parotid area, left side, large ruminants.

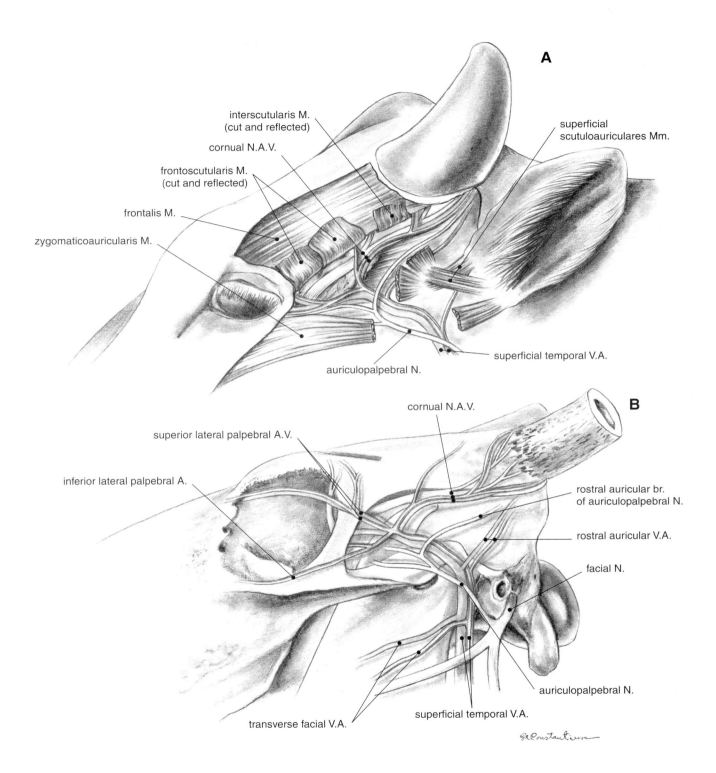

Fig. R7.9. Structures in the region of temporal fossa, large ruminants. **A.** Structures between the eye, ear, and horn. **B.** Vessels and nerves between the eye, ear, and horn.

The muscular fibers of the **mylohyoideus M.** are oriented in different directions. The tendon of the digastricus M. does not pass through the tendon of the stylohyoideus M., as it does in the horse.

*Remember!* The stylohyoideus M. has the tendon at the proximal end, and it is not split.

There is no **alar canal** in the ruminants, therefore the only nerve crossing the lateral aspect of the **maxillary A.** is the **buccal N.** The other branches of the **mandibular N. (V3)** (the **lateral and medial pterygoid**, **lingual**, **inferior alveolar**, and **mylohyoid Nn.**) cross the medial aspect of the artery. The **masticatory** and **auriculotemporal Nn.** don't cross the maxillary A.

Table R7.2. The Cranial Nerves in the Horse and Large Ruminants

| Nerve | Leaves Skull Through | Motor | Sensory | Mixed | Para-sympathetic | Observations |
|---|---|---|---|---|---|---|
| I. Olfactory | Cribriform plate ethmoid | | SVA | | | Terminal ggl. |
| II. Optic | Optic canal | | SSA | | | |
| III. Oculomotor | Foramen orbitorotundum (Ru) Orbital fissure (eq) | GSE | | | GVE | Ciliary ggl. (parasymp.); short ciliary Nn. postggl. fibers |
| IV. Trochlear | Foramen orbitorotundum (Ru) Orbital fissure/Foramen trochleare (eq) | GSE | | | | |
| V. Trigeminal | | | | * | | |
|   1. Ophthalmic | Foramen orbitorotundum (Ru) Orbital fissure (eq) | | GSA | | | |
|   2. Maxillary | Foramen orbitorotundum (Ru) Foramen rotundum (eq) | | GSA | | | Trigeminal ggl. (sens.) |
|   3. Mandibular | Foramen ovale | SVE | GSA | | | |
| VI. Abducent | Foramen orbitorotundum (Ru) Orbital fissure (eq) | GSE | | | | |
| VII. Facial | Enters facial canal Leaves stylomastoid foramen | SVE | GSA | * | GVE | Geniculate ggl. (sens.) Pterygopalatine ggl. (parasymp.) |
| | Leaves petrotympanic fissure for chorda tympani N. | | | | | Greater petrosal N. preggl. fibers Mandibular ggl. (parasymp.) Chorda tympani N. preggl. fibers |
| VIII. Vestibulocochlear | Enters internal acoustic meatus | | SP | | | Vestibular ggl. |
| | | | SSA | | | Spiral ggl. |
| IX. Glossopharyngeal | Jugular foramen | SVE | | | | Proximal ggl. |
| | | SVA | | * | | Distal ggl. |
| | | GVA | | * | | |
| | | GSA | | * | | |
| | | | | | GVE | Lateropharyngeal ggl. (bo, ov) Otic ggl. (parasymp.) Lesser petrosal N. preggl. fibers |
| X. Vagus | Jugular foramen | SVE | GSA | * | | Proximal ggl. (sens.) |
| | | | GVA | | | Distal ggl. (sens.) |
| | | | SVA | | | |
| XI. Accessory | Jugular foramen | SVE | | | GVE | |
| XII. Hypoglossal | Hypoglossal canal | GSE | | | | |

*Note:* GSE = general somatic efferent; GVE = general visceral efferent; GSA = general somatic afferent; GVA = general visceral afferent; SVA = special visceral afferent; SVE = special visceral efferent; SSA = special somatic afferent; SP = special proprioception.
  * = mixed nerves.

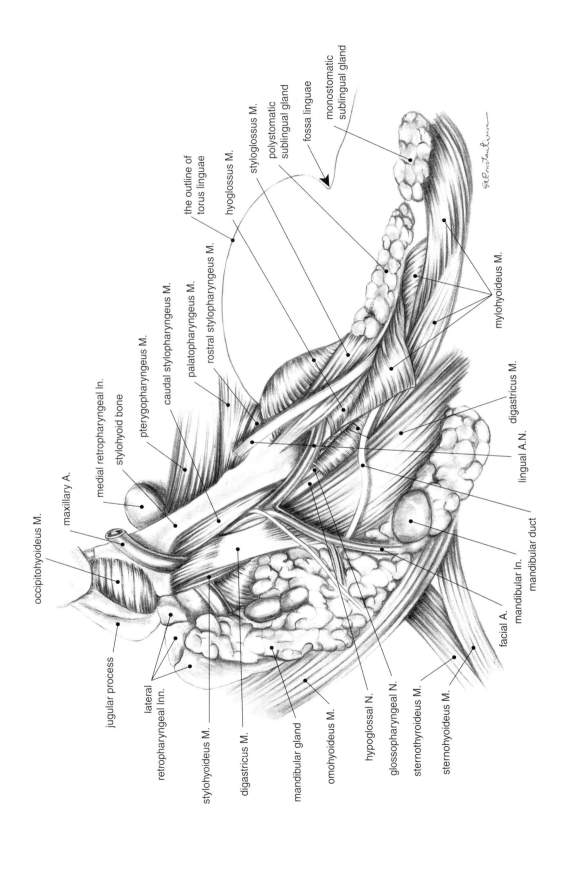

occipitohyoideus M.

maxillary A.

medial retropharyngeal ln.

stylohyoid bone

pterygopharyngeus M.

caudal stylopharyngeus M.

palatopharyngeus M.

rostral stylopharyngeus M.

the outline of
torus linguae

hyoglossus M.

styloglossus M.

polystomatic
sublingual gland

fossa linguae

monostomatic
sublingual gland

mylohyoideus M.

digastricus M.

lingual A.N.

mandibular duct

mandibular ln.

facial A.

jugular process

lateral
retropharyngeal lnn.

stylohyoideus M.

digastricus M.

mandibular gland

omohyoideus M.

hypoglossal N.

glossopharyngeal N.

sternothyroideus M.

sternohyoideus M.

Fig. R7.l0. Structures within the area of hyoid apparatus of the large ruminants, right lateral aspect. (Mandible has been removed.)

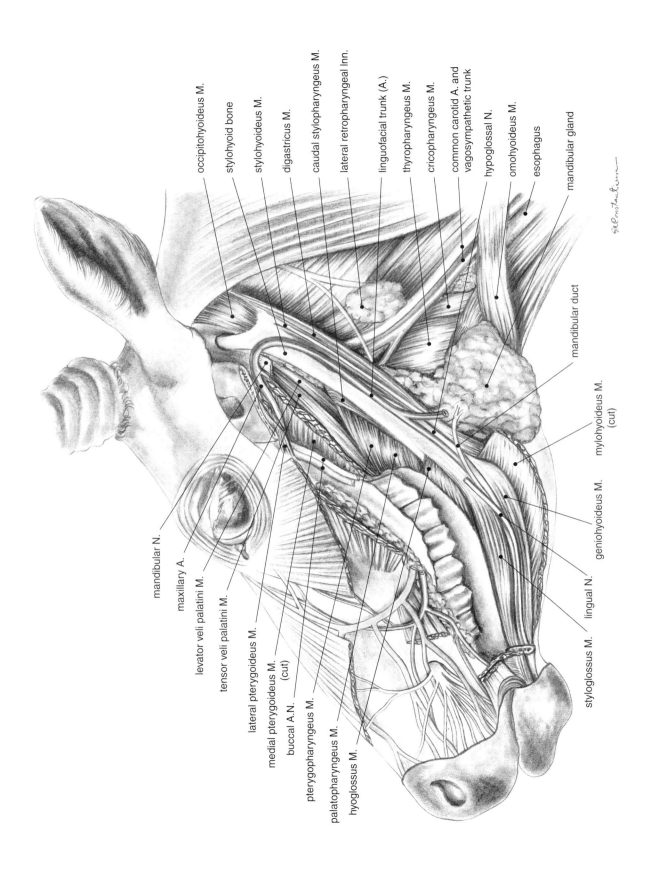

occipitohyoideus M.

stylohyoid bone

stylohyoideus M.

digastricus M.

caudal stylopharyngeus M.

lateral retropharyngeal lnn.

linguofacial trunk (A.)

thyropharyngeus M.

cricopharyngeus M.

common carotid A. and
vagosympathetic trunk

hypoglossal N.

omohyoideus M.

esophagus

mandibular gland

mandibular duct

mylohyoideus M.
(cut)

geniohyoideus M.

lingual N.

styloglossus M.

hyoglossus M.

palatopharyngeus M.

pterygopharyngeus M.

buccal A.N.

medial pterygoideus M.

lateral pterygoideus M. (cut)

tensor veli palatini M.

levator veli palatini M.

maxillary A.

mandibular N.

Fig. R7. 11. Deep structures of the head, lateral aspect, large ruminants.

There are **rostral** and **caudal stylopharyngeus Mm.** in the ruminants. The former is a constrictor (part of the first pharyngeal constrictor), whereas the latter is *the* dilator of the pharynx.

In the ruminants there are no venous sinuses in the head, as in the horse, except the brain cavity.

Transect the **hyoglossus** and the **hyo-, thyro-,** and **cricopharyngeus Mm.**, reflect the stumps, and expose the lateral aspects of the **hyoid apparatus** and the **larynx.** The **lingual A.** and the **hypoglossal N.** are now widely exposed, running parallel to the **ceratohyoideus M.**

Follow the **recurrent laryngeal N.** in a cranial direction toward the larynx, where it becomes the **caudal laryngeal N.**, and identify the **thyroid** and the **parathyroid glands.** The latter are very small, usually embedded into the thyroid gland, and may be difficult to see grossly. Pulling the **common carotid A.** and the external jugular V. caudally, dissect the **cranial** and **caudal thyroid, cranial laryngeal**, and **ascending pharyngeal Aa.** and **Vv.**

Identify the **occipital** and **internal carotid Aa.** at the level of transition between the common carotid A. and external carotid A., and the **ascending palatine A.** supplying the **soft palate.** Identify the **vagosympathetic trunk**, consisting of the **vagus N.** and the **cervical sympathetic trunk**; the **cranial cervical ggl.**; and the **accessory N.**, with the dorsal and ventral divisions of the external branch.

*Note.* In the adult ruminants the extracranial segment of the internal carotid A. is regressed, and nonpatent.

Turn the head with the split (median) side up and examine, step by step, the **nasal cavity**, the **oral cavity**, the **pharynx**, the **esophagus**, and the **larynx** (see Fig. R7.12).

Remove the **nasal septum** with a knife, if necessary. Explore the three conchae, and the three meatuses separating the conchae from each other and from the roof and the floor of the nasal cavity. There is a **common meatus** on either side of the nasal septum in addition to the **dorsal, middle, and ventral meatuses.** *Remember!* The dorsal, middle, and ventral meatuses communicate with the common meatus. Observe that the **middle nasal concha** is very large in comparison to that of the horse. With a knife, make small windows in the rostral and caudal parts of the **dorsal** and **ventral nasal conchae** and compare the internal configuration of the rostral and caudal parts; they are very different from each other.

Focus your attention on the **hard palate** and identify the large **palatine sinus**, the **palatine ridges** and the **palatine raphe** of the mucosa of the hard palate, the **incisive papilla**, and the **venous plexus** of the **major palatine Vv.** On both sides of the incisive papilla, identify the oral openings of the **incisive** ducts of the **vomeronasal organ.**

*Notice* that in all ruminants there is a **dental pad**, a tough plate of oral mucosa that replaces the missing upper incisors.

Examine the mucosal papillae of the **lips and cheeks**; they are conical and cornified.

Identify the **torus linguae** (the prominence on the dorsal aspect of the **tongue**) and the **fossa linguae** (at the rostral end of the torus linguae). The **lingual papillae** are the following: **filiform**, cornified; **conical**; **fungiform**; **lentiform**; and **vallate**; there are 8–17 vallate papillae on each side. Identify the **genioglossus, geniohyoideus**, and **mylohyoideus Mm.** and the **lingual process** of the **basihyoid bone.**

*Notice* that there are *no* **foliate papillae** in ruminants.

Pull the tongue off the **oral cavity proper**, causing the **glossoepiglottic folds** and the **palatoglossal arch** to tense. *Notice* that the **apex of the tongue** is pointed. Identify the **lingual frenulum**, and the **sublingual caruncle**; the latter protects the openings of the mandibular and major sublingual salivary ducts. Find the **parotid papilla** at the level of the upper second molar (location is specific to the large ruminants), at the mucosa of the oral vestibulum.

The pharynx has the same three compartments as in the horse. The following are the specific features of the pharynx in the large ruminants.

There is an incomplete **pharyngeal septum** on the roof (**fornix**) of the **nasopharynx**, which is a membranous continuation of the nasal septum.

The **pharyngeal opening of the auditory tube** is not located on the lateral wall of the nasopharynx, but in the caudal part of the fornix; it is hidden by the pharyngeal septum and tonsil.

The **pharyngeal tonsil** is located on the caudal end of the pharyngeal septum.

There is a branching **tonsillar sinus**, surrounded by numerous follicles of the **palatine tonsil**, located within the lateral wall of the **oropharynx**, ventral to the **soft palate** (see Fig. R7.13).

In the horse and the large ruminants, the **tensor veli palatini M.** is located lateral to the **levator veli palatini M.**, in an oblique rostroventral position. The tendon of the tensor surrounds the **pterygoid hamulus.** To expose the tensor and levator veli palatini Mm. and the **pterygopharyngeus** and **palatopharyngeus Mm.**, it is necessary to remove the mucosa of the nasopharynx, after palpating the hamulus as a landmark (see Fig. R7.12).

There is *no* **laryngeal ventricle** in the large ruminants. Therefore, the **thyroarytenoideus M.** is not divided into the **vocalis** and **ventricularis Mm.** Also, there is *no* **vestibular fold**, even though the **vestibular lig.** is present. The **hyoepiglottic lig.** is very thin.

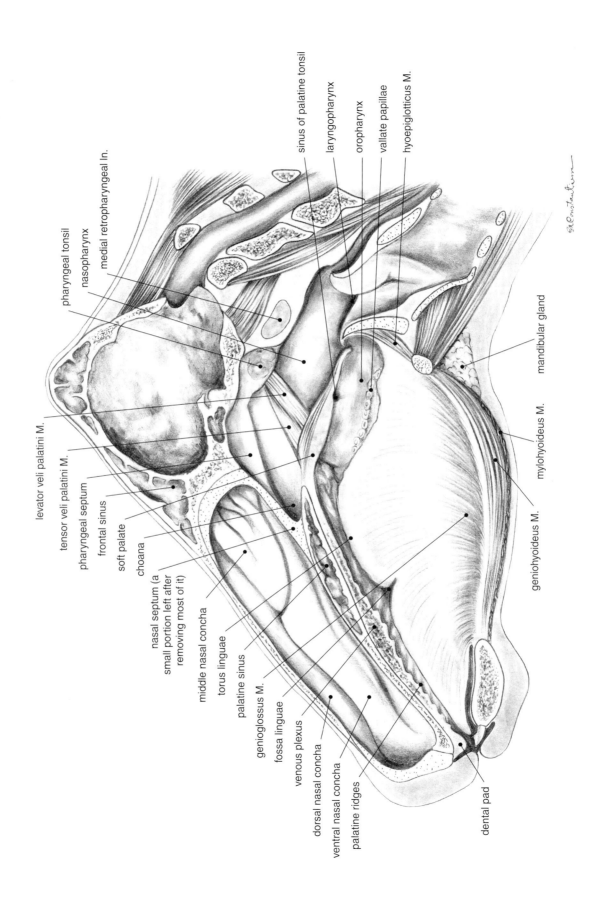

pharyngeal tonsil

nasopharynx

medial retropharyngeal ln.

sinus of palatine tonsil

laryngopharynx

oropharynx

vallate papillae

hyoepiglotticus M.

mandibular gland

levator veli palatini M.

tensor veli palatini M.

pharyngeal septum

frontal sinus

soft palate

choana

nasal septum (a
small portion left after
removing most of it)

middle nasal concha

torus linguae

palatine sinus

genioglossus M.

fossa linguae

venous plexus

dorsal nasal concha

ventral nasal concha

palatine ridges

dental pad

geniohyoideus M.

mylohyoideus M.

Fig. R7.12. Head, median aspect, large ruminants.

The **epiglottis** has no **cuneiform processes,** as it does in the horse. In a manner similar to that used in the horse (see page 245), proceed to the removal of the hyoid apparatus, the tongue, and the larynx. Free the stylohyoid bone from the **styloid process (of the temporal bone)** by transecting the **tympanohyoid bone/cartilage**. Section the **occipitohyoideus M.,** free the mylohyoideus, geniohyoideus, genioglossus, and digastricus Mm. from the mandible, free the lingual mucosa from the oral cavity, free the vessels of the esophagus and pharynx, transect the cranial laryngeal N., and free the larynx from any other attachment. Remove the hyoid apparatus, tongue, pharynx, and larynx and place them on a tray for further examination. Free the hyoid bones and cartilages and the laryngeal cartilages from muscles, ligaments, membranes, and mucosa and examine them separately.

Examine the **teeth** (see Fig. R7.14). The components of a tooth are similar to those described in the horse (see page 239). The ruminants are **selenodont** species in contrast to the horse, which is a lophodont species.

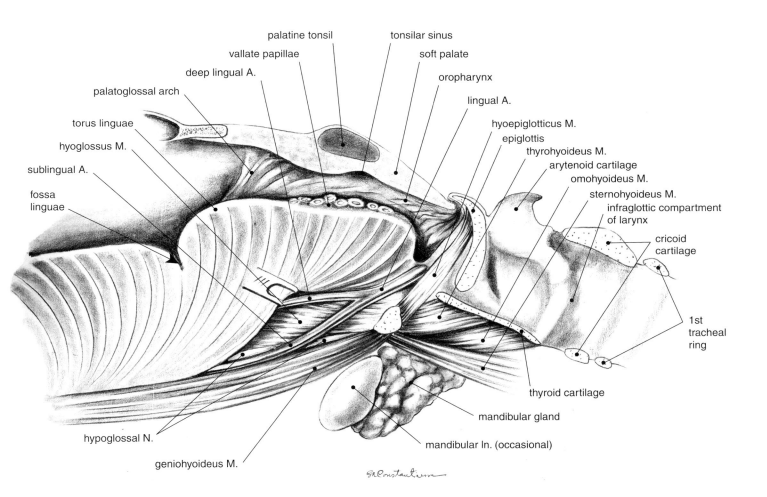

Fig. R7.13. Tongue, oropharynx, and larynx, medial aspect of the right half, large ruminants.

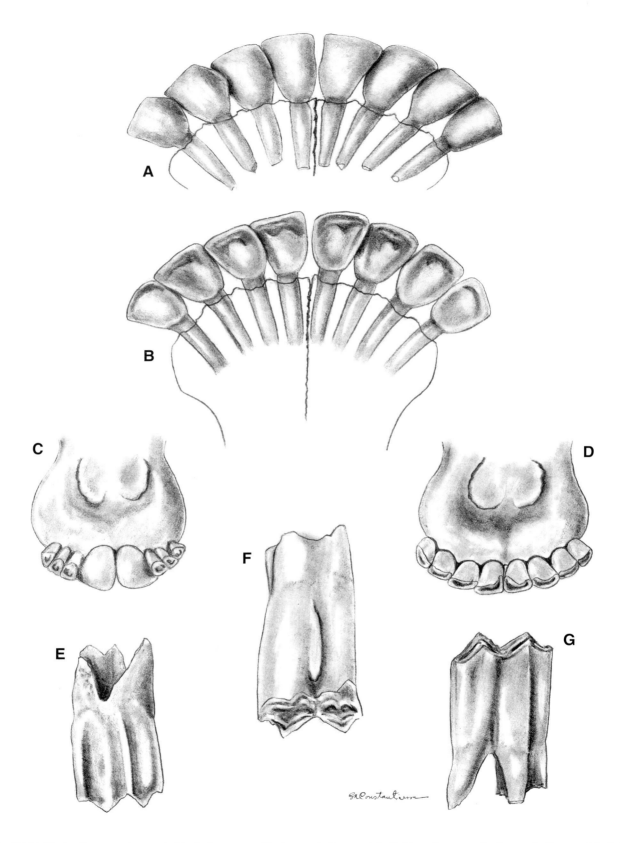

Fig. R7.14. Teeth of large ruminants. **A.** Vestibular aspect of incisor teeth (5 years old). **B.** Lingual aspect of incisor teeth (5 years old). **C.** Lingual aspect of incisor teeth (2 years old). **D.** Lingual aspect of incisor teeth (6 years old). **E.** Vestibular aspect of superior third molar (permanent). **F.** Lingual aspect of superior third molar (permanent). **G.** Vestibular aspect of inferior third molar (permanent).

The dental formula of the large ruminants is the following:

The **deciduous dentition**:
2(Di0/4 Dc0/0 Dp3/3) = 20 teeth
The **permanent dentition**:
2(I0/4 C0/0 P3/3 M3/3) = 32 teeth

The (only lower) incisors, in mediolateral order are called the **central, first intermediate, second intermediate**, and **corner incisors**. Again, the corner incisors are **canine teeth** that have migrated rostrally. Differences exist between the deciduous and permanent incisors. However, only the apical halves of all incisors' roots are enclosed in the (large) alveoli; in addition, the **periodontium** is loose and allows for a slight movement of the teeth. An incisor tooth generally has a shovel-shaped **crown** that is separated from the thin rounded or squared **root** by a distinct **neck**. The deciduous incisors are set in a divergent position.

The free edge of the incisors, corresponding to the level at which the **vestibular** and **lingual surfaces** meet, is sharp on both deciduous and permanent teeth. The crown is covered with **enamel**. No **infundibulum** is found in ruminants. The enamel is worn from the free edge in a caudal direction, exposing the **dentine** on the **occlusal surface**. The **dental cavity** and the **root canal** are very large in the deciduous incisors. In the middle of the occlusal surface, a small **dental star** appears in specimens that are between 5 and 12 years of age. In these specimens, **secondary dentine** obliterates the dental cavity.

The **premolars** and **molars** resemble those of the horse. However, the vestibular ridges of the upper cheek teeth are more prominent and the grooves separating them are deeper than those of the horse. The lingual surface of these teeth is convex (single for premolars and separated into two halves by a vertical groove in molars). Both the vestibular and lingual surfaces of the lower cheek teeth are convex and are provided with vertical grooves. The occlusal surface of all the cheek teeth is very irregular and shows dentine, enamel, and cementum.

In the ruminants, the premolars are considered as the P2, P3, and P4 on both dental arcades.

Table R7.3 shows the eruption and replacement of the teeth in the large ruminants.

The **paranasal sinuses** in the large ruminants are the **medial rostral frontal, middle (intermediate) rostral frontal, lateral rostral frontal, caudal frontal, maxillary, lacrimal, sphenoid, palatine** (see Fig. R7.12), and

Table R7.3. Eruption and Replacement of Teeth in Large Ruminants

| Teeth | Time of Eruption | Teeth | Time of Eruption |
|---|---|---|---|
| Di 0/1 | Before birth | I 0/1 | 14–25 months |
| Di 0/2 | Before birth | I 0/2 | 17–33 months |
| Di 0/3 | Before birth—up to 2–6 days | I 0/3 | 22–40 months |
| Di 0/4 | Before birth—up to 2–14 days | I 0/4 | 32–42 months |
| Dp 2/2 | Before birth—up to 14–21 days | P 2/2 | 24–28 months |
| Dp 3/3 | Before birth—up to 14–21 days | P 3/3 | 24–30 months |
| Dp 4/4 | Before birth—up to 14–21 days | P 4/4 | 28–34 months |
| M 1/1 | 5–6 months | | |
| M 2/2 | 15–18 months | | |
| M 3/3 | 24–28 months | | |

Source: After Nickel, Schummer, Seiferle, Sack 1979.

**dorsal conchal, middle conchal**, and **ventral conchal sinuses**.

On the midsagittal surface of the head of your specimen, identify the external and internal plates (laminae) of the frontal bone. A **median septum** separates the two symmetrical bones. The **frontal sinuses** are sculptured within the frontal, parietal, interparietal, temporal, and occipital bones. Take a hammer and a chisel and remove the external plate of the frontal bone to expose all the frontal sinuses. The **caudal frontal sinus**, separated by an **oblique septum** from the **rostral frontal sinuses**, is divided into the three diverticula, the **cornual, nuchal**, and **postorbital**. The rostral frontal sinuses are three, the **lateral, middle**, and **medial** (see Fig. R7.15).

**Clinically, we have access only to the frontal and maxillary sinuses. By trepanation (trephination), these sinuses can be inspected, cleaned, and medicated in case of sinusitis or parasites. The landmarks and approaches to these sinuses will be exposed in Modlab R4.**

Turn the head lateral side up and focus on the eye. Examine the two **eyelids**, their **commissures**, and the **palpebral fissure**, which starts and ends in the **lateral/medial angles of the eye** (called by the clinicians **canthi—sing. canthus**); inside the medial canthus identify the **lacrimal caruncle** and the two **lacrimal puncta**, which are located dorsal and ventral to the caruncle and are sometimes difficult to identify in the large ruminants (see Fig. R7.16A).

Everting the eyelids, examine the **palpebral** and **bulbar conjunctivae**, the **conjunctival fornix**, and the **conjunc-**

A

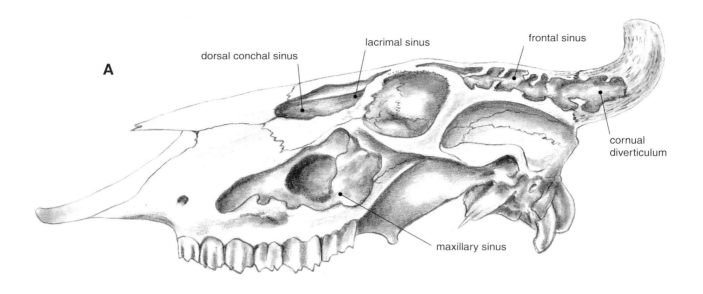

dorsal conchal sinus

lacrimal sinus

frontal sinus

cornual diverticulum

maxillary sinus

B

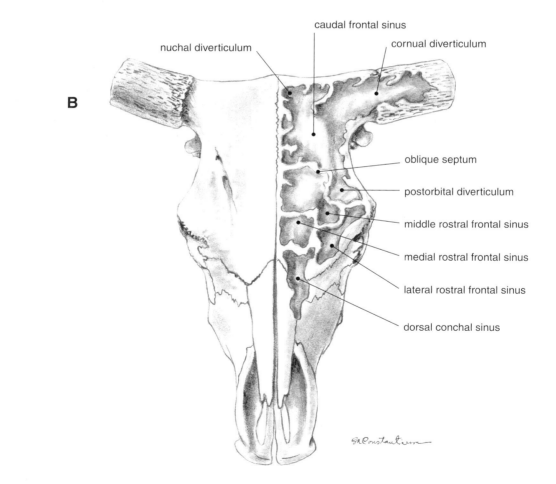

nuchal diverticulum

caudal frontal sinus

cornual diverticulum

oblique septum

postorbital diverticulum

middle rostral frontal sinus

medial rostral frontal sinus

lateral rostral frontal sinus

dorsal conchal sinus

Fig. R7.15. Paranasal sinuses in the large ruminants. **A.** Lateral aspect. **B.** Frontal aspect.

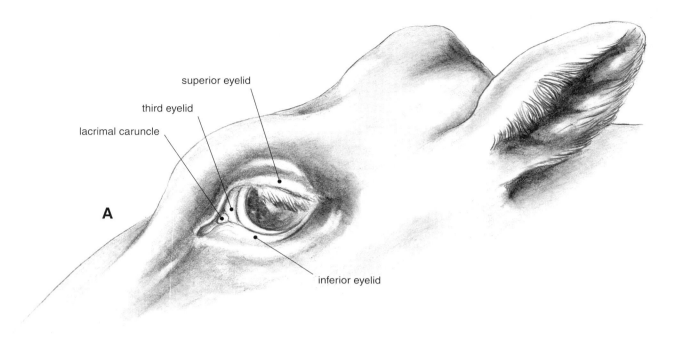

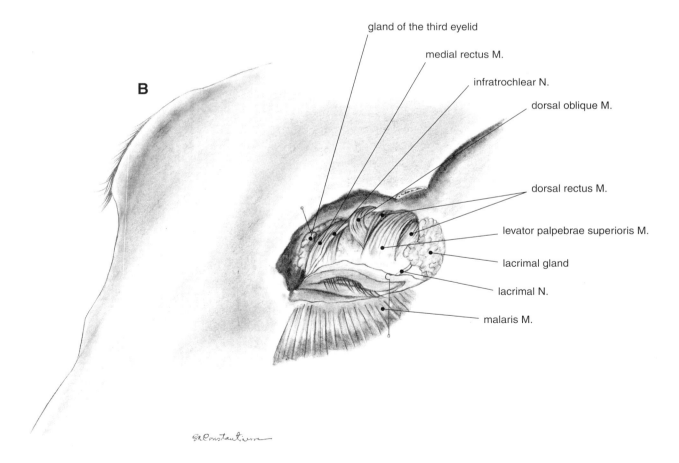

Fig. R7.16. The eye of the large ruminants. **A.** External features. **B.** Structures of the eye within the orbita, dorsal view.

tival sac. Make a transverse incision in the eyelids and identify the **tarsus**, the **tarsal glands**, the **orbicularis oculi M.**, the **orbital septum**, and for the upper eyelid, the **levator palpebrae superioris M.**

Examine the **semilunar fold (the third eyelid, nictitating membrane)**, the T-shaped **cartilage**, and the **superficial** and **deep glands** of the **third eyelid**.

Remove the large amount of **extraperiorbital fat** and expose the **periorbita**. Transect the periorbita in its long axis, free its rostral attachment from the **orbital septum** and the caudal attachment from the **pterygoid crest**, and reflect the stumps. The fat found on the deep aspect of the periorbita is part of the **intraperiorbital fat**. Save the **lacrimal gland** and try to identify the most superficial structures within the periorbita (see Fig. R7.16B). The most superficial structures (muscles, arteries and nerves) are illustrated in Figure R7.17A. The deep structures, including the **rete mirabile ophthalmicum**, which is specific to ruminants, are illustrated in Figure R7.17B. The technique for dissecting these structures is similar to that shown for the horse (starting page 229).

Turn the head midsagittal side up and examine the **spinal cord** and the **brain** (see Fig. 7.18).

Identify the gray and the white matter and the **central canal** of the spinal cord. Separate and identify the **pia mater** from the **arachnoid** and the **dura mater**. Probe the **subarachnoid**, **subdural**, and **epidural spaces** (the latter only in the vertebral canal).

*Remember!* The pia mater and the archnoid are called the **leptomeninges**. The dura mater is the **pachymeninx**.

Identify the meninges of the brain, especially the **falx cerebri**, the **tentorium cerebelli membranaceum**, and the **diaphragma sellae**.

Remove the brain from the cranial cavity and systematically identify the same structures of the brain as were described for the horse in Chapter H7 (starting page 248) and compare these structures with those on the dorsal, ventral, and lateral perspectives (see Figs. R7.18 and R7.19).

A few significant differences must be mentioned. In ruminants, the **cavernous sinus** (venous), which surrounds the **hypophysis**, does not enclose the internal carotid A. In the ruminants there is an arterial network protected within the cavernous sinus, called the **rete mirabile epidurale**, which consists of the **rostral rete mirabile epidurale** and the **caudal rete mirabile epidurale**, which are continuous with each other (see Fig. R7.20). In the pig, there are two retia (pl. of rete) mirabile epidurale, separated from each other.

## MODLAB R4

The following landmarks and approaches to the paranasal sinuses may be helpful.

1. **Frontal sinuses** (see Fig. R7.15)

α. The **caudal frontal sinus** (see Fig. R7.15B)
  A. *Landmarks*: lateral canthus of the eye, temporal line, supraorbital foramen, middorsal line of the head, base of the horn
  B. *Approach*:
    a. 4 cm caudal to the lateral canthus, between the temporal line and the supraorbital foramen, through the skin and external plate of the frontal bone (into the postorbital diverticulum)
    b. Halfway between the middorsal line of the head and the base of the horn, through the skin and the external plate of the frontal bone (into the nuchal diverticulum)
    c. Lateral to the previous approach, into the cornual diverticulum

β. The **rostral frontal sinuses** (see Fig. R7.15B)
  A. *Landmarks*: dorsal rim of the orbita, middorsal line of the head
  B. *Approach*: halfway between the dorsal rim of the orbita and the middorsal line of the head
    *Note*. (1) In all instances avoid damage to the frontal V. (2) The caudal frontal sinus is completely separated from the rostral frontal sinuses by the oblique septum.

2. **Maxillary sinus** (see Fig. R7.15A)
  A. *Landmarks:* lateral and medial canthi of the eye, zygomatic arch, ventral border of maxilla rostral to the premolars, the upper P3 or P4 (***Remember*** that in the ruminants the numbering of the premolars starts with P2.), the upper M4
  B. *Approach:* within the triangular area outlined by the zygomatic arch along the lateral and medial canthi of the eye, and a line in continuation to the ventral border of maxilla, from P3 or P4 to the M4

**The sites for the nerve block of the head** are shown in Figure R7.21.

**The sites for the nerve block of the spinal cervical nerves supplying the ox head** are illustrated in Figure R7.22.

**The cutaneous innervation of the bovine head** is shown in Figure R7.23.

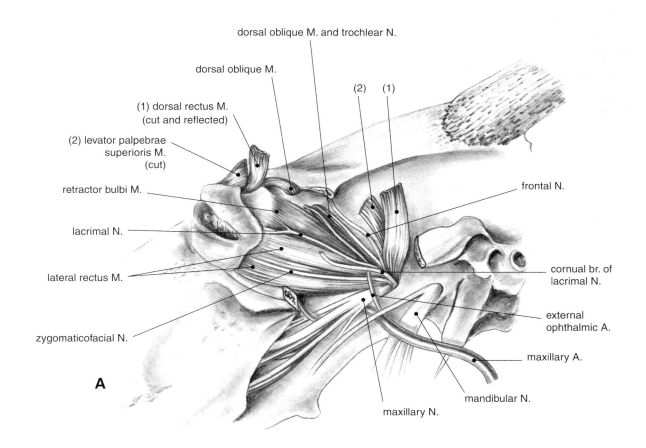

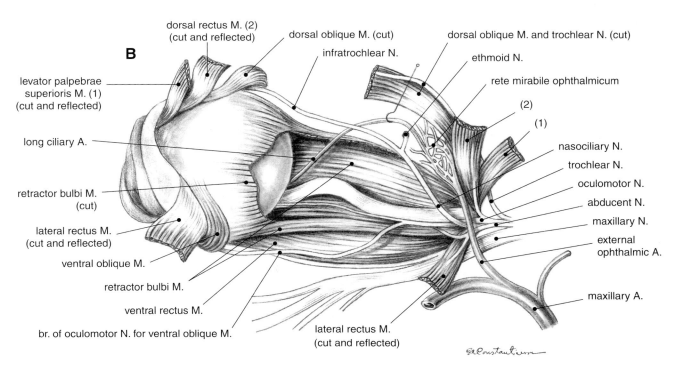

Fig. R7.17. Structures of the eye, large ruminants. **A.** Structures in the orbital area, lateral view. **B.** Deep structures in the orbital area, lateral view.

The lobules of vermis
1–lingula
2–lobulus centralis
3-3'–culmen
4–declive
5–folium vermis
6–tuber vermis
7–pyramis
8–uvula
9–nodulus

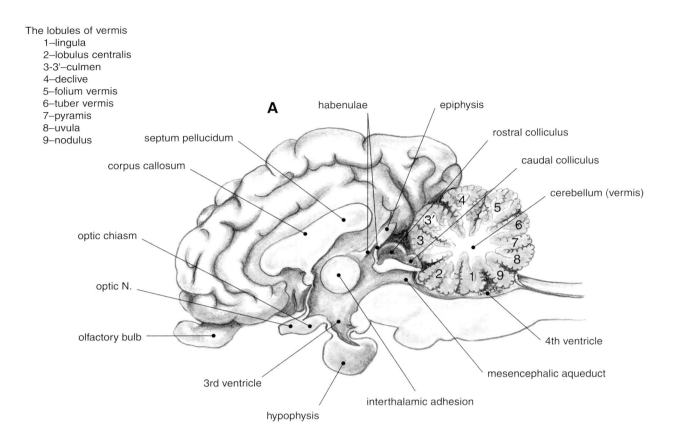

A

habenulae

epiphysis

rostral colliculus

caudal colliculus

cerebellum (vermis)

septum pellucidum

corpus callosum

optic chiasm

optic N.

olfactory bulb

3rd ventricle

hypophysis

interthalamic adhesion

mesencephalic aqueduct

4th ventricle

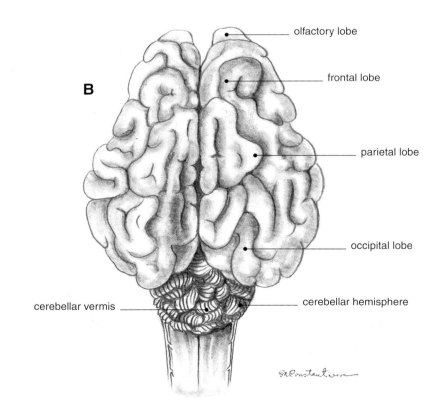

B

olfactory lobe

frontal lobe

parietal lobe

occipital lobe

cerebellar vermis

cerebellar hemisphere

Fig. R7.18. The brain of the large ruminants. **A.** Median aspect. **B.** Dorsal aspect.

**A**

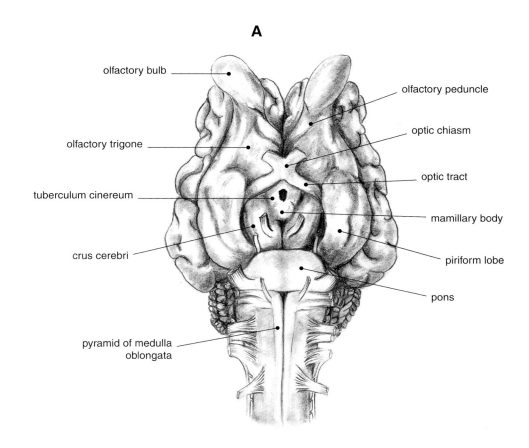

olfactory bulb

olfactory peduncle

optic chiasm

olfactory trigone

optic tract

tuberculum cinereum

mamillary body

crus cerebri

piriform lobe

pons

pyramid of medulla
oblongata

**B**

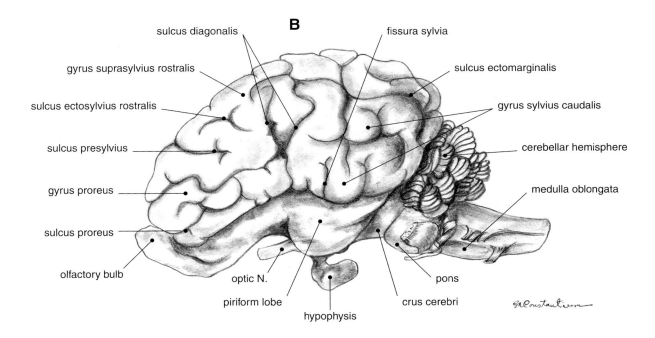

sulcus diagonalis

fissura sylvia

gyrus suprasylvius rostralis

sulcus ectomarginalis

sulcus ectosylvius rostralis

gyrus sylvius caudalis

sulcus presylvius

cerebellar hemisphere

gyrus proreus

medulla oblongata

sulcus proreus

olfactory bulb

optic N.

pons

piriform lobe

crus cerebri

hypophysis

Fig. R7.19. The brain of the large ruminants. **A.** Ventral aspect. **B.** Lateral aspect.

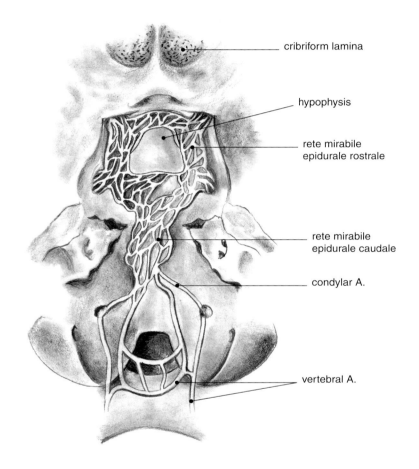

cribriform lamina

hypophysis

rete mirabile
epidurale rostrale

rete mirabile
epidurale caudale

condylar A.

vertebral A.

Fig. R7.20. Arteries of the floor of the brain cavity, large ruminants.

1–mental N.
2–infraorbital N.
3–zygomaticofacial N.
4–infratrochlear N.
5–frontal N.
6–lacrimal N.
7–cornual N.
8–optic N.
9–ophthalmic, maxillary, and motor Nn. of the eye
10–auriculopalpebral N.
11–inferior alveolar N.

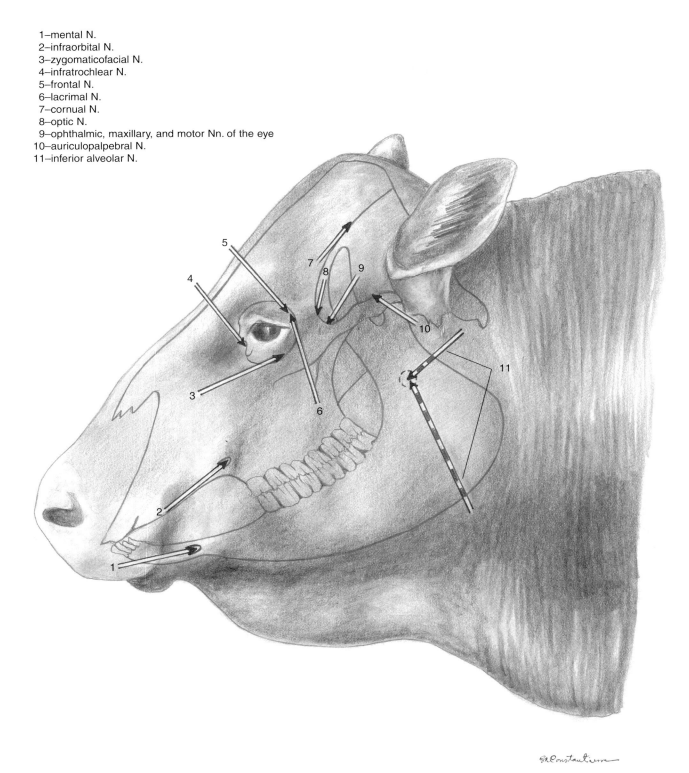

Fig. R7.21. Sites for nerve block in the ox head.

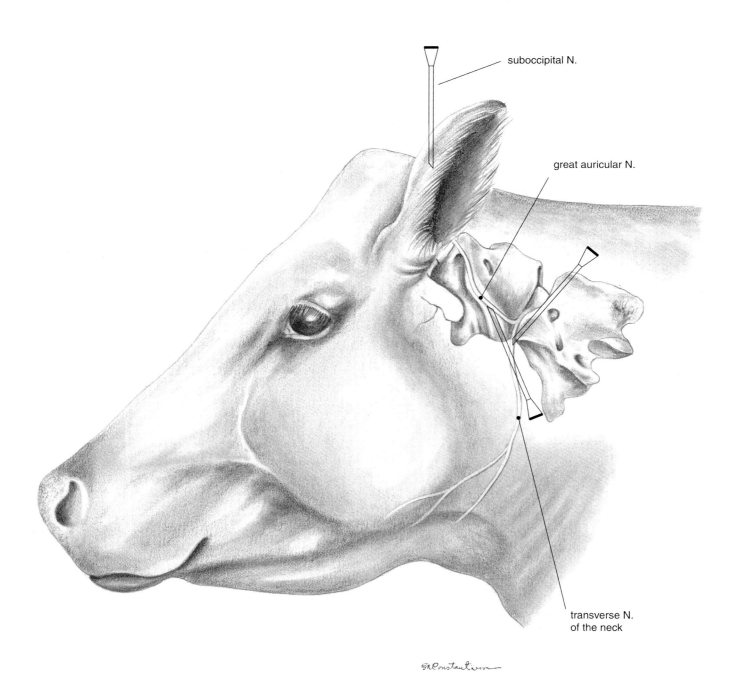

Fig. R7.22. Sites for nerve block of the spinal cervical nerves supplying the ox head.

1–infraorbital N.
2–mental N.
3–infratrochlear N.
4–frontal N.
5–zygomaticofacial N.
6–lacrimal N.
7–cornual N.
8–auriculotemporal N.
9–suboccipital
10–internal auricular br. of facial N.
11–great auricular N.
12–transverse N. of the neck

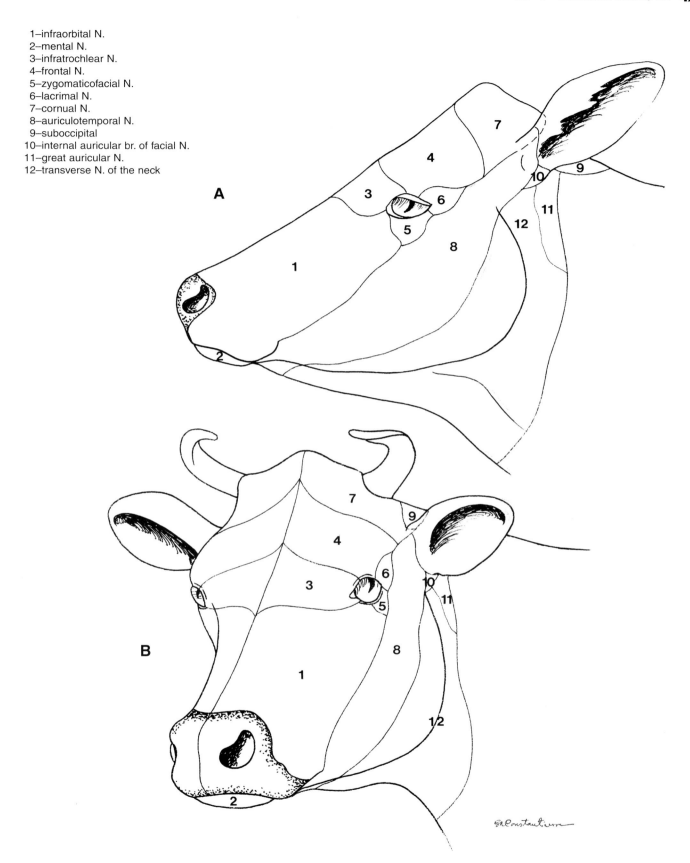

Fig. R7.23. Cutaneous innervation of the bovine head. **A.** Lateral view. **B.** Anterolateral view.

Table R7.4 shows the average age of fusion of the epiphyses of all bones. This table is helpful for radiological, clinical, and necropsy purposes.

Table R7.4. The Revised Table with the Average Age of Fusion of the Epiphyses

| The Bone | The Ossification Center, which Is Fused | Species | | | | |
|---|---|---|---|---|---|---|
| | | Horse | Ox | Small Ruminant | Pig | Dog |
| Occipital | Exoccipital-basioccipital | 3–6 mo. | 10–12 mo. | 6 mo. | 8–10 mo. | 2½–3 mo. |
| | Exoccipital-squama | 12–15 mo. | | | | 3–4 mo. |
| | Interparietal-squama | 1–2 yr. | b.b. | a.b. | absent | b.b. |
| Presphenoid | Body + wings | b.b. | | | | |
| Basisphenoid | Body + wings | 6 mo. | 6 mo. | 3–4 yr. | 12 mo. | 3–4 yr. |
| | Pre- and Basisphenoid | 2–4 yr. | 2½–4 yr. | 4–5 yr. | 6–12 mo. | 1–2 yr. |
| | Spheno-occipital | 3–5 yr. | 2 yr. | 1–2 yr. | 1–2 yr. | 8–10 mo. |
| Parietal | Interparietal suture | 15–36 mo. | 6 mo. | 1 mo. | 6–15 mo. | 2–3 yr. |
| Frontal | Interfrontal suture | 5–7 yr. | Incomplete | 5–7 yr. | 1–2 yr. | 3–4 yr. |
| Temporal | Petrotympanic | 2–4 mo. | At birth | Never or very late | 6 mo. | |
| | Petrosquamous | Never or very late | 2–4 mo. | 4–6 mo. | At birth | 2–3 yr. |
| Mandible | Centers of each bone | b.b. | | | | |
| | Fusion of the two bones | 6 mo. | Never complete | | After birth | Never or very late |
| Vertebrae | Body epiphyses | 4½–5 yr. | 4½–5 yr. | 4–5 yr. | 4–7 yr. | 1½–2 yr. |
| Scapula | Coracoid center | 10–12 mo. | 7–10 mo | 10–11 mo | 1 yr | 5–8 mo |
| Humerus | Proximal extremity | 42 mo. | 42–48 mo. | 30–40 mo. | 42 mo. | 12–15 mo. |
| | Distal extremity | 15–18 mo. | 15–20 mo. | 9–11 mo. | 12 mo. | 7–8 mo. |
| Radius | Proximal extremity | 15–18 mo. | 12–15 mo. | 8–10 mo. | 12 mo. | 9–10 mo. |
| | Distal extremity | 42 mo. | 40–48 mo. | 40–60 mo. | 42 mo. | 10–12 mo. |
| Ulna | Proximal extremity | 42 mo. | 42 mo. | 20–40 mo. | 42 mo. | 7–8 mo. |
| | Distal extremity | 2–3 mo. to radius | 3 yr. | 35–40 mo. | 3 yr. | 9–12 mo. |
| Metacarpals | Distal extremity | 15 mo. | 24–30 mo. | 30–36 mo. | 2 yr. | 6–7 mo. |
| Prox. phalanx | Proximal extremity | 12–15 mo. | 20–24 mo. | 10–16 mo. | 13 mo. | 6–7 mo. |
| Middle phalanx | Proximal extremity | 10–12 mo. | 15–18 mo. | 12–18 mo. | 1 yr. | 6–7 mo. |
| Coxal | Main centers + acetabular | 10–12 mo. | 7–10 mo. | 10 mo. | 1 yr. | 6 mo. |
| | Ischiatic tuberosity | 4–5 yr. | 5 yr. | 4–5 yr. | 6–7 yr. | 10–12 mo. |
| | Iliac crest | 4½–5 yr. | 5 yr. | 4½–5 yr. | 6–7 yr. | 2–3 yr. |
| Femur | Proximal extremity | 3 yr. | 3 yr. | 36–40 mo. | 3 yr. | 9–12 mo. |
| | Distal extremity | 42 mo. | 42 mo. | 40–42 mo. | 42 mo. | 9–12 mo. |
| Tibia | Proximal extremity | 42 mo. | 4 yr. | 50–55 mo. | 42 mo. | 10–12 mo. |
| | Distal extremity | 2 yr. | 24–30 mo. | 25–35 mo. | 2 yr. | 9–10 mo. |
| Fibula | Proximal extremity | | 42 mo. to tibia | | 42 mo. | 10–12 mo. |
| Calcaneus | Tuberosity | 3 yr. | | | 24–30 mo. | 6–7 mo. |

*Source:* After Barone 1999.

*Note:* mo. = month(s); yr. = year(s); b.b. = before birth; a.b. = after birth.

# References

Adams, S.B. 1999. Biology and treatment of specific muscle disorders. In J.A. Auer and J. A. Stick, (eds.), *Equine Surgery,* 2nd ed., 720–727. Philadelphia: W.B. Saunders.

Adams, S.B., and J.F. Fessler. 2000. Castration. In S.B. Adams and J.F. Fessler (eds.), *Atlas of Equine Surgery,* 209–214. Philadelphia: W.B. Saunders.

Ashdown, R.R., and S. Done. 1987. *Color Atlas of Veterinary Anatomy—The Horse.* Baltimore: University Park Press, Gower Medical Publishing.

_____. 1996. *Color Atlas of Veterinary Anatomy— The Ruminants.* London: Mosby-Wolfe.

Barber, S.M. 1999. Diseases of the guttural pouches. In P.T. Colohan, I.G. Mayhew, A.M. Merritt, and J.N. Moore (eds.), *Equine Medicine and Surgery,* 501–512. St. Louis: Mosby.

Barone, R. 1968–2000. *Anatomie comparée des mammifères domestiques,* vols. 1–5. Laboratoire École Nationale Vétérinaire, Lyon and Vigot.

Berg, R. 1988. *Angewandte und topographische Anatomie der Haustiere,* 3rd ed. Jena: VEB Gustav Fischer Verlag.

Bohanon T.C. 1995. Developmental musculoskeletal disease. In C. Kobluck, T. Ames, and R. Goer (eds.), *The Horse Diseases and Clinical Management,* 815–855. Philadelphia: W.B. Saunders.

Bonen, C.G., J. Bryant, J. Hernandez, et al. 1999. Sternothyroideus tenectomy or sternothyroideus tenectomy with staphylectomy for the treatment of soft palate displacement. *Proceedings of the American Association of Equine Practioners* 45:85–86.

Budras, K.-D., W.O. Sack, and S. Roeck. 1994. *Anatomy of the Horse. An Illustrated Text,* 2nd ed. London: Mosby-Wolfe.

Clayton, H.M., and P.F. Flood. 1996. *Color Atlas of Large Animal Applied Anatomy.* London: Mosby-Wolfe.

Constantinescu, D.M., and G.M. Constantinescu. 2000. Feto-maternal ethology during parturition in the cow, with neurophysiological arguments for using adequate obstetrical techniques. *Analele Institutului de Cercetare și Producție pentru Creșterea Bovinelor* 17:201–214.

Constantinescu, G.M. 1962. The mechanical structure of the hock in horse (*Equus caballus* L.). Stamps of the mechanical function on the organization and structure. Ph.D. Thesis, Bucharest, Romania.

_____. 1979. Critical considerations on the veterinary anatomical nomenclature of the arteries of the thoracic limb in domestic mammals with proposals of improvement of the nomenclature. *The Second Symposium of Anatomy,* 29–30 June, Cluj-Napoca, Romania.

_____. 1988. A controversial problem: Is the M. iliocostalis cervicis a fictitious structure? Personal observations in goat and critical review of the literature. *Anatomia, Histologia, Embryologia* 17:34.

_____. 1988. How many cervical intertransversarii Mm. are there in domestic mammals? A special study in goat and a critical review of the literature. *Anatomia, Histologia, Embryologia* 17:34.

_____. 1991. New concepts and directions for dissecting large animals. *Second Annual College of Veterinary Medicine Teaching Techniques Competition,* Columbia, MO, no.6, p.6.

_____. 1991. *Clinical Dissection Guide for Large Animals.* St. Louis, MO: Mosby-Year Book.

_____. 1994. Concepts and principles in the teaching of anatomy, histology and embryology. *Romania and Romanians in Contemporary Science* (International Conference), Sinaia, Romania, 25.

_____. 1994. Role of modern anatomy in veterinary medicine. *The Sixth National Congress of Veterinary Medicine,* Sinaia, Romania, 177.

_____. 1995. The cutaneous areas and the clinical applications of the nerve block anesthesia of the cranial nerves in the horse. *Revista Română de Medicină Veterinară* 5(1): 57–66.

_____. 1995. Block anesthesia of cranial nerves in the ruminants. Anatomy, landmarks, and approaches. *Revista Română de Medicină Veterinară* 5(3): 279–294.

_____. 1996. Landmarks and approaches of the main anatomic structures of the horse susceptible to clinical intervention. *Anatomia, Histologia, Embryologia* 25:202.

_____. 1996. Reconsideration and comparative view of the internal cremaster M. in stallion, bull, goat, boar and dog. *Anatomia, Histologia, Embryologia* 25:218.

_____. 1998. The scalenus system in goat and a critical review of the literature of the scalene in domestic animals. *Anatomical Record* 220(4): 25A.

_____. 1999. Clinical anatomy—The future of anatomy. *Surgical and Radiologic Anatomy—Journal of Clinical Anatomy* 52: 29.

_____. 1999. Clinical anatomy of the equine fetlock. *Topical Interests in Animal Breeding Pathology,* 3–8. Cluj-Napoca, Romania: Risoprint Press.

_____. 2000. Illustrations. In *The Merck Veterinary Manual,* 8th ed. (CD-ROM 2000).

_____. 2001. *Guide to Regional Ruminant Anatomy Based on the Dissection of the Goat.* Ames: Iowa State University Press.

Constantinescu, G.M., E.M. Brown, and R.C. McClure. 1988. Accessory parotid lymph nodes and hemal nodes in the temporal fossa in three oxen. *Cornell Veterinarian* 78:147–154.

Constantinescu, G.M., and I. Constantinescu. 1980. Comments on the nomenclature of veins of thoracic limb in horse. *The Third Symposium of Anatomy,* 30 June–1 July, Craiova, Romania.

_____. 2001. Clinical anatomy and clinical concepts taught in the first semester to the VM1 students in Columbia, Missouri (USA). *The Sixth International Congress of the European Association of Clinical Anatomy,* 13–15 September, Montpellier, France.

Constantinescu, G.M., I.A. Constantinescu, J.Z. March, J. Gottdenker, and T. Nieuwenhuizen. 2002. Concepts of teaching clinical anatomy in the veterinary curriculum at the University of Missouri—USA. *The 17th International Symposium on Morphological Sciences,* 11–15 September, Timişoara, Romania.

Constantinescu, G.M., I. Constantinescu, C. Radu, and R. Palicica. 1979. The homologizing of the arteries of clinical importance in the thoracic limb of ruminants and horses. *Probleme de ameliorare, de tehnologie de creştere şi de patologie la taurine şi ovine—Lucrările secţiei de patologie,* Cluj-Napoca, Romania, 128–132.

Constantinescu, G.M., J. Cosoroabă, and D. Constantinescu. 1969. The pelvis minor in cow. *Symposium, 12–14 December,* Timişoara, Romania.

Constantinescu, G.M., and V. Coţofan. 1958. The fasciae of the autopodium in ruminants. *Caiet documentar de medicină veterinară—10 ani de comunicări ştiinţifice în învăţămîntul superior veterinar, 1948–1958,* no. 705.

Constantinescu, G.M., B.L. Frappier, and G.E. Brimer. 1996. Retrospective and modern considerations about the pharynx in the domestic animals: Gross anatomical and histological correlations. *Anatomia, Histologia, Embryologia* 25:202–203.

Constantinescu, G.M., and E.M. Green. 1987. Transrectal palpation of the horse: A clinically oriented comprehensive review. *Abstracts—23rd World Veterinary Congress,* Montreal, Canada, paper 1.2.9:29.

Constantinescu, G.M, E.M. Green, and R.C. McClure. 1986. Nerve blocks in the horse head—Landmarks, topographic anatomy, clinical applications. *Proceedings of 62nd Annual Conference for Veterinarians,* Columbia, MO, 123–126.

_____. 1994. Block anesthesia of cranial nerves in the horse (landmarks, approaches, topographic anatomy and the technique of anesthesia). *Revista Română de Medicină Veterinară* 4(1): 48–67.

Constantinescu, G.M., H.E. König, D.A. Wilson, and K. Keegan. 1997. Clinical anatomy of the parotid region in the horse. *Wiener Tierärztliche Monatschrift* 84:144–148.

Constantinescu, G.M., and R.C. McClure. 1995. Clinical approach on anatomic structures—Nerve block anesthesia in the thoracic limb of the horse. *Proceedings of the American Association of Veterinary Anatomists,* Philadelphia, PA, 16.

Constantinescu, G.M., R.C. McClure, and B.L. Frappier. 1998. Anatomical terminology—Are we finished? *Abstract of the Annual Meeting of the American Association of Veterinary Anatomists,* 23–25 July, Blacksburg, VA, 7–8.

Constantinescu, G.M., R.C. McClure, and H.E. König. 1997. Clinical approach to nerve block anesthesia of horse limbs. *Anatomia, Histologia, Embryologia* 26:239.

Constantinescu, G.M., G. Nappert, I.A. Constantinescu, B.L. Frappier, and R.B. Miller. 2000. An anatomoclinical review of the landmarks for physical examination and clinical approach in the thoracic limb of the large ruminants. I. Nerve block anesthesia, arthroscopy, arthrocentesis and intraarticular analgesia. *21st World Buiatrics Congress* (CD-ROM), Punta del Este, Uruguay.

Constantinescu, G.M., G. Nappert, B.L. Frappier, I.A. Constantinescu, and R.B. Miller. 2000. An anatomo-clinical review of the landmarks for physical examination and clinical approach in the pelvic limb of the large ruminants. I. Nerve block anesthesia, arthroscopy, arthrocentesis and intraarticular analgesia. *21st World Buiatrics Congress* (CD-ROM), Punta del Este, Uruguay.

Constantinescu, G.M., and R. Palicica. 1979. Comparison between the veterinary anatomical nomenclature of the arteries of limbs in horse. *The Second Symposium of Anatomy,* 29–30 June, Cluj-Napoca, Romania.

_____. 1981. Comparative view on the nomenclature of arteries of postdiaphragmatic digestive tube of the abdominal cavity. *Scientific Session,* 10–11 April, Timișoara, Romania.

_____. 1981. Comparative evolutive aspects of irrigation of the postdiaphragmatic digestive tube in domestic mammals. *Symposium,* 10–11 April, Iași, Romania.

Constantinescu, G.M., V. Pintea, and J. Cosoroabă. 1972. Quelques considérations de dynamique musculaire au niveau du membre pelvien. *The Eighth Congress of European Association of Veterinary Anatomists,* Wien, Austria.

Constantinescu, G.M., C. Radu, and V. Coțofan. 1997. Retrospective and comments on the acropodial fasciae in the horse. *Anatomia, Histologia, Embryologia* 26:64.

Constantinescu, G.M., C. Radu, and R. Palicica. 1979. Contributions to the topographic anatomy of thoracic limb in the large ruminants through serial transverse sections of zeugopodium and autopodium. *Probleme de ameliorare, de tehnologie de creștere și de patologie la taurine și ovine—Lucrările secției de patologie,* Cluj-Napoca, Romania, 132–136.

_____. 1979. Landmarks and topography for intraarterial injections of the pelvic limb in the large ruminants. *Probleme de ameliorare, de tehnologie de creștere și de patologie la taurine și ovine—Lucrările secției de patologie,* Cluj-Napoca, Romania, 136–138.

_____. 1979. The relationship among vessels, nerves, and osteomuscular substratum of the thoracic zeugopodium in the large ruminants. *Probleme de ameliorare, de tehnologie de creștere și de patologie la taurine și ovine—Lucrările secției de patologie,* Cluj-Napoca, Romania, 139–144.

_____. 1982. Peculiarities of peritoneum of the abdominal cavity in some domestic animals. *Symposium,* 2–3 April, Timișoara, Romania.

_____. 1982. The topography of the visceral aspect of liver in some species of domestic animals. *Symposium,* 2–3 April, Timișoara, Romania.

_____. 1982. The impressions of the surface of the lungs in some species of domestic mammals. *Symposium,* 2–3 April, Timișoara, Romania.

Constantinescu, G.M., C. Radu, R. Palicica, and C. Trandafir. 1980. Comparative view on the reticular groove in large and small ruminants. *Symposium,* 16–17 May, Cluj-Napoca, Romania.

Constantinescu, G.M., and D. Theodorescu. 1977. Practical aspects concerning the topography, and the pre- and post-ganglionic branches of the pelviperineal plexus in cow. *Symposium,* 22–23 January, Timișoara, Romania.

Constantinescu, G.M., D. Theodorescu, and O. Fuciu. 1977. L'anatomie clinique du plexus pelvi-périnéal chez la vache et le mouton. *Zentralblatt für Veterinär Medizin C,* G:367.

Constantinescu, G.M., and L.M. Wallace. 1995. The cutaneous innervation, the technique and clinical applications of nerve block anesthesia of the cranial nerves in ruminants. *Revista Română de Medicină Veterinară* 5(4): 383–394.

_____. 1995. The cutaneous innervation, the technique and clinical applications of nerve block anesthesia of the cranial nerves in ruminants. *Proceedings of Pathology in Ruminants* (Symposium with International Participation), Timișoara, Romania, 39–40.

Constantinescu, G.M., and D.A. Wilson. 1999. Clinical anatomy of the equine tarsus. *Surgical and Radiologic Anatomy, Journal of Clinical Anatomy, Abstract book of the Fifth European Association of Clinical Anatomy Congress,* 3–5 June, Constanța, Romania, 29 (no. 53).

_____. 1999. Clinical anatomy of the equine carpus. *26th World Veterinary Congress* (CD-ROM), Lyon, France.

Cornelissen B.P.M. 1997. The equine proximal sesamoid bone. Vascular and neural characteristics. Ph.D. Thesis, Utrecht, The Netherlands.

De Lahunta, A., and R.E. Habel. 1986. *Applied Veterinary Anatomy.* Philadelphia: W.B. Saunders.

Diaconescu, I., and G.M. Constantinescu. 1981. Evolutive comparative aspects on the vascularization of the digestive tube (Canalis alimentarius) and of its annex glands. *The Fourth Symposium of Anatomy,* 11–12 September, Timișoara, Romania.

Diesem, C.D. 1973. *A Guide for Bovine Dissection.* Copyright Charles D. Diesem.

Dyce, K.M., W.O. Sack, and C.J.G. Wensing. 2000. *Textbook of Veterinary Anatomy,* 3rd ed. Philadelphia: W.B. Saunders.

Ellenberger, W., and H. Baum. 1943. *Handbuch der vergleichenden Anatomie der Haustiere,* 18th ed. Berlin: Springer.

Evans, T.J., G.M. Constantinescu, and V.K. Ganjam. 1997. Clinical reproductive anatomy and physiology of the mare. In B.S. Youngquist (ed.), *Theriogenology,* 1st ed., 43–70. Philadelphia: W.B. Saunders.

Firth, E.C. 1980. Bilateral ventral accessory neurectomy in windsucking horses. *Veterinary Record* 106(2): 30–32.

Foreman, J.H. 1998. The exhausted horse syndrome. *Veterinary Clinics of North America: Equine Practice* 14(1): 205–219.

Freeman D.E. 1999. Guttural pouch. In J.A. Auer and J. A. Stick (eds.), *Equine Surgery,* 2nd ed., 368–376. Philadelphia: W.B. Saunders.

Garner, H.E., and G.M. Constantinescu. 1999. Heart. In J.A. Auer and J. A. Stick (eds.), *Equine Surgery,* 2nd ed., 387–393. Philadelphia: W.B. Saunders.

Garrett, P.D. 1987. Urethral recess in male goats, sheep, cattle, and swine. *Journal of American Veterinary Medical Association,* 191(6): 689–691.

Getty, R. 1975. *Sisson and Grossman's the Anatomy of the Domestic Animals,* vol. 1, 5th ed. Philadelphia: W.B. Saunders.

Gheţie, V. 1967. *Anatomia animalelor domestice.* Bucureşti: Editura Didactică şi Pedagogică.

Gheţie, V., and G.M. Constantinescu. 1960. Die morphophysiologischen Grundlagen der Sexualreflexe beim Stier. *Zuchthygiene* 4:285–291.

Gheţie, V., and A. Hillebrand. 1971. *Anatomia animalelor domestice,* vol. 1. Bucureşti: Editura Academiei Republicii Socialiste Româna.

Gheţie, V., E. Paştea, I. Atanasiu, and Z. Paştea. 1962. *Sistemul neurovegetativ la mamiferele si păsările domestice.* Bucureşti: Editura Academiei Republicii Socialiste Româna.

Goshal, N.G., T. Koch, and P. Popesko. 1981. *The Venous Drainage of the Domestic Animals.* Philadelphia: W.B. Saunders.

Green, E.M., G.M. Constantinescu, and R.A. Kroll. 1992. Equine cerebrospinal fluid: Physiologic principles and collection technique. *Compendium on Continuing Education for the Practicing Veterinarian* 14(2): 229–238.

Greet, T.R. 1982. Windsucking treated by myectomy and neurectomy. *Equine Veterinary Journal* 14(4): 299–301.

Habel, R.E. 1956. A source of error in the bovine pudendal nerve block. *Journal of the American Veterinary Medical Association* 128:16–17.

_____. 1966. The topographic anatomy of the muscles, nerves and arteries of the bovine female perineum. *American Journal of Anatomy* 119:79–96.

_____. 1989.*Guide to the Dissection of Domestic Ruminants,* 4th ed. Ithaca, NY: R.E. Habel.

Hahn, C.N., I.G. Mayhew, and R.J. Mackay. 1999. Diseases of the brainstem and cranial nerves (autonomic and somatic). In P.T. Colohan, I.G. Mayhew, A.M. Merritt, and J.N. Moore (eds.), *Equine Medicine and Surgery,* 937–938. St. Louis: Mosby.

Hardy J. 1995. Disease of soft tissue. In C. Kobluck, T. Ames, and R. Goer (eds.), *The Horse Diseases and Clinical Management,* 719–814. Philadelphia: W.B. Saunders.

Hardy J., M. Minton, J.T. Robertson, W.L. Beard, and L.A. Beard. 2000. Nephrosplenic entrapment in the horse: A retrospective study of 174 cases. *Equine Veterinary Journal Supplement* 32:95–97.

Harrison, I.W. 1988. Sternothyroideus myectomy in horses: 17 cases 1984–1985. *Journal American Veterinary Medical Association* 193:1299.

Holcombe S.J., F.J. Derksen, J.A. Stick, and N.E. Robinson. 1999. Pathophysiology of dorsal displacement of the soft palate in horses. *Equine Veterinary Journal Supplement* 30:45–48.

Holcombe, S.J., and N.G. Ducharme. 1999. Pharynx. In J.A. Auer and J.A. Stick (eds.), *Equine Surgery,* 2nd ed., 337–349. Philadelphia: W.B. Saunders.

Horney, F.D. 1960. Surgical drainage of the pericardial sac. *Canadian Veterinary Journal* 1:363.

Johnson, P.J., and G.M. Constantinescu. 2000. Collection of cerebrospinal fluid in horses. *Equine Veterinary Education* 12(1): 7–12.

Johnson P.J., and L.L. Kellam. 2001. The vestibular system. Part II: Differential diagnosis. *Equine Veterinary Education Journal* 13(3): 141–150.

Klochnen A., A.M. Vachon, and A.T. Fischer, Jr. 1996. Use of diagnostic ultrasonography in horses with signs of acute abdominal pain. *Journal American Veterinary Medical Association* 209(9): 1597–1601.

König, H.E., and H.-G. Liebich. 1999. *Anatomie der Haussäugetiere. Lehrbuch und Farbatlas für Studium und Praxis,* vols. 1 and 2. Stuttgart: Schattauer.

Kriz, N.G., D.R. Hodgson, and R.J. Rose. 2000. Prevalence and clinical importance of heart murmurs in racehorses. *Journal of the American Veterinary Medical Association* 216(9): 1441–1445.

Larson, L.L. 1953. The internal pudendal nerve block for anesthesia of the penis and the relaxation of the retractor penis muscle. *Journal of the American Veterinary Medical Association* 123:18–27.

Marks, D., M.P. Mackay-Smith, L.S. Cushing, and J.A. Leslie. 1970. Use of a prosthetic device for surgical correction of laryngeal hemiplegia in horses. *Journal of the American Medical Association* 157(2): 157–163.

Martin, M.T., M.T. Martin, W.L. Scrutchfield, and J.R. Joyce. 1999. A systematic approach to estimating the age of a horse. *Proceedings for the 45th AAEP Annual Convention,* 273–275.

McClure, R.C., and G.M. Constantinescu. 1985. Local anesthesia—Ox head—"Nerve blocks." *Proceedings of the 61st Annual Conference for Veterinarians,* Columbia, MO, 38.

Moyer, W., and J. Schumacher. 2002. *A Guide to Equine Joint Injection,* 3rd ed. Yardley, PA: Veterinary Learning Systems.

Mueller, P.O.E., and W.P. Hay. 1999. Ancillary diagnostic aids. In P.T. Colohan, I.G. Mayhew, A.M. Merritt, and J.N. Moore (eds.), *Equine Medicine and Surgery,* 1292–1306. St. Louis: Mosby.

Muir, W.W., III, J.A.E. Hubbell, R.T. Skarda, and R.M. Bednarski. 1995. *Handbook of Veterinary Anesthesia,* 2nd ed. St. Louis, MO: Mosby.

Murray, R.C., E.M. Green, and G.M. Constantinescu. 1992. Equine enterolithiasis. *Compendium on Continuing Education for the Practicing Veterinarian.* 14(8): 1104–1113.

Nickel, R., A. Schummer, E. Seiferle, et al. 1979-1984. *The Anatomy of the Domestic Animals,* vols. 1–4. Berlin: Paul Parey.

Noordsy, J.L. 1994. *Food Animal Surgery,* 3rd ed., 41–45; 49–50. Trenton, NJ: VSL Books.

Owen R., F.J. McKeating, and D.W. Jagger. 1980. Neurectomy in windsucking horses. *Veterinary Record* 106(6): 134–135.

Paştea, E., E. Mureşianu, G.M. Constantinescu, and V. Coţofan. 1978. *Anatomia comparativă şi topografică a animalelor domestice.* Bucureşti: Editura Didactică şi Pedagogică.

Pavaux, C. 1982. *Atlas en couleurs d'anatomie des bovins—Splanchnologie.* Paris: Maloine.

Peterson, D.R. 1951. Nerve block of the eye and associated structures. *Journal of the American Veterinary Medical Association* 118: 145–148.

Pintea, V., and G.M. Constantinescu. 1980. The lymphoid system in domestic mammals. *Third Symposium of Anatomy,* 30 June–1 July, Craiova, Romania.

Pintea, V., G.M. Constantinescu, S. Botărel, and M. Sincai. 1980. Vascular and neuromuscular structures in the interosseous medius of horse. *Symposium,* 7–8 November, Timişoara, Romania.

Popescu, P., V. Paraipan, and V. Nicolescu. 1958. Anestezia subsacralâ la taur şi la cal. *Probleme Zootehnice şi Veterinare,* no. 3, 46–50.

Rebhun, W.C. 1995. *Diseases of Dairy Cattle.* Philadelphia: Lea and Febiger.

Robertson, J.T. 1998. Dorsal displacement of the soft palate. In N.A. White and J.N. Moore (eds.), *Current Techniques in Equine Surgery and Lameness,* 131–135. Philadelphia: W.B. Saunders.

Schaller, O., G.M. Constantinescu, R.E. Habel, W.O. Sack, P. Simoens, and N.R. de Vos. 1992. *Illustrated Veterinary Anatomical Nomenclature.* Stuttgart: Ferdinand Enke.

Schumacher, J. 1999. The testis and associated structures. In J.A. Auer and J.A. Stick (eds.), *Equine Surgery,* 2nd ed., 515–540. Philadelphia: W.B. Saunders.

Schumacher J., J. Schumacher, J.S. Spano, J. McGuire, W.L. Scrutchfield, and R.G. Feldman. 1988. Effects of castration on peritoneal fluid in the horse. *Journal of Veterinary Internal Medicine* 2(1): 22–25.

Short, C.E. 1987. *Principles and Practice of Veterinary Anesthesia.* Baltimore: Williams and Wilkins.

Short, C.E., H.E. Garner, and J.R. Coffman. 1988. Local anesthesia. In F.W. Oehme (ed.), *Textbook of Large Animal Surgery,* 2nd ed. Baltimore: Williams and Wilkins.

Skarda, R.T. 1987. Local and regional anesthesia. In *Principles and Practice of Veterinary Anesthesia.* Baltimore: Williams and Wilkins.

Soma, L.R. 1972. *Textbook of Veterinary Anesthesia.* Baltimore: Williams and Wilkins.

Stashak, T.S. 2002. Local anesthesia. In T.S. Stashak (ed.), *Adams' Lameness in Horses,* 5th ed., 160–180. Philadelphia: Lippincott Williams and Wilkins.

Step D.L., J.F. Cummings, A. de Lahunta, B.A. Valentine, B.A. Summers, P.H. Rowland, H.O. Mohammed, R.H. Eckerlin, and W.C. Rebhun. 1993. Motor neuron degeneration in a horse. *Journal of American Veterinary Medical Association* 202(1): 86–88.

Streeter, R.N. 2000. Abdominal ultrasound in cattle. *Proceedings of the ACVIM (American College of Veterinary Internal Medicine) Forum.*

Theodorescu, D., G.M. Constantinescu, N. Cociu, C. Stock, I. Garboni, E. Giurginca, and I. Maywurm. 1977. The utilization of procaine in veterinary obstetrique and gynecology. *Referatele primului simpozion al medicamentului de uz veterinar,* Bucureşti, 158–161.

Theodorescu, D., G.M. Constantinescu, I. Garboni, and N. Corin. 1977. A practical approach proceeding in the interventions upon the ovary in cow. *Symposium,* 16–17 December, Bucharest.

Theodorescu, D., G.M. Constantinescu, and E. Mlelwa. 1978. Some researches concerning the technique of the direct puncture of the ovary in cow. *Scientific Session,* 15 December, Timişoara, Romania.

Theodorescu, D., G.M. Constantinescu, and R. Silaghi. 1977. A practical method of relaxation of the cervix and other viscera in the pelvic cavity in cow. *Probleme de Patologie Veterinară,* Timişoara, Romania 1:331–335.

Turner, A.S., and C.W. McIlwraith. 1989. *Techniques in Large Animal Surgery,* 2nd ed., 263–288. Philadelphia: Lea and Febiger.

Van Metre, D.C., J.K. House, B.P. Smith, L.W. George, S.M. Angelos, J.A. Angelos, and G. Fecteau. 1996. Obstructive urolithiasis in ruminants. In *Medical Treatment and Urethral Surgery, Compendium on Continuing Education for the Practicing Veterinarian* 18:317–328.

Waibl, H., J. Hermann, J. Rehage, P. Lorenzi, and G.M. Constantinescu. 2001. Zur angewandten Anatomie des distalen "Vinculum tendinis" in der Fesselbeugesehnenscheide der Beckengliedmasse des Rindes. *Deutsche Tierärztliche Wochenschrift* 108 (6): 233–280.

Waibl, H., P. Lorenzi, J. Rehage, and G.M. Constantinescu. 2000. Clinical/applied anatomy of the bovine fetlock tendon sheath in the hindlimb. *21st World Buiatrics Congress* (CD-ROM), Punta del Este, Uruguay.

Wethues, M., and R. Fritsch. 1964–1965. *Animal Anesthesia,* vols. 1 and 2. Edinburgh and London: Oliver and Boyd [The English Translation].

Wheat, J.D. 1950. New landmark for cornual nerve block. *Veterinary Medicine* 45:29–30.

White, N.A., and K.E. Sullins. 1990. Surgical exploration and manipulation of the intestinal tract during abdominal surgery. In N.A. White (ed.), *The Equine Acute Abdomen,* 216–237. Philadelphia: Lea and Febiger.

Wilson, D.A., and G.M. Constantinescu. 1999. Spleen. In J.A. Auer and J.A. Stick (eds.), *Equine Surgery* 2nd ed., 394–399. Philadelphia: W.B. Saunders.

Wilson, D.A., and G.M. Constantinescu. 1999. Lymph nodes and lymphatics. In J.A. Auer and J.A. Stick (eds.), *Equine Surgery* 2nd ed., 399–403. Philadelphia: W.B. Saunders.

Wilson D.A., and K.G. Keegan. 1995. Pathophysiology and diagnosis of musculoskeletal disease. In C. Kobluck, T. Ames, and R. Goer (eds.), *The Horse Diseases and Clinical Management,* 607–685. Philiadelphia: W.B. Saunders.

# Index

Page references in *italics* refer to illustrations.

Abdomen
  horse
    anatomical regions, *57*
    cavity of, 54–56, *63*
    flank, 50
    landmarks and approaches, *50, 74*
    muscles of, 51–53, 289
    nerve supply to, *52*
    viscera of. *See* Abdominal viscera
    wall of, *51, 52, 56, 57*
  large ruminants
    muscles of, 51, 289, 292, *293*
    nerve supply to, *290, 291*
    viscera of. *See* Abdominal viscera
    wall of, *290, 293*
Abdominal vein, subcutaneous, large
    ruminants, 324
Abdominal viscera
  horse, 53–74
    blood supply to, 62, *65, 71, 72*
    cecum, 53–54, *55, 56, 58, 59, 68,
      69, 74*
    colon. *See* Colon, horse
    duodenum, 53, *55, 56, 59, 60, 68*
    esophagus. *See* Esophagus, horse
    ileum, 53, *69*
    intestine, *70,* 71–72
    jejunum, 53, *55, 56, 58, 68, 70*
    kidney. *See* Kidney, horse
    left aspect, *55, 61*
    liver, 50, 54, *55, 56, 59, 61,* 66–68
    mesoduodenum, 53, *59*
    pancreas, 54, *55, 56, 60, 67*
    pylorus, 66
    removal of, 62–66
    right aspect, *55, 59, 60*
    spleen, 50, *55, 56, 71*
    stomach, 53, 56, *59, 61, 67,* 71
    ventral aspect, *58*
  large ruminants, 292–312
    abomasum, 294–296, *297, 299,*
      301, *307*
    blood supply to, *303, 309*
    cecum, 294, *297, 299, 300,* 301,
      302
    colon. *See* Colon, large ruminants
    duodenum, 294, 296, *297, 299,
      300,* 301
    esophagus. *See* Esophagus, large
      ruminants

gall bladder, *297,* 301, *308*
ileum, 294
jejunum, 294, *299,* 301
kidney. *See* Kidney, large ruminants
liver, 279, 295, *297, 298, 299, 300,
  301, 308, 311*
mesoduodenum, 280, *297, 299*
omasum, 294, *297,* 301, *307*
omentum, *299*
pancreas, 280, 294, 295, *297, 299,
  300,* 301, *311*
pylorus, 296, *297, 299,* 301, 306,
  *307*
reticulum, 294, 301, *304, 307, 310*
right aspect, *299, 300*
rumen, 292, *305*
spleen, 295, *295, 296, 308*
stomach, 292, 306, *307, 309, 310*
topography, *297*
Abducent nerve
  horse, 225, 234, *251, 252, 254*
  large ruminants, 225, *419*
Abductor pollicis longus
  horse, *173,* 175, *176, 177, 205*
  large ruminants, *381, 382, 386*
Abomasal groove, 306, *310*
Abomasum, 294, *297, 299,* 301, *307*
  displacement of, 296
  fundus of, 295
  greater curvature, 297
Accessoriocarpoulnar ligament, horse,
  *163*
Accessoriometacarpal ligament, horse,
  *163,* 182
Accessorioquartal ligament, horse, *163*
Accessorioulnar ligament, horse, *163*
Accessory carpal bone, large ruminants,
  *362, 366, 386*
Accessory cephalic vein, large ruminants, *377, 378, 379*
Accessory gluteal line, horse, 96
Accessory groove, large ruminants, 295,
  306, *307*
Accessory ligament, horse, 128, *131,
  132,* 140
  femur, *79*
  hip joint, *100*
Accessory muscle
  horse, *175, 176*

large ruminants, *382*
Accessory nerve
  horse
    head, *222, 225, 227, 231, 251, 252,
      254*
    neck, *7, 9,* 11, *13*
    neurectomy of, 10
  large ruminants
    head, 225, *404, 405, 406,* 411
    neck, 268, *269, 270, 271*
Accessory pancreatic duct, large ruminants, 306
Accessory pillar, large ruminants, *310*
Accessory tendon. *See* Check tendon
Acetabular ligament
  horse, *79,* 140
  large ruminants, *332, 344*
Acetabulum
  horse, 75, *76, 122*
  large ruminants, *314,* 344
Acoustic meatus, external
  horse, *209, 210, 212,* 229
  large ruminants, *398, 400, 401*
Acoustic meatus, internal, horse, *212*
Acromion, large ruminants, *359*
Acropodium
  horse, *117, 155*
  large ruminants, 383
Adductor major, horse, *97,* 98, 128, *131,
  132, 133, 134*
Adductor minor, horse, 128, *131, 132,
  133*
Adductor muscle, large ruminants, 324,
  *329, 343, 344*
Adenohypophysis, horse, *249, 250*
Aditus laryngis, horse, 238, 245
Aditus pharyngis, horse, 238
Adrenal glands
  horse, 62, *64, 65, 67*
  large ruminants, 302, 306, *311*
Aerophagia, 10, 13
Alar canal, horse, *209,* 234
Alar cartilage, horse, *215,* 216
Alar foramen
  horse, *3,* 16, *209, 210, 211,* 234
  large ruminants, *268*
Albuginea
  horse, 91, *91*
  large ruminants, *320*
Alveolar artery or vein, horse, 224, 234

Alveolar nerve
  horse, *223, 224, 235*
    landmarks and approaches,
      257–258
  large ruminants, 408
Alveoli, maxillary, horse, 240
Ammon's horn, horse, 252, *255*
Ampullae, colic, horse, *70*
Analgesia. *See also* Nerve blocks
  digital
    horse, *202*
    large ruminants, 350, *354, 392, 395*
  epidural block, horse, 108, *110*
  intraarticular
    horse, 150–154, 199–201
    large ruminants, 350, *356, 357,
      391, 393–395*
  intravenous regional, large ruminants,
    350, *355*, 393
  paravertebral/paralumbar, large rumi-
    nants, 289
  pelvic limb
    horse, 146–154
    large ruminants, 350, *356, 357*
  subsacral
    horse, 108, *110*
    large ruminants, 313, *317*, 334
  thoracic limb
    horse, 197–205
    large ruminants, 391–395
Anal sphincter
  horse, 99, 101, *101, 102*
  large ruminants, *327, 328, 332*
Anconeal process
  horse, *158*
  large ruminants, *361*
Anconeus, horse, *174, 175, 176*
Anemia, large ruminants, 279
Anesthesia. *See* Analgesia; Nerve blocks
Angularis oculi artery or vein
  horse, *217*
  large ruminants, *402*
Angular notch, horse, *67, 71*
Anisognathous, 239
Annular cartilage, horse, 229
Annular ligament
  horse, 182, *185–189, 191*
  large ruminants, *367, 388, 389*
Ansa cervicalis
  horse, 222
  large ruminants, *405, 406*
Ansa subclavia
  horse, *33*, 34–35
  large ruminants, *281, 282*
Antebrachial artery or vein, large ruminants, *378, 379*
Antebrachial fascia
  horse, 166, *167, 175, 176, 179*
  large ruminants, *372, 377*
Antebrachial interosseous space, large
  ruminants, *361*
Antebrachial nerve
  horse, *169*, 172, *173, 174, 175, 177*
    landmarks and approaches, 197,
      *198*
  large ruminants, 371, *373, 374, 375,*

*376, 377, 378, 379*, 380, *381*
  blocking, 391, 392
Antebrachii, horse, *167*
Antebrachiocarpometacarpal joint. *See*
  Carpal joint
Antimesenteric ileal branch artery, large
  ruminants, 302, *303*
Anus
  horse, *106*
  large ruminants, *336*
Aorta
  abdominal
    horse, 59, 61, *81, 100*
    large ruminants, *308, 319*
  thoracic
    horse, 35, *39, 43*
    large ruminants, *281, 282, 285*
Aortic arch, horse, 35
Aortic bulb, horse, 44
Aortic hiatus
  horse, 36, 62
  large ruminants, 306
Aortic sinuses, horse, 44
Aortic valve, horse, *40*
  auscultation of, *47*
Apical ligament, large ruminants, 318,
  *320*
Aqueous humor, horse, 236
Arachnoid
  horse, *127*, 248
  large ruminants, 418
Arcus inguinalis, horse, 82, *83, 85, 89*
Arcus terminalis, large ruminants, 387
Area cribosa, horse, *233*, 236
Arm
  horse, 170
  large ruminants, 368, 369, *377*
Arthrocentesis
  horse, 150–152, 197–205
  large ruminants, 350, *356, 357,
    393–395*
Arthroscopy
  horse, 150–152, 165
  large ruminants, 350, *356, 357,
    393–395*
Articular bursae, horse, *149*, 150
Articularis coxae, horse, 135, 140
Aryepiglottic fold, horse, *230*, 238, 245,
  *245, 246*
Arytenoid cartilage, horse, *237*, 244,
  *245, 246*
Arytenoideus transversus, horse, *231,
  245*
Atlantal fossa, horse, *3*
Atlantoaxial joint, horse, *4*
Atlantoaxial ligament, horse, *4*
Atlantoaxial membrane, horse, *4*
Atlantooccipital joint, horse, *4*
Atlantooccipital membrane, horse, *4*
Atlantooccipital space, horse, 22
Atlas
  horse, *3*, 5, 6, *6, 17*
  large ruminants, 268
Atrioventricular valve
  horse, *40, 41, 47*
    cusps of, *40, 42, 42, 43, 43*

large ruminants, *286, 287*
Atrium
  left, large ruminants, *286*
  right
    horse, *36, 39, 41*
    large ruminants, *285, 286, 288*
  ruminal, 294, *295, 304, 305, 310*
Auditory tube
  horse, 7, 220, *227, 231, 237*, 238
  large ruminants, 411
Auricula
  horse, *36, 39, 41*
  large ruminants, *281, 285, 286, 288*
Auricular artery or vein
  horse, *218, 219*, 220, *222, 232*
  large ruminants, *404, 405, 406, 407*
Auricular nerve
  horse, 7, 10, *12, 15, 218, 219, 221*
    landmarks and approaches, 262,
      *263*
  large ruminants, 268, *269, 404, 405*
    nerve block, *424*
Auriculopalpebral nerve
  horse, *219*
    landmarks and approaches, *259,*
      260
  large ruminants, *405, 406, 407*
Auriculotemporal nerve
  horse, *217, 218, 219, 227*, 259
    landmarks and approaches, 258,
      *259*
  large ruminants, *402, 404*, 408
Autopodium
  horse, *117, 147, 155*
  large ruminants, 344, 368, 383
AV valve. *See* Atrioventricular valve
Axial tendon, large ruminants, *367, 388,
  389*
Axillary artery or vein
  horse, *18*, 30, *32, 33, 167, 169*, 172
  large ruminants, *276, 277, 278, 281,
    282, 371, 372*
Axillary fascia
  horse, 13, *172*
  large ruminants, 371
Axillary loop
  horse, *172*
  large ruminants, *370*, 371, *372*
Axillary nerve
  horse, *167, 169*, 172, 175
  large ruminants, *370, 372, 374*
Axis, horse, *3, 17*
Azygos vein
  horse, 36, *36, 39*
  large ruminants, 281, *281, 282, 285*

Basal nuclei, horse, 252
Basihyoid bone
  horse, 13, *214*, 216, *237*, 244
  large ruminants, 411
Basilar artery, horse, *249, 250*
Basilary groove, horse, 252
Basipodium
  horse, *117, 155*
  large ruminants, 383
Basisphenoid, horse, *212*

Bicarotid trunk artery, horse, 35
Biceps brachii
  horse, 166, *168, 173, 174, 176, 177*
    nerve supply to, 172
    tendon of, *196*
  large ruminants, 371, *372, 373, 374, 376–379,* 380
    tendon of, *365*
Biceps femoris
  horse, 95, 96, *97, 101, 102, 132, 136*
  large ruminants, *330,* 343, 344, *348*
Bicipital artery or vein
  horse, *169,* 172
  large ruminants, 371, *373, 379*
Bicipital tuberosity, horse, *118*
Bijugular trunk vein, horse, 32, 35
Bile duct
  horse, 53, 62
  large ruminants, *308*
Blind sacs, rumen, 292, 295, *295, 305, 307,* 310
Blood samples, venous. *See* Venipuncture
Brachial artery or vein
  horse, *169,* 172, 175, *177, 179*
  large ruminants, *370,* 371, *372, 373, 377, 378, 379,* 380
Brachial fascia, horse, 166
Brachialis
  horse, 166, *168, 173, 174, 176, 177, 179*
  large ruminants, 371, *373–377, 379, 380, 381*
Brachial nerve, large ruminants, *373, 379*
Brachial plexus
  horse, 11, *18,* 30, *30, 32, 33,* 166, *167, 169*
  large ruminants, 276, *277, 278, 370, 372*
    blocking, *391,* 393
Brachiocephalic trunk artery
  horse, 35
  large ruminants, *288*
Brachiocephalicus
  horse, 166
  large ruminants, 368, *370,* 371
Brain
  horse, 248–255
  large ruminants, 418, *420–422*
Brain cavity
  horse, *249*
  large ruminants, 397, 403, *422*
Brain stem, horse, *254, 255*
Broad ligament
  horse, 86, 98, *106*
  large ruminants, 318, *319*
Bronchoesophageal artery, horse, 35, 36, *71*
Bronchopneumonia, large ruminants, 279
Bronchus, horse, 37
Buccal artery or vein
  horse, *223,* 234, *256*
  large ruminants, *410*
Buccal nerve

  horse, *223, 225, 235*
  large ruminants, 408, *410*
Buccinator muscle
  horse, *217, 223*
  large ruminants, *402*
Bulboglandularis, large ruminants, *335*
Bulbospongiosus
  horse, 89, *90, 91, 101*
  large ruminants, *321, 327, 333,* 334
Bulbourethral gland
  horse, *103,* 104
  large ruminants, *321, 332, 333, 334, 335*
Bulbus olfactorius, horse, *249*
Bulbus penis
  horse, 89, 105
  large ruminants, *332*
Bulbus urethralis, large ruminants, *332*
Bulbus vestibuli, horse, 101, 105
Bursae
  horse, landmarks and approaches, *148–150,* 201, *203,* 204
  large ruminants, 371

C1 nerve
  horse, 16, *222, 232*
  large ruminants, *405, 406*
C2 nerve
  horse, 7, 11, *16, 218, 232*
  large ruminants, 269, *272*
C3 nerve
  horse, 7, 10, 11, *12, 16, 218*
  large ruminants, *272, 404*
C4 nerve
  horse, 7, 10, 11, *12, 16*
  large ruminants, *272*
C5 nerve
  horse, 7, 10, 11, *12, 16*
  large ruminants, *272*
C6 nerve, horse, 11, *16*
C7 nerve, horse, 11
C8 nerve, horse, 11
Calcanean tendon
  horse, 134, 135, *136, 137, 139,* 140, *145*
  large ruminants, 344
Calcanean tuber, large ruminants, *341*
Calcaneus
  horse, *120,* 140
  large ruminants, *341*
Calices, large ruminants, 306
Canine tooth
  horse, 239, *243*
  large ruminants, 397, 415
Caninus muscle
  horse, *217*
  large ruminants, *402,* 430
Canon bone, horse, *121, 160*
Canthi
  horse, 220, 229, *233*
  large ruminants, 415
Capitulum
  horse, *157*
  large ruminants, *360*
Capsula externa, horse, 252
Capsula extrema, horse, 252, 255

Capsula interna, horse, 252, *254, 255*
Cardia
  horse, *67,* 71
  large ruminants, 302, *304, 305, 310*
Cardiac fold, horse, 71
Cardiac nerves, horse, 34–35, 36
Cardiac notch
  horse, 34, *37, 38, 67,* 71
  large ruminants, *284*
Cardiac sphincter, horse, 71
Cardiac vein, horse, *39, 41*
Carotid artery, common
  horse
    head, 220, *222,* 227, 229, *231*
    neck, 6, *9,* 13, *14, 18, 21*
    thorax, 32, *33*
  large ruminants
    head, *405, 406, 410,* 411
    neck, 269, *270–272*
    thorax, 276, 277, *277, 278*
Carotid artery, external
  horse, 220, *221*
  large ruminants, *405,* 430
Carotid artery, internal
  horse, *222, 227,* 229, *231*
  large ruminants, *406,* 411
Carotid groove, horse, *212*
Carotid notch, horse, *212,* 229
Carotid sheath
  horse, 6, 9, 32
  large ruminants, 269, 277
Carotid sinus, 229
Carpal artery or vein, large ruminants, *386*
Carpal bones
  horse, *155, 159*
  large ruminants, *362*
Carpal canal
  horse, 178
  large ruminants, 383
Carpal chips, horse, 165
Carpal hygroma, horse, 165
Carpal joint
  horse, *163,* 195
  large ruminants, *366*
    nerve block sites, *394*
Carpometacarpal ligaments
  horse, *163*
  large ruminants, *366*
Carpus, horse, *180, 181, 183*
  landmarks and approaches, 200, 201, *203*
Caruncles
  sublingual, 411
  uterine, 334, *336*
Castration
  horse
    closed, 92
    inguinal approach, 108
    median approach, 111
    open, 92
    paramedian approach, 111
  large ruminants
    closed, 318
    open, 318

Catheterization, urinary bladder, large
  ruminants, 334
Cauda equina, 127
Caudal artery or vein, horse, 98, 108,
  *109*
Caudal commissure, horse brain, 250
Caudal fascia, horse, 96
Caudal nerve, horse, 108, *109*
Caudal recess, large ruminants, 297
Caudal vertebrae
  horse, *78*
  large ruminants, *78, 316*
Cavernous sinus, large ruminants, 418
Cecal artery
  horse, 72, *72*
  large ruminants, *303*
Cecal sphincter, horse, 68
Cecocentesis, horse, 50, 73, *74*
Cecocolic fold, horse, 54, *59, 68,* 69–70
Cecocolic ostium, horse, 68, *69*
Cecocolic valve, horse, 69
Cecotomy, horse, 50, 73, *74*
Cecum
  horse, 53–54, *55,* 56, *58, 59, 68, 68,
    69*
    approaches to, *74*
  large ruminants, 294, 297, 299, 300,
    301, 302
Celiac artery
  horse, 62, *65,* 68, 71, *71*
  large ruminants, 306, *309*
Celiotomy, horse, 50, 70, 73, *74*
Cementum, horse tooth, 239, *240, 243*
Central nervous system, horse, 248–255
Centrifugal coils, 294, 302
Centripetal coils, 294, 302
Centrum tendineum, 56
Cephalic vein
  horse
    neck, 6, *14,* 15, *18, 21*
    thoracic inlet, *32*
    thoracic limb, 166, 175, *177, 179,
      180, 181*
  large ruminants
    elbow, *373*
    shoulder, *374*
    thoracic inlet, 276, 277, 278
    thoracic limb, 371, *377, 378, 379,
      381, 383, 386*
Ceratchyoid, horse, *214*
Ceratohyoideus
  horse, 228, 229
  large ruminants, 411
Cerebellar arteries, *251,* 252
Cerebellar peduncle, horse, 252, *254,
  255*
Cerebellum
  horse, 248, *249,* 250, *251, 253*
  large ruminants, *420, 421*
Cerebral arterial circle, horse, *251,* 252
Cerebral arteries, horse, *249,* 250, *251,*
  252
Cerebral peduncle, horse, 250, 252, *254*
Cerebri magna, horse, *249*
Cerebri magna vein, horse, 250
Cerebrospinal fluid

horse, 248
  collection of, 6, *6, 80,* 108
Cerebrum, horse, 248
Cervical artery or vein
  horse, 6, 13, 15, *16, 18, 21, 35,* 166
    deep, *33,* 36
    superficial, 32, *32, 33*
  large ruminants, superficial, 270, *276,
    277, 278, 281*
Cervical fascia
  horse, *9*
  large ruminants, 268
Cervical spinal nerves
  horse, 15, *19*
    cutaneous, *10*
  large ruminants, *269*
    nerve block sites, *424*
Cervical sympathetic trunk
  horse, 13, 32, 229
  large ruminants, 277, 411
Cervical vertebrae
  horse, *3*
  large ruminants, 268
Cervicoauricularis, horse, *232*
Cervicoscutularis
  horse, *232*
  large ruminants, *402*
Cervix
  horse, 105, *106*
  large ruminants, 334, *336, 337*
Cesarian section, large ruminants, 296
Chabert-Fromage approach, horse, 262,
  *263*
Check ligament
  horse, 178, *179,* 182, *183*
    landmarks and approaches, 205
  large ruminants, *367*
Check tendon, horse, *196*
Cheeks, large ruminants, 411
Cheek tooth
  horse, 244
  large ruminants, 415
Chestnut, horse, 165
Chin, horse, *215,* 216
Choana
  horse, *210,* 236
  large ruminants, 397, *401, 412*
Chondrocompedale ligament, horse, *187,
  188*
Chondrocoronale ligament, horse, *161,
  189*
Chondrosesamoid ligaments, horse, *187,
  189*
Chondroungulare ligament, horse, *161,
  189*
Chordae tendinae, horse, 42, *42, 43, 43*
Chorda tympani nerve, horse, 226, *227*
Chorionic villi, large ruminants, 334
Choroid, horse, *233,* 236
Choroid plexus, horse, 248, 250
Ciliary artery, large ruminants, *419*
Ciliary body, horse, *233,* 236
Ciliary muscle, horse, *233,* 236
Ciliary nerves, horse, *235,* 236
Ciliary processes, horse, *233,* 236
Ciliary zonule, horse, *233,* 236

Cingulum, horse, *117, 155*
Claustrum, horse, 252
Clavicle, horse, 13
Cleidobrachialis
  horse, *12,* 13, *14,* 15
  large ruminants, 371, *373, 374*
Cleidocephalicus, large ruminants, 268
Cleidomastoideus
  horse
    neck, 6, *9,* 11, *12,* 13, *14,* 15, *15,*
      head, *218, 219,* 220
  large ruminants
    neck, 268, *269, 270, 271, 272*
    head, *404, 405, 406*
Cleidooccipitalis, large ruminants, 268,
  *269, 270, 271, 272, 404, 405*
Cleidotransversarius, horse, *7, 12*
Cleidotransversus, horse, 13
Clinical crown, horse tooth, 239, *240*
Clinical root, horse tooth, 239, *240*
Clitoris
  horse, 105, *106, 107*
    artery or vein of, 101, *132*
    nerves of, 101
  large ruminants, *328, 336, 337*
Club foot, horse, 182, 190
Clunial nerves, horse, *95*
Coccygeus
  horse, *95, 97,* 98, *99, 100,* 102, *134*
  large ruminants, *327–332*
Cochlea tibiae, large ruminants, *340*
Coffin joint, horse, *161, 163, 164,* 197
  landmarks and approaches, 201, *202*
Colic arteries
  horse, 68, 72, *72,* 82
  large ruminants, 302, *303*
Collateral ligament
  horse
    carpal joint, *163*
    coffin joint, *187, 189*
    digital, 195
    elbow, *162, 173, 174,* 175, *176,
      177,* 178, *179*
    fetlock, *164, 189*
    hock, 144
    navicular, *187, 189*
    stifle, *123, 124, 136*
    tarsal joint, *126*
  large ruminants, *351, 356*
    carpal joint, *366*
    digit, *367*
    elbow, *366, 374, 381, 382*
    stifle joint, *347*
Collateral sesamoid ligament, large
  ruminants, *367*
Colliculus, large ruminants, *420*
Colliculus caudalis, horse, 250, *255*
Colliculus rostralis, horse, 250, *255*
Colliculus seminalis, horse, 104, *104*
Collum glandis, horse, *89*
Colon
  horse
    ascending, 54, *55*
    descending, 54, *55,* 56, *70*
    left dorsal, *55,* 56, *61, 68, 69, 70*
    left ventral, *55,* 56, *58, 61, 68,* 69, *70*

right dorsal, *55, 56, 59, 60, 68,* 69, *70*

right ventral, *55,* 56, 58, *59, 60,* 68, *69, 70*

transverse, 54, 70

large ruminants

ascending, 294, 297, *297,* 298, *298, 299, 300,* 301, 302

descending, 294, *297, 299, 300,* 301, 302

distal loop, 294

proximal loop, 294

sigmoid, 295, 302

spiral loop, 294

transverse, 294

Communicating branch nerve, horse, *180, 181, 184*

Conchae, nasal

horse, 236, 238

large ruminants, 411, *412*

Conchal septa, horse, 238

Conchal sinus, horse, 238

Conchofrontal sinus, horse, *230,* 238, *247,* 248

Condylar artery, large ruminants, *422*

Condylar process, horse, *213*

Conjugate diameter, large ruminants, 313

Conjunctivae

horse, *233,* 234

large ruminants, 415

Conjunctival fornix

horse, *233,* 234

large ruminants, 415

Conjunctival sac

horse, 234

large ruminants, 418

Constrictors, pharynx, horse, *228,* 229

Constrictor vaginae, horse, 101, *102*

Constrictor vestibuli, horse, *99,* 105

Constrictor vulvae

horse, *99,* 101, *102, 106*

large ruminants, *328*

Contagious equine metritis, 91

Conus arteriosus

horse, *39,* 42

large ruminants, *286*

Conus medullaris, horse, *127*

Coracobrachialis

horse, 166, *168,* 172

large ruminants, 365, 371, *372, 373, 377*

Coracohumeral ligament, *162*

Coracoid process

horse, *156*

large ruminants, *359, 365*

Cordis magna vein, large ruminants, *285*

Corium

horse, *187,* 190, *192*

large ruminants, *390,* 391

Cornea, horse, *233, 236*

Corniculate process, horse, 244, *245*

Cornual artery or vein, 403, *407*

Cornual nerve, *407*

Cornual process, 397, *398, 400*

Corona glandis, horse, *89, 90, 90*

Coronal artery or vein

horse, *185,* 190, *191*

large ruminants, *387*

Coronary artery

horse, *39, 40,* 43

large ruminants, *285, 288*

Coronary border, large ruminants, *364*

Coronary groove

heart

horse, 190, *193,* 195

large ruminants, *285, 292, 302, 306, 307*

hoof

horse, 39

large ruminants, *390,* 391

Coronary ligament

horse, 59, *59,* 62

large ruminants, 301, *308*

Coronary pillars, 292, 306, *310*

Coronary sinus, horse, 41, *41*

Coronet, horse, 182

Coronoid process

horse, *158, 213*

large ruminants, *361, 399*

Corpus callosum

horse, 248, *249,* 250

large ruminants, *420*

Corpus cavernosum penis

horse, *89, 90,* 91, *91,* 105

large ruminants, 334

Corpus lentiformis, horse, *254*

Corpus spongiosum glandis, horse, 91

Corpus spongiosum penis

horse, *91*

large ruminants, 334

Corpus striatum, horse, 252, *254*

Costal arch

horse, *23,* 24, *25, 50, 52,* 55

large ruminants, 273

Costal fovea, large ruminants, *274*

Costal notches, large ruminants, *274*

Costal pleura, horse, 34

Costal sulcus/groove, horse, 33

Costoabdominal nerve

horse, 51, *52,* 53

large ruminants, 289, *291, 293, 295*

Costocervical trunk artery or vein

horse, *33, 35, 36, 36*

large ruminants, *277, 278, 281, 282*

Costochondral junction

horse, 25

large ruminants, 273

Costodiaphragmatic recess, horse, 34

Costotransverse ligament, horse, *24*

Costovertebral joint

horse, *24, 36*

large ruminants, 273

Cotyledons, large ruminants, 334

Coxal bones

horse, *75, 76, 117*

large ruminants, *314*

Coxofemoral joint. *See* Hip joint

Cranial cavity, horse, *212,* 236

Cranial flexure, horse, 60

Cranial fossa, horse, *212*

Cranial nerve I (Olfactory)

horse, 225, 250, *251, 253*

large ruminants, 225

Cranial nerve II (Optic)

horse, 225, *233, 235,* 236, 250, *251, 252, 253, 254*

large ruminants, 225, *420*

Cranial nerve III (Oculomotor)

horse, 225, 234, *235, 251,* 252

landmarks and approaches, *259,* 260

large ruminants, 225, *419*

Cranial nerve IV (Trochlear)

horse, 225, 234, *235, 251,* 252

large ruminants, 225, *419*

Cranial nerve V (Trigeminal)

horse, 225, *251,* 252

large ruminants, 225

Cranial nerve VI (Abducent)

horse, 225, 234, *251,* 252, *254*

large ruminants, 225, *419*

Cranial nerve VII (Facial)

horse, 7, 11, *217, 218,* 225, 227, *251, 252, 254*

branches of, *219,* 220

landmarks and approaches, 258, *259,* 260

large ruminants, 225, *402,* 403, *404, 405, 406,* 407

Cranial nerve VIII (Vestibulocochlear)

horse, 225, *251, 252, 253, 254*

large ruminants, 225

Cranial nerve IX (Glossopharyngeal)

horse

head, 220, *221, 222, 223,* 225, 227, *229, 231, 251, 252, 254*

neck, 13

thorax, 32, *33,* 35, *35,* 36, *36*

large ruminants, 225

head, *405, 406, 409,* 411

thorax, 277, 278, 281, 282

Cranial nerve X (Vagus)

horse

head, 222, 225, 227, 231, *251,* 252, *254*

neck, 13

thorax, 32, *33,* 35, *35,* 36, *36*

large ruminants, 225, 306

head, *405, 406,* 411

thorax, 277, 278, 281, 282

Cranial nerve XI (Accessory)

horse

head, *222,* 225, 227, 231, *251,* 252, *254*

neck, 7, 9, 10, 11, 13

large ruminants

head, 225, *404, 405, 406,* 411

neck, 268, *269, 270,* 271

Cranial nerve XII (Hypoglossal)

horse, 220, *221–223,* 225, 227, *228, 229, 230, 231,* 238, *251, 252, 254*

large ruminants, 225, *405, 406, 409, 410,* 411, *413*

Cranial nerves
  horse, 225, *227*, 408. *See also under*
    individual nerve
  large ruminants, 225, 408, *419*. *See*
    *also under* individual nerve
Cremasteric artery, horse, *81*, 82
Cremasteric fascia, large ruminants, 318
Cremaster muscle
  horse, *81*, *84*, *85*
  large ruminants, 318, *321*, *322*
Cribbing, 10, 13
Cribiform lamina
  horse, *212*
  large ruminants, *422*
Cricoarytenoideus, horse, *231*, *237*, *245*,
    *246*, 247
Cricoarytenoid ligament, horse, *245*
Cricoesophageus, horse, *246*
Cricoid cartilage, horse, 13, *231*, *237*,
    244, *245*
Cricopharyngeus
  horse, *18*, 229, *246*, 247
  large ruminants, *410*, 411
Cricothyroideus, horse, *228*, *246*
Cricothyroid ligament, horse, *237*, 244
  landmarks and approaches, *256*
Crista galli, horse, *212*
Crista terminalis
  horse, *41*
  large ruminants, *286*
Croup, large ruminants, *329*
Crown, ruminant teeth, 415
Cruciate ligament
  horse, *124*, *125*, 143, *187*
  large ruminants, *356*, *367*
Crura, cerebral, horse, 250, 252
Crurae, penis, horse, 102, 105
Crural fascia
  horse,135–138
  large ruminants, 344
Crural interosseous membrane, horse,
    *123*, *124*
Crus
  horse, 135, *135*, *136*, *137*, *139*, *142*
  large ruminants, *347*, *349*, *351*
    muscles of, 344, 345
Crus cerebri
  horse, *249*, 250, *251*, 252, *253*
  large ruminants, *421*
Cubital artery or vein
  horse, 172, 175, *177*
  large ruminants, 371, *373*, *378*, *379*,
    *381*
Cubital nerve, large ruminants, *377*
Cunean tendon, horse, *39*, *137*, *138*
Cuneiform process, 244
Cup, horse tooth, 239, 244
Curb, 140
Cutaneous colli muscle, horse, 8, *8*, *9*,
    216
Cutaneous colli nerve, horse, 7
Cutaneous faciei, horse, *8*, 216, *218*
Cutaneous omobrachialis, horse, *8*, 26
Cutaneous trunci
  horse, *8*, 26, 51, *95*
  large ruminants, 292

Cystic duct, large ruminants, *308*

Dartos, horse, 92
Deltoideus
  horse, *26*, *28*, 172, *173*, *174*
  large ruminants, 371, *374*, *375*, *376*
Deltoid tuberosity
  horse, *157*, 175
  large ruminants, *360*, 371
Dens
  horse, *3*
  large ruminants, *268*
Dental arch, horse, 239
Dental cavity, large ruminants, 415
Dental pad, large ruminants, 411, *412*
Dental star
  horse, 239, *243*
  large ruminants, 415
Denticulate ligaments, 248
Dentin, horse, 239, *240*, *243*
Dentine, secondary
  horse, 239
  large ruminants, 415
Dentition
  horse, 239–244
  large ruminants, 413–415
Depressor anguli oris, horse, 216, *217*
Depressor labii inferioris
  horse, *217*, 220
  large ruminants, *402*
Depressor labii superioris, large rumi-
    nants, *402*, 430
Dewclaws, large ruminants, 350, 391
Diaphragm
  horse, *27*, 34, *35*, 36, 59
  large ruminants, 279, *281*, 294, 295,
    *308*, *311*
Diaphragma sellae
  horse, 248, *249*, 250
  large ruminants, 418
Diaphragmatic flexure, horse, 54, *55*, 56,
    *58*, *59*, *61*, 69, *70*
Diaphragmatic pleura, horse, 34
Diastema, horse, *209*, *213*, *215*, 239
Diencephalon, horse, 248, 250, 252
Diestrus, horse, 106, *107*
Digastricus
  horse, 11, *18*, *219*, 220, *221*, *223*, *231*
  large ruminants, *405*, *406*, 408, *409*,
    *410*, 430
Digit
  horse, 170, *185*–192
    blood supply to, *185*. *See also* Dig-
      ital arteries or veins
    corium of, *192*
    cushion. *See* Digital cushion
    fascia of, 182, *186*
    ligaments of, *187*, *189*
    muscles of, 170
    nerve block sites, *202*
    nerves of, 170, *185*, *191*. *See also*
      Digital nerves
    tendons of, *186*, *187*, *188*, *189*
  large ruminants, *384*, *385*, *387*–389
    bones of, *364*
    ligaments of, *367*

  nerve block sites, 350, *354*, *392*,
    *395*
  nerves of, 369. *See also* Digital
    nerves
  tendons of, *367*
Digital arteries or veins
  horse, *139*, 140, *141*, 182, *184*, 190
    landmarks and approaches, 146,
      *147*
    palmar, *185*, *191*
    palmar common, 178, *180*, *181*,
      182, *184*
  large ruminants, *352*, 383, *385*, *386*,
    387
    axial/abaxial, 383
Digital cushion
  horse, *85*, 182, *188*, *191*, *192*
    fascia of, *185*, *187*
  large ruminants, *387*, 388
Digital extensors
  horse, *205*
    pelvic limb, *123*, 136, *136*, *137*,
      138, *139*, *141*
    tendons of, 139, *164*, *185*, *186*,
      *187*, *189*, *196*
    thoracic limb, *173*–176
  large ruminants
    pelvic limb, 344, *347*–349, 350
    tendons of, 343, *349*, *352*, *367*,
      383, *384*, *385*
    thoracic limb, *374*, *380*, *381*, *382*
Digital fascia, horse, 182, *186*
Digital flexors
  deep
    horse, 140, *145*, *173*, *176*, *177*,
      178, *179*, *181*, 182, *183*
    tendon of, *141*, *180*, *184*, *185*, *186*,
      *187*, *188*, *191*, *196*
    large ruminants, *374*, *379*, 380,
      *380*, *381*, *382*, *384*
    tendon of, *352*, *367*, 383, *386*
  lateral
    horse, *136*, *137*, 140, *142*, *143*
    large ruminants, *347*, *348*, *351*
  medial
    horse, *132*, *139*, 140
    large ruminants, *351*
  superficial
    horse, 140, 178, *179*, *180*, *181*, 182
    tendon of, *141*, *145*, *180*, *181*, *184*,
      *185*, *187*, *188*, *191*, *196*
    large ruminants, *348*, *377*, *378*,
      *379*, 380, *380*, *382*, *384*, *386*
    tendon of, *347*, *349*, *352*, 383,
      *386*
Digital nerves
  horse, 182
    landmarks and approaches, 199
    palmar, *184*, *185*, 190, *191*
    plantar, *141*
  large ruminants, 383, *385*, *386*
    axial/abaxial, 383
    blocking sites, 350, *354*, *392*, *395*
Dilator maris apicalis, horse, 216
Diphyodonts, 240
Dorsalis nasi vein, horse, *217*

Dorsalis pedis artery or vein, horse, *136*, 139

Dorsalis penis artery or vein, large ruminants, *332*

Dorsalis penis nerve, large ruminants, *332*

Dorsal ligament, large ruminants, *367*

Dorsoscapular artery or vein
  horse, *33, 35, 36*
  large ruminants, *277*

Dorsoscapular ligament
  horse, 30–31, *31, 44*
  large ruminants, 278

Ducts of Gärtner, large ruminants, *336*

Ductus arteriosus, horse, 35

Ductus deferens
  horse, *81*, 82, *83, 84, 85, 93, 103, 113*
    ampullae of, 102, *103, 113*
    artery of, 92
  large ruminants, *321, 322, 323, 333, 335*

Duodenal ampulla, *67*

Duodenocolic fold, 59

Duodenojejunal flexure
  horse, 59–60
  large ruminants, 294

Duodenorenal ligament, horse, 59

Duodenotransverse ligament, horse, 59

Duodenum
  horse, 53
    ascending, 59
    cranial flexure, 60, *60*
    descending, *55, 56, 59, 59, 68*
    sigmoid loop, 60
    transverse, 59
  large ruminants, 294
    ascending, 294, *300*
    caudal flexure, 294, *297, 300*, 301
    cranial flexure, 294, 297, *297, 299*
    descending, 294, 296, *297, 300*, 301
    sigmoid loop, 294, 297, *299*

Dural nerve, horse, *95, 132*

Dura mater
  horse, *127*, 248
  large ruminants, 418

Dystocia, large ruminants, 313

Ear
  horse, *215*, 216, 229, *232*
    muscles of, 216
  large ruminants, 430
    muscles of, 403

Ejaculatory orifice, horse, 104, *104*

Elbow
  horse, 162, 175, 195
    landmarks and approaches, 199, *200*
  large ruminants, *366, 372, 378*
    nerve block sites, *394*

Emasculator, 92

Enamel
  horse tooth, 239, *240, 243*
  ruminant tooth, 415

Enamel spot, horse tooth, 239, *243*

Encephalon, horse, *249*

Endoabdominal fascia, horse, 34, 53, 82

Endometrium, large ruminants, 334

Endoscopy
  nasopharynx, horse, 236, 238
  peritoneal cavity, horse, 55

Endothoracic fascia, horse, 9, 34

Epaxial muscles
  horse, *81*
  large ruminants, 278

Epicondyles
  horse, *118, 157*
  large ruminants, *339, 360*

Epididymis
  horse, *84, 92, 93, 103*
  large ruminants, 318, *321, 323*

Epidural space, large ruminants, *343*, 418

Epigastric artery or vein
  horse, *81, 82, 83, 85, 89, 133*
  large ruminants, *290, 319, 322*, 324, *325, 326*

Epiglottis
  horse, *230, 237, 244, 245, 246*
  large ruminants, 413

Epihyoid, horse, *214*

Epiphyses, fusion of
  horse, 264
  large ruminants, 426

Epiphysis
  horse, *249, 250, 252, 254, 255*
  large ruminants, *420*

Epiploic foramen
  horse, 60
  large ruminants, *300*

Episiotomy, horse, *109*, 111

Epithalamus, horse, 250

Equine motor neuron disease, 10

Erector spinae, *27*

Ergot
  horse, 182, *185*
    ligament of, *189*, 190
  large ruminants, ligament of, *388, 389*

Eruption, horse teeth, 242

Esophageal branch artery, large ruminants, *309*

Esophageal hiatus
  horse, 36
  large ruminants, 306

Esophageal vestibule, horse, 238

Esophagus
  horse
    abdomen, 53, *59, 67*
    head, 220, *230, 231, 237, 246*
    neck, 9, 13, *18, 19, 21*
    thorax, 33, *35*
  large ruminants
    abdomen, 292, *304, 305*, 306, *307, 308*
    head, *410*, 411
    neck, 269, *270, 271*
    thorax, *276, 277, 278, 281, 282*

Estrus, horse, 106, *107*

Ethmoidal foramen
  horse, *211*, 236
  large ruminants, 397

Ethmoid artery, horse, *235*, 236

Ethmoid bone, horse, *212*

Ethmoid nerve
  horse, *235*, 236
  large ruminants, *419*

Eustachian tube, horse, 7, 220

Exenteration
  horse, 66
  large ruminants, 302

Exercise intolerance, horse, 229, 238

Extensor carpi radialis
  horse, *173, 174*, 175, *176, 177, 179*, 205
    tendon of, *196*
  large ruminants, *372–375, 377–382*, 386

Extensor carpi ulnaris
  horse, *173, 176, 184*
  large ruminants, *374*, 380, *380, 381*, 382

Extensor digitalis brevis, horse, *138, 141*

Extensor fossa, horse, *118*

Extensor groove
  horse, *137*, 143
  large ruminants, *340*

Extensor processes, large ruminants, 383

Extensor retinaculum
  horse, 135–136, 138, *139, 141*, 175
  large ruminants, 344, *347, 348, 349, 351, 352*, 383

Extensors, digital. *See* Digital extensors

Extensor sulcus, horse, *123, 125*

Eye
  horse, 229, *233, 234, 235*, 236
    chambers of, *233*, 236
  large ruminants, 415–416, *417, 419*

Eyeball, horse, *235*, 236

Eyelid
  horse, 216, 229, *233, 234*, 236
  large ruminants, 415, *417*, 418

Face, muscles of
  horse, 216
  large ruminants, 403

Facial artery or vein
  horse, 216, *217, 218, 219*, 220, *223, 227, 228*, 229
    landmarks and approaches, *256*
  large ruminants, *402, 404, 405, 407, 409*

Facial crest
  horse, *208, 209, 215*, 220, 248
  large ruminants, 397

Facial nerve
  horse, 7, 11, *217, 218*, 225, *227, 251, 252, 254*
    branches of, *219*, 220
    landmarks and approaches, 258, *259*, 260
  large ruminants, 225, *402*, 403, *404, 405, 406, 407*

Facial tubercle
  horse, *209, 210*
  large ruminants, 397, *398, 400, 401*

Facies aspera, large ruminants, *339*

Facies infraspinatus, large ruminants, *360*, 371

Facies lunata, large ruminants, *314*
Falciform ligament
    horse, 62, *67*
    large ruminants, 301, *308*
Falx cerebri, horse, 248, *249*, 250
Farquharson method, 289, *291*
Fasciae
    antebrachial, horse, 166, *167*, 175,
        *176*
    axillary
        horse, 13, 172
        large ruminants, 371
    brachial, horse, 166
    caudal, horse, 96
    cervical
        horse, *9*
        large ruminants, 268
    cremasteric, large ruminants, 318
    crural
        horse, 135–138
        large ruminants, 344
    digital, horse, 182, *186*, *188*
    digital cushion
        horse, *185*, *187*
        large ruminants, 388
    endoabdominal, horse, 34, 53, 82
    endothoracic, horse, 34
    gluteal, horse, 96
    iliac, horse, 82
    palmar
        horse, 178, *181*, *183*
        large ruminants, 383
    pharyngeal, horse, *246*, 247
    proper antebrachial
        horse, 175, *179*
        large ruminants, *372*, *377*
    spermatic
        horse, 92
        large ruminants, 318, *322*
    thoracolumbar, horse, 26, 51
    transverse
        horse, 34, 53, 82
        large ruminants, 292
Fascia lata, large ruminants, *329*
Fasciculus cuneatus, horse, 252, *255*
Fasciculus gracilis, horse, 252, *255*
Fauces, horse, 238
Femoral artery or vein
    horse
        landmarks and approaches, 146
        pelvic limb, 128, *131*, *132*, *133*,
            *136*, *142*
        pelvis, 82, *83*, *85*, *89*, *91*, *100*
        large ruminants, *319*, *329*, *330*, 344,
            *346*, *348*, 350
Femoral canal, horse, 128, *131*
Femoral head, horse, 140
Femoral lamina, horse, 82, 128
Femoral nerve
    horse, 52, *95*, *97*, *98*, *99*, *100*, *133*,
        *134*
    large ruminants, 292, 324, *330*, *331*,
        *333*, 344, *346*
Femoral triangle
    horse, 128, *131*
    large ruminants, 344

Femoral trochlea, horse, 144
Femoropatellar ligaments, horse, 142
Femorotibial menisci, horse, 143
Femur
    horse, *117*, *118*, *123*
    large ruminants, *339*
Fetlock
    horse, *164*, 195–197
        landmarks and approaches, 201,
            *202*
        nerve supply to, 182
    large ruminants, 383, *385*
        nerve block sites, *395*
Fibropapillomatosis, penile, large rumi-
    nants, 318
Fibrous band, large ruminants, *405*, *406*
Fibula
    horse, *117*, *119*, *124*, *125*
    large ruminants, *340*
Fibularis longus, large ruminants, 343,
    344, *347*, *348*, *349*, 352
Fibularis tertius
    horse, *123*, 137, *137*, *138*, *139*, *141*
    large ruminants, *347*, *348*, *349*, 352
Fibular nerve
    horse, *97*, *132*, 134, *136*, 137, 138,
        *141*
        landmarks and approaches, 146,
            *147*
    large ruminants, *329*, 344, *347*, *348*,
        *349*, 352
        nerve block site, 350, *353*, *354*
Filum terminale
    horse, 127
    large ruminants, *343*
Fissura sylvia, horse, *253*
Flank
    horse, *50*
    large ruminants, 289, 292, 298
Flax cerebri, large ruminants, 418
Flexor carpi radialis
    horse, 175, *177*, *179*, 205
    large ruminants, 371, *372*, *377*, *378*,
        *379*, *380*, 386
Flexor carpi ulnaris
    horse, *173*, 175, *176*, *177*, *179*
    large ruminants, *372*, *377*, *378*, *379*,
        *380*, *380*, 386
Flexor retinaculum
    horse, 135, 178, *180*, *181*
    large ruminants, *377*, 383, *386*
Flexors, digital. *See* Digital flexors
Foramen lacerum, horse, *209*, *212*, 229
Foramen magnum
    horse, *6*, *210*
    large ruminants, *401*
Foramen orbitorotundum, large rumi-
    nants, 397
Foramen rotundum, horse, *211*, 234
Forearm
    horse, 170
        landmarks and approaches, *203*
        lateral aspect, *176*
        medial aspect, *177*, *179*
        muscles of, 170
        nerves of, 170

    tendons of, 175
    large ruminants, *377*, *378*, *380*, *381*
        muscles of, 368
        nerve block sites, 392
        nerves of, 369
Forelimb. *See* Thoracic limb
Fornix, horse, 229, 248, *249*
Forssell's procedure, 13
Fossa glandis, horse, *89*, 90, *90*
Fossa linguae, large ruminants, 411, *412*
Fossa ovalis
    horse, *41*
    large ruminants, *286*
Fovea capitis
    horse, *118*, 140, *158*
    large ruminants, *339*, *361*
Frenulum, horse, *107*
Frog
    horse, 182, *186*, *187*, *188*, 190, *193*,
        195
        corium of, *192*
Frontal bone
    horse, *208*
    large ruminants, *397*, *398*, *400*, 415
Frontalis muscle, large ruminants, *402*,
    *407*
Frontal lobe, large ruminants, *420*
Frontal nerve
    horse, 234, *235*, 236
    large ruminants, *419*
Frontal sinus
    horse, 238, 248
    large ruminants, *412*, 415, 418
Frontoscutularis
    horse, *232*
    large ruminants, *402*, *407*
Fundus, horse, *67*
Funiculus nuchae
    horse, 5, 6, *9*, 15, *15*, *17*, *19*, 31, *31*
    large ruminants, *272*

Galavayne's groove, 243
Gall bladder, large ruminants, *297*, 301,
    *308*
Ganglia
    celiac
        horse, 36, 62, 65
        large ruminants, 306
    cervical
        horse, 32, 33, *33*, 34, 36, *36*, 222,
            227, 229, 231
        large ruminants, 277, *277*, 278,
            *281*, *282*, *406*, 411
    cervicothoracic
        horse, *33*, 34, *36*
        large ruminants, 277, *277*, 278,
            *281*, *282*
    ciliary, horse, *235*, 236
    mandibular, horse, *223*, 226
    mesenteric
        horse, 36, 62, *65*, 82, 98
        large ruminants, 333
    otic, horse, 226
    pelvic, large ruminants, *332*, 333
    pterygopalatine, horse, *235*, 236
    renal, horse, 63

stellate, horse, 34, 36
  sympathetic, horse, 35
  thoracic, horse, 36
Gärtner's ducts, large ruminants, 334, *336*
Gastric artery
  horse, 61, *71*
  large ruminants, 306, *309*
Gastric groove, large ruminants, 294, 306
Gastric impression, horse, *67*
Gastric tube, passing, horse, 207, 236, 238
Gastrocnemius
  horse, *97, 101*, 128, *132, 134, 136, 137*
  large ruminants, *329, 347, 348, 349, 351*
Gastroduodenal artery
  horse, *71*
  large ruminants, *309*
Gastroepiploic artery
  horse, *71*
  large ruminants, 306, *309*
Gastrophrenic ligament, horse, 59, 61
Gastrosplenic ligament, horse, 61
Gemelli muscles
  horse, *97, 98, 134*
  large ruminants, *329, 331*, 344
Genicular artery or vein
  horse, 128, *131*
  large ruminants, *346*
Geniculate bodies, horse, 252, *254, 255*
Genioglossus
  horse, *228, 229, 230, 237*
  large ruminants, 411, *412*
Geniohyoideus
  horse, *223, 228, 229, 230*, 238
  large ruminants, *410*, 411, *412, 413*, 430
Genital apparatus
  bull, *321, 333*
  cow, 334, *336*
  mare, 81, *87, 88, 102, 106*
  stallion, 81, *89–91, 101, 110*
Genital fold, horse, 98, *103*
Genital glands, horse, *103*
Genital tract
  mare, 92, *94*, 101, *101, 102*, 105, *106, 107, 109*
  stallion, *89–93, 101, 103, 104, 110*
Genitofemoral artery, horse, 85
Genitofemoralis, horse, *100*
Genitofemoral nerve
  horse, *81, 82, 132*
  large ruminants, *291, 322, 324, 325, 346*
Gingiva, horse, 240
Glans penis
  horse, *89, 90, 90*, 91–92
  large ruminants, 318, *320, 321*
    physical examination, 313
Glenoid cavity
  horse, *156*
  large ruminants, *359*
Glenoid notch, horse, *156*

Glomus caroticum, horse, *222, 229*
Glossoepiglottic fold
  horse, 238, *245*
  large ruminants, 411
Glossopharyngeal nerve
  horse
    head, 220, *221, 222, 223, 225, 227, 228, 229, 231, 251, 252, 254*
    neck, 13
    thorax, 32, *33*, 35, *35*, 36, *36*
  large ruminants, 225
    head, *405, 406, 409*, 411
    thorax, 277, *278, 281, 282*
Glottis, horse, 245
Gluteal artery or vein
  horse, *97, 98, 99, 100*, 134
  large ruminants, *328, 329, 330, 331*
Gluteal fascia, horse, 96
Gluteal muscles
  horse, *95, 96, 97, 99, 101*, 134
  large ruminants, 324, *329, 330, 331*, 343, 344
Gluteal nerve
  horse, *97, 99, 100*, 134
  large ruminants, *330, 331*, 333
Gluteobiceps, large ruminants, 324, *327, 329, 330, 331*, 343
Gluteus medius, horse, 51
Gracilis
  horse, *100, 101*, 128, *131, 132, 133*
  large ruminants, 324, *327, 332*, 343, 344, *346*
Gray matter, horse brain, 250, 252
Greater tubercle, humerus, horse, *157*, 165, 166
Gubernaculum testis, 92
Guttural pouch
  horse, 220, *222, 227, 230*
    landmarks and approaches, 207, 262, 263
    surgical approach, 6–7
Gyri
  centrifugal, 302, *303*
  centripetal, *303*
Gyri cerebri
  horse, *249, 250, 253*
  large ruminants, *421*

Habenulae
  horse, *249*, 250
  large ruminants, *420*
Hanulus, horse, *209*
Haustrae, horse, 68, *69*
Head
  horse
    blood supply to, *217–231*
    bones of, 207-*214*
    landmarks and approaches, 207, *215*, 256–263
    lateral aspect, *217*
    muscles of, 216–*231*
    nerves of, *217–231*
  large ruminants, *402, 410*
    blood supply to, *402–411*
    bones of, 397-*401*
    landmarks and approaches, *398*

lateral aspect, *402, 410*
  muscles of, *402*–411
  nerve block sites, *423*
  nerves of, *402–411, 425*
Heart
  horse, *34, 35, 36*, 39–43
    auscultation and percussion of, 24, 45, *47*
    blood supply to, 40
    left ventricle, *42*
    right atrium, *41*
    right ventricle, *42*
  large ruminants, *280, 281, 282, 285–288*
    blood supply to, 40
Heel
  horse, 182, *186*, 190, *193, 194*, 195
  large ruminants, *390*
Hemoptysis, large ruminants, 279
Hepatic artery
  horse, *67, 71*
  large ruminants, 306, *308, 309*
Hepatic duct, horse, 66, *67*
Hepatoduodenal ligament
  horse, 60
  large ruminants, 297, 298
Hepatogastric ligament, large ruminants, 297
Hepatopancreatic ampulla, horse, 66
Hepatorenal ligament
  horse, 59
  large ruminants, 302, *308, 311*
Hernia
  inguinal, large ruminants, 334
  omental, horse, 60
Hilus, horse, *67*
Hip joint
  horse, *79*, 98, *122*, 140
    accessory ligament, *100*
    landmarks and approaches, 151
  large ruminants, *122*, 344
    nerve block sites, *356*
Hippocampus, horse, 248, *249*, 252, *255*
Hock
  horse, 135, 140, 144
    landmarks and approaches, 152
  large ruminants, *347, 350*
    nerve block sites, *357*
Hoof
  horse, *185, 188, 193, 194*, 195
    cartilage of, 182, *185, 186, 187*
    horny lamellae of, 190, *193*, 195
  large ruminants, *390*
Horny lamellae, horse hoof, 190, *193*, 195
Horse
  abdominal muscles, 51–53, 289
  abdominal viscera, 53–74. *See also under* individual organ
  central nervous system, 248–255
  cervicothoracic area, *30*
  cranial cavity, *212*
  cranial nerves, 225, 227. *See also under* individual nerve
  crus, *142*
  cutaneous muscles, *8*

Horse (*continued*)
digit, *185–192*
dorsoscapular structures, *28*
ear, *215*, 216, 229, *232*
eye, 229, *233, 234, 235, 236*
flank of, 50
genitalia
mare, 92, *94*, 101, *101, 102*, 105, *106, 107, 109*
stallion, 89–93, *101, 103, 104, 110*
guttural pouch, 6–7, 207, 220, *222, 227, 230*, 262, *263*
head. *See* Head, horse
heart, *34, 35, 36*, 39–43
auscultation and percussion of, 24, 45, *47*
hip joint, *79*, 98, *100, 122*, 140, 151
hock, 135, 140, 144, 152
hyoid apparatus, *214*, 228, *231*, 245, 247
iliac artery. *See* Iliac artery or vein
large intestine, *114. See also* Colon, horse
larynx, *5, 21*, 220, 228, *231*, 237, 244–246, 257
lungs, 24, *34*, 36, *37, 38*, 45, *47*
mandible, *213, 215*, 220, *224, 230*
neck, 3–22
orbit, *208, 209, 211, 215*, 234
palpable structures, rectal examination, 113–115
parotid region, *218, 219, 221*
pelvic limb, 117–154
pelvis. *See* Pelvis, horse
penis, *89, 90, 91*, 111
perineal region, *101, 102, 109, 110*
pharynx, 220, 228, *231, 237*, 238
sacroiliac joint, *79*
sacrum, *75, 76, 77*, 98
sternum, *24*
stifle, *123, 124*, 140, *142*, 144, 151
suspensory apparatus, *44*
tail, *78, 96*
tarsal joint, *126*
teeth of, *209, 210, 213*, 239–244, 261
thoracic limb, 155–205
thoracic viscera, 34–44. *See also under* individual organ
thorax
landmarks and approaches, *25*, 45, *46, 47*
muscles of, *26–29*, 273
nerves of, *27*
thoracic cavity, 34–37
thoracic inlet, 18, 31, *32, 33*
tongue, 220, 228, *239, 245*
vertebrae
caudal, *78*
cervical, *3*
lumbar, *49*, 80
thoracic, *23*
Humeral artery or vein
horse, *169*, 172, 175
large ruminants, 371, *372, 374, 376*
Humeral crest, horse, 13, 166
Humeroradioulnar joint, horse, *162*

Humerus
horse, *155, 157*
greater tubercle, *157*, 165, 166
large ruminants, *359, 360, 373*
greater tubercle, *360*, 371
Hymen, horse, 105, *106*
Hyoepiglottic ligament
horse, *230*, 238, 244, *245*
large ruminants, 411
Hyoepiglotticus
horse, *230*, 237, 244, *245*
large ruminants, *412, 413*
Hyoglossus
horse, *223*, 228, 229, *230*, 238
large ruminants, *409, 410, 411, 413*
Hyoid apparatus
horse, *214*, 228, *231*, 245, 247
large ruminants, *409*, 411
Hyoideus, horse, 228, 229
Hyopharyngeus
horse, 228, 229, *246*
large ruminants, *405, 406*
Hyovertebrotomy, horse, 262, *263*
Hypochondrium, horse, *25, 50*
Hypogastric nerves
horse, 82, 98
large ruminants, 333
Hypoglossal canal
horse, *209, 210, 212*
large ruminants, *401*
Hypoglossal nerve
horse, 220, *221–223*, 225, *227*, 228, *229, 230, 231*, 238, *251, 252, 254*
large ruminants, 225, *405, 406, 409, 410*, 411, *413*
Hypophyseal fossa, horse, *212*
Hypophysis
horse, 248, 250, *253*
large ruminants, 418, *420, 421, 422*
Hypothalamus, horse, 250
Hysterectomy, horse, *46*, 73

Ileal artery
horse, *72*
large ruminants, *303*
Ileal sphincter, horse, 68
Ileocecal fold
horse, 53, 54, 70
large ruminants, 302
Ileocolic artery, *72, 72*
large ruminants, *303*
Ileum
horse, 53, *69*
large ruminants, 294
Iliac artery or vein
horse, *81*, 82, *83*, 92, *100, 105, 131, 133*
circumflex, 52, *52*, 53, *81*, 82, *97*, 98, *100, 131, 133, 134*
large ruminants, 292, 318, *319, 331*, 344, *346*
Iliac bursa, horse, *148*
Iliac crest
horse, *75, 76*
large ruminants, *314*

Iliac fascia, horse, 82
Iliacofemoral artery or vein, horse, *97, 99, 133, 134*
Iliacus
horse, *83, 97*, 98, *99, 100*, 128, *134*
large ruminants, *330*
Iliocecal ostium, horse, 68, *69*
Iliocostalis cervicis
horse, *14*, 18–19, *30, 32, 33*
large ruminants, *271, 272, 276*
Iliocostalis thoracis, horse, *18, 29, 29, 44*
Iliocostalis thoracolumbar muscle, horse, 51
Iliohypogastric nerve
horse, *95*
large ruminants, *291*, 324
Iliohypogastricus, horse, *100*
Ilioinguinalis, horse, *100*
Ilioinguinal nerve
horse, *95*
large ruminants, *291*, 324
Iliolumbar artery or vein
horse, 98, *99*
large ruminants, *330*
Iliolumbar ligament, horse, *79*
Iliopsoas, horse, 86, 133
Iliopubic eminence
horse, *75, 76*
large ruminants, *314*
Ilium
horse, wing of, 96
large ruminants, wing of, *314*
Impaction sites, horse, 70
Impressions
abdominal viscera, large ruminants, *308*
liver, horse, 66, *67*
lungs
horse, *37–38*
large ruminants, *283, 284*
Incisive bone
horse, *208, 209, 215*, 238
large ruminants, *398, 400, 401*
Incisive papilla, horse, *230*, 239
Incisors
horse, *209, 210, 213, 215*, 239, 240, *240, 242, 243*
eruption of, 244
large ruminants, 397, *399, 414, 415*
Infraglenoid tubercle, large ruminants, *359*
Infraglottic cavity, 245
Infraorbital artery, horse, 234
Infraorbital canal, horse, *247*
Infraorbital foramen
horse, *208, 209, 215*, 234
large ruminants, *397, 398*
Infraorbital nerve
horse, 234
landmarks and approaches, 257, *258*
Infraspinatus
horse, 28, *28, 173*
subtendinous bursa, *174*, 175
large ruminants, *275*, 371, *374, 375, 376*

Infraspinous fossa
  horse, *156*
  large ruminants, *359*
Infratrochlear nerve
  horse, *235*, 236
    landmarks and approaches, *259*, 260
  large ruminants, *417*, *419*
Infratrochlear notch
  horse, *208*, *211*
  large ruminants, *398*, *400*
Infundibulum
  hypothalamic, horse, 250
  tooth, horse, 239, *240*, *243*
  uterine tube
    large ruminants, *336*
    mare, 86, *87*, *88*
Inguinal canal, horse, 82, *85*
Inguinal ring
  horse, 82, *83*
  large ruminants, 324, *325*
Insula, large ruminants, *305*, 306, *307*, *310*
Interarcual space
  horse, *3*
  large ruminants, *268*, *290*
Interatrial septum, horse, 41
Intercapital ligament, horse, *24*
Intercarpal ligaments
  horse, *163*, 195
  large ruminants, *366*
Intercondylar eminence, large ruminants, *340*
Intercornual ligament, 318, *319*, *336*
Intercornual process, 397, *400*
Intercornual protuberance, 267
Intercostal artery or vein
  horse, 33, 36, *36*, 45, *46*
  large ruminants, *277*
Intercostal muscles
  horse, *26*, 28–29, *29*, 53
  large ruminants, 295
Intercostal nerves, horse, 27, 33, 45, *46*
Intercostal space, horse, 53
Intercostobrachial nerve, horse, *26*, *27*
Interdigital artery, large ruminants, 383
Interdigital ligaments, large ruminants, *367*, *388*, *389*
Interdigital phalangosesamoid ligament, large ruminants, *367*
Interflexorii, large ruminants, 343, 380, *380*
Interhemispheric fissure, horse, *253*
Interincisive canal, horse, *210*, *230*
Interincisive fissure, large ruminants, *401*
Intermammary groove, horse, 92
Intermammary sulcus, large ruminants, 324
Intermediate nerve, horse, 226
Intermediate tendon, horse, *18*, 135, *145*
Intermediofacial nerve, horse, *251*, 252, *254*
Interossei muscles
  large ruminants, 343, *352*, *367*, *384*, *385*, *386*, *388*, *389*

accessory ligament of, *386*, *388*
Interosseous antebrachial membrane, large ruminants, *366*
Interosseous artery
  horse, 175, *176*, 178, *179*
  large ruminants, *378*, *379*, *380*, *382*, *385*
Interosseous ligaments, horse, *126*
Interosseous medius
  horse, *126*, *141*, *145*, *164*, *181*, *184*, *185*, *189*, *196*, 197
  large ruminants, 383
Interparietal bones, horse, *208*, 248
Interpeduncular fossa, horse, *251*, 252
Interphalangeal joint, horse, *164*, 182, *191*
Interscutularis
  horse, *232*
  large ruminants, *402*, *407*
Intersesamoid ligament, large ruminants, *367*
Interspinales, 27
Interspinal ligament, horse, *79*
Interthalamic adhesion
  horse, 248, *249*
  large ruminants, *420*
Intertransversarii
  horse, *99*, 101
  large ruminants, *329*
Intertransversarii cervicis, 19, *19*
  large ruminants, 270, *272*
Intertransversarii lumborum, large ruminants, 292
Intertransversarii thoracis, horse, 27, 29, *29*
Intertransverse ligaments, large ruminants, 292
Intertrochanteric crest, horse, 96, *118*
Intertrochanteric line, large ruminants, *339*
Intertrochlear notch, large ruminants, *363*, *364*, *384*
Intervenous tubercle
  horse, *41*
  large ruminants, *286*
Interventricular foramen, horse, 248
Interventricular septum
  horse, 40, *42*
  large ruminants, *288*
Intervertebral foramina
  horse, *3*, 11, *49*
  large ruminants, *268*, *274*, *290*, 292
Intestine, horse, *70*. *See also under* individual organ
  blood supply to, 71–72
  large, 53–54, *114*
  small, 53
Intraabdominal tunics, horse, 86
Intramuscular injections, horse, sites for, *5*, 7
Intrapharyngeal ostium, horse, 238
Intravenous injections, horse, sites for, 6
Iridocorneal angle, horse, *233*, 236
Iridocorneal spaces, horse, *233*, 236
Iris, horse, *233*, 236
Ischial arch, horse, *75*, *76*, 105, 111

Ischial tuberosity, horse, *75*, *76*
Ischiatic bursa, horse, 96, *148*, *153*
Ischiatic foramina
  horse, *79*, 98
  large ruminants, 313, *329*
Ischiatic notch, external, *328*
Ischiatic spine, horse, 96
Ischiatic symphysis, horse, *89*
Ischiatic tuberosity, large ruminants, *327*
Ischiocavernosus
  horse, 89, 101, *101*
  large ruminants, *327*, *332*, *333*, *335*
Ischiourethralis, large ruminants, *321*
Ischium, large ruminants, *314*
Isognathous, 239
Isthmus faucium, horse, 238
Its sleeve
  horse, *186*, *188*
  large ruminants, *386*

Jejunal ansae, 58
Jejunal arteries
  horse, 68, *70*, 72, *72*
  large ruminants, *303*
Jejunum
  horse, 53, *55*, 56, *58*, 68, *70*
  large ruminants, 294, 297, 299, 301
Jugular foramen
  horse, *209*
  large ruminants, 397, *401*
Jugular fossa, horse, 5, 6
Jugular groove
  horse, 5, *5*, 6
  large ruminants, 269
Jugular (paracondylar) process
  horse, *210*, 215
  large ruminants, *398*, *401*, *409*
Jugular vein, external
  horse
    clinical approach, *5*, *21*, *22*
    head, *217*, *219*, *221*, *222*
    neck, 7, *9*, 11, *14*, *15*, *18*
    thorax, *30*, *32*, 36
  large ruminants,
    head, *402*, *405*, 411
    neck, 268, *269*, *270*
    thorax, *276*, *277*, *278*, *281*, *282*
Jugular vein, internal, large ruminants, 269, *271*, 281

Kidney
  horse
    biopsy of, 50
    left, 56, 62, *64*, *65*, 67
    right, *55*, 56, *59*, *60*, 62, *64*, *65*, 67
  large ruminants
    left, *300*, 302, 306, *312*
    right, 297, 299, *300*, 301, 302, 306, *308*, *311*, *312*
Knuckling, large ruminants, 350

L1 nerve, large ruminants, 292, *293*, 295
L2 nerve, large ruminants, 292, *293*, 295
L3 nerve, large ruminants, 295

L4 nerve
  horse, 98, *99*
  large ruminants, *295*
L5 nerve, large ruminants, *295*
L6 nerve, horse, *80*
Labia
  horse, 105, *106*
  large ruminants, *336*
Labial artery or vein
  horse, *217*
  large ruminants, 324, *325, 326, 328, 346, 402*
Labial nerves
  horse, 101
  large ruminants, *328*
Lacertus brachii, horse, *196*
Lacertus fibrosus
  horse, *173*, 175, *176, 177, 179*
  large ruminants, *371, 372, 377, 378, 379*
Lacrimal bone
  horse, *208, 209*
  large ruminants, *398, 400*
Lacrimal bulla, large ruminants, 397, *398, 401*
Lacrimal canaliculi, horse, 229
Lacrimal caruncle
  horse, 229
  large ruminants, 415
Lacrimal fossa, horse, 234
Lacrimal gland
  horse, 234, *235*, 236
    landmarks and approaches, *256,* 257
  large ruminants, *417*, 418
Lacrimal nerve
  horse, 234, *235*, 236
    landmarks and approaches, 260
  large ruminants, *417, 419, 430*
Lacrimal process
  horse, *211*
  large ruminants, *398, 400*
Lacrimal punta
  horse, 229
  large ruminants, 415
Lacrimal sac, horse, *211*, 229
Lactiferous ducts
  horse, 92, *94*
  large ruminants, 324, *325*
Lactiferous sinus
  horse, 92, *94*
  large ruminants, 324, *325*
Lacuna musculorum, horse, 86
Lacuna vasorum, horse, 86
Lamellae, horny, large ruminants, *390,* 391
Lameness, large ruminants, 350, 391
Lamina dura, horse, 240
Laminae of cervical fascia
  horse, *9*
  large ruminants, 268
Laminae of suspensory apparatus, large ruminants, 324, *325*
Lamina nuchae
  horse, *9*, 15, *15, 16, 17, 19*
  large ruminants, *272*

Lamina quadrigemina, horse, 250
Laminitis, horse, 190
Laparoscopy, horse, 50
Laparotomy, horse, 50, 73
Large ruminants. *See* Ruminants, large
Laryngeal artery or vein
  horse, *246, 247*
  large ruminants, 411
Laryngeal hemiplegia, horse, 245
Laryngeal nerve
  horse
    head, 220, *222, 223, 227, 228, 246*
    neck, 6, *9*, 13, *21*
    thorax, 32, *33*, 35–36
  large ruminants, 269, *278, 406*, 411
Laryngeal recess, horse, *231*, 245, *245*
Laryngeal ventricle
  horse, *230, 231*, 245, *246*
    landmarks and approaches, *256,* 257
Laryngeal vestibule, horse, 245
Laryngopharynx
  horse, *230, 237*, 238
  large ruminants, *412*
Laryngoplasty, horse, 262, *263*
Larynx
  horse, *5, 21*, 220, *228, 231, 237,* 244–246
    landmarks and approaches, 257
  large ruminants, 411, *413*
Lateral ligament, horse, *4*
Latissimus dorsi
  horse, 26, *26, 28*, 29, *51, 167, 169*
    aponeurosis of, 51, *168, 169*, 172
  large ruminants, *370, 371, 372, 374*
    aponeurosis of, *274, 275*
Lens, horse eye, *233*, 236
Leptomeninges
  horse, 248
  large ruminants, 418
Lesser tubercle, horse, *157*, 166
Levator anguli oculi medialis, horse, *217*
Levator ani
  horse, 98, *99*, 101, *101, 102*
  large ruminants, *327, 328, 329, 330, 331, 332, 333*
Levator costae, horse, 29, *29*, 44
Levator labii superioris
  horse, 216, *217*
  large ruminants, *402, 430*
Levator nasolabialis
  horse, *217*
  large ruminants, *402, 430*
Levator palpebrae superioris
  horse, *233*, 234, *235*
  large ruminants, *417*, 418, *419*
Levator veli palatini
  horse, 229, *230, 231, 235*
  large ruminants, *410*, 411, *412*
Ligament of the ergot
  horse, 182, *189*, 190
  large ruminants, *388, 389*
Ligamentum arteriosum
  horse, 13, 35
  large ruminants, *285*
Ligamentum nuchae, horse, 15, 229

Ligamentum pectinatum, horse, *233*
Linea alba, horse, 53, *81, 82*
Line of peritoneal reflection, large ruminants, *321*
Line of pleural reflection, horse, 34, 45, *46*
Lingual artery or vein
  horse, *228, 230*, 299
  large ruminants, *409*, 411, *413*
Lingual frenulum
  horse, *230*, 239
  large ruminants, 411
Lingual nerve
  horse, *223, 226, 228*, 229
  large ruminants, 408, *409, 410*
Lingual papillae, horse, 238
Lingual process, horse, *214*
Linguofacial artery, horse, *221, 223, 227,* 229
Linguofacial nerve, horse, *5, 7*
Linguofacial trunk artery, large ruminants, *406, 410*
Linguofacial vein
  horse
    head, *215, 217, 218, 219, 221, 222*
    landmarks and approaches, 262, *263*
    neck, 6, 7, 11, *12, 14, 15, 18*
  large ruminants, *404, 405*
Lips
  horse, *215*, 216
  large ruminants, 411
Liver
  horse, 54, *55, 56*, 59, *59, 61*, 66–68
    biopsy of, 50
  large ruminants, 295, *297, 298, 299, 300, 301, 308, 311*
    biopsy of, 279
Lobus piriformis, horse, *251*, 252
Locking mechanism, stifle, 144
Longis capitis, large ruminants, *406*
Longissimus atlantis
  horse, 15, *16, 18*
  large ruminants, *271, 272*
Longissimus capitis
  horse, 15, *16, 18*
  large ruminants, 270, *271, 272*
Longissimus cervicis, horse, 15, *16, 18, 19*
Longissimus thoracis, horse, *18*, 29, *29*
Longissimus thoracolumbar, horse, *44*
Longitudinal groove, large ruminants, 292, 295, 306, *307*
Longitudinal ligament, horse, *24, 79*
Longitudinal ligament of dens, horse, *4*
Longitudinal pillar, large ruminants, *310*
Longus atlantis, large ruminants, 270, *271, 272*
Longus capitis
  horse, *17*, 18, *231*
  large ruminants, *271, 405*
Longus colli, horse, *9, 18*, 19
Longus piriformis, horse, *253*
Lophodonts, 239
Lou Gehrig's disease, horse, 10
Lumbar arteries, horse, 62

Lumbar spinal nerves
  horse, 27, 51, 52, *52*, 53, 98
    cutaneous, *10*
  large ruminants, 289, *291*
Lumbar vertebrae
  horse, *49*, 80
  large ruminants, *290*
Lumbosacral cistern, *80*
Lumbosacral plexus
  horse, 128
  large ruminants, 333
Lumbricalis, horse, *185*
Lungs
  horse, *34, 37, 38, 47*
    accessory lobe, 36
    auscultation and percussion of, 24, 45
  large ruminants, *280, 283–285*
    auscultation and percussion of, 279
    cranial lobe, *281, 283*
    lobes of, *283, 284*
Lymphadenitis
  horse, 6
  large ruminants, 267
Lymph nodes
  abomasal, 306
  axillary
    horse, *169*
    large ruminants, 368, *370*
  cecal, horse, 70
  cervical
    horse, *5*, 6, 13, *14, 21, 32, 33, 219, 222*
    large ruminants, 267, 269, 270, *271, 276, 277, 278*
  colic, horse, 70
  cubital, horse, *169, 172*
  gastric, horse, 68
  hepatic, large ruminants, *308*
  iliac, horse, 82
  iliofemoral, horse, 128
  inguinal
    horse, *89*, 146, *147*
    large ruminants, *319, 322, 324, 325*
  ischiatic
    horse, *97, 134*
    large ruminants, *329, 331*
  jejunal, horse, 68, *70*
  lumbar, horse, 82
  mammary, large ruminants, 324, *325, 326*
  mandibular
    horse, 216, 220, *256*
    large ruminants, *402, 404, 405, 409, 413*
  mediastinal, large ruminants, *282*
  mesenteric, horse, *70*
  omasal, 306
  parotid, large ruminants, *402*, 403, *404*
  popliteal
    horse, 134
    large ruminants, *329*
  portal
    horse, 66
    large ruminants, 306

proper axillary
  horse, *167, 172*
  large ruminants, *370*, 371
pulmonary, horse, 37
renal
  horse, 62
  large ruminants, 302
reticular, 306
retropharyngeal
  horse, *219*, 220, *222, 231*
  large ruminants, *405, 406, 409, 410, 412*
ruminal, 306
sacral, horse, 82
splenic, horse, 71
subiliac
  horse, *46, 51, 52*, 73
  large ruminants, *290*, 292, *330*
tracheobronchial, horse, *37*

Magda's method, 289, *291*
Malaris artery, horse, *235*, 236
Malaris muscle
  horse, *217*
  large ruminants, *402, 417*
Malleolar bone, large ruminants, *340*
Malleolus, horse, *118*
Mamillary body
  horse, 250, *251, 252, 254*
  large ruminants, *421*
Mammary artery or vein
  horse, *89*
  large ruminants, 324, *326, 328, 346*
Mammary glands
  horse, 92
  large ruminants, 324, *325*
Mammary papilla
  horse, 92, *94*
  large ruminants, 324
Mammary suspensory apparatus, large ruminants, 324, *325*
Mandible
  horse, *213, 215, 230*
    removing, 220, *224*
  large ruminants, 397, *399*
Mandibular duct
  horse, *230*, 238
  large ruminants, *409, 410*
Mandibular foramen
  horse, *213*, 224
  large ruminants, *399*
Mandibular fossa, horse, *209*
Mandibular nerve
  horse, *225, 227*
  large ruminants, 408, *410, 419*
Mandibular notch, horse, *213*
Mane, horse, *5, 7, 215*
Manubrium sterni
  horse, *5*, 6, *7*, 13, *24, 25*
  large ruminants, 267, 273, *274*
Margo plicatus, horse, 53, 71
Masseteric artery or vein
  horse, *217, 218, 219*, 220, *221, 222, 228*
  large ruminants, *404, 405*
Masseteric fossa, large ruminants, *399*

Masseteric nerve, horse, *223, 225, 228*
Masseter muscle
  horse, 216, *217*, 220, *223*, 224
  large ruminants, *402*, 403, *404*
Mastication, muscles of
  horse, 216
  large ruminants, 403
Masticatory nerve
  horse, *223, 225, 235*
  large ruminants, 408
Mastoid process
  horse, *209, 210*
  large ruminants, 397
Maxilla
  horse, *209*, 238, 298
  large ruminants, *398, 400, 401*
Maxillary artery or vein
  horse, *218, 219*, 220, *221, 222, 223*, 225, 227, 228, *234, 235*
  large ruminants, *405, 406*, 408, *409, 410, 419*
Maxillary foramen
  horse, *211*, 234
  large ruminants, 397, *401*
Maxillary groove, horse, *212*
Maxillary nerve
  horse, 234, *235*
    landmarks and approaches, *256*
  large ruminants, *419*
Maxillary septum, *247*, 248
Maxillary sinus
  horse, 238, *247*, 248
  large ruminants, landmarks and approaches, 418
Meatuses, nasal
  horse, *230*, 236
  large ruminants, 411
Median artery or vein
  horse, 178, *179, 180, 181, 183, 184*
    landmarks and approaches, 197, *198*
  large ruminants, *378*, 380, 383, *385, 386*, 387, *387*
Median fissure, horse, *251, 252*
Median nerve
  horse, *167, 169*, 172, *179, 180, 181*
    landmarks and approaches, 197, *198*
  large ruminants, 371, *372, 373, 377, 378, 379*, 380, 383, *385, 386*
    blocking, *391, 392*
Median raphe of scrotum, 86
Mediastinum
  horse, 35
  large ruminants, 279
Medius gluteus, large ruminants, *356*
Medulla oblongata
  horse, 250, 252, *253, 255*
  large ruminants, *421*
Medullary canal, large ruminants, *343*
Medullary velum, horse, 250
Meibomian glands, horse, 234
Melena, large ruminants, 279
Membrane tectoria, horse, *4*
Meningeal artery, horse, *227*, 234

Meniscofemoral ligament, horse, *124, 125*, 143
Meniscotibial ligament, horse, *124, 125*, 143
Meniscus
 horse, *123, 124, 125, 144*
 large ruminants, *356*
Mental foramen
 horse, *213, 215*, 220, *224*
 large ruminants, *399*
Mental nerve, horse, *258*
Meridians, horse eye, 236
Mesencephalic aqueduct
 horse, *249, 250*
 large ruminants, *420*
Mesencephalon, horse, 250, 252
Mesenteric arteries
 horse, 62, *65, 72, 82*
 large ruminants, 302, *303*
Mesenteric ileal branch artery, large ruminants, 302, *303*
Mesentery, large ruminants, 302
Mesocolon
 horse, 59, *59, 60*, 61, *68, 70, 82*
 large ruminants, 302
Mesoductus deferens
 horse, 82, *84, 85, 93*
 large ruminants, *322*, 323
Mesoduodenum
 horse, 53, 59
 large ruminants, 280, 297, *299*
Mesoepididymis, horse, 92
Mesofuniculus
 horse, 84, *84, 85*
 large ruminants, *322*, 323
Mesojejunum, horse, *60*
Mesometrium
 horse, 86, *88*
 large ruminants, *336*
Mesonephronic ducts, 334
Mesorchium
 horse, 84, *84, 85*, 92, *93*
 large ruminants, *322*, 323
Mesorectum
 horse, *81, 87*, 98
 large ruminants, *319*
Mesosalpinx
 horse, 86, *87, 88, 106*
 large ruminants, *336*
Mesovarium
 horse, 86, *87, 88*
 large ruminants, 318, *336*
Metacarpal artery or vein
 horse, 182, *183, 184*
 large ruminants, 383, *385*, 387, *387*
Metacarpal bones
 horse, *155, 160, 184*
 large ruminants, *362, 363*, 383, *384*
Metacarpal canal, large ruminants, *384*
Metacarpal nerves, horse, 182, *185*, 199
Metacarpointersesamoid ligament, horse, *189*
Metacarpophalangeal joint, horse, *164*
Metacarpus, horse, *183*
Metapodium
 horse, *117, 155*

large ruminants, 383
Metatarsal artery or vein
 horse, 139, *141*
  landmarks and approaches, 146, *147*
 large ruminants, *355*
Metatarsal bones, horse, *117, 121*
Metatarsal nerves
 horse, 139, 140, 148
 large ruminants, blocking sites, *354*
Metatarsal retinaculum, horse, 138
Metatarsus, horse, *141*
Metathalamus, horse, 252, *254*
Metencephalon, horse, 250, 252
Metritis, equine, 91
Milk vein, large ruminants, 324
Milk well, large ruminants, 324
Molars
 horse, *209, 210, 213, 215*, 239, *241, 243*, 244
 large ruminants, *399, 414*, 415
Monophyodonts, 240
Multifidi cervicis
 horse, *15*, 16, *16, 17*, 19, *19*
 large ruminants, *272*
Multifidus thoracis, horse, 29, *29*
Muscle of Phillips, horse, 175
Muscle of Thiernesse, horse, 175
Muscular bursae, horse, 152, *153*
Muscular lacuna, horse, 128
Muscular process, large ruminants, *398, 401*
Muscular tubercle, large ruminants, 397
Musculocutaneous nerve
 horse, *167, 169*, 172
 large ruminants, 371, *372, 373, 377, 379*
Myelencephalon, horse, *249*, 250, 252
Mylohyoideus
 horse, 216, 220, *223*, 228, *230*, 238
 large ruminants, *402*, 408, *409, 410*, 411, *412*, 430
Mylohyoid nerve
 horse, 220, *223*, 224
 large ruminants, 408

Nasal aperture, horse, *215*, 216
Nasal bone
 horse, *208, 209*
 large ruminants, *398, 400*
Nasal cavity
 horse, 236
 large ruminants, 411
Nasal conchae
 horse, *230*
 large ruminants, 411, *412*
Nasal diverticulum, horse, 216, *217*
Nasal glands, horse, 236
Nasal meatus, horse, landmarks and approaches, 260, *261*
Nasal muscle, horse, 216, *217*
Nasal nerve, horse, 234, *235*
Nasal planum, large ruminants, 279
Nasal process, large ruminants, *398*
Nasal septum
 horse, *230*, 236

large ruminants, 411, *412*
Nasociliary nerve
 horse, *235*, 236
 large ruminants, *419*
Nasoincisive notch, horse, *215*
Nasolacrimal duct, horse, 229
Nasopharynx
 horse, 229, *230, 237*, 238
 large ruminants, 411, *412*
Navicular bone
 horse, *161, 182, 187, 191*
 large ruminants, *384*, 390
Navicular disease, horse, 165, 190
Navicular ligament, horse, *164, 187, 189*, 190, *191*
Neck
 horse
  cervical vertebrae, *3*
  deep structures, *14–18*
  fasciae, 9
  joints of, 4
  landmarks and approaches, 5–7, 20, *21, 22*
  muscles of, *11*
  spinal nerves, 7, 10–12
  superficial structures, 7, *12*
 large ruminants
  cervical vertebrae, 268
  deep structures, *270–272*
  muscles of, *11*, 267, 269–272
  spinal nerves, 269–272
  superficial structures, 269
Nephrosplenic ligament, 61
Nerve blocks
 cervical spinal nerves, large ruminants, *423, 424*
 digital nerves, horse, 182
 epidural, horse, 108
 fibular nerve, large ruminants, 350, *353*
 great auricular nerve, horse, 6
 of interosseous medius, horse, 182
 intraarticular
  horse, 150–154, 199–201
  large ruminants, 350, *356, 357, 391, 393–395*
 paravertebral/paralumbar, large ruminants, 289, *291*
 pelvic limb
  horse, 146–154
  large ruminants, 350, *356, 357*
 regional, large ruminants, 350, *355*, 393
 subsacral, horse, 75
 thoracic limb
  horse, 197–205
  large ruminants, 391–395
 tibial nerve, large ruminants, 350, *353*
 udder, large ruminants, *291*
 ulnar nerve, large ruminants, *391, 392, 392*
Neurohypophyseal recess, horse, 248
Neurohypophysis, horse, *249*, 250
Nictitating membrane, large ruminants, 418
Nostril, horse, *215*, 216

Nuchal bursae, horse, 6, 16, *17, 21*
Nuchal ligament, horse, 7, *9, 15, 17*
Nucleus caudatus, horse, 248, *249, 254, 255*
Nucleus lentiformis, horse, 252, *255*

Oblique muscle of abdomen
  external
    horse, 26, *26, 28, 29, 51, 52,* 82
      aponeurosis, 128
      transverse section, *44*
    large ruminants, 276, *290, 292, 325*
  internal
    horse, *81,* 82, *89, 99, 100, 134*
    large ruminants, 292, *293, 319*
Oblique muscle of eye
  horse, 234, *235,* 236
  large ruminants, *417, 419*
Obliquus capitis caudalis
  horse, *15,* 16, *16, 17, 18, 19*
  large ruminants, *272*
Obliquus capitis cranialis, horse, 16, *17*
Obturator
  external
    horse, 98, *132, 133*
    large ruminants, *328, 329, 333,* 344
  internal
    horse, *100*
    large ruminants, 344
Obturator artery or vein, horse, 89, 98, *100,* 101, 128, *131, 132, 133*
Obturator canal, horse, *79*
Obturator foramen
  horse, *75, 76*
  large ruminants, *314,* 344
Obturator membrane
  horse, *79*
  large ruminants, 313
Obturator nerve, horse, *100,* 128, *131, 133*
Obturator tendon, horse, *97,* 98
Occipital artery or vein
  horse, 16, *17,* 222, 227, 229, *231*
  large ruminants, *404, 405, 406,* 411
Occipital bone
  horse, *17,* 208, 248
  large ruminants, 397
Occipital condyle
  horse, 6, *209, 210*
  large ruminants, *398, 401*
Occipital lobe, large ruminants, *420*
Occipital protuberance, horse, 6, *208, 215*
Occipitohyoideus
  horse, 220, *221,* 222, 228, 229, *231,* 245
    landmarks and approaches, 262, *263*
  large ruminants, *405, 406, 409, 410, 413*
Oculomotor nerve
  horse, 225, 234, *235, 251,* 252
    landmarks and approaches, *259,* 260
  large ruminants, 225, *419*
Olecrannon

horse, 24, *25, 51, 158,* 165
  large ruminants, 273, *361*
Olecrannon fossa
  horse, *157*
  large ruminants, *360*
Olecrannon tuber
  horse, *158*
  large ruminants, *361*
Olfactory bulb
  horse, 248, 250, *251,* 252, *253*
  large ruminants, *420, 421*
Olfactory groove, horse, 250, *251,* 252
Olfactory lobe, large ruminants, *420*
Olfactory nerve
  horse, 225, 250, *251, 253*
  large ruminants, 225
Olfactory peduncle
  horse, 250, *251,* 252
  large ruminants, *421*
Olfactory tract, horse, 250, *251,* 252
Olfactory trigone, large ruminants, *421*
Olfactory tubercle, horse, 250
Omasal folds, 306, *310*
Omasal groove, 294, 306, *310*
Omasal pillar, 306
Omasoabdominal orifice, *310*
Omasoabdominal ostium, 294
Omasum, 294, *297,* 301, *307*
Omental bursa, 280, 297
Omental foramen
  horse, 60
  large ruminants, 280, 297
Omentum
  greater
    horse, 60, 61
    large ruminants, *295, 296, 299*
  lesser
    horse, 60
    large ruminants, 297
Omohyoideus
  horse
    head, *217, 218, 219,* 220, *222,* 228
    neck, 6, *7, 9, 12,* 13, *14, 15, 18*
    large ruminants, 269, *269,* 270, *271, 409, 410, 413, 460*
Omotransversarius
  horse, 6, *7, 9,* 11, *12,* 13, *14,* 15, *15*
  large ruminants, 269, *269,* 270, *271, 272, 370*
Ophthalmic artery
  horse, 234, *235,* 236
  large ruminants, *419*
Ophthalmic groove, horse, *212*
Ophthalmic nerve
  horse, 236
    landmarks and approaches, *259,* 260
Optic canal
  horse, *211*
  large ruminants, 397
Optic chiasm
  horse, 250, *251,* 252, *254*
  large ruminants, *420, 421*
Optic disc, horse, *233,* 236
Optic nerve
  horse, 225, *233, 235,* 236, 250, *251,*

*252, 253, 254*
  large ruminants, 225, *420*
Optic recess, horse, 248
Optic tract
  horse, 250, *254*
  large ruminants, *421*
Oral cavity
  horse, 238–239
  large ruminants, 411
Oral cleft, horse, *215*
Ora serrata, horse, *233,* 236
Orbicularis oculi
  horse, *217, 233,* 234
  large ruminants, *402,* 418
Orbicularis oris, horse, 216, *217*
Orbita
  horse, *208, 209, 211, 215,* 234
  large ruminants, 397, *398, 400*
Orbital fissure, horse, *211*
Orbital septum
  horse, 234
  large ruminants, 418
Oropharynx
  horse, *228,* 230, 238
  large ruminants, 411, *412, 413*
Os ilium, horse, *75, 76*
Os ischium
  horse, *75, 76*
  large ruminants, *314*
Os pubis
  horse, *75, 76*
  large ruminants, *314*
Osteochondrosis, horse, 144
Ostium
  cardiac, 53
  cecocolic, 54
  ileocecal, 54
  pyloric, 53
Oval foramen, large ruminants, 397, *398, 401*
Oval notch, horse, *212*
Ovarian artery, horse, 62, 86
Ovarian bursa
  horse, 86, *87, 88*
  large ruminants, 318
Ovarian fossa, horse, 86, *87, 88*
Ovariectomy, horse, 86
Ovary
  horse, 86, *87, 88, 106*
  large ruminants, 318, *319, 336*

P I
  horse, *117, 155, 161,* 188
  large ruminants, *364, 384*
P II
  horse, *117, 155, 161,* 188, 190
  large ruminants, *364, 384*
P III
  horse, *117, 155, 161, 187,* 190, *191*
  large ruminants, *364, 384*
Pachymenix
  horse, 248
  large ruminants, 418
Palate, hard
  horse, *210,* 229, *230,* 238
  large ruminants, 397, *401,* 411

Palate, soft
horse, *230, 237, 245*
displacement of, 13, 229, 238
large ruminants, 411, *412, 413*
Palatine artery or vein
horse, *228*, 229, 234, *235*
large ruminants, 411
Palatine bone
horse, *210*, 238
large ruminants, 397, *401*
Palatine fissure
horse, *208, 210*
large ruminants, *400, 401*
Palatine foramen
horse, *210, 211*
large ruminants, 397, *401*
Palatine nerve, horse, 234, *235*
Palatine raphe
horse, 239
large ruminants, 411
Palatine rugae, horse, 239
Palatine sinus
horse, 238
large ruminants, 411
Palatinus muscle, horse, 229
Palatoglossal arch
horse, *37*, 238
large ruminants, 411, *413*
Palatopharyngeal arch, horse, *237*, 238, 245
Palatopharyngeus
horse, *228*, 229, *230, 231*
large ruminants, *409, 410*, 411
Pallidum, horse, 252, *255*
Palmar arch artery or vein
horse, 178, *183, 184*
large ruminants, *386, 387, 387*
Palmar fascia
horse, 178, *181*, 183, *183*
large ruminants, 383
Palmar ligaments
horse, *164*, 182, *189*
large ruminants, *367*
Palmar nerves
horse, 178, *180, 181*, 182, *183, 184*
landmarks and approaches, 199
large ruminants, *386*
Palpebral artery or vein, large ruminants, *407*
Palpebral commissures, horse, 229
Palpebral fissure
horse, 229
large ruminants, 415
Palpebral ligaments, horse, 234, 236
Palpebral limbus, horse, 229
Pampiniform plexus, large ruminants, *322, 323*
Pancreas
horse, 54, *55*, 56, *60, 67*
large ruminants, 280, 294, 295, *297, 299, 300*, 301, *311*
Pancreatic duct
horse, 53, 54, 62, 66, *67*
large ruminants, *311*
Pancreatic notch, large ruminants, 302
Pancreaticoduodenal artery

horse, *71, 72, 72*
large ruminants, 302, *303*, 306, *309*
Papillae
duodenal
horse, 66, *67*
large ruminants, 306
ileal, horse, 68
incisive, large ruminants, 411
lingual
horse, *230, 237*
large ruminants, 411
mammary, horse, *94*
parotid, large ruminants, 411
Papillary ducts
horse, 92, *94*
large ruminants, 324, *325*
Papillary muscles
horse, 42, *42, 43*
large ruminants, *286, 287*
Papillary veins, large ruminants, *326*
Papillary venous plexus, large ruminants, *326*
Papillomavirus, bovine, 318
Papple shape, 306
Paraconal interventricular branch artery, horse, 39, *40*
Paraconal interventricular groove
horse, 39
large ruminants, *285, 286*
Parallels, horse eye, 236
Paralumbar fossa
horse, *50*
large ruminants, approaches to, 289, 292
Paranasal sinuses
horse, *247*
landmarks and approaches, 260, *261*
trephination of, 207
large ruminants, 415, *416*
landmarks and approaches, 418
Pararectal fossa
horse, *81*, 98
large ruminants, *328*
Parathyroid gland, large ruminants, 411
Parietal bones
horse, *208*, 248
large ruminants, 397, *398*
Parietal lamina, large ruminants, 323
Parietal lobe, large ruminants, *420*
Parietoauricularis, horse, *232*
Parotid duct
horse, 216, *217, 218*
landmarks and approaches, *256*
large ruminants, *402, 404*
Parotid gland
horse, *7*, 11
large ruminants, *402, 404*, 430
Parotidoauricularis
horse, *7*, 11, *217, 218*
large ruminants, *402, 404*
Parotid region
horse, *218, 219, 221*
large ruminants, *404–406*
Parturition, large ruminants, 313
Passive-stay apparatus, horse

pelvic limb, 145–146
thoracic limb, 195, *196*, 197
Pastern
horse, *164*, 197, 201, *202*
large ruminants, *388*
Patella
horse, *50*, 52, 96, *117, 118, 123, 124, 125*
locking mechanism, 144
large ruminants, *339, 356*
Patellar ligaments
horse, *123, 124, 125, 136, 137*, 140, 142, *144, 145*
landmarks and approaches, 150
large ruminants, *347, 348, 356*
Pecten
horse, 75, *76*
large ruminants, *314, 317*
Pectinate ligament, horse, 236
Pectinate muscle
horse, 41, *41*
large ruminants, *286, 287*
Pectineus
horse, *100*, 128, *131, 132*
large ruminants, 344, *346*
Pectoral groove, horse, 5, 6, 15, *21*, 165, 166
Pectoral muscles
horse, *14*, 15, *26*, 28, *29, 30, 32, 51*, 166
large ruminants, *275, 276, 276*, 368, *370, 371, 374, 376*
Pectoral nerves, horse, *167, 169*, 172
Pelvic axis, large ruminants, 313
Pelvic cavity, large ruminants, 318
Pelvic diaphragm, horse, 98
Pelvic flexure, horse, 53, *55*, 61, *61*, 68, 69, *70*
Pelvic inclination, large ruminants, 313, *317*
Pelvic inlet
large ruminants, 313, *319*
mare, 86, *87*
stallion, *81, 83*
Pelvic limb
horse
blood supply to, *131–136*, 139–143
bones of, *117–126*
bursae of, *148–150*
landmarks and approaches, 127, *147*
lateral aspect, *134*
ligaments of, *123–126*, 140–146
locking mechanism, 144
medial aspect, *131–133*
muscles of, 128–143
nerve supply to, 128, *129, 130, 131–136, 137–141*
passive stay apparatus, 145–146
large ruminants
blood supply to, 344, *346–352*
bones of, 339–342
landmarks and approaches, 343, 350
ligaments of, 344, *348*, 351
muscles of, *344–352*

nerve blocking sites, 350, *353–357*
nerve supply to, 345, *346–355*
tendons of, *347, 349*
Pelvic nerves, large ruminants, *331, 332*
Pelvic plexus
  horse, 82
  large ruminants, *332*, 333
Pelvic symphysis
  horse, *79, 100*
  large ruminants, 313, *314*
Pelvimetry, cow, *317*
Pelvis
  horse
    blood supply to, 82–85, *97,*
      *99–102, 105*
    bones of, 75–80
    genitalia
      mare, 87–88, 92, *94, 101, 101, 102,*
        105, *106, 107, 109*
      stallion, *84–86, 89–93, 101, 103,*
        *104, 110*
    landmarks and approaches, *80,*
      *92–93*, 108, *109*
    lateral aspect, *95, 97, 99*
    muscles of, 82–84, *95–102*
    nerve supply to, 95, *97–102*
    pelvic inlet, *81, 83*, 86, *87*
    perineal region, *101, 102, 109, 110*
    right aspect, *100*
  large ruminants
    blood supply to, 313, 318, *319,*
      324, *330–332*
    bones of, *314, 315, 317*
    genitalia
      bull, *320–323, 327*, 333, *335*
      cow, 324–326, *328*, 334, 336, *336,*
        *337*
    internal measurements, 313
    lateral aspect, *330, 331*
    medial aspect, *332*
    muscles of, 313, *319*, 324, *330–332*
    nerve supply to, *317*, 324,
      *330–332*, 333
    palpable structures, 334
    pelvic cavity, 318
    pelvic inlet, 313, *319*
    perineal region, 324, *327, 328*
Penis
  horse, *89, 90, 91*, 111
    artery or vein of, 89, *89*, 91, 98,
      101
    nerves of, *89*, 91, 101
  large ruminants, 318, *321, 322, 332,*
    *335*
    artery or vein of, *332*
Pericarditis, large ruminants, 279
Pericardium
  horse, 34, 39
  large ruminants, 279, *280*
Perineal artery or vein, large ruminants,
  324, *327, 328, 332*
Perineal muscles, horse, 101, *101*
Perineal nerve
  horse, 101, 108
  large ruminants, *328*
Perineal region

bull, *327*
cow, 324, *328*
mare, *102, 109*
stallion, *101, 109, 110*
Perineal septum, horse, 101
Periodontium
  horse, 240
  large ruminants, 415
Perioplic groove, horse hoof, *193*, 195
Periorbita
  horse, 234
  large ruminants, 418
Peritoneal cavity
  horse, 53, 55
  large ruminants, 292
Peritoneal recess, large ruminants, *337*
Peritoneum
  horse, 53, 62, 82
  large ruminants, 292
Peritonitis, horses, 92
Peroneal nerves
  horse, landmarks and approaches, 146
  large ruminants, 344
Persistent penile frenulum, 318
Petrooccipital fissure, large ruminants,
  397, *401*
Petrosal crest, horse, *212*
Petrosal nerve, horse, 226, 236
Phalanges
  horse, *117, 155, 161, 187*, 188, 190,
    191
  large ruminants, *364, 384*
Pharyngeal artery or vein
  horse, *246*
  large ruminants, *405, 406*, 411
Pharyngeal constrictor, horse, *223*
Pharyngeal fascia, horse, *246*, 247
Pharyngeal recess, horse, 238
Pharyngeal septum, large ruminants, *412*
Pharyngotympanic tube, horse, 7, 220
Pharynx
  horse, 220, *228, 231, 237*, 238
  large ruminants, 411
Philtrum, horse, *215*
Phrenic nerve
  horse, 11, *18*, 32, *32, 33*, 35, 36, *36*
  large ruminants, *272, 277, 278, 281,*
    *282*
Phrenicosplenic ligament
  horse, 60
  large ruminants, 295, *308*
Pia mater
  horse, *127*, 248
  large ruminants, 418
Pillars, ruminal, 292, *304, 305*, 306, *310*
Pineal body, horse, 250
Pineal recess, horse, 248
Piriformis
  horse, 96, *97, 99, 134*
  large ruminants, *329, 330, 331*
Piriform lobe
  horse, 250
  large ruminants, *421*
Piriform recess, horse, *237*, 238
Pituitary gland, horse, 250
Placenta, large ruminants, 334

Placentomes, large ruminants, 334
Plantar artery or vein
  horse, *136, 139*, 140, *141*
  large ruminants, *347, 351, 352*
Plantar fascia, horse, 135, 140
Plantar ligaments, horse, *126*, 140
Plantar metatarsal nerve, horse, *141*
Plantar nerves
  horse, *136, 139*, 140
    landmarks and approaches, 146,
      *147*
  large ruminants, *347, 351, 352*
    digital anesthesia, *354*
Plantar tarsometatarsal ligament, horse,
  140
Pleurae
  costal, 34
  diaphragmatic, 34
Pleural cavity, horse, 34, 35, 37
Pleurocentesis, horse, 24, 34
Plexus brachialis, large ruminants, *272*
Plica vena cava, horse, 36
Pneumothorax, large ruminants, 279
Poll, horse, 7
Pons
  horse, *249*, 250, *251, 252, 253, 254*
  large ruminants, *421*
Popliteal artery or vein
  horse, 128, *132*, 142, 143, *143*
  large ruminants, *348*, 350, *351*
Popliteal fossa, horse, *118*, 143
Popliteal line, horse, 143
Popliteal notch
  horse, *119, 124, 125*, 143
  large ruminants, *340*
Popliteal surface, large ruminants, *339*
Popliteus
  horse, *123, 124, 132, 137, 139*, 143
  large ruminants, *348, 351, 352*
Portal vein
  horse, 54, 60, *60*, 65, 67
  large ruminants, 280, *299, 300*, 302,
    *308*
Pouches, of horse digit, *202*
Pregnancy, horse, *107*
Premature spiraling, 318
Premolars
  horse, *209*, 210, *213, 215*, 239, *241,*
    *243*, 244
  large ruminants, *399*, 415
Prepubic tendon
  horse, *79, 81, 122*, 128
  large ruminants, *321*
Prepuce
  horse, 85, 89, 105
  large ruminants, 318, *320, 321*
Preputial cavity, horse, 89, *90*
Preputial fold, horse, 89, *90*
Preputial muscles, large ruminants, 318
Preputial orifice, horse, *90*
Preputial ostium, horse, 89
Preputial ring, horse, 89, *90*
Presphenoid, horse, *212*
Proestrus, horse, 106
Promontory, large ruminants,
  *314, 317*

Pronator teres
    horse, *177*, 178, *179*
    large ruminants, *366*, 371, *372*, *373*,
        *377*, *378*, *379*, *380*
Proper ligament of ovary
    horse, 86, *87*, *88*
    large ruminants, *336*
Proper ligament of testicle
    horse, 92, *93*
    large ruminants, *323*
Prostate gland
    horse, *103*, 104
    large ruminants, *321*, *333*, *335*
Prostatic artery or vein, horse, 98
Proventriculis, large ruminants, 294
Psoas major
    horse, *81*, 82, *100*
    large ruminants, 292, *295*, *319*
Psoas minor
    horse, *81*, 82, *100*
    large ruminants, 292
Pterygoid bone, horse, *210*, 229
Pterygoid crest
    horse, 234
    large ruminants, 397, 418
Pterygoideus
    horse, *223*, 224, *235*
    large ruminants, *410*
Pterygoid fossa
    horse, *213*, 224
    large ruminants, *399*
Pterygoid fovea
    horse, *213*, 224
    large ruminants, *399*
Pterygoid hamulus
    horse, 229, *230*, *231*
    large ruminants, *398*, 411
Pterygoid nerve
    horse, 226
    large ruminants, 408
Pterygoid process, large ruminants, *398*,
    *401*
Pterygopalatine fossa, large ruminants,
    397
Pterygopalatine nerve, horse, 234
Pterygopharyngeus
    horse, *228*, 229, *230*, *231*
    large ruminants, *409*, *410*, 411
Pubic symphysis, horse, *89*
Pubovesical pouch
    horse, 98
    large ruminants, *337*
Pudendal artery or vein
    horse, 73, *74*, *81*, 85, *89*, 92, 97, 98,
        *100*, *133*, *134*
    large ruminants, *319*, *322*, 324, *325*,
        *326*, *328*, *332*
Pudendal nerve
    horse, 98, *99*, *100*, 101
        blocking, 108
    large ruminants, 324, *325*, 327, *330*,
        *331*, *332*, 333
        blocking, 313, *317*, 334
Pudendoepigastric trunk artery
    horse, *81*, *83*, 85, *89*, *100*, 128,
        *133*

large ruminants, *319*, *322*, *346*
Pulmonary embolic disease, large rumi-
    nants, 279
Pulmonary trunk artery
    horse, 13, *35*, *39*
    large ruminants, *281*, *285*, *286*, 288
Pulmonary valve
    horse, *40*, 42
        auscultation of, *47*
    large ruminants, *285*, 286
Pulmonary vein, horse, *39*
Pulp cavity, horse tooth, *240*, *243*
Pupil, horse, *233*, 236
Putamen, horse, 252
Pyelonephritis, large ruminants, 334
Pyloric folds, horse, 71
Pyloric sphincter, horse, *67*, 71
Pylorus
    horse, 66
    large ruminants, 296, *297*, *299*, 301,
        306, *307*
Pyramid of medulla oblongata
    horse, *251*, 252
    large ruminants, *421*

Quadratus femoris
    horse, 97, 98, *132*, *133*, *134*
    large ruminants, *329*, 344
Quadratus lumborum, large ruminants,
    292
Quadriceps femoris, horse, 135
Quarter, horse hoof, *193*

Radial artery or vein
    horse, *174*, 175, 178, *179*, *180*, *181*,
        *183*, *184*
    large ruminants, 371, *375*, *377*, *378*,
        *379*, *380*, 383, *386*, *387*
Radial nerve
    horse, *167*, *169*, 172, *174*, 175, *176*
        landmarks and approaches, 199
    large ruminants, *370*, 371, *372*, *375*,
        *377*, *378*, *380*, *382*, 383, *385*
Radial tuberosity, *157*, *158*
Radiocarpal joint, 199
Radiocarpal ligament, large ruminants,
    *366*
Radius
    horse, *155*, *158*, *176*, *177*, *179*
    large ruminants, *361*, *362*, *372*, *378*,
        *379*, *382*, *386*
Ramus mandibulae, horse, 5, *5*, 6
Raphe penis, large ruminants, *320*
Rectal artery, horse, 98, 101
Rectal examination, horse, 111–113
Rectal nerve
    horse, 98, *99*, *100*
        blocking, 108
    large ruminants, *330*, *331*, *332*, 333
        blocking, 313, *317*, 334
Rectococcygeus
    horse, 98, *101*
    large ruminants, *327*, *332*
Rectogenital pouch
    horse, 98
    large ruminants, *337*

Rectum
    horse, *81*, 87
    large ruminants, *319*, *321*, *328*, *331*,
        *337*
Rectus abdominis
    horse, 33, 52, *81*, 82
    large ruminants, *293*, *319*
Rectus capitis dorsalis major
    horse, 16, *16*, 17
    large ruminants, *272*
Rectus capitis dorsalis minor, horse, 16,
    *17*
Rectus capitis lateralis, horse, 19
Rectus capitis ventralis
    horse, *18*, 19, *222*
    large ruminants, *405*, *406*
Rectus femoris
    horse, 97, *99*, *100*, *131*, 133,
        *134*, 135
    large ruminants, 344, *346*, *351*
Rectus muscles of eye
    horse, 234, *235*, 236
    large ruminants, *417*, *419*
Rectus sheath, horse, 52, 53, 82
Rectus thoracis
    horse, *30*, *32*, 33
    large ruminants, *276*
Renal artery or vein
    horse, 60, *64*, *65*, 86
    large ruminants, 306
Renal capsule, horse, 62
Renal cortex, horse, 62, *64*
Renal medulla, horse, 62, *64*
Renal pelvis, horse, 62, *64*
Renal sinus, horse, 62
Renosplenic ligament, 61
Reproductive tract, cattle, palpation of,
    334
Rete mirabile epidurale
    large ruminants, 418
    pig, 418
Rete mirabile ophthalmicum, 418, *419*
Reticular artery, *309*
Reticular groove, 302, *304*, 305, *305*,
    306
Reticuloomasal orifice, *310*
Reticulo-peritonitis, 279
Reticulum, 292, 294, 295, 296, *297*, 301,
    *304*, *307*, *310*
Retina, horse, *233*, 236
Retractor bulbi
    horse, 234, *235*
    large ruminants, *419*
Retractor clitidoris
    horse, 98, *99*
    large ruminants, *328*
Retractor costae
    horse, 51, *52*
    large ruminants, *290*, 292, *293*
Retractor penis
    horse, *89*, *91*, 98, *101*
    large ruminants, 318, *321*, *322*, 327,
        *332*, *333*, *335*
Retroarticular process
    horse, *209*, *210*
    large ruminants, *398*

Retroperitoneal space, horse, 98
Rhinencephalon, horse, 250
Rhomboideus cervicis
    horse, *7, 9*, 11, *14, 15*, 28, *28*, 166
    large ruminants, *269*, 270, *272, 278*
Rhomboideus thoracis
    horse, 28, *28*, 29, *29, 44*, 166
    large ruminants, *275*, 278
Ribs
    horse, 23, 24, *24*
        removing, 34
    large ruminants, 273, *274*
Rima glottidis, horse, 245
Root, ruminant teeth, 415
Root canal
    horse, 240
    large ruminants, 415
Rostral commissure, horse, 248,
    *249*
Rostral communicating artery, horse,
    *251*, 252
Round ligaments, horse
    liver, 68
    urinary bladder, 82
    uterus, *87*
Rugae palati, horse, *230*
Rumen, 292, 295, 296, *305*
    artery of, *309*
    atrium, 292
    distention of, 306
    grooves of, 292
    recess of, 292, *295, 305, 310*
    sacs of, 295, *310*
Ruminants, large
    abdomen
        muscles of, 51, 289, 292, *293*
        viscera of, 292–312
        wall of, *290, 293*
    brain, 418, *420–422*
    brain cavity, 397, 403, *422*
    cranial nerves, 225. *See also under*
        individual nerve
    eye, 415–416, *417, 419*
    genitalia of
        bull, *320–323, 321, 327, 333, 335*
        cow, 324–326, *328, 334, 336, 337*
    head, 397–411, *423, 425*
    heart, *280, 281, 282, 285–288*
    hip joint, *122, 344, 356*
    hyoid apparatus, *409*, 411
    lungs, 279, *280, 283, 284, 285*
    mandible, 397, *399*
    neck, *11*, 267–272
    parotid region, *404–406*
    pelvic limb, 339–357
    pelvis, 313–*319, 329–332*
        viscera of, 320–328, 333–337
    skull, 397, *398–401*
    teeth, 413–415
    thoracic limb, 359–395
    thorax, 273–278
        muscles of, 27, 273, *275*
        thoracic cavity, *280–282*
        thoracic inlet, *276–278*
        viscera, 279–288. *See also under*
            individual organ

vertebrae
    caudal, *78*
    cervical, 267, *268*
    lumbar, *290*
    thoracic, 273, *274*
Ruminoreticular fold, *304, 305*, 306
Ruminoreticular groove, 292, 295, *295,*
    *307*

S2, horse, *80*
Saccus cecus, horse, 53, *67*
Sacral crest, large ruminants, *314, 315*
Sacral foramina, horse, 98
Sacrocaudales
    horse, 96, *97*, 98, *99*, 101, *101, 102,*
        *134*
    large ruminants, *329, 330*
Sacrococcygei ventrales, large rumi-
    nants, *327*
Sacroiliac joint
    horse, *79*
    large ruminants, 313
Sacroiliac ligament
    horse, *79*, 98, *99*
    large ruminants, 313
Sacrorectal pouch
    horse, 98
    large ruminants, *337*
Sacrosciatic ligament
    horse, *79*, 96, *97*, 98, *99, 100, 134*
    large ruminants, 313, 324, *329, 331,*
        *333*
Sacrum
    horse, *75, 76, 77*, 98
    large ruminants, *314, 315, 329, 332*
Sagittal crest, horse, *208*
Sagittal sinus, hors, 250
Salivary glands
    mandibular
        horse, *219*, 220, *223*, 228
        large ruminants, *402*, 403, *404,*
            *409, 410, 412, 413*
    sublingual
        horse, *223*, 228, *230*, 238
        large ruminants, *409*, 430
Salpinx, horse, 86, *87, 88*
Saphenous artery or vein
    horse, *97*, 128, *131, 132, 133*, 134,
        *134, 136*, 139, 140, *141, 143*
        landmarks and approaches, 146,
            *147*
    large ruminants, *329*, 344, *346, 347,*
        *348, 349, 351, 352*
        injections, 350, *355*
Saphenous nerve
    horse, 128, *131, 133*, 139
    large ruminants, *346*, 350, *351*
Sartorius
    horse, 86, *100*, 128, *131, 132*
    large ruminants, *319*, 344, *346*
Scalenus dorsalis, large ruminants, *271,*
    *272, 276, 277*
Scalenus medius
    horse, 18, *18*, 30, *30, 32*
    large ruminants, 271, *272, 277, 277,*
        *278*

Scalenus ventralis
    horse, *14*, 18, *18*, 30, *30, 32*
    large ruminants, *270, 271, 276, 277,*
        *277, 278*
Scapula
    horse, 29, 30–31, *155, 156*, 165, 172
        cartilage of, *44*
        as percussion landmark, 24
        spine of, 24, *25*, 28
    large ruminants, 273, 278, *359*
Scapular artery, circumflex, horse, 172
Scapular nerve, horse, *167, 169*
Scapulohumeral joint, horse, *21, 162.*
    *See also* Shoulder, horse
Sciatic nerve
    horse, 134
    horse, *97*, 98, *99, 134*
    large ruminants, *330, 331*, 333
Sclera, horse, *233*, 236
Sclerocorneal limbus, horse, *233*
Scrotal artery or vein
    horse, *89*
    large ruminants, *322*
Scrotal nerves, horse, 101
Scrotum
    horse, 85, 86, 92, *101*
    large ruminants, 318, *322, 327*
Scutiform cartilage
    horse, *229, 232*
    large ruminants, *402*
Scutuloauricularis
    horse, *232*
    large ruminants, *402, 407*
Scutum
    horse, *164*, 182, *188, 189*, 190, *191,*
        *196*
    large ruminants, *367, 388, 389,*
        390
Selenodonts, 413
Semilunar fold
    horse, 234
    large ruminants, 418
Semilunar line, horse, 190, *191*
Semilunar valvule, horse, 42, 43, *43*
Semimembranosus
    horse, *97*, 98, *99, 100, 101, 102*, 128,
        *131, 134*
    large ruminants, *327, 329, 332*, 344,
        *346, 348, 351*
Seminal vesicles, horse, 102, *103*
Semispinalis
    horse, *44*
    large ruminants, 270
Semispinalis capitis
    horse, 15, *15*, 16, *16, 17, 31*
    large ruminants, 272
Semispinalis thoracis, horse, 29, *29*
Semitendinosus
    horse, 95, 96, *97, 101, 102, 131, 134,*
        *136*
        aponeurosis of, *139*
    large ruminants, 324, *327, 329, 330,*
        344, *346, 351*
Septum pellucidum
    horse, 248
    large ruminants, *420*

Serratus dorsalis caudalis, horse, 29, *29,*
  *44, 52*
Serratus dorsalis cranialis
  horse, 29, *29, 30, 44*
  large ruminants, *275,* 278
Serratus ventralis cervicis
  horse, *7, 14, 16,* 18, *26, 28,* 166
  large ruminants, *269, 270, 272, 370*
Serratus ventralis thoracis
  horse, *26, 28, 28, 29, 30, 30,* 31, *44,*
    *51, 52*
  large ruminants, *275, 276, 370, 374*
Sesamoid bones
  horse, *155, 161,* 182, 190, 197
  large ruminants, *364, 384,* 390
Sesamoidean nerves, horse, landmarks
  and approaches, 199
Sesamoid ligaments
  horse, 145, *164, 186, 187,* 188, *188,*
    *189, 196*
  large ruminants, *367, 388, 389*
Short ligaments, horse, *187*
Shoulder
  horse, 25, *162, 167, 168,* 170, 172,
    195
    landmarks and approaches, 199,
      *203*
    muscles of, 29, 170
    nerves of, 170
    slipped, 172
  large ruminants, 273, *365*
    muscles of, *275, 368, 372, 374–376*
    nerve block sites, *393*
    nerves of, 369, *372, 374–376*
    vessels of, *372, 374–376*
Sigmoid arteries, large ruminants, *303*
Sigmoid flexure, bull penis, 318, *321,*
  *322*
Sinus caroticus, horse, *222*
Sinusectomy, horse, 105
Sinuses
  nasal, horse, 238
  paranasal, horse, *247,* 260, *261*
  venous, horse brain, *249*
Sinusitis, large ruminants, 415
Sinus rectus, horse, 250
Skull
  horse, *208–210*
  large ruminants, 397, *398–400*
    landmarks and approaches, *401*
Solar border, large ruminants, *364*
Solar canal, horse, 190
Solar foramen, horse, *191*
Sole
  horse hoof, *187,* 190, *193, 194,* 195
  ruminant hoof, *390*
Soleus
  horse, *136,* 137, *137*
  large ruminants, *347, 348*
Spermatic cord
  horse, 82, *84, 85,* 92, *103,* 108
  large ruminants, 318, *322,* 323
Spermatic fascia
  horse, *84, 86,* 92
  large ruminants, 318, *322*
Sphenoid bone, horse, 234

Sphenopalatine artery, horse, 234, *235*
Sphenopalatine foramen
  horse, *211*
  large ruminants, 397, *401*
Sphenopalatine sinus, horse, *230,* 238,
  248
Spinal artery, horse, *251,* 252
Spinal cord
  horse, *127,* 248
  large ruminants, 418
Spinalis capitis, large ruminants, *272*
Spinalis cervicis
  horse, 15, *15, 16, 19*
  large ruminants, *272*
Spinalis thoracis, horse, 29, *29, 44*
Spinal nerves. *See under* Cervical, Lumbar, and Thoracic spinal nerves
Spinous notch, horse, *212*
Splanchnic nerve
  horse, *35,* 36, *65*
  large ruminants, 306
Spleen
  horse, *55,* 56, *71*
  biopsy of, 50
  large ruminants, *295, 295, 296, 308*
Splenic artery
  horse, 61, *71*
  large ruminants, 306, *309*
Splenius muscle
  horse, *7, 9, 13, 14,* 15, *15, 16, 28,* 219
  large ruminants, *269, 270, 270, 271,*
    *272, 404*
Splenorenal ligament, 60, 61
Splint bone, horse, *121, 160,* 178, 182
Sternal crest, horse, 30
Sternal flexure, horse, 54, *55,* 56, *59, 61,*
  *69, 70*
Sternal ligament, horse, *24*
Sternebrae
  horse, *24*
  large ruminants, *274*
Sternocephalicus
  horse, 5, 6, *7, 9,* 11, 12, *12,* 13, *14,*
    *15, 18, 30*
  large ruminants, *268, 276*
Sternocostal joint
  horse, *24*
  large ruminants, *273*
Sternocostal ligament, horse, *24*
Sternohyoideus
  horse
    head, 220, 228
    neck, 6, *9, 12,* 13, *14, 18*
  large ruminants, *269, 270, 404, 409,*
    *413*
Sternomandibularis
  horse, 5, *7,* 11, *218, 219,* 220, *221,*
    222
    tendon for, *5*
  large ruminants, *269, 270, 271, 402,*
    *404, 405*
Sternomastoideus, large ruminants, *269,*
  *270, 404*
Sternopericardial ligament, horse, 38
Sternothyroideus
  horse

head, *228, 246*
  neck, 6, *9, 12,* 13, *14, 18*
  large ruminants, *269, 270, 276, 404,*
    *406, 409*
Sternum
  horse, *24*
  large ruminants, *274*
Stifle joint
  horse, *123, 124,* 140, *142,* 144
    landmarks and approaches, 151
    locking mechanism, 144
  large ruminants, 344, 350
    nerve block sites, *356*
Stomach
  horse, 53, 56, 59, *61, 67,* 71
  large ruminants, 292, 306, *307*
    arterial supply to, *309*
    compartments of, *307, 310*
Striate body, horse, 252
Stria terminalis, horse, *255*
Stringhalt, 139
Styloglossus
  horse, *223, 228,* 229
  large ruminants, *409, 410,* 430
Stylohyoid bone
  horse, *214, 215,* 220, *221, 223,* 229,
    *231,* 245
  large ruminants, *405, 406, 409, 410,*
    430
Stylohyoideus
  horse, 220, *221, 222, 223,* 228, *231*
  large ruminants, *405, 406,* 408, *409,*
    *410,* 430
Styloid process
  horse, *158, 209, 210*
  large ruminants, *361, 362,* 397, *401*
Stylomastoid foramen
  horse, *209*
  large ruminants, 397
Stylomastoid process, horse, *210*
Stylopharyngeus
  horse, 229, *231*
  large ruminants, *406, 409, 410,* 411
Stylopodium, horse, *117, 155*
Subarachnoid space, large ruminants,
  418
Subclavian artery or vein
  horse, 13, 32, 35
  large ruminants, 281, *281, 282*
Subclavian nerve, horse, *167, 169*
Subclavius
  horse, 6, 13, *14, 26, 30, 32,* 166, *167*
  large ruminants, 368, *370*
Subcutaneous bursae, horse, landmarks
  and approaches, *148,* 201, *203*
Subdural space, large ruminants, 418
Subfascial bursae, horse, *149,* 150
Sublingual artery or vein
  horse, *228,* 229
  large ruminants, *413*
Sublingual caruncles, horse, 239
Sublingual fold, horse, 239
Sublingual nerve, horse, 226
Sublingual recess, horse, 239
Suboccipital nerve, large ruminants,
  *424*

Subparotid aponeurosis, horse, *219*, 220, *221*
Subscapular artery or vein
    horse, *167*, *169*, 172
    large ruminants, *370*, 371, *372*
Subscapularis
    horse, 30, 166, *167*, *168*, 172
    large ruminants, *370*, 371, *372*
Subscapular nerve
    horse, *167*, *169*, 172
    large ruminants, *370*, 371, *372*
Subsinuosal interventricular branch
        artery, horse, *39*, *40*
Subsinuosal interventricular groove
    horse, 39
    large ruminants, *285*
Substantia negra, horse, 250
Subtendinous bursae, horse, *149*, 150
    landmarks and approaches, 201, *203*
Suburethral diverticulum, large rumi-
        nants, *334*, *337*
Sulci, of medulla oblongata, horse, *251*,
        252
Sulci cerebri
    horse, *249*, 250, *253*
    large ruminants, *421*
Sulcus chiasmatis, horse, *212*
Sulcus terminalis, large ruminants, *288*
Supracondylar fossa
    horse, *118*, *124*
    large ruminants, *339*
Supracondylar tuberosity, horse, *118*
Supraglenoid tubercle, horse, *156*, 165
Supraglenoid tuberosity, large ruminants,
        *365*
Supraomental recess, large ruminants,
        297
Supraorbital artery, horse, *235*, 236
Supraorbital canal, large ruminants, 397,
        *401*
Supraorbital foramen
    horse, *208*, *209*, *215*, 234
    large ruminants, *400*
Supraorbital groove, large ruminants,
        397, *398*, *400*
Supraorbital nerve, horse, 234, *235*
    landmarks and approaches, *259*, 260
Suprapineal recess, horse, 248
Suprascapular artery or vein
    horse, *167*, *169*, 172
    large ruminants, 371
Suprascapular nerve
    horse, *167*, *169*, 172
    large ruminants, *370*, 371, *372*
Supraspinatus
    horse, 26, 28, *28*, *167*, *168*, 172, *173*,
        *174*
    large ruminants, 368, *370*, 371, *372*,
        *374*, *376*
Supraspinous bursa, horse, *31*, 32, 45, *46*
Supraspinous fossa
    horse, *156*
    large ruminants, *359*
Supraspinous ligament
    horse, 31, *31*, *44*, 79
    large ruminants, 276

Supratrochlear nerve, horse, 234
    landmarks and approaches, *259*, 260
Supreme intercostal artery or vein, horse,
        *33*, *35*
Sural nerve
    horse, *97*, 134, *134*, *136*, *141*, *142*
    landmarks and approaches, 146
    large ruminants, 324, *329*, 344, *347*,
        *348*, *352*
Suspensory apparatus
    horse, *44*
    large ruminants, mammary gland,
        324, *325*
Suspensory ligament of ovary, horse, 86
Sustentaculum tali, horse, *120*
Sweeney, 165, 172
Symphyseal tendon
    horse, *132*
    large ruminants, 324, *332*
Synovial sacs, horse, *151*
Synovial tendon sheaths, horse, land-
        marks and approaches, 204, *205*

T12 spinal nerve, large ruminants, *293*
T13 spinal nerve, large ruminants, *293*
Tail
    horse, muscles of, *78*, *96*
    large ruminants, 313, *316*
Talocrural joint, horse, 144
Talus
    horse, *120*
    large ruminants, *357*
Tapetum lucidum, horse, 236
Tarsal artery, horse, *136*, 139
Tarsal bones
    horse, *117*, *120*
    large ruminants, *341*
Tarsal glands, horse, *233*, 234
Tarsal joint, horse, *126*
Tarsocrural joint, horse, landmarks and
        approaches, 152
Tarsometatarsus, large ruminants, *352*
Tarsometatarsal ligament, horse, *126*
Tarsus
    eye, horse, *233*, 234
    large ruminants, 418
    forelimb, horse, *138*, *141*
*Taylorella equigenitalis,* 91, 105
Teat
    horse, 92, *94*
    large ruminants, 324
Teat canal, large ruminants, 324
Teat sinus, large ruminants, 324
Tectum, horse, *249*, 250, 252, *254*
Teeth
    brachydont, 239
    horse, 209, *210*, *213*, 239–244
        landmarks and approaches, *261*
    hypsodont, 239
    large ruminants, 413, 414, 415
Tegmentum, horse, *249*, 250
Tela choroidea, horse, 248, 250
Telencephalon, horse, 248, 250, 252
Temporal artery or vein
    horse, *219*, 220, *221*, *222*, 227, *232*,
        234, *235*

large ruminants, *405*, *406*, *407*
Temporal bone
    horse, 208, *209*, 224
    large ruminants, *398*
Temporal fossa
    horse, *208*, *215*
    large ruminants, 397, *398*, *401*, *407*
Temporalis muscle, horse, 224, *232*
Temporal line, large ruminants, 397,
        *398*, *400*, 403
Temporal nerve, horse, 225, *235*
Temporal process, horse, 220
Temporal sinus, horse, 250
Temporomandibular disc, horse, *223*,
        224
Temporomandibular joint, horse, *215*
Tendon sheaths, horse, landmarks and
        approaches, *151*, 152–154, 204
Teniae, horse, 68, *69*
Tensor fasciae antebrachii
    horse, 30, *167*, *168*, *169*, *173*, *174*
    aponeurosis of, *168*, *169*, 172
    large ruminants, 274, *370*, 371, *372*,
        *374*, *377*
Tensor fasciae latae
    horse, *51*, *95*, *96*, *98*, *131*
    large ruminants, 324, *329*, *330*, 343,
        *346*, *351*
Tensor tympani nerve, horse, 226
Tensor veli palatini muscle
    horse, 229, *230*, *231*, *235*
    large ruminants, *410*, 411, *412*
Tensor veli palatini nerve, horse, 226
Tentorium cerebelli membranaceum
    horse, 248, *249*, 250
    large ruminants, 418
Tentorium cerebelli osseum, horse, 248,
        250
Teres major
    horse, *167*, *168*, 172
    large ruminants, *275*, *370*, 371, *372*,
        *374*
Teres major tuberosity, horse, *157*
Teres minor
    horse, 172, *173*, *174*
    large ruminants, 371, *375*, *376*
Teres minor tuberosity, horse, *157*
Testicle
    horse, 84, 85, 86, 92, *103*
    large ruminants, 318, *321*, *322*
Testicular artery or vein
    horse, 62, *81*, *83*, 84, 92, *93*, *103*
    large ruminants, *321*, *323*
Tete mirabile epidurales, *422*
Thalamus, horse, 248, 255
Thigh
    horse, *95*, *97*
    large ruminants, 329, 344, 345,
        *346*
Thoracic artery or vein
    horse, 26, 28, *29*, 32, *33*, *35*, 45, *46*,
        166, *167*, 172
    large ruminants, *276*, *277*, 324
Thoracic cavity
    horse, *34*, *35*, *36*, 37
    large ruminants, *280–282*

Thoracic duct
   horse, *33, 35*
   large ruminants, *277, 281*
Thoracic inlet
   horse, 18, 31, *32, 33*
   large ruminants, *276–278*
Thoracic limb
   horse
      blood supply to, 166–169, 172,
         174–185, 190, *191*
      bones of, 155–161
      carpal joint, *163*, 195
      digit, *185–192*
      elbow, *162*, 175, 195, 199, *200*
      hoof, *193, 194*, 195
      joints of, 162–164
      landmarks and approaches, 165,
         197–205
      lateral aspect, *173, 174*
      ligaments of, *163, 164*
      muscles of, 166–190
      nerve supply to, *167*, 169–185
      passive-stay apparatus, 195, *196*,
         197
      removing, 29–32
      shoulder. See Shoulder, horse
      tendons of, *162, 186*
   large ruminants
      arteries of, *387*
      blood supply to, *370–382, 385–387*
      bones of, 359–366
      carpal joint, *366*
      digit, *364, 367, 384, 385, 387–389*
      elbow, *366, 372, 378, 394*
      landmarks and approaches, 368,
         391–395
      ligaments of, *366, 367, 382, 388*
      muscles of, 368–383, *388, 389*
      nerve supply to, 369–383, *391, 392*
      shoulder. *See* Shoulder, large rumi-
        nants
      tendons of, *365, 367, 384, 385,
        386, 389*
Thoracic spinal nerves
   horse, *10*, 27, 53
      lateral, *29*, 31, *32*, 166, *167, 169*
      long, 31, *32, 167*
   large ruminants, 278
      lateral, *276*
      long, *276*
Thoracic sympathetic trunk, horse, 35,
   36
Thoracic vertebrae, horse, *23*, 24, 25
Thoracodorsal artery or vein
   horse, *167, 169*, 172
   large ruminants, *370, 372*
Thoracodorsal nerve, horse, *167, 169*,
   172
Thoracolumbar fascia, horse, 26, 51
Thoracolumbar nerves, large ruminants,
   289, *290*
Thorax
   horse
      landmarks and approaches, 25, 45,
        *46, 47*
      muscles of, *26–29*, 273

      nerves of, *27*
      thoracic cavity, *34, 35, 36*, 37
      thoracic inlet, 18, 31, *32, 33*
      viscera, 34–43
   large ruminants
      muscles of, 27, 273, *275*
      thoracic cavity, *280–282*
      thoracic inlet, *276–278*
      viscera, 279–288
Thyroarytenoideus
   horse, 245
   large ruminants, 411
Thyrohyoid, horse, *214*
Thyrohyoideus
   horse, *223, 228*, 246
   large ruminants, *406, 413*
Thyroid artery or vein
   horse, *228, 246*, 247
   large ruminants, *406*, 411
Thyroid cartilage
   horse, *237*, 244, *245, 246, 256*
      wing of, *247*
Thyroid gland
   horse, 13, *18, 228, 246*
   large ruminants, 269, 411
Thyroid notch, horse, *256*
Thyropharyngeus
   horse, *223, 228, 229, 246*, 247
   large ruminants, *404, 405, 406, 410*
Tibia
   horse, *117, 119, 125, 139*, 140, *142,
      143*
   large ruminants, *340, 341, 351, 352*
Tibial artery or vein, 350
   horse, *136*, 138, *139*, 140, *141, 142,
      143*
      landmarks and approaches, 146,
        *147*
   large ruminants, *347, 348, 349*
Tibial muscles
   horse, *136*, 137, *137*, 138, *139*, 140,
      *141*
   large ruminants, *347, 348, 349, 351*,
      352
Tibial nerve
   horse, *97, 132*, 134, *139, 141, 142,
      143*
      landmarks and approaches, 146,
        *147*
   large ruminants, 324, 329, 348, 350,
      *351, 352*
      nerve block sites, 350, *353*
Tibial tendons, horse, 138, *138*
Tibiotarsal joint, large ruminants, *357*
Toe, horse, *193*
Tongue
   horse, 220, *228, 239, 245*
   large ruminants, 411, *413*
Tonsils
   horse, *230, 237*, 238
   large ruminants, 411, *412, 413*
Torus levatorius, horse, 238
Torus linguae, large ruminants, 411, *412*
Torus pyloricus, large ruminants, 294,
   306
Torus tubarius, horse, 238

Trabeculae carneae
   horse, 42, *42*, 43, *43*
   large ruminants, *286, 287*
Trabeculae of corpus cavernosum, horse,
   91
Trabeculae septomarginalis
   horse, 42, *42*
   large ruminants, *286, 287*
Trachea
   horse, *5, 9, 13, 14, 21*, 33, *35*, 212
   large ruminants, 269, *270, 271, 276,
      277, 278*
Tracheal bronchus, large ruminants, 279
Tracheal cartilage, horse, 244
Tracheal duct, horse, 13
Trachealis, horse, 13
Tracheal rings, horse, *237*
Transverse cervical nerve
   horse, 7, 10, *12*, 13, *15, 218*
   large ruminants, 268, *269, 404, 424*
Transverse fascia
   horse, 34, 53, 82
   large ruminants, 292
Transverse humeral retinaculum, large
   ruminants, *364*, 371
Transverse lamina, horse, *145*
Transverse sinus, horse, 250
Transversospinalis, *27*
Transversus abdominis
   horse, 52, 53, 82, *89, 100*
   large ruminants, 292, *293*, 319
Transversus arytenoideus, horse, 246
Trapezius muscle pars cervicalis
   horse, *7, 9*, 11, *14*, 15, *15*, 26, *28*
   large ruminants, 269, *269, 270, 271,
      272, 275, 404*
Trapezius muscle pars thoracica
   horse, *14, 26, 28, 44, 51*
   large ruminants, 274, *275*, 276
Trapezoid body, horse, *251*, 252,
   *254*
Trepanation, of sinuses
   horse, 207, 244
   large ruminants, 415
Trephination. *See* Trepanation
Triangular ligament
   horse, 59, 62, *67*
   large ruminants, 301, *308*
Triceps brachii
   horse, *51*
      thoracic limb, *168*, 172, *173, 174*,
        175, 178
      thorax, 24, *25*, 26, *26*
   large ruminants, *381*
      thoracic limb, *370*, 371, *372, 374,
        375, 376, 379*
      thorax, 273, 274
Triceps surae, horse, 140
Trigeminal nerve
   horse, 225, *251*, 252
   large ruminants, 225
Trochanter
   greater
      horse, 96, *118*
      large ruminants, *339*
   lesser

horse, *118*
  large ruminants, *339*
Trochanteric bursae, horse, 96, *99, 148*
  landmarks and approaches, 152, *153*
Trochlea
  horse, *118, 123, 137,* 144, *157*
  large ruminants, *339*
Trochlear foramen, horse, *209*
Trochlear groove, horse, *212*
Trochlear nerve
  horse, 225, 234, *235, 251,* 252
  large ruminants, 225, *419*
Trochlear notch
  horse, *158*
  large ruminants, *361*
Truncus bicaroticus, 32
Tuber cinereum, horse, 250, *251,* 252,
  *254*
Tuber coxae
  horse, 24, *25, 50, 75, 76,* 80, *97, 134*
  large ruminants, *314*
Tuberculin, 267
Tuberculum cinereum, large ruminants,
  *421*
Tuber sacrale
  horse, *75, 76, 80*
  large ruminants, *314*
Tunica albuginea
  horse, *91*
  large ruminants, *318*
Tunica dartos, horse, 92
Tunica flava abdominis
  horse, 28, *44,* 52
  large ruminants, 276, 292, 324, *325*
Tunics, intraabdominal/extraabdominal,
  horse, 86
Tympanic artery, horse, 234
Tympanic bulla
  horse, *210*
  large ruminants, 397, *398, 401*
Tympanohyoid bone
  horse, *214,* 245
  large ruminants, *413*
Typhlotomy, horse, 73

Udder
  large ruminants, 318, 324, *325*
    blood supply to, *326*
  mare, 86
Ulna
  horse, *155, 158,* 165
  large ruminants, *361, 362, 382*
Ulnar artery or vein
  horse, *169,* 172, 178, *180, 181*
  large ruminants, 371, *373, 377, 379*
Ulnar nerve
  horse, *167, 169,* 172, *173,* 175, 178,
    *180, 181, 183, 184*
    landmarks and approaches, 197,
      *198,* 199
  large ruminants, 371, *372, 373, 377,
    379,* 380, *380, 381,* 383, *385,
    386*
    nerve block sites, *391,* 392, *392*
Ultrasound, abdominal viscera, large
  ruminants, 296

Umbilical artery or vein, horse, 82, 92,
  98
Umbilicus
  horse, 62, 82
  large ruminants, 301
Urachus, horse, 82
Ureter
  horse, 62, *64, 67, 81, 103*
    mare, *87*
    stallion, *81*
  large ruminants, *300,* 306, *311,* 335
    bull, *321, 333*
    cow, *319*
Urethra
  horse, 89, 90, *90, 91,* 104, *104,* 105,
    111
  large ruminants, 318, *320, 321, 332,
    334, 335, 336*
Urethral calculi, large ruminants, 334
Urethral diverticulum, large ruminants,
  334, *335*
Urethral groove, horse, *91*
Urethralis
  horse, 101, *101, 103,* 104
  large ruminants, *321, 333, 335*
Urethral isthmus, horse, 104
Urethral ostium, large ruminants, *337*
Urinary bladder
  horse, 82, 87, 92, *104*
  large ruminants, *319, 321, 333, 337*
    catheterization of, 334
Urogenital fold, horse, *81*
Uterine artery or vein, horse, 82, 86, *87*
Uterine fundus, horse, *106*
Uterine tube
  horse, 86, *87, 88*
  large ruminants, 318
Uterus
  horse, 86, *87, 88, 106*
    horns of, *87, 88*
    torsion of, 50, 86
  large ruminants, *336, 337*
    approaches to, 296
    horns of, 318, *319, 336, 337*
Uterus masculinus, horse, 102, *103*

Vagal indigestion syndrome, cattle, 306
Vagal trunk, horse, 36
Vagina
  horse, 105, *106, 107*
  large ruminants, *336, 337*
Vaginal artery or vein, horse, 87, 98, 101
Vaginal canal
  horse, 84, *85,* 92
  large ruminants, *322,* 323
Vaginal cavity
  horse, 85, 92
  large ruminants, *322,* 323
Vaginal fornix
  horse, 105, *106, 107*
  large ruminants, 334, *336*
Vaginal ring
  horse, *81,* 82, 89, *103, 113*
  large ruminants, *321*
Vaginal tendon sheaths, horse, landmarks
  and approaches, 204, *205*

Vaginal tunic
  horse, *84, 85,* 92
  large ruminants, *322*
Vagosympathetic trunk
  horse
    head, 220, 222, 227, 229, *231*
    neck, 6, *9, 13, 21*
    thoracic, 32, *33*
  large ruminants
    head, *406, 410,* 411
    neck, 269, *270, 271*
    thorax, *276, 277, 277, 278*
Vagus nerve
  horse
    head, 222, 225, 227, *231, 251, 252,
      254*
    neck, 13
    thorax, 32, *33, 35, 35,* 36, *36*
  large ruminants, 225, 306
    head, *405, 406,* 411
    thorax, 277, *278, 281, 282*
Valleculae epiglotticae, horse, 238
Valves, horse heart, 40
Valvules, horse heart, *40, 42*
Vascular lacuna, horse, 128
Vascular notch, horse, *215*
Vastus lateralis
  horse, *97, 99, 134*
  large ruminants, *329, 330, 348*
Vastus medialis
  horse, *100,* 128, *131,* 133
  large ruminants, 344, *346, 351*
Vena cava
  caudal
    horse, 36, *36, 39,* 41, *41, 64, 65,
      81, 100*
    foramen of, 36, 62
    large ruminants, *282, 285, 286,
      288, 299, 300,* 301, *308, 311,
      319*
    abscessation of, 279
  cranial
    horse, 32, 35, *36, 39,* 41
    large ruminants, *282, 285, 286,* 288
Venipuncture, horse, jugular vein, 6
Venograms, horse, 190
Venous angle, 35
Venous plexus
  horse, *230*
  large ruminants, 411, *412*
Venous sinuses, horse, 220
Ventricle
  cerebral
    horse, 248, *249,* 250
    large ruminants, *420*
  heart
    horse, *39,* 40, *42, 43*
    large ruminants, *285, 286*
Ventricular groove, large ruminants,
  302
Ventricularis, horse, 245, *245, 246,*
  247
Ventrotomy, horse, 73
Vermis
  horse, *249,* 250, *253*
  large ruminants, *420*

Vertebrae
  caudal
    horse, *78*
    large ruminants, *78*
  cervical
    horse, *3*
    large ruminants, 267, *268*
  lumbar
    horse, *49*, 80
    large ruminants, *290*
  thoracic
    horse, 23, 24, 25
    large ruminants, 273, *274*
Vertebral artery or vein
  horse, *17, 19, 33, 35, 36, 251*, 252
  large ruminants, *277, 278, 281, 422*
Vertebral foramen, horse, *3*, 16
Vertebral nerve
  horse, *33*
  large ruminants, *277, 278*
Vesical arteries, horse, 82, 92, 98,
  *103*
Vesical ligament
  horse, *81*, 82, *87*
  large ruminants, *319, 333*
Vesical trigone, horse, *104*
Vesicogenital pouch
  horse, 98
  large ruminants, *337*
Vesicular gland, large ruminants, *321,
  333, 334, 335*
Vestibular fold, horse, *230*, 245
Vestibular gland, large ruminants, 334,
  *336*

Vestibular ligament
  horse, 245, *245*
  large ruminants, 411
Vestibule, omental bursa, 297
Vestibulocochlear nerve
  horse, 225, *251*, 252, *253, 254*
  large ruminants, 225
Vestibulum
  horse, 105, *106*
  large ruminants, *336, 337*
Viborg's triangle, horse, 6, 207
  landmarks and approaches, 262, *263*
Vitreous body, horse, 236
Vitreous chamber, horse, *233*, 236
Vitreous humor, horse, 236
Vocal cords, horse, *237*, 245
Vocal fold, horse, *230, 231*, 245
Vocalis muscle, horse, *245, 246*, 247
Vocal ligament, horse, *245*
Vocal process, horse, 244
Vomer
  horse, *210*, 236
  large ruminants, *401*
Vomeronasal organ, large ruminants,
  411
Vulva
  horse, 105, *106*
  large ruminants, *336, 337*

Whitehouse approach, 7, 262, *263*
White matter, horse brain, 250
White zone
  horse, 195
  large ruminants, *390*

Windsucking, 10
Withers, horse, *5, 7, 25*
Wolf tooth, horse, 244

Xiphoid cartilage
  horse, *24*
  large ruminants, *274*
Xiphoid process, large ruminants, 318

Zeugopodium, horse, *117, 155*
Zonule of Zinn, horse, 236
Zygomatic arch
  horse, *208, 209, 210, 224*
  large ruminants, *398, 401*
Zygomatic bone
  horse, *208, 210*
  large ruminants, *398, 400*
Zygomatic nerve
  horse, 234, *235*, 236
  large ruminants, *419*, 430
Zygomaticoauricularis, large ruminants,
  *407*
Zygomaticofacial nerve, horse, 234
  landmarks and approaches, 259, 260
Zygomaticotemporal nerve, horse, 234
  landmarks and approaches, 259,
  260
Zygomatic process, horse, 220
Zygomaticus
  horse, *217*
  large ruminants, *402*, 430
Zygomatoauricularis
  horse, *232*
  large ruminants, *402, 404*